JACQUELINE BRINKMAN ARNETT
JOSEANN HELMES DEWITT

STUDY GUIDE FOR

MEDICAL-SURGICAL NURSING

*Critical Thinking
in Client Care*

THIRD EDITION

LEMONE ■ BURKE

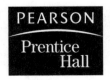

PEARSON
Prentice
Hall

Upper Saddle River, New Jersey

Pearson Education LTD.
Pearson Education Australia PTY, Limited
Pearson Education Singapore, Pte. Ltd
Pearson Education North Asia Ltd
Pearson Education Canada, Ltd.

Pearson Educación de Mexico, S.A. de C.V.
Pearson Education—Japan
Pearson Education Malaysia, Pte. Ltd
Pearson Education, Upper Saddle River, NJ

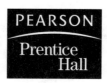

10 9 8 7 6 5 4 3

ISBN 0-13-113666-6

CONTENTS

PREFACE

A career in nursing is filled with opportunities for lifelong learning. Nurses today must be able to grow and evolve in a rapidly changing environment. This concise study guide has been developed to help you learn and apply key concepts and hone critical thinking skills based upon *Medical-Surgical Nursing: Critical Thinking in Client Care, Third Edition* by LeMone and Burke.

At the beginning of each chapter in this study guide, you will find a MediaLink box. Just as in the main textbook, this box identifies for you, the student, all the specific media resources and activities available for each chapter on the Student CD-ROM found in the main textbook and on the Companion Website at www.prenhall.com/lemone. You will find reference to video clips and animations from the Student CD-ROM to help you visualize and comprehend difficult concepts. On the Companion Website, you will find a variety of activities, such as case studies and care plans, to help you apply these concepts in clinical scenarios.

In addition, each chapter of this Study Guide provides a variety of questions and activities that help you comprehend difficult concepts and reinforce basic knowledge gained from textbook reading assignments. Following is the list of features included in this edition that will enhance your learning experience:

- **Learning Outcomes** and **Key Topics** highlight the key concepts that are reinforced by completing the study guide exercises.
- **Lecture Outline** helps you to follow lectures and organize your notes.
- **Focused Study Tips** help you recall the important nursing concepts from each chapter.
- **NCLEX Test Questions** provide you with additional review of key nursing topics.
- **Case Studies** provide clinical settings for critical thinking and the application of learned processes and procedures.
- **Care Plan Critical Thinking Activities** apply concepts from the textbook to real nursing scenarios and ask you to identify the steps of the nursing processes.
- An **Answer Key** with rationales for NCLEX test questions is provided in the back of the study guide.

We hope that you will benefit from using this study guide and that it will help prepare you to provide quality-nursing care based on knowledge and clinical judgment.

CHAPTER 1

THE MEDICAL SURGICAL NURSE

LEARNING OUTCOMES

After completing this chapter, you will be able to:

- Describe the activities and characteristics of the nurse as caregiver, educator, advocate, leader and manager, and researcher.
- Discuss the attitudes, mental habits, and skills necessary for critical thinking.
- Discuss the relationship between critical thinking and the nursing process in client care.
- Describe the importance of nursing codes and standards as guidelines for medical-surgical nursing care.
- Discuss the effect of legal and ethical dilemmas on nursing care.
- Discuss selected trends and issues in health care that affect medical-surgical nursing care.

KEY TOPICS

- Roles of the professional nurse
- Trends in health care
- Nursing codes and standards
- Effects of legal and ethical dilemmas on nursing care

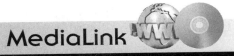

MediaLink

www.prenhall.com/lemone

Additional resources for this chapter can be found on the Student CD-ROM accompanying this textbook, and on the Companion Website at www.prenhall.com/lemone. Click on Chapter 1 to select the activities for this chapter.

CD-ROM
- Audio Glossary
- NCLEX Review

Companion Website
- More NCLEX Review
- Case Study
  Advance Directive
- Care Plan Activity
  Nursing Process

LECTURE OUTLINE

I. Critical Thinking
   A. Definition: self-directed thinking focused on how to respond to specific situation
   B. Includes own attitude, skills, experience
   C. Learned skill—needs practice; dynamic (will change with time, experience)
   D. Needed attitudes/mental habits
      1. Independent thinking: based on reason, knowledge

2. Intellectual courage: open to other's beliefs, ideas
3. Intellectual empathy: able to mentally place own self in a similar situation and understand client's point of view
4. Intellectual sense of justice and humility: consideration of views of others and ability to delay giving answer while getting assistance from other resources

5. Disciplined: logical decision making
6. Creative: looking for other improved ways to provide nursing care

E. Skills involved
1. Divergent thinking: determining relevance of assessment data
2. Reasoning: ability to discriminate facts
3. Clarifying: defining terms noting similarities and differences

F. Close relationship to **Nursing Process**: the 5-phase framework for nursing practice
1. **Assessment**: collection of information organized, communicated
   a. Subjective Data: information perceived by person experiencing it
      Example: client's pain, feeling of nausea
   b. Objective Data: sensual data verified by another person
      Example: blood pressure reading
   c. Types of assessment:
      1. Initial: admission: includes nursing history and physical examination
      2. Focused: ongoing and continuous, with each client interaction; nurse continually evaluates, notes changes in condition and interprets significance and need for action
2. **Diagnosis**: identification of actual or potential health alterations
   a. Nursing diagnosis according to NANDA system
   b. Written as PES [Problem, Etiology (probable cause), Signs and symptoms (the evidence)]
3. **Planning**: development of action plan of nursing interventions and client outcomes that promotes health and decreases unhealthy responses with client participation
   Client problems are 2 types:
   a. **Nursing Diagnoses** which require nursing interventions
   b. **Collaborative (Clinical) problems** include pathophysiologic, treatment-related, personal, environmental, or maturational situations
4. **Implementation**: nursing actions, which include setting priorities, and consider the individual client
   a. Implementation involves the action of giving care by nurse or client
   b. Documentation is the final component of implementation and is legally required
5. **Evaluation**: ongoing process in which the nurse decides to continue, revise, or terminate the plan of care that was established

II. Guidelines for nursing practice and protect the consumer
A. Codes of ethics: part of a profession; established principles of conduct
B. Ethical behavior: concerned with moral duty, values, obligations, rights and wrongs of practice
C. Codes utilized are:
1. The International Council of Nurses (ICN) Code
2. American Nurses Association (ANA) Code
3. Standards of Nursing Practice Standard: statement used by profession and general public to measure quality of practice
D. Nurses face ethical dilemmas in practice
1. Dilemma: choosing between 2 unpleasant, ethically troubling actions
   Examples:
   a. Client right to privacy and confidentiality vs. Nurse's right to information and safety. (Clients with communicable diseases such as HIV infected clients)
   b. Client's right to refuse treatment: development of laws concerning advanced directives, living wills, durable power of attorney

III. Roles of the Nurse
A. All roles include practice within the legal definition of nursing
B. All roles must be client-focused (client is a person (or community) requiring health care
C. Caregiver
1. Traditional role associated with nursing
2. Includes nursing and collaborative care planned by nurses and other health care team members such as physician interventions
3. Art (caring) and science (knowledge based)
4. Holistic care: includes physical, psychosocial, cultural, spiritual, environmental needs, but must include client as unique individual

D. Educator
   1. Maintains health and well-being of client including health promotion and illness prevention
   2. Is competent in teaching-learning process
      a. Assesses learning needs
      b. Plans and implements teaching methods
      c. Evaluates effectiveness
   3. Creates a positive learning environment:
      a. Effective interpersonal skills
      b. Adult learning principles
   4. Performs discharge planning
      a. Begins upon admission to health care setting
      b. Makes appropriate referrals
      c. Identifies resources (client's, community)
      d. Arranges for equipment/supply needs for home care
      e. Updates care plans
E. Advocate
   1. Promotes client's right to autonomy, free choice
      Individual client; assess need
      Communicate client's concerns to health care team members
      Provide teaching to client and family members
      Accepts client decisions differing from nurse preference
   2. Interacts with health care system
      Serves as agent of change
      Formulates health policy
F. Leader and Manager
   1. Works within health care environments (hospitals, clinics, physician offices, home, community sites such as schools, prison)
   2. Manages resources, people, time, environment where care provided
   3. Models of Care Delivery
      a. **Primary Nursing**: nurse provides individualized direct care to small number of clients during inpatient stay
         Advantage: decrease fragmentation of care; promote continuity for client
      b. **Team Nursing**: health care team provides care with various levels of education; registered nurse is leader and utilizes delegation

      Advantage: teamwork with each member performing tasks within their preparation: efficiency
      c. **Case Management**: health care team provides care with case manager (clinical specialist or experienced nurse) managing clients often with similar health care needs
         Advantage: Maximize positive outcomes and cost containment
   4. Care Delivery Terms or Terminology
      a. **Delegation**: nurse assigns appropriate and effective work activities to health team members; nurse assigns nursing care activities to team member but retains accountability; nurse must consider legality, matching care involved to competence level of team member, appropriate communication, feedback, and evaluation
      b. **Evaluating Outcomes of nursing care**
         1. **Critical Pathways**: a model in which the care path and client outcome are mapped on a predetermined time line; usually used with specific client medical-surgical diagnoses, e.g., Joint replacement surgery
         2. **Quality Assurance**: program within institution used to evaluate nursing care provided actual care given to client is compared to established standards of care for client
G. Researcher
   1. Developer of science of nursing
   2. Clinical research findings to allow nurses to provide evidence-based nursing care
IV. Medical Surgical Nursing
A. Health promotion, health care and illness to adult clients aged late teens to early hundreds
B. Trends and Issues facing medical-surgical nurses
   1. Aging population
   2. HIV infection continues
   3. Diagnosis and treatment of diseases genetic in origin
   4. Physical and mental illnesses in medically indigent and homeless populations

FOCUSED STUDY TIPS

- When in the clinical setting, observe a professional nurse functioning as an educator, advocate, manager, leader, researcher, and caregiver. Identify one behavior he/she demonstrates for each role.
- Clip an article from the newspaper regarding health care. Does the story reflect national or local health-care trends?
- Obtain the address and phone number of the state board of nursing in the state in which you wish to be licensed. Request copies of nursing standards of practice and become familiar with them.

NCLEX TEST QUESTIONS

1. The American Nurses Association (ANA) standards of clinical nursing practice allow:
   a. ethical guidelines for nursing practice.
   b. legal resolution of moral actions.
   c. objective evaluation of nursing licensure and certification.
   d. a framework for "right" and "wrong" decision making.

2. A document in which a client formally states preferences for health care in the event that he or she later becomes mentally incapacitated is called:
   a. living will.
   b. durable power of attorney.
   c. informed consent.
   d. code status.

3. A major component of the nurse educator's role today is:
   a. mediation.
   b. discharge planning.
   c. delegation.
   d. critical pathways.

4. The fifth cause of death among 25- to 44-year-olds in the United States today is:
   a. cancer.
   b. heart disease.
   c. accidents.
   d. HIV infection.

5. What goal is a component of the nurse's role as a manager?
   a. performing ROM (range-of-motion) exercises
   b. obtaining informed consent for procedures
   c. providing privacy and maintaining confidentiality
   d. delegating responsibilities for client care to others

6. Chronic problems affecting the health of the homeless are:
   a. high blood pressure, malnutrition, tuberculosis.
   b. diabetes, obesity, unemployment.
   c. unemployment, diabetes, advanced age.
   d. advanced age, high blood pressure, lack of hygiene.

7. A client tells the nurse that he is terminating his hemodialysis treatment for ESRD (end-stage renal disease). What does the nurse do first?
   a. ask the client's family if they agree
   b. establish whether or not the client has a living will or advance directive
   c. notify the physician
   d. establish the client's competency

CHAPTER 2

THE ADULT CLIENT IN HEALTH AND ILLNESS

LEARNING OUTCOMES

After completing this chapter, you will be able to:

- Compare and contrast the physical status, risks for alterations in health, assessment guidelines, and healthy behaviors of the young adult, middle adult, and older adult.
- Discuss the definitions, functions, and developmental stages and tasks of the family.
- Define health, incorporating the health-illness continuum and the concept of high-level wellness.
- Identify factors affecting health status.
- Discuss the nurse's role in health promotion.
- Describe the primary, secondary, and tertiary levels of illness prevention.
- Compare and contrast illness and disease.
- Describe illness behaviors and needs of the client with acute illness and chronic illness.
- Discuss the role of the nurse in providing care as a part of rehabilitation.

KEY TOPICS

- Client behaviors and needs in acute vs. chronic illnesses
- The nurse's role in health promotion
- Definition and application of wellness concepts at each developmental stage
- The nurse's role in rehabilitation

LECTURE OUTLINE

I. Concept of Health Definitions
   A. World Health Organization
   B. Health-illness continuum (dynamic, changes with time)

MediaLink

www.prenhall.com/lemone

Additional resources for this chapter can be found on the Student CD-ROM accompanying this textbook, and on the Companion Website at www.prenhall.com/lemone. Click on Chapter 2 to select the activities for this chapter.

CD-ROM
- Audio Glossary
- NCLEX Review

Companion Website
- More NCLEX Review
- Case Study
   Developing Teaching Programs
- Care Plan Activity
   The Family and Chronic Illness
- MediaLink Application
   The Older Adult and Preventive Health

C. Concept of high-level wellness including holism
D. National Goals (Healthy People 2010, U.S. Dept HHS):

5

1. Increase quality and years of healthy life
Life expectancies in years: 73.6 male;
79.4 female
2. Eliminate health disparities
II. Factors Affecting Health Status (can they be modified?)
   A. Genetic makeup (predisposition to specific illnesses: genome project)
   B. Cognitive abilities and education (response to health teaching)
   C. Race, ethnicity, cultural background
   D. Age, gender, developmental level
   E. Life style, environment
   F. Socio-economic status
   G. Geographic area
III. Health and the Nursing Process
   A. Assessment of client's health status and identifiable health risks related to factors affecting health status
   B. Interventions include client teaching regarding status and preventative actions
   Example: overweight 35-year-old woman with a strong family history of Diabetes Type II changes to low fat diet and adds 3 thirty-minute walks per week
   C. Evaluation: improvement of leading indicators Healthy People 2010
IV. Concept of Illness
   A. Differentiation from disease
   B. Illness behaviors measured in stages
   Progression through stages halts if reverts to healthy state
   1. Experiencing symptoms
   2. Assuming the sick role
   3. Seeking medical care
   4. Assuming dependent role
   5. Achieving recovery and rehabilitation
   C. Acute illness: characteristics: rapid onset, self-limiting
   D. Chronic illness: characteristics: requires long period of care, includes permanent disability
   1. 3-fold increase in incidence in future
   2. Client's adaptation to illness
   3. Effect on family members and developmental tasks
   4. Nursing interventions focus on education to promote client independence, improved quality of life, rehabilitation
V. Nurse's Role in Health Promotion
   A. Client's achievable high-level wellness

B. Prevention of illness
   1. Primary prevention key concept: healthy living to prevent disease
   Example: Dietary intake: 5–9 servings of fruits and vegetables daily
   2. Secondary prevention key concepts: early diagnosis, treatment of disease
   Example: Blood pressure screening
   3. Tertiary prevention key concepts: prevention of complications; rehabilitation
   Example: Exercise program post hip fracture
VI. Adult Client Health Status and Risks: Divided according to age
   A. Young adult (age 18 to 40)
   1. Peak physiologic development to age 25
   2. Specific age health risks: accidents, sexually transmitted diseases, substance abuse, physical and psychosocial stressors
   3. Developmental tasks
   B. Middle adult (age 40 to 65)
   1. Physical changes
   2. Specific age health risks: obesity, cardiovascular disease, cancer, substance abuse (nicotine, alcohol, prescribed drugs), psychosocial stressors
   3. Developmental tasks
   C. Older adult (over age 65)
   1. Population increasing at faster rate than any other
   2. Physical changes
   3. Specific age health risks:
      a. Chronic illness (includes arthritis, hypertension, hearing impairments, cardiovascular diseases, cataracts), obesity, cancer
      b. Injuries mainly falls, fires, motor vehicle accidents
      c. Pharmacologic effects due to predisposition to drug toxicity
      d. Physical and psychosocial stressors
   4. Developmental tasks
VII. Family of an Adult Client: Structure and function affected by health
   A. Establishing interdependence
   B. Maintaining boundaries
   C. Adapting to change
   D. Performing family tasks

FOCUSED STUDY TIPS

- Identify the developmental tasks of members of your family. Using health assessment guidelines described in the chapter, identify two healthy behaviors demonstrated by each family member.
- Identify factors affecting the health status of your family.
- What does your family do to prevent illness? Identify behaviors to promote wellness within your family setting.

NCLEX TEST QUESTIONS

1. Which of the following is a tertiary prevention measure?
   a. preoperative teaching
   b. work training programs following illness or injury
   c. identifying risk factors for disease and illness
   d. formulating critical pathways

2. A handicap is best defined as:
   a. disturbance in structure or function resulting from physiological or psychological abnormalities.
   b. the degree of observable and measurable impairment.
   c. total adjustment to disability that limits functioning at a normal level.
   d. loss of physiological function only.

3. The leading cause of illness in Native Americans in the United States is:
   a. hypertension.
   b. eye disorders.
   c. ESRD (end-stage renal disease).
   d. tuberculosis and diabetes.

4. The older adult is at increased risk for:
   a. alcohol abuse.
   b. homelessness.
   c. chronic illness.
   d. malnutrition.

5. Accidents are the leading cause of injury and death in people between the ages of:
   a. 0–12.
   b. 35–50.
   c. 15–24.
   d. 60–75.

6. The middle-aged adult is at increased risk for cancer as a result of:
   a. psychosocial stressors related to occupation.
   b. inadequate health prevention and maintenance routines.
   c. increased length of exposure to environmental carcinogens.
   d. increased sexual activity during this age span.

7. You have been asked to present a health-related program for freshman college students. What topic would be most appropriate?
   a. obesity
   b. substance abuse
   c. abstinence
   d. heart disease

CHAPTER 3

COMMUNITY AND HOME CARE OF THE ADULT CLIENT

LEARNING OUTCOMES

After completing this chapter, you will be able to:

- Define community-based nursing care.
- Discuss factors affecting health status in the community.
- Describe community-based health care services.
- Describe home health nursing and the roles of the home health nurse.
- Describe the components of the home health care system, including agencies, clients, referrals, physicians, reimbursement, and legal considerations.
- Discuss the effect of the home setting on nursing practice.
- Apply the nursing process to care of the client in the home.

KEY TOPICS

- Home-health care system
- Community based health-care services
- Factors affecting health in the community

LECTURE OUTLINE

   I. Community-based Nursing
      A. Definition: Direct health care services to individuals to manage health problems and promote self-care
      B. Care for clients where they are: in local community, culturally competent, and family centered
      C. Factors affecting health of community:
        1. Social Support Systems

Inclusive of client and family, friends, neighbors, church, organizations, self help groups, professional providers
2. Community health structure: urban vs. rural, financial basis of area
3. Environmental factors: air, water, safety, transportation

4. Economic resources: financial and insurance resources
   a. Private health insurance policies
   b. Social Security Act amendments (1965) health care services through Medicare (over 65); Medicaid (low-income)
II. Community-based Health Care Services
   A. Home care (home, hospice, respite)
   B. Community centers, Clinics
   C. Senior Centers
   D. Parish and block nursing
   E. Variety organizations and services
III. Home Health Nursing: health services provided in home include recovery, chronically ill; hospice, respite
   A. Roles of nurse
      1. Advocate
      2. Provider of direct care
      3. Educator/motivator of client; hospital nurse starts process
      4. Coordinator of services
   B. Standards
   C. Home Care Bill of Rights: given to each client on first visit
   D. Agency types
   E. Clients: includes client and family
   F. Referrals: preparation done while in hospital, may be planned in critical pathway; self-referral; need signature of physician referral
   G. Reimbursements
      1. Medicare (largest reimbursement source) mandates:
         a. Signed physician referral and plan of care
         b. Client requires skilled intermittent nursing care, physical, speech, or occupational therapy

c. Client is homebound
d. Home care agency is Medicare-approved
      2. May be part of employee insurance; also some private pay
   H. Legal considerations:
      1. Client consents to treatment and allows agency personnel into home
      2. Nurse maintains client privacy and confidentiality
      3. Care is consistent with standards
IV. Nursing Practice in Home Setting
   A. Establish trust and rapport with client
   B. Perform mutual goal setting with client; plan for discharge; set boundaries
   C. Assess home situation: address safety, describe infection control and establish emergency plan
   D. Teach medications, client physical state, and progression of recovery or disease process
   E. Meet standards of care according to visit guidelines set by Medicare
V. Nursing Process in Home Setting
   A. Assessment: nurse receives referral with some chart information; new written orders for admission to home health agency; assessment on first visit
   B. Diagnosis: identifies client learning needs
   C. Planning: develops plan of care within 48 hours including plan of visit frequency and goals, which is shared with client
   D. Implementation: contracting; work within the realm of client's home environment so long as meets reasonable safety and no harm
   E. Evaluation: continuous, formative and summative

FOCUSED STUDY TIPS

- Identify a community-based health-care service in your local area. Contact the staff and determine their effect on meeting a specific health-care need in your community.
- Identify a client that has utilized home-health nursing services. Discuss the impact such care had on the client's family and lifestyle. What were the benefits?
- Work with a nurse in the clinical setting making a referral to a community-based health-care agency. What steps in the nursing process are utilized to make the referral? Who will pay for the services?

CASE STUDY

Sarah Barnes is a 35-year-old mother dying of AIDS. She lives at home with her husband and two children, ages 4 and 12. What type of care and skills would a nurse employ in caring for Sarah? What type of community resources might be available for her care?

CARE PLAN CRITICAL THINKING ACTIVITY

Describe how teaching is designed and implemented in the home-care setting.

NCLEX TEST QUESTIONS

1. Medicare coverage provides:
   a. coverage for OTC (over-the-counter) medications and adaptive devices.
   b. state health insurance for all people with limited incomes.
   c. all home care services needed for those clients over 65 and collecting Social Security.
   d. health assistance for acutely ill or disabled clients over 65 years of age.

2. Home care's largest single source of reimbursement is:
   a. Medicaid.
   b. private insurance such as Blue Cross/Blue Shield.
   c. public funding.
   d. Medicare.

3. The nurse understands that the primary predictors of need for home care services are:
   a. gender and socioeconomic level.
   b. age and functional disability.
   c. educational level and functional disability.
   d. cognitive level and age.

4. The nurse's primary focus when discharging client's to the home setting is:
   a. safety.
   b. availability of community resources.
   c. medication compliance.
   d. follow-up medical appointments.

5. Most of the home health nurse's time is spent:
   a. procuring medical supplies.
   b. documenting care.
   c. limiting distractions.
   d. teaching.

6. The hospice nurse provides palliative care, which is best described as:
   a. supportive care.
   b. curative care.
   c. holistic care.
   d. symptom-controlled care.

CHAPTER 4

NURSING CARE OF CLIENTS IN PAIN

LEARNING OUTCOMES

After completing this chapter, you will be able to:

- Describe the neurophysiology of pain.
- Compare and contrast definitions and characteristics of acute, chronic, central, phantom, and psychogenic pain.
- Discuss factors affecting individualized responses to pain.
- Clarify myths and misconceptions about pain.
- Discuss collaborative care for the client in pain, including medications, surgery, and transcutaneous electrical nerve stimulation, and complementary therapies.
- Use the nursing process as a framework for providing individualized nursing care for clients experiencing pain.

KEY TOPICS

- Theories and neurophysiology of pain
- Types and characteristics of pain
- Factors affecting responses to pain
- Myths and misconceptions about pain
- Nursing care of clients experiencing pain

LECTURE OUTLINE

I. Significance of Pain
   A. Subjective response: only felt by the person
   B. Negative: discomfort
   C. Protective role: warning of potential threat to health (sometimes a life-threatening condition); prompt for person to seek medical attention
   D. *Fifth vital sign* according to JCAHO

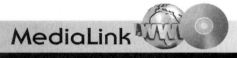

MediaLink

www.prenhall.com/lemone

Additional resources for this chapter can be found on the Student CD-ROM accompanying this textbook, and on the Companion Website at www.prenhall.com/lemone. Click on Chapter 4 to select the activities for this chapter.

CD-ROM
- Audio Glossary
- NCLEX Review

Animations
- Components of a Reflex Arc
- Morphine

Companion Website
- More NCLEX Review
- Case Study
     Assessing the Client in Pain
- Care Plan Activity
     Nursing Care for the Client in Pain
- MediaLink Application
     Complementary Therapies

II. Definition: "pain is whatever the person experiencing it says it is, and exists whenever the person says it does" (McCaffery, 1979)
   A. Pain has personal meaning to individual experiencing pain
   B. All pain is real

C. Dimensions of pain include physical, emotional, cognitive, sociocultural, spiritual aspects

D. Response to and warning of actual or potential trauma

III. Neurophysiology of Pain
  A. Gate control theory:
     Dorsal horns of spinal cord; impulses of touch and pain mediate each other
     Inhibitory system in brain stem; cells activated by opiates, psychologic factors
  B. Stimuli: nociceptors: nerve receptors for pain ends; located in numerous skin and muscles; stimulated by direct cellular damage or local release of biochemicals from cellular damage such as bradykinin
  C. Pain pathway
  D. Endorphins (endogenous morphines) bind with opiate receptors on neuron to inhibit pain impulse transmission

IV. Classifications of Pain and Definitions
  A. Acute: sudden onset, usually sharp and localized; less than 6 months; significant of actual or potential injury to tissues; initiates flight or fight stress response
     1. Somatic: arises from skin, close to surface of body; sharp or dull; often with nausea and vomiting
     2. Visceral: arises from body organs; dull and poorly localized; with nausea and vomiting; may radiate or is referred
     3. Referred: pain perceived in area distant from stimuli
  B. Chronic: prolonged pain; more than 6 months; often dull, aching, diffuse; not always associated with specific cause, often unresponsive to conventional treatment; most common is lower back pain
     1. Recurrent acute pain
     2. Ongoing time-limited pain
     3. Chronic nonmalignant pain
     4. Chronic intractable nonmalignant pain
  C. Common chronic pain conditions:
     1. Neuralgias: pain from peripheral nerve damage
     2. Dystrophies: pain from peripheral nerve damage characterized by continuous burning pain
     3. Hyperesthesias: state of oversensitivity to touch and painful stimuli
     4. Phantom Pain: post amputation, the person experiences sensations and pain in the missing body part
     5. Psychogenic pain: pain without a physiologic cause or event

V. Factors Affecting Response to Pain
  A. Pain threshold: Point at which a stimulus is experienced as pain; same for all persons, but individuals have different perceptions and reactions to pain
  B. Pain tolerance: amount of pain a person can endure before outwardly responding to it
     1. Decreased by repeated pain episodes, fatigue, anger, anxiety, sleep deprivation
     2. Increased by alcohol, hypnosis, warmth, distraction, spiritual practices
  C. Age
  D. Sociocultural influences
     1. Family beliefs, e.g., males don't cry
     2. Cultural: some persons of ethnic groups handle pain in similar manner
  E. Emotional status, e.g., anxiety
     1. Fatigue and/or lack of sleep
     2. Depression: decreased amount of serotonin, a neurotransmitter, thus increased amount of pain sensation
  F. Past experiences with pain
  G. Source and meaning
  H. Knowledge about pain

VI. Common Fallacies and Myths about Pain
  A. Chronic pain is really a masked form of depression
     1. Depression and pain are both affected by levels of serotonin
     2. Depression and pain can co-exist
  B. Narcotic medication is too risky to be used with chronic pain
  C. Wait until pain is present before administering medication
  D. Many clients lie about existence or severity of pain
  E. Pain after surgery is best treated with intramuscular injections

VII. Collaborative Care of Clients in Pain
  A. Medications: most common approach to pain management
  B. Nurse needs to know for each medication: classification; physiologic action; peak effect, adverse effects, antidote, nursing implications
     Classifications of meds:
     1. Non-narcotic analgesics: (e.g., acetaminophen) mild to moderate pain
     2. NSAIDs: (aspirin, ibuprofen) peripheral nerve endings; interfere with prostaglandin synthesis
     3. Narcotics (e.g., morphine) or Synthetic narcotics (Oxycodone): act within and outside CNS (central nervous system)

4. Antidepressants: (such as tricyclic antidepressants) promote serotonin and inhibit pain, promotes sleep
5. Local anesthetics

C. Duration of Action: evaluate effectiveness according to individualized dosing schedule
   1. Around the clock (ATC)
   2. As necessary (PRN)
   3. Give analgesics before pain begins or becomes severe

D. Route: affects how much medication is needed to relieve pain; dosages differ with route
   Most common routes
   1. Oral: simplest method
   2. Transdermal: delivers continuous level of medication
   3. Intravenous: provides most rapid onset (but short duration) unless available as PCA (patient controlled analgesia administration)

E. Surgery: different types done to alter nerve transmission; may alter sensation or movement as well as pain; used after other methods not effective

F. TENS: (Transcutaneous electrical nerve stimulation) nerve conducts electrical current and so cannot conduct pain

G. Complementary therapies
   1. Acupuncture
   2. Biofeedback
   3. Hypnotism

4. Relaxation (guided imagery, meditation)
5. Distraction
6. Cutaneous stimulation (massage)

VIII. Nursing Process in Care of Client Experiencing Pain
   A. Assessment: 4 aspects
      1. Client's perception of pain
         Pain rating scale; location; quality; pattern; precipitating and relieving factors; impact of pain; physiologic and behavior changes
      2. Physiologic response to acute pain: tachycardia, increased blood pressure, muscle tension, dilated pupils, sweating
      3. Behavioral responses to acute pain: guarding, facial expressions, withdrawing
      4. Client's management of pain and administration effectiveness
         Denial of pain: due to fear, misconceptions
   B. Diagnosis: acute or chronic pain
   C. Nursing interventions:
      1. Acknowledges and documents pain
      2. Administers prescribed analgesics
      3. Utilizes non-pharmacologic methods and comfort measures
      4. Teaches clients and family about pain, medications, comfort measures
      5. Suggests referrals as necessary
   D. Evaluation: utilizes client perception and pain rating scale to document changes in pain

FOCUSED STUDY TIPS

- Evaluate your personal responses to pain. Compare and contrast them to a classmate's responses. What factors can you identify that influence your responses to pain?
- Assess a family member the next time he or she complains of pain. What type of pain is being experienced?
- Compare and contrast pharmaceuticals used in the hospital and in the home setting to treat pain. What are the differences in the types of medications prescribed and the routes of administration?

CASE STUDY

Joseph is a recent immigrant to the United States. He has no family or friends in this country. Postoperatively, the physician has ordered meperidine 100 mg IM q4h as needed for pain relief.

The client is experiencing considerable pain, 9/10 on the pain scale 2 hours after being medicated. What would you do? What type of pain is he most likely experiencing? What factors may be influencing his response to pain?

CARE PLAN CRITICAL THINKING ACTIVITY

When assessing a client with postoperative pain, what questions would the nurse ask to understand the client's level of distress? How would your questions differ when assessing a client with chronic pain from osteoarthritis?

NCLEX TEST QUESTIONS

1. Which of the following nursing interventions has been found *most* helpful when caring for clients in pain?
   a. leaving the client to rest in a quiet, darkened room
   b. asking the client's opinion as to the origin of pain
   c. asking family members to remain with the client
   d. allowing client to describe the nature of their pain

2. Hospice nurses provide narcotic analgesics for clients experiencing pain. One of the most common side effects of narcotic analgesics is:
   a. constipation
   b. anorexia
   c. muscle cramping
   d. nausea

3. Autonomic responses to pain may result in:
   a. decreased blood pressure and pinpoint pupils.
   b. increased blood pressure and decreased respirations.
   c. increased blood pressure and increased pulse and respirations.
   d. muscle weakness and decreased level of consciousness.

4. TENS (transcutaneous electrical nerve stimulation) is most commonly used to control:
   a. chronic, malignant pain.
   b. burn pain.
   c. psychogenic pain.
   d. acute postoperative pain.

5. Precipitating factors of pain include:
   a. anxiety, fear, and depression.
   b. inactivity, isolation, and insomnia.
   c. temperature extremes, loneliness, and fear.
   d. low self-esteem, fear, and loneliness.

6. The client refuses to take ordered pain relief medication. The nurse tells the client:
   a. "The physician has ordered this medication; you really need it."
   b. "You have the right to refuse this. I will respect your right."
   c. "Let me give you this medicine now and in a while I will call your physician to see if we can hold it in the future."
   d. "You do not have to take this medicine, but let me explain what this medicine is for and why the doctor has prescribed it for you."

7. In planning for the pain management of a 1-day postoperative client, the nurse should instruct the client to inform him/her of the need for pain medication:
   a. as the sensation of pain begins.
   b. when the pain is 5 or above on a 10-point pain scale.
   c. every time she is able to have a dose of medication, even if it is before awareness of pain.
   d. when pain is perceived, if the prescribed time interval period between medications has passed.

CHAPTER 5

NURSING CARE OF CLIENTS WITH ALTERED FLUID, ELECTROLYTE, AND ACID-BASE BALANCE

LEARNING OUTCOMES

After completing this chapter, you will be able to:

- Discuss the functions and regulatory mechanisms that maintain water and electrolyte balance in the body.
- Compare and contrast the causes, effects, and care of the client with fluid volume or electrolyte imbalance.
- Describe the pathophysiology and manifestations of imbalances of sodium, potassium, calcium, magnesium, and phosphorus.
- Discuss the causes and effects of acid-base imbalances.
- Identify laboratory and diagnostic tests used to diagnose and monitor treatment of fluid, electrolyte, and acid-base disorders.
- Recognize normal and abnormal values of electrolytes in the blood.
- Use arterial blood gas findings to identify the type of acid-base imbalance present in a client.
- Provide teaching about diet and medications used to treat or prevent electrolyte disorders.
- Use the nursing process as a framework to provide individualized nursing care to clients with fluid, electrolyte, and acid-base disorders.

KEY TOPICS

- Normal fluid and electrolyte balance
- Fluid and electrolyte imbalances
- Acid-base disorders
- Nursing care of clients with fluid and electrolyte imbalances and acid-base imbalances

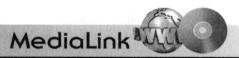

MediaLink

www.prenhall.com/lemone

Additional resources for this chapter can be found on the Student CD-ROM accompanying this textbook, and on the Companion Website at www.prenhall.com/lemone. Click on Chapter 5 to select the activities for this chapter.

CD-ROM
- Audio Glossary
- NCLEX Review

Animations
- Membrane Transport
- Acid-Base Balance
- Fluid Balance

Companion Website
- More NCLEX Review
- Case Study
    Hypernatremia
- Care Plan Activity
    Fluid Volume Deficit
    Hypocalcemia
- MediaLink Application
    Metabolic Acidosis and Type 1
    Diabetes

LECTURE OUTLINE
FLUIDS IN HUMAN BODY

I. Fluid Status of Human Body
  A. Homeostasis: state of the body when maintaining a state of balance in the presence of constantly changing conditions
  B. Includes balance of fluid, electrolytes, and acid-base balance
  C. Body water intake and output approximately equal (2500 mL/24 hr.)

II. Body Fluid Composition
  A. Water: 60% of body weight
  B. Electrolytes: substances that become charged particles in solution
    1. Cations: positively charged (e.g., Na^+, K^+)
    2. Anions: negatively charged (e.g., Cl^-)
    3. Both are measured in milliequivalents per liter (mEq/L)
  C. Osmolality: concentration of a solution measured in milliosmoles per liter
  D. Balance of hydrostatic pressure and osmotic pressure regulates movement of water between intravascular and interstitial spaces

III. Body Fluid Distribution
  A. 2 body compartments:
    1. Intracellular fluids (ICF): fluids within cells of body [major intracellular electrolytes: Potassium (K^+), Magnesium(Mg^{+2})]
    2. Extracellular fluids (ECF): fluid outside cells [major extracellular electrolytes: Sodium (Na^+), Chloride(Cl^-)]; this is where transportation of nutrients, oxygen, and waste products occurs
  B. Locations of ECF:
    1. Interstitial: fluid between most cells
    2. Intravascular: fluid within blood vessels; also called plasma
    3. Transcellular: fluids of body including urine, digestive secretion, cerebrospinal, pleural, synovial, intraocular, gonadal, pericardial

IV. Mechanisms of Body Fluid Movement (i.e., movement of solutes, solvents across different extracellular locations)
  A. **Osmosis:** water is mover; water moves from lower concentration to higher concentration
    1. Normal osmolality of ICF and ECF: 275–295 mOs/kg (milliliters osmolality per kilogram)
    2. Types of solutions according to osmolality
      a. Isotonic: all solutions with osmolality same as that of plasma

Body cells placed in isotonic fluid: neither shrink nor swell
      b. Hypertonic: fluid with greater concentration of solutes than plasma Cells in hypertonic solution: water in cells moves to outside to equalize concentrations: cells will shrink
      c. Hypotonic: fluid with lower concentration of solutes than plasma Cells in hypotonic solution: water outside cells moves to inside of cells: cells will swell and eventually burst (hemolyze)
    3. Different intravenous solutions, used to correct some abnormal conditions, categorized according to osmolality:
      a. Hypertonic: 5% glucose/.45% NaCl solution
      b. Isotonic: 9% NaCl, Lactated Ringers solution
      c. Hypotonic: 45% NaCl
  B. **Diffusion:** solute molecules move from higher concentration to lower concentration
    1. Solute, such as electrolytes, is the mover; not the water
    2. Types: simple and facilitated (movement of large water-soluble molecules)
  C. **Filtration:** water and solutes move from area of higher hydrostatic pressure to lower hydrostatic pressure
    1. Hydrostatic pressure is created by pumping action of heart and gravity against capillary wall
    2. Usually occurs across capillary membranes
  D. **Active Transport:** molecules move across cell membranes against concentration gradient; requires energy, e.g., Na^+–K^+ pump

V. Mechanisms that Regulate Homeostasis: How the body adapts to fluid and electrolyte changes
  A. **Thirst:** primary regulator of water intake (thirst center in brain)
  B. **Kidneys:** regulator of volume and osmolality by controlling excretion of water and electrolytes
  C. **Renin-angiotension-aldosterone mechanism:** response to a drop in blood pressure; results from vasoconstriction and sodium regulation by aldosterone
  D. **Antidiuretic hormone:** hormone to regulate water excretion; responds to osmolality and blood volume
  E. **Atrial natriuretic factor:** hormone from atrial heart muscle in response to fluid

excess; causes increased urine output by blocking aldosterone

FLUID AND ELECTROLYTE IMBALANCES

I. Fluid Volume Deficit (FVD) (too little fluid in body)
  A. Common Stimuli:
    1. Excessive fluid loss, e.g., hemorrhage, excess loss of GI fluids (vomiting, diarrhea, or wound drainage)
    2. Insufficient fluid intake, e.g., no access to fluid, unable to drink
    3. Failure of regulatory mechanisms, fluid shifts
  B. Terminology:
    1. Dehydration: technically loss of water alone (but usually any state of low fluid)
    2. Hypovolemia: decreased circulating blood volume
    3. Third Spacing: shift of fluid from vascular space (inside blood vessels) to another area such as abdomen/bowels, soft tissues (like swelling that occurs with a severe injury—like a twisted ankle)
  C. Signs/Symptoms
    More rapid fluid loss, equals more rapid development of symptoms
    1. Weight loss (liter fluid = 2.2 lb or 1 kg)
    2. Diminished skin turgor, tongue turgor (more reliable in elderly)
    3. Postural (orthostatic) hypotension: drop of 15mm Hg of systolic BP with position change from lying to standing
    4. Flat neck veins when recumbent
    5. Diagnostic test findings (usual, not absolute):
      a. Electrolytes: isotonic fluid loss: sodium is within normal limits; if loss of water only, sodium is elevated
      b. Serum Osmolality: isotonic fluid loss: osmolality is within normal limits; loss of water alone, osmolality is elevated
      c. Urine specific gravity, urine osmolality: both elevated as urine becomes more concentrated as kidneys conserve water
      d. Increased hematocrit due to hemoconcentration
      e. Possible elevated blood urea nitrogen (BUN)
      f. CVP (mean pressure in right atrium of heart) sub normal
  D. Compensatory Mechanisms (how the body responds to restore homeostasis)

Goal: to conserve water and sodium; to maintain circulation
    1. Tachycardia (may lead to hypotension)
    2. Vasoconstriction as evidenced by pale, cool skin
    3. Decrease in urinary output with rise in urine specific gravity
  E. Collaborative Care
    1. Prevent deficits in clients at risk: especially aged; anyone with increased fluid loss, such as persons with prolonged vomiting and diarrhea; during hot weather, those under physical exertion without adequate fluid replacement
    2. Correct the deficits and treat the underlying cause
      a. Replacement of fluids and electrolytes by oral, IV, or enteral route; Isotonic electrolyte IV solutions for hypotensive clients and those with abnormal losses
      b. Fluid challenge: physician orders a specific amount of IV fluid over short period of time (e.g., 300 mL of isotonic solution over 10 minutes). Obtain baseline assessment of vital signs, breath sounds, output, mental status before initiation; compare results after fluid challenge completed; physician re-evaluates response and orders fluids accordingly
      c. Assess parameters pertinent to the signs and symptoms, vital signs, and level of consciousness; reassess lab results
      d. Notify physician if urine output < 30 mL/hr (client has a foley catheter with hourly output as monitoring)
    3. Pertinent nursing diagnoses
      a. Fluid Volume Deficit
      b. Ineffective Tissue Perfusion
      c. Risk for Injury
II. Fluid Volume Excess (FVE) (too much fluid in body)
  Water and sodium are proportionately excessive and in extracellular compartment
  A. Common Stimuli (one or combination of conditions)
    1. Pathophysiology: mechanisms that should maintain homeostasis are impaired:
      a. Heart failure
      b. Kidney failure
      c. Cirrhosis of liver
      d. Adrenal disorders or corticosteroid administration
      e. Stress conditions causing release of ADH and aldosterone

2. Excessive intake of sodium and fluid
   a. Excessive intake of foods high in sodium (salt)
   b. Excessive intake of IV fluids containing sodium (0.09% NaCl)
B. Terminology
   1. Hypervolemia: excess intravascular fluid
   2. Edema: excess interstitial fluid
C. Signs/Symptoms
   1. Weight gain: > 5% of body weight over short time
   2. Circulatory overload: bounding pulse; S3 heart sound; neck and peripheral vein distention; increased CVP, i.e., mean pressure in right atrium of heart; cough; dyspnea; orthopnea; breath sounds, moist crackles; pulmonary edema; polyuria; ascites
   3. Peripheral edema worse in most dependent body part: pedal, sacral for bed-bound client; anasarca (severe generalized over all body edema); possibly cerebral edema, i.e., altered mental status
   4. Diagnostic test findings:
      a. Chest x-ray: variable degrees of pulmonary edema
      b. Serum sodium and osmolality: usually within normal range
      c. Hematocrit and hemoglobin: usually slightly decreased
      d. Decreased blood urea nitrogen (BUN), in some cases
D. Compensatory Mechanisms
   Heart failure results when heart is unable to increase workload to handle excess blood volume
   1. Left-side heart failure: pulmonary edema
   2. Right-side heart failure: peripheral edema
E. Collaborative Care
   1. Prevent fluid volume excess in at risk populations (those receiving IV fluids, significant at risk health histories, elderly)
   2. Effective fluid management:
      a. Assessment of signs/symptoms of fluid overload, lab results
      b. Fluid restrictions as ordered
      c. Dietary management: sodium-restricted diets
      d. Monitor intake and output, daily weights
   3. Treatment with diuretic medications
      a. Loop diuretics (e.g., Furosemide (Lasix))
      b. Thiazide-type diuretics (e.g., Hydrochlorothiazide (HCTZ))
   c. Potassium-sparing diuretics (e.g., Triamterene (Dyrenium))
F. Nursing Diagnoses
   1. Fluid Volume Excess
   2. Risk for Impaired Skin Integrity (related to peripheral edema)
   3. Risk for Impaired Gas Exchange (related to pulmonary congestion and/or edema)
   4. Activity Intolerance
III. Electrolyte Imbalances
   One electrolyte or several; often treat underlying cause; careful observation as over treatment may cause additional imbalances
   A. Sodium
      1. Characteristics:
         a. Mainly in ECF
         b. Blood normal values: 135–145 mEq/L
         c. Actions:
            1. Regulates volume
            2. Regulates osmolality
            3. Maintains neuromuscular activity
         d. Sources: dietary intake, prescription drugs, and self-remedies
         e. Compensatory mechanisms: kidney excretes or conserves sodium in response to changes in vascular volume, e.g., drop in blood pressure
            1. Stimulates renin-angiotensin-aldosterone system
            2. Regulates ADH secretion
            3. Modulates glomerular filtration rate
            4. Controls atrial natriuretic peptide release (sodium excretion)
      2. Hyponatremia
         Serum sodium is lower than normal (Serum Na^+ < 135 mEq/L)
         a. Common Stimuli
            1. Water shifts to ECF; osmolality changes and cells swell
            2. Loss of sodium (without water)
               a. Excessive through urine (e.g., diuretics, kidney disease)
               b. GI (e.g., vomiting, diarrhea, GI suction)
               c. Skin (e.g., sweating, burns)
               d. Water gain to dilute ECF
            3. Diseases: heart or renal failure; cirrhosis; Syndrome of Inappropriate secretion of Anti-Diuretic Hormone (SIADH); excessive hypotonic IV fluids
         b. Signs and Symptoms (depend on rapidity and severity of onset)
            1. Early: (Na^+ at 125)
               a. Muscle cramps, weakness, fatigue

  b. GI: anorexia, vomiting, diarrhea, nausea, abdominal cramping
  2. Later ($Na^+ < 120$)
    a. Cerebral edema symptoms (brain cells swell)
    b. Headache, depression, personality changes
    c. Lethargy, muscle twitching, tremors
    d. Further progress to convulsions and coma with severely low levels
  3. Diagnostic test findings
    a. Decreased serum Na^+ (< 135 mEq/L)
    b. Serum Osmolality (< 275 mOsm/kg)
    c. 24-hour urine collection for Na^+ used to differentiate cause
  c. Collaborative Care
  Restoration of blood volume and sodium levels
    1. Medications
      a. Isotonic IV solution (Ringer's, 0.9% NaCl)
      b. Hypertonic IV Na^+ solution (3% NaCl) is used to treat the client with severe hyponatremia (Na^+ : 110–115 mEq/L)
      c. Loop diuretics (e.g., Furosemide) to promote isotonic diuresis
    2. Fluid and Dietary Management
      a. Increase foods high in sodium
      b. Restrict fluid in volume
    3. Assessment of signs/symptoms of hyponatremia, especially
      a. Continual mental status assessment
      b. Seizure precautions
      c. Strict intake and output and monitoring weight daily
      d. Reassess lab results
  d. Nursing Diagnoses
    1. Risk for Impaired Fluid Volume
    2. Risk for Decreased Intracranial Adaptive Capacity
3. Hypernatremia
  Serum sodium is higher than normal (Serum sodium > 145 mEq/L)
  Hyperosmolality of ECF; may occur with fluid volume deficit or excess
  a. Common Stimuli
    1. Sodium gained in excess of water, e.g., excessive salt intake or hypertonic IV solutions, clients

with heat stroke, near drowning in seawater
    2. Water lost in excess of sodium, e.g., clients unable to respond to thirst as with altered mental status or physical disability; diabetes insipidus
  b. Signs and Symptoms (depend on rapidity and severity of onset)
    1. Initially: thirst
    2. If not responded to: altered neurologic function; lethargy; irritability; seizures; coma; death
    3. Diagnostic test findings:
      a. Serum sodium is greater than 145 mEq/L
      b. Serum Osmolality (> 295 mOsm/kg)
  c. Collaborative Care
    1. Treatment according to cause with slow correction of sodium to avoid development of cerebral edema
    2. Medications
      a. Oral or intravenous water replacement (hypotonic IV solutions such as 5% dextrose or 0.45% NaCl)
      b. Diuretics for sodium excretion
    3. Assessment
      a. Nursing history for precipitating factors as stimuli
      b. Vital signs, including temperature
      c. Mental status
      d. Signs/symptoms consistent with fluid volume deficit or excess
      e. Reassess lab results
  d. Nursing Diagnoses: Risk for Injury
B. Potassium (K^+)
  1. Characteristics
    a. Primary intracellular cation
    b. Normal serum potassium level 3.5–5.0 mEq/L
    c. Actions: vital role in cellular metabolism, heart function, and neuromuscular function
    d. Need daily intake of potassium, usually through food
    e. Kidneys eliminate potassium from body under regulation by aldosterone
    f. Shifts in and out of cells in response to concentration of hydrogen ion (pH) in the blood
  2. Hypokalemia
  Serum potassium is lower than normal (< 3.5 mEq/L)
    a. Common Stimuli

1. Excessive loss of potassium
   a. Through kidneys: secondary to drugs, hyperaldosteronism, diabetes mellitus
   b. Through GI tract: severe vomiting, gastric suction, diarrhea or ileostomy drainage
2. Inadequate intake
   a. Unable or unwilling to eat, anorexia nervosa
   b. Alcoholism
3. Shift from extracellular to intracellular space
b. Signs and Symptoms
   1. Abnormal heart rhythms including atrial and ventricular, potentiates digitalis toxicity (medication to treat heart failure)
   2. Muscle weakness, including leg cramps
   3. Slowed abdominal peristalsis
   4. Diagnostic test findings:
      a. Serum K^+: if K^+ = 2.5–3.0, moderate; if < 2.5, severe and probably symptomatic
      b. Arterial blood gases (hypokalemia associated with alkalosis, elevated pH)
      c. Electrocardiogram changes: flattened or inverted T waves, U waves
c. Collaborative Care
   1. Medications
      a. Potassium supplements, oral or parenteral
      b. Never give potassium IV push, only as IV infusion
   2. Dietary management
      Potassium rich foods (fruits and vegetables)
   3. Health promotion: Prevention of hypokalemia
      a. Using balanced electrolyte fluids with GI loss
      b. Diet teaching and/or potassium supplements with meds that predispose to hypokalemia
      c. Regular monitoring of serum potassium levels
   4. Assessment
      a. Nursing history for precipitating factors as stimuli
      b. Mental status
      c. Vital signs
      d. Reassess lab results

e. Nursing Diagnoses
   1. Activity Intolerance
   2. Decreased Cardiac Output
   3. Risk for Imbalance Fluid Volume
   4. Acute Pain (Potassium can be irritating to veins even when diluted; never give IV push)
3. Hyperkalemia
   Serum potassium is higher than normal (> 5.0 mEq/L)
   a. Common Stimuli
      1. Inadequate excretion of potassium
         a. Impaired renal excretion of potassium (untreated renal failure, adrenal insufficiency)
         b. Medications that impair K^+ excretion by kidneys (e.g., K^+ sparing diuretics)
      2. Excessively high intake of potassium
         a. Excess oral potassium by supplement, salt-substitute
         b. Rapid IV administration of potassium, transfusion of aged blood
      3. Shift from intracellular to extracellular space
         May occur with acidosis, severe tissue trauma
   b. Signs and Symptoms
      1. Abnormal heart function: slowing of heart rate and conduction; ventricular dysrhythmias progress to cardiac arrest
      2. Skeletal muscle irritability, tremors progress to weakness, and paralysis
      3. GI disturbances: initially, diarrhea and colic
      4. Diagnostic test findings
         a. Serum K^+: > 5.0 mEq/L
         b. Electrocardiogram: peaked T waves, prolonged conduction P-R, QRS
         c. Arterial blood gases to determine presence of acidosis
   c. Collaborative Care
      1. Medications
         a. Stop all potassium supplements orally and IV, if receiving
         b. Medications to lower serum potassium and stabilize conduction system of heart, including
            1. Intravenous Calcium Gluconate

2. Intravenous 50 gm of glucose and regular insulin (Moves K^+ intracellularly)
3. Sodium polystyrene sulfonate (Kayexalate), orally or rectally (binds K^+ in GI tract)
   c. Loop diuretics (e.g., Furosemide (Lasix)), if adequate renal function
2. Dialysis "artificial kidney" removes excess potassium
3. Health promotion: Teach clients at risk to read food and dietary supplements for potassium
4. Assessment
   a. Nursing history for precipitating factors as stimuli
   b. Cardiac status with continuous cardiac monitoring
   c. Vital signs
   d. Reassess lab results
   e. Hemolyzed blood sample: if serum K^+ is very high and client does not appear ill enough to have a potassium that high, blood should be redrawn and re-tested. First blood sample may have been hemolyzed.
   d. Nursing Diagnoses
   1. Risk for Activity Intolerance
   2. Risk for Decreased Cardiac Output
   3. Risk for Imbalanced Fluid Volume
C. Calcium (Ca^{+2})
   1. Characteristics
   a. Abundant in body
   b. Normal serum calcium level 8.5–10.0 mEq/L
   c. Body's source is from diet; 20% of calcium ingested is absorbed
   d. 99% calcium is in bones and teeth and is bound to phosphorus
   e. Extracellular, and only ionized form is active
   f. Actions:
   1. Regulates muscle contraction and relaxation, including respiratory muscles
   2. Maintains cardiac function
   3. Acts in blood clotting process
   g. Calcium levels are affected by acid-base balance
   2. Hypocalcemia
   Total serum calcium level < 8.5 mg/dL

Systemic effects caused by decreased levels of ionized Ca^{+2} in extracellular fluid
   a. Common Stimuli
   1. Hypoparathyroidism (neck surgery 24–48 hr post op)
   2. Acute pancreatitis
   3. Electrolyte imbalances (low magnesium, high phosphate), alkalosis
   4. Malabsorption disorders
   5. Certain medications, e.g., loop diuretics (Furosemide) anticonvulsants (phenytoin—generic for Dilantin)
   6. Massive transfusion of banked blood
   b. Signs and Symptoms
   1. Neuromuscular:
      a. Most serious is tetany (tonic muscle spasm) and convulsions
      b. Earlier: numbness and tingling around mouth, in hands and feet advancing to muscle spasms of face and extremities, hyperactive deep tendon reflexes (DTR's)
      c. Positive Chvostek's sign: face spasm with cheek tapping; positive Trousseau's sign: carpal spasm with inflation of BP cuff on arm
   2. Respiratory status: muscle spasms can lead to laryngeal spasms
   3. Cardiac: hypotension, bradycardia, ventricular dysrhythmias and cardiac arrest
   4. Diagnostic test findings
      a. Total serum Ca^{+2} < 8.5 mg/dL
      b. Serum albumin affects Ca^{+2}
      c. Serum magnesium: low, < 1.6 mg/dL is associated with low Ca^{+2}
      d. Serum phosphate: elevated, > 4.5 mg/dL is inversely related to Ca^{+2}
      e. Parathryoid hormone (PTH) to detect hyperparathyroidism
      f. Electrocardiogram: evaluate cardiac conduction: such as prolonged ST segment
   c. Collaborative Care
   1. Medications
      a. Calcium supplements
      b. Severe hypocalcemia: intravenous (CaChloride or CaGluconate)

      c. Chronic asymptomatic; oral forms, sometimes with Vitamin D

  2. Dietary management includes calcium in diet (milk, figs, salmon)

  3. Health promotion: Teaching to include prevention of osteoporosis (calcium moves from bones; not measured by serum Ca^{+2})

  4. Assessment:
    a. Nursing history for precipitating factors as stimuli
    b. Neuro assessment, cardiac status and vital signs
    c. Continuous cardiac monitoring and airway support, if indicated;
    d. Reassess lab results

 d. Nursing Diagnoses: Risk for Injury

3. Hypercalcemia
Total serum calcium level > 10.0 mg/dL
Systemic effects caused by increased levels of ionized Ca^{+2} in extracellular fluid
  a. Common Stimuli
    1. Increased reabsorption of calcium from bones
      a. Hyperparathyroidism
      b. Malignancies: cancers with metastasis (bone destruction by the tumor)
      c. Result of immobility and lack of weight-bearing
    2. Diminished elimination of calcium Occurs with medications (e.g., thiazide diuretics, lithium)
  b. Signs and Symptoms
    1. Decreased neuromuscular irritability: muscle weakness, depressed deep tendon reflexes (DTR's), advances to confusion, lethargy to coma
    2. GI: anorexia, nausea, vomiting, constipation
    3. Cardiac: heart conduction disturbances: bradycardia, heart block
    4. Polyuria and increased thirst
    5. Complications: peptic ulcer disease, pancreatitis, renal calculi (kidney stones)
    6. Hypercalcemic crisis; acute Ca^{+2} excess, can lead to cardiac arrest
    7. Diagnostic test findings
      a. Serum calcium > 10.0 mg/dL
      b. Serum Parathyroid level

      c. Electrocardiogram: changes including shortened QT, bradycardia, heart blocks

 c. Collaborative Care
Goal: to promote Ca^{+2} elimination by kidneys; to reduce Ca^{+2} reabsorption from bone
  1. Medications
    a. Intravenous fluids: usually isotonic saline
    b. Loop diuretic (e.g., Furosemide (Lasix) Calcitonin)
    c. For hypercalcemic crisis: IV sodium phosphate or potassium phosphate
    d. For inhibiting bone reabsorption: Plicamycin (Mithracin)
    e. Glucocorticoids
  2. Dietary Management: Increase intake of acid ash foods, fiber, fluid intake
  3. Health Promotion
    a. Identify persons at risk
    b. Encourage weight-bearing activity
    c. Fluids up to 3–4 quarts, if not contraindicated
    d. Limit calcium foods and supplements and calcium containing antacids
  4. Assessment
    a. Nursing history for precipitating factors as stimuli
    b. Vital signs
    c. Neuro assessment
    d. Cardiac status, continuous cardiac monitoring if indicated
    e. Reassess lab results (increased risk for digitalis toxicity)
 d. Nursing Diagnoses
  1. Risk for Injury
  2. Risk for Excess Fluid Volume

D. Magnesium
 1. Characteristics
  a. Mainly intracellular and in bone
  b. Normal serum level 1.6–2.6 mg/dL
  c. Obtained through diet (green vegetables, meat, grains, nuts)
  d. Excreted by kidneys
  e. Vital to cellular processes, enzyme, protein synthesis
  f. Sedative effect on neuromuscular junction
  g. Affected by potassium and calcium levels

2. Hypomagnesemia
   Magnesium level < 1.6 mg/dL
   Common in critically ill patients
   a. Common stimuli
      1. Usually occurs along with K^+ and Ca^{+2} deficiencies
      2. Loss of GI fluids as with diarrhea, ileostomy
      3. Impaired nutrition absorption from gut; starvation, NPO (nothing by mouth) status
      4. Chronic alcoholism
      5. Medications such as loop or thiazide diuretics, some antibiotics
   b. Signs and Symptoms
      1. Increased neuromuscular excitability: tremors, hyperactive reflexes, tetany, mood changes
      2. Cardiac: dysrhythmias and sudden death; increased risk of digitalis toxicity
      3. GI: nausea, vomiting, diarrhea, anorexia, abdominal distention
      4. Diagnostic test findings:
         a. Electrolyte levels; low magnesium often with low Ca^{+2} and K^+
         b. Electrocardiogram: delayed conduction with dysrhythmias, cardiac arrest, sudden death
   c. Collaborative Care
      1. Medications: if symptomatic, treated with IV Magnesium Sulfate, and/or oral supplements
      2. Dietary Management: encourage balanced diet including green vegetables, meat, grains, nuts, seafood
      3. Health Promotion
         a. Identify persons at risk (post-surgery clients, clients with malnutrition, alcoholics)
         b. Encourage well-balanced nutrition
      4. Assessment
         a. Nursing history for precipitating factors as stimuli
         b. Vital signs
         c. Neuro status
         d. Cardiac status, continuous cardiac monitoring
         e. GI assessment
         f. Reassess lab results (increased risk for digitalis toxicity)
   d. Nursing Diagnoses: Risk for Injury
3. Hypermagnesemia
   Magnesium level > 2.6 mg/dL
   Less common
   a. Common Stimuli: renal failure, especially clients receiving parenteral or oral supplements
   b. Signs and Symptoms
      1. Neuromuscular: weakness, lethargy leading to weak or absent deep tendon reflexes (DTR), drowsiness as level rises
      2. Cardiovascular: hypotension, flushing, sweating, brady-dysrhythmias leading to heart block, cardiac arrest as level rises; respiratory depression with high levels
      3. GI: nausea and vomiting
      4. Diagnostic test findings
         a. Magnesium level elevated
         b. Electorcardiogram: changes with bradycardia, heart block
   c. Collaborative Care
      1. Medications
         a. Withhold medications containing magnesium
         b. Dialysis for clients with renal failure
         c. Calcium Gluconate IV for reversal or neuro and cardiac effects
      2. Health Promotion
         a. Identify clients at risk (those with renal failure, receiving magnesium supplements)
         b. Teach to avoid laxatives, antacids, and enemas containing magnesium
      3. Assessment
         a. Nursing history for precipitating factors as stimuli
         b. Neuromuscular assessment
         c. Cardiac assessment, continuous cardiac monitoring and airway support if indicated
         d. Reassess lab results
   d. Nursing Diagnoses
      1. Decreased Cardiac Output
      2. Risk for Ineffective Breathing Pattern
      3. Risk for Injury
E. Phosphate
   1. Characteristics
      a. Mostly in bone; intracellular anion
      b. Normal serum level 2.5–4.5 mg/dL
      c. Essential to intracellular processes, including muscle contraction and nerve conduction, metabolism, acid base balance

d. Source is from diet, excreted by kidneys

e. Inverse relationship with calcium

2. Hypophosphatemia

Serum phosphorus < 2.5 mg/dL

Total body deficit or cellular shift

a. Common Stimuli

1. Usually iatrogenic (related to treatment)

2. Refeeding syndrome: occurs with beginning enteral or total parenteral feedings to malnourished clients

3. Medications: intravenous glucose solutions, diuretics, aluminum or magnesium-based antacids

4. Alcoholism

5. Hyperventilation with respiratory alkalosis

b. Signs and Symptoms

1. Neuromuscular: irritability, weakness, paresthesias, confusion, and seizures leading to respiratory failure

2. Cardiac: dysrhythmias, chest pain

3. GI: anorexia, dysphagia, nausea, vomiting, decreased GI motility

4. Diagnostic test findings: serum phosphate is < 2.5 mg/dL

c. Collaborative Care

1. Medications

a. Oral phosphate supplements (Neutra-Phos)

b. Intravenous phosphorus such as sodium phosphate, potassium phosphate

c. Eliminate phosphate depleting medications, if possible

2. Dietary Management: stress well-balanced diet

3. Health Promotion

a. Identify clients at risk

b. Teach, including avoidance of phosphorus-binding antacids

4. Assessment

a. Nursing history for precipitating factors as stimuli

b. Neuromuscular

c. GI

d. Cardiac with cardiac monitoring and respiratory support if indicated

e. Reassess lab results, especially electrolytes

d. Nursing Diagnoses

1. Impaired Physical Mobility

2. Ineffective Breathing Pattern

3. Decreased Cardiac Output

4. Risk for Injury

3. Hyperphosphatemia

Serum phosphorus > 4.5 mg/dL

Impaired excretion, total body excess or cellular shift

a. Common Stimuli

1. Acute or chronic renal failure

2. Excess or rapid intake of phosphates

3. Phosphate shifts from chemotherapy, trauma, heat stroke

4. Accompanies altered calcium concentrations

b. Signs and Symptoms

1. Neuromuscular: muscle cramps, paresthesias, muscle spasms, tetany

2. Calcification of soft tissues

3. Diagnostic test findings: serum phosphate is > 4.5 mg/d/L

c. Collaborative Care

1. Treat cause

2. Promote renal excretion by IV saline or dialysis for client in renal failure

3. Dietary Management: eliminate phosphate rich foods, such as organ meats, milk, and milk products

4. Health Promotion

a. Identify clients at risk

b. Teach, including avoidance of phosphate sources, foods or medications

5. Assessment

a. Nursing history for precipitating factors as stimuli

b. Neuromuscular

c. Reassess lab results, especially electrolytes

d. Nursing Diagnoses: Risk for Injury

ACID-BASE BALANCE

I. Background

A. Facts and Definitions

1. Acid-base homeostasis is necessary to maintain life.

2. Acid base balance must be within a definite range for cellular function to occur.

3. The acidity of a substance, determined by the hydrogen ion (H^+) concentration, is expressed as pH.

4. Acids

a. Release hydrogen ions into solution

b. Have pH < 7
5. Alkalines (bases)
  a. Accept hydrogen ions into solution
  b. Have pH > 7
B. Body fluids
  1. Normally slightly alkaline
  2. Normal range is narrow: 7.35–7.45 (pH of 7 is neutral)
  3. Arterial blood pH < 7.35 is considered acid
  4. Arterial blood pH > 7.45 is considered alkaline
C. Acids and Bases in the body
  1. Body functions constantly produce acids
  2. Most acids and bases in the body are weak
  3. Acids include
    a. Carbonic acid, which is eliminated as a gas, carbon dioxide
    b. Lactic, hydrochloric, phosphoric, sulfuric acids, which are metabolized or excreted as fluids
  4. Bicarbonate is the major base
II. Body regulation of acid-base balance
Constant response to changes in pH to maintain the pH in the normal range
3 systems in the body, with various response times, to maintain acid-base balance
A. Buffer System
  1. Responds immediately, but has limited capacity to maintain
  2. Buffers: substances that bind or release hydrogen ions
    a. When body fluid becomes acid, buffers bind with hydrogen ions to raise pH
    b. When body fluid becomes alkaline, buffers release hydrogen ions to lower pH
  3. Buffer systems
    a. Bicarbonate-carbonic acid buffer system

$$CO_2 + H_2O \leftrightarrow H_2CO_3 \leftrightarrow H^+ + HCO_3$$
weak acid   weak base

Process is reversible but the ratio of 20 (bicarbonate) to 1 (hydrogen) must be maintained
    b. Protein buffer system (intracellular and plasma)
    c. Phosphates buffer system
B. Respiratory System
  1. Responds within minutes
  2. Includes respiratory center of brain stem and lungs
  3. Occurs automatically, not under voluntary control
  4. Adjusts the depth and frequency of respiration according to the pH of the blood; increases or decreases the amount of carbon dioxide in the blood; controls the amount of carbonic acid formed and adjusts the pH of the blood
    a. Hyperventilation: increased depth and frequency of respiration; blows off more CO_2 in response to an acid pH
    b. Hypoventilation: decreased depth and frequency of respiration; retains more CO_2 in response to an alkaline pH
C. Renal (Metabolic) System
  1. Responds within hours to days
  2. Adjusts the amounts of hydrogen and bicarbonate ions
    a. Kidneys excrete H^+ ions, or generate and reabsorb bicarbonate ions, in response to an acid pH
    b. Kidneys retain H^+ ions, or generate and excrete bicarbonate ions, in response to an alkaline pH
III. Determination of Acid-Base Balance: Analysis of Arterial Blood Gases (ABG's)
A. pH
  1. Normal: 7.35–7.45
  2. Acidic: < 7.35
  3. Alkaline: > 7.45
B. pCO_2
Pressure of carbon dioxide; respiratory component
  1. Normal: 35–45 mm Hg
  2. Acidic: > 45 mm Hg (carbon dioxide forms carbonic acid)
Hypercapnia: elevated levels of carbon dioxide in blood
  3. Alkaline: < 35 mm Hg
Hypocapnia: decreased levels of carbon dioxide in blood
C. HCO_3
Bicarbonate; renal or metabolic component
  1. Normal: 22–26 mEq/L
  2. Acidic: < 22 mEq/L
  3. Alkaline: > 26 mEq/L
D. Base Excess
  1. Calculated value for buffer base capacity: the amount of acid or base added to blood to obtain a pH of 7.4
  2. Normal: −3 to +3
E. pO_2
Pressure of oxygen in blood
  1. Gives data about level of oxygenation; not used to calculate acid-base status of blood

2. Normal: 80–100 mm Hg
3. Hypoxemia: < 80 mm Hg
IV. Acid-Base Imbalance
  A. Classifications
    1. Acidosis or alkalosis
      a. Acidosis: Hydrogen ion concentration in blood increases above normal and pH is below 7.35
      b. Alkalosis: Hydrogen ion concentration in blood decreases below normal and pH is above 7.45
    2. Origin of the problem
      a. From the respiratory system
      b. From the metabolic system
  B. Disorders: Simple or Combined
    1. Primary disorders
      a. Simple
      b. One cause, either respiratory or metabolic
    2. Combined disorders
      a. More severe
      b. Both the respiratory and metabolic systems are the cause of the same imbalance
  C. Compensation
    1. Only occurs with primary disorders
    2. Response by the system not causing the imbalance to correct the pH Example: with respiratory acidosis, the kidneys would eliminate hydrogen ions in urine to offset the acidosis caused by hypoventilation of lungs.
    3. Complete compensation occurs if the pH is corrected to the normal range (7.35–7.45).
    4. Partial compensation occurs if there is improvement in the pH but not to the normal range.
    5. Compensation can be determined by analysis of the arterial blood gas results.
  D. Treatment
    1. Urgency
      a. Mental ability and level of consciousness is often affected
      b. Brain function usually affected; brain cells need proper conditions to perform cellular functions
      c. Cells cannot function properly if significant acidosis or alkalosis occurs
    2. Indirect treatment
      a. Treating and correcting the precipitating condition often corrects the acid-base imbalance
      b. Directly treating the acid-base imbalance, by adding or removing hydrogen or bicarbonate ions, may lead to further imbalances
      c. Not usually first line of treatment
V. Types of Acid-Base Imbalances
  A. Respiratory Acidosis
    pH < 7.35
    pCO_2 > 45 mm Hg (excess carbon dioxide in the blood)
    Respiratory system impaired and retaining CO_2; causing acidosis
    1. Common Stimuli
      a. Acute respiratory failure from airway obstruction
      b. Over-sedation from anesthesia or narcotics
      c. Some neuromuscular diseases that affect ability to use chest muscles
      d. Chronic respiratory problems, such as advanced Chronic Obstructive Lung Disease
    2. Signs and Symptoms
      a. Compensation: kidneys respond by generating and reabsorbing bicarbonate ions, so HCO_3 > 26 mm Hg
      b. Respiratory: hypoventilation, slow or shallow respirations
      c. Neuro: headache, blurred vision, irritability, confusion
      d. Respiratory collapse leads to unconsciousness and cardiovascular collapse
    3. Collaborative Care
      a. Early recognition of respiratory status and treat cause
      b. Restore ventilation and gas exchange; CPR for respiratory failure with oxygen supplementation; intubation and ventilator support if indicated
      c. Treatment of respiratory infections with bronchodilators, antibiotic therapy
      d. Reverse excess anesthetics and narcotics with medications such as naloxone (Narcan)
      e. Chronic respiratory conditions
        1. Breathe in response to low oxygen levels
        2. Adjusted to high carbon dioxide level through metabolic compensation (therefore, high CO_2 not a breathing trigger)
        3. Cannot receive high levels of oxygen, or will have no trigger to breathe; will develop carbon dioxide narcosis

4. Treat with no higher than 2 liters O_2 per cannula
   f. Continue respiratory assessments, monitor further arterial blood gas results
4. Nursing Diagnoses
   a. Impaired Gas Exchange
   b. Ineffective Airway Clearance
B. Respiratory Alkalosis
   pH > 7.45
   pCO_2 < 35 mm Hg
   Carbon dioxide deficit, secondary to hyperventilation
   1. Common Stimuli
      a. Hyperventilation with anxiety from uncontrolled fear, pain, stress (e.g., women in labor, trauma victims)
      b. High fever
      c. Mechanical ventilation, during anesthesia
   2. Signs and Symptoms
      a. Compensation: kidneys compensate by eliminating bicarbonate ions; decrease in bicarbonate
         HCO_3 < 22 mm Hg
      b. Respiratory: hyperventilating: shallow, rapid breathing
      c. Neuro: panicked, light-headed, tremors, may develop tetany, numb hands and feet (related to symptoms of hypocalcemia; with elevated pH more Ca^{+2} ions are bound to serum albumin and less ionized "active" calcium available for nerve and muscle conduction)
      d. May progress to seizures, loss of consciousness (when normal breathing pattern returns)
      e. Cardiac: palpitations, sensation of chest tightness
   3. Collaborative Care
      a. Treatment: encourage client to breathe slowly in a paper bag to rebreathe CO_2
      b. Breathe with the patient; provide emotional support and reassurance, anti-anxiety agents, sedation
      c. On ventilator, adjustment of ventilation settings (decrease rate and tidal volume)
      d. Prevention: pre-procedure teaching, preventative emotional support, monitor blood gases as indicated
C. Metabolic Acidosis
   pH < 7.35
   Deficit of bicarbonate in the blood $NaHCO_3$
   < 22 mEq/L

Caused by an excess of acid, or loss of bicarbonate from the body
1. Common Stimuli
   a. Acute lactic acidosis from tissue hypoxia (lactic acid produced from anaerobic metabolism with shock, cardiac arrest)
   b. Ketoacidosis (fatty acids are released and converted to ketones when fat is used to supply glucose needs as in uncontrolled Type 1 Diabetes or starvation)
   c. Acute or chronic renal failure (kidneys unable to regulate electrolytes)
   d. Excessive bicarbonate loss (severe diarrhea, intestinal suction, bowel fistulas)
   e. Usually results from some other disease and is often accompanied by electrolyte and fluid imbalances
   f. Hyperkalemia often occurs as the hydrogen ions enter cells to lower the pH displacing the intracellular potassium; hypercalcemia and hypomagnesemia may occur
2. Signs and Symptoms
   a. Compensation: respiratory system begins to compensate by increasing the depth and rate of respiration in an effort to lower the CO_2 in the blood; this causes a decreased level of carbon dioxide: pCO_2 < 35 mm HG.
   b. Neuro changes: headache, weakness, fatigue progressing to confusion, stupor, and coma
   c. Cardiac: dysrhythmias and possibly cardiac arrest from hyperkalemia
   d. GI: anorexia, nausea, vomiting
   e. Skin: warm and flushed
   f. Respiratory: tries to compensate by hyperventilation: deep and rapid respirations known as Kussmaul's respirations
   g. Diagnostic test findings:
      1. ABG: pH < 7.35, HCO_3 < 22
      2. Electrolytes: Serum K^+ > 5.0 mEq/L
      3. Serum Ca^{+2} > 10.0 mg/dL
      4. Serum Mg^{+2} < 1.6 mg/dL
3. Collaborative Care
   a. Medications: Correcting underlying cause will often improve acidosis
   b. Restore fluid balance, prevent dehydration with IV fluids
   c. Correct electrolyte imbalances

  d. Administer sodium bicarbonate IV, if acidosis is severe and does not respond rapidly enough to treatment of primary cause. (Oral bicarbonate is sometimes given to clients with chronic metabolic acidosis) Be careful not to overtreat and put client into alkalosis
  e. As acidosis improves, hydrogen ions shift out of cells and potassium moves intracellularly. Hyperkalemia may change to hypokalemia and potassium replacement will be needed.
  f. Assessment
    1. Vital signs
    2. Intake and output
    3. Neuro, GI, and respiratory status
    4. Cardiac monitoring
    5. Reassess repeated arterial blood gases and electrolytes
  4. Nursing Diagnoses
    a. Decreased Cardiac Output
    b. Risk for Fluid Volume Excess (FVE)
    c. Risk for Injury
D. Metabolic Alkalosis
  pH > 7.45
  HCO_3 > 26 mEq/L
  Caused by a bicarbonate excess, due to loss of acid, or a bicarbonate excess in the body
  1. Common Stimuli
    a. Loss of hydrogen and chloride ions through excessive vomiting, gastric suctioning, or excessive diuretic therapy
    b. Response to hypokalemia
    c. Excess ingestion of bicarbonate rich antacids or excessive treatment of acidosis with sodium bicarbonate
  2. Signs and Symptoms
    a. Compensation: Lungs respond by decreasing the depth and rate of respiration in effort to retain carbon dioxide and lower pH
    b. Neuro: altered mental status, numbness and tingling around mouth, fingers, toes, dizziness, muscle spasms (similar to hypocalcemia due to less ionized calcium levels)
    c. Respiratory: shallow, slow breathing
    d. Diagnostic test findings
      1. ABG's: pH > 7.45, HCO_3 > 26
      2. Electrolytes: Serum K^+ < 3.5 mEq/L
      3. Electrocardiogram: as with hypokalemia
  3. Collaborative Care
    a. Correcting underlying cause will often improve alkalosis
    b. Restore fluid volume and correct electrolyte imbalances (usually IV NaCl with KCL).
    c. With severe cases, acidifying solution may be administered.
    d. Assessment
      1. Vital signs
      2. Neuro, cardiac, respiratory assessment
      3. Repeat arterial blood gases and electrolytes
  4. Nursing Diagnoses
    a. Impaired Gas Exchange
    b. Ineffective Airway Clearance
    c. Risk for Injury

FOCUSED STUDY TIPS

- While in your clinical setting, obtain a lab requisition form for serum electrolytes. Become familiar with normal values.
- Request to care for a client experiencing fluid and electrolyte imbalance. What treatments can you identify that are being utilized to correct the imbalances?
- Find an abnormal serum electrolyte value while caring for a client in the clinical setting. Assess the client for manifestations of the abnormal value.

CASE STUDY

Mrs. Babcock is a diabetic and has a history of chronic alcoholism and heart disease. She is admitted to the emergency room for treatment of diabetic ketoacidosis and hypomagnesemia. The physician orders a digitalis preparation for treatment of her heart disease. What specific observation should be made regarding the administration of a digitalis preparation when the client has hypomagnesemia? What nursing interventions must be initiated? What diagnostic tests can be anticipated?

CARE PLAN CRITICAL THINKING ACTIVITY

An 84-year-old male is admitted in a very confused state from home. His neighbor states he has been ill for several days. What would you do to assess the patient for dehydration and electrolyte imbalance?

NCLEX TEST QUESTIONS

1. Isotonic solutions have:
   a. greater concentration of solutes than plasma.
   b. lower concentration of solutes than plasma.
   c. the same concentration of solutes as plasma.
   d. 0 .45% concentration of solutes.
2. Early manifestations of hyperkalemia include:
   a. diarrhea, colic, anxiety, and muscle tremors.
   b. flaccid paralysis, bradycardia, and headache.
   c. confusion, anxiety, and constipation.
   d. polyuria, diarrhea, and anorexia.
3. The diagnostic test instrumental in the diagnosis of respiratory or metabolic acidosis or alkalosis is:
   a. serum electrolytes.
   b. arterial blood gases.
   c. pulmonary function tests.
   d. serum chemistry profile.
4. Whenever possible, administer intravenous potassium:
   a. via IV piggyback over 6 hours.
   b. as a bolus dose for rapid effects.
   c. as an IV push for 5 minutes duration.
   d. via a central line.
5. Clients who take digitalis and need IV calcium should:
   a. hold the digitalis for 24 hours prior and after the administration of IV calcium.
   b. have serial calcium levels drawn q 1 hour until the dose is completed.
   c. be monitored via continuous ECG monitoring to detect digitalis toxicity.
   d. have an EKG before and after the calcium administration to detect digitalis toxicity.
6. Clients most at risk for hypocalcemia are clients:
   a. who are elderly.
   b. experiencing hyperthyroidism.
   c. have undergone neck surgery.
   d. postoperative who become dehydrated.
7. Fluid challenges are utilized to evaluate:
   a. fluid volume overload.
   b. shock.
   c. dehydration.
   d. questionable cardiac or renal functioning.

CHAPTER 6

NURSING CARE OF CLIENTS EXPERIENCING TRAUMA AND SHOCK

LEARNING OUTCOMES

After completing this chapter, you will be able to:

- Describe the components and types of trauma.
- Discuss causes, effects, and initial management of trauma.
- Discuss diagnostic tests used in assessing clients experiencing trauma and shock.
- Describe collaborative interventions for clients experiencing trauma and shock, including medications, blood transfusion, and intravenous fluids.
- Discuss organ donation and forensic implications of traumatic injury or death.
- Discuss cellular homeostasis and basic hemodynamics.
- Discuss the risk factors, etiologies, and pathophysiologies of hypovolemic shock, cardiogenic shock, obstructive shock, and distributive shock.
- Use the nursing process as a framework for providing individualized care to clients experiencing trauma and shock.

KEY TOPICS

- Components and types of trauma
- Nursing care of the client experiencing trauma
- Types and pathophysiology of shock
- Nursing care of the client experiencing shock

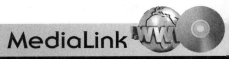

MediaLink

www.prenhall.com/lemone

Additional resources for this chapter can be found on the Student CD-ROM accompanying this textbook, and on the Companion Website at www.prenhall.com/lemone. Click on Chapter 6 to select the activities for this chapter.

CD-ROM
- Audio Glossary
- NCLEX Review

Animation
- Hypovolemic Shock

Companion Website
- More NCLEX Review
- Case Study
    A Client Experiencing Trauma
- MediaLink Applications
    Organ Donation
    Injury Prevention

LECTURE OUTLINE
TRAUMA

I. Analysis of Trauma
   A. Definition and Impact
      1. Definition: sudden accidents or purposeful acts leading to injury, disability, or death
      2. Impact: initial physical injuries and long term effects; rehabilitation and psychosocial effects on clients and family members
   B. Components of trauma
      1. Host: person or group at risk of injury
      2. Mechanism: source of energy that causes trauma
         Most common: mechanical energy from motor vehicles in accidents
      3. Intention: deliberate or unintentional
      4. Environment: location and under what circumstances
   C. Types of trauma
      1. Blunt: no communication between damaged tissue and outside environment; injuries are internal and can be minor to lethal
      2. Penetrating: actual tissue damage to body structures, obvious from outside
      3. Often combination of blunt and penetrating
II. Prehospital Care
   A. Injury identification
      1. Rapid comprehensive trauma assessment
      2. Determine need for trauma center and rapid transport
      3. Airway, Breathing, Circulation
      4. Level of consciousness/possible spinal cord injuries
      5. Any obvious injuries
   B. Critical interventions
      1. Life support
      2. Immobilize cervical spine
      3. Airway management (intubation)
      4. Treat hemorrhage and shock
      5. Apply direct pressure over wounds
   C. Rapid Transport
III. Hospital Care: Emergency Department Care
   A. Support above critical interventions
   B. Determine extent of injuries/plan of treatment through common diagnostic tests
      1. Blood type and crossmatch: determine client's blood type; ready donor blood for transfusion
      2. Blood alcohol level: alters level of consciousness and pain response
      3. Urine drug screen: alters level of consciousness and pain response
      4. Pregnancy test for women of child-bearing age: treatment concerns
      5. Diagnostic peritoneal lavage: test for presence of blood in peritoneal cavity; determine hemorrhaging internally (catheter placed in lower abdomen and aspiration for free blood; infuse warm isotonic solution rapidly and drain by gravity; check for presence of blood)
      6. Computerized Tomography (CT Scan) special x-ray of body area in layers with computerized views; brain, chest, abdomen
   C. Medications
      1. May have been initiated at scene
      2. Intravenous (IV) access and fluids, blood components
      3. Cardiovascular support with inotropic agents, vasopressors
      4. Pain control
      5. Tetanus immunization, if indicated
   D. Blood Transfusions
   E. Emergency surgery
   F. Organ Donation
      1. Client will not recover; client meets brain death criteria
      2. Uniform Anatomical Gift Act (1968, 1987): client be informed about options for organ donation; address option with next of kin
      3. Care given to maintain circulation and perfuse organs, if organs will be harvested
      4. Supportive care to family member; assist with grief
   G. Forensic Considerations
      1. Trauma may have occurred in illegal activity
      2. Determine if client is under influence of alcohol, illegal drugs
      3. Maintain chain of custody, i.e., preserve, label, document, dispose, evidence
IV. Prevention of Trauma
   Educate the public about trauma prevention and safety, e.g., seatbelts, bicycle helmets
V. Common Nursing Diagnoses for Trauma Clients
   A. Ineffective Airway Clearance
   B. Risk for Infection
   C. Impaired Physical Mobility
   D. Spiritual Distress: Client and Family
   E. Risk for Post-Trauma Syndrome
      1. Intense emotional response to disastrous event

2. Impaired coping mechanisms
3. Nurses assist client and family to express feelings
4. Referrals for counseling, support groups

SHOCK

I. Definition and Pathophysiology
  A. Definition
    1. Clinical syndrome, systemic imbalance between oxygen supply and demand
    2. Inadequate blood flow to body organs and tissue causing life-threatening cellular dysfunction
  B. Pathophysiology
    1. Stimulus leads to alteration in hemodynamics within the body
    2. Body responds by maintaining perfusion to vital organs, heart and brain
    3. Results in inadequate tissue and cellular perfusion; if not reversed, body develops acidosis and if untreated, progresses to organ hypoxia, ischemia and death
    4. Alteration in hemodynamics results in a drop in arterial blood pressure by one of these mechanisms
      a. Decrease in cardiac output (ability of heart to supply adequate circulation)
      b. Decrease in circulating blood volume
      c. Increase in size of vascular bed

II. Hemodynamic Terms
  A. Stroke Volume (SV): amount of blood pumped into aorta by contraction of left ventricle
  B. Cardiac Output (CO): amount of blood pumped into aorta by contraction of left ventricle in one minute
  C. Mean arterial pressure (MAP): product of cardiac output and systemic vascular resistance

III. Stages of Shock
  A. Early reversible and compensatory shock
    1. Mean arterial pressure drops 10–15 mm Hg
    2. Decrease in circulating blood volume (25–35%) 1000 ml
    3. Sympathetic nervous system stimulated; release of catecholamine
    4. To maintain blood pressure: increase in heart rate and contractility; increase in peripheral vasoconstriction
    5. Circulation maintained, but can only be sustained short time without harm to tissues
    6. Underlying cause of shock must be addressed and corrected or will progress to next stage
  B. Intermediate or progressive shock
    1. Further drop in MAP (20%)
    2. Increase in fluid loss (1800–25 400 ml)
    3. Vasoconstriction continues and leads to oxygen deficiency
    4. Body switches to anaerobic metabolism forming lactic acid as a waste product
    5. Body increases heart rate and vasoconstriction
    6. Heart and brain become hypoxic
    7. More severe effects on other tissues which become ischemic and anoxic
    8. State of acidosis with hyperkalemia develops
    9. Needs rapid treatment
  C. Refractory or irreversible shock
    1. Tissues are anoxic, cellular death widespread
    2. Even with restoration of blood pressure and fluid volume, there is too much damage to restore homeostasis of tissues
    3. Cellular death leads to tissue death; vital organs fail and death occurs

IV. Effects of Shock on Body Systems
  A. Cardiovascular
    1. Initially: slight tachycardia, normal blood pressure
    2. Progresses to weak, rapid pulse with dysrhythmias
    3. Progressive decrease in systolic and diastolic blood pressures with narrowing of pulse pressure; blood pressure becomes inaudible
  B. Respiratory
    1. Initially: Increased respiratory rate, but gas exchange is impaired; leads to anaerobic metabolism and development of acidosis
    2. *Acute Respiratory Distress Syndrome (ARDS):* complication of decreased lung perfusion
  C. Gastrointestinal and Hepatic
    1. GI organs become ischemic, with blood circulation shunted to heart and brain
    2. Complications
      a. *Stress Ulcers:* GI mucosa becomes ischemic, prone to rapid ulceration
      b. *Paralytic Ileus:* decreased gastrointestinal motility with decreased blood flow
    3. Altered liver metabolism: initially glucose made available, then hypoglycemia, fat

breakdown leads to ketones and metabolic acidosis
  D. Neurologic
    1. Develops cerebral hypoxia
    2. Restlessness initially, then altered level of consciousness, lethargy, coma
  E. Renal: Decreased kidney perfusion leads to *oliguria* (urine output < 20 ml/°)
  F. Skin, temperature, thirst
    1. Skin: cool, pale, hypothermic
    2. Thirsty from dehydration
V. Types of Shock (categorized according to underlying causes)
  A. Hypovolemic
    1. Decrease in intravascular volume > 15%
    2. Most common: occurs with other types of shock
    3. Common stimuli: hemorrhage, burns, severe dehydration, third spacing
    4. Progresses through stages of shock without restoration of fluid volume
  B. Cardiogenic
    1. Pumping ability of heart compromised to a degree that cannot maintain cardiac output and adequate tissue perfusion
    2. Common stimuli: myocardial infarction, cardiac arrest
    3. Develops left and right sided heart failure
    4. Cyanosis occurs with this type of shock
  C. Obstructive
    1. Heart or great vessels obstructed; venous return or cardiac pumping action impeded
    2. Common stimuli: pulmonary embolism, pneumothorax
  D. Distributive (Vasogenic)
    1. Widespread vasodilatation
    2. Decreased peripheral resistance
  E. Septic Shock
    1. Leading cause of death in intensive care units
    2. Common stimuli: Gram negative bacterial infections (pseudomonas, *E coli*); Gram positive bacterial infections (staphylococcus and streptococcus)
    3. Increased risk: clients with chronic illness, poor nutritional status, invasive procedure or tubes, such as foley catheters
    4. Course
      a. Septicemia develops (pathogens and their toxins in the blood)
      b. Endotoxins disrupt circulation
      c. Normal coagulation mechanisms
      d. Inflammatory response triggered
    5. Phases of Septic Shock
      a. Warm Phase (early): skin flushed, warm due to vasodilatation
      b. Cold Phase (late): skin cool due to fluid deficit with shock
  F. Neurogenic Shock
    1. Imbalance between parasympathetic and sympathetic nervous stimulation of vascular smooth muscle, resulting in sustained vasodilatation
    2. Common stimuli: head injury, spinal cord trauma, insulin reactions, anesthesia
  G. Anaphylactic Shock
    1. Result of widespread hypersensitivity (anaphylaxis)
    2. Vasodilatation occurs leading to hypovolemia and altered cellular metabolism
    3. Sensitized in past, re-contact with the allergen (medication, bee sting, food allergen)
    4. Allergic reaction with large amounts of histamine released
    5. Histamine leads to increased permeability and massive vasodilatation
    6. Develops respiratory distress with bronchospasm and laryngospasm
VI. Collaborative Care
  A. Focus on treating underlying cause to stop progression through stages of shock
  B. Rapid shock identification; rapid diagnosis of cause; rapid aggressive treatment: better outcome for client
  C. Goal: improving arterial oxygenation and tissue perfusion
  D. Determine type of shock
  E. Diagnostic tests and purpose used with clients in shock
    1. Blood hemoglobin and hematocrit: hypovolemic shock
    2. Arterial Blood Gases: identify body compensatory mechanisms, such as acidosis
    3. Electrolytes
    4. BUN and creatinine, osmolality: renal function
    5. Blood cultures: identify causative organism in septic shock; treatment
    6. White blood count and differential: septic shock
    7. Cardiac enzymes: diagnosis of cardiogenic shock (cardiac enzymes are: lactate dehydrogenase (LDH); Creatine phosphokinase (CPK); serum glutamic-oxaloacetic transaminase (SGOT):
    8. Other tests may be ordered
  F. Medications
    1. Inotropic agents: improve cardiac contractility

2. Vasoactive agents: drugs causing vasoconstriction or vasodilatation according to client symptoms
3. Other meds according to cause such as antibiotics, steroids

G. Oxygen Therapy
   1. Patent airway and adequate oxygenation critical interventions
   2. Monitor with ABG, pulse oximetry (more accurate in early stage)
   3. Mechanical ventilation assistance may be needed

H. Fluid Replacement
   1. Essential for hypovolemic shock; also with other types as symptoms indicate
   2. Types of Intravenous Fluids
      a. Crystalloid solutions
         1. Dextrose or electrolyte solutions
         2. Increase intravascular and interstitial fluid volume
         3. Examples: Isotonic (0.9% NaCl, lactated Ringers) Hypotonic (5% dextrose in water, .45% NaCl)
      b. Colloids
         1. Do not diffuse easily through capillary walls
         2. Fluids stay in vascular compartment; increase osmotic pressure
         3. Examples: albumin, hetastarch, plasma protein fraction, dextran
      c. Blood and blood products
         1. Treatment of hemorrhage
         2. Restore coagulation properties

VII. Blood Transfusion
   A. Background
      1. Four blood types; categorized according to antigens on red blood cells
         a. Type A: A antigens
         b. Type B: B antigens
         c. Type O: no antigens (universal donor)
         d. Type AB: A and B antigens (universal recipient)
      2. D antigen, third antigen; may be present on the red blood cells
         a. Rh factor positive: D antigen is present
         b. Rh factor negative: D antigen is not present
   B. Type and Crossmatch (T & C)
      1. Performed on blood to be transfused
      2. Donated blood is matched to the recipient's blood according to type and Rh factor status.
   C. Blood transfusion reactions

1. Occur when there is some degree of incompatibility between the donor and recipient blood
2. Nurses administering blood need to be aware and observant for signs of transfusion reactions
3. Types of blood transfusion reactions
   a. Febrile
      1. Recipient's antibodies are directed against donor's white blood cells, causing fever and chills
      2. Occurrence: within first 15 minutes of transfusion
   b. Hypersensitivity
      1. Recipient's antibodies react against proteins in donor's blood causing urticaria (hives) and itching
      2. Occurrence: during or after transfusion
   c. Hemolytic
      1. Most dangerous; ABO incompatibility causing red blood cells to clump and block capillaries, decreasing blood flow to vital organs; hemoglobin is released which blocks renal tubules and can cause renal failure.
      2. Signs and symptoms: lumbar, abdominal and/or chest pain, fever, chills, urticaria, nausea and vomiting
      3. Occurrence: after 100–200 ml of incompatible blood infused
4. Nursing interventions with transfusions and reactions:
   a. Follow policy of institution for blood transfusion which includes
      1. Procedure to establish client and unit of blood are correctly matched (verification by 2 nurses)
      2. Assessment of vital signs prior to transfusion
      3. Direct observation of client during first 15 minutes of infusion
      4. Take vital signs according to protocol
   b. Established procedure if transfusion reaction is suspected
      1. Stop transfusion immediately and do not transfuse the blood in the tubing
      2. Continue IV infusion with fluid
      3. Notify physician of client's signs and symptoms
      4. Provide care for client as indicated

5. Complete reaction form according to institution protocol.
6. Obtain urine specimen from client and send for free hemoglobin.

VIII. Nursing Process with clients experiencing shock
    A. Nurse assesses and analyzes client situation and any change in condition
    B. Notification of physician: early treatment before shock is advanced and less responsive to treatment
    C. Care of client in shock: constant assessment with modification of treatment
    D. Transferred to intensive care unit for hemodynamic monitoring and respiratory support
    E. Complexities of changing status of fluid, acid-base, cardiovascular function
    F. Support of client and family

IX. Common Nursing Diagnoses
    1. Decreased Cardiac Output
    2. Altered Tissue Perfusion
    3. Anxiety

FOCUSED STUDY TIPS

- Have you or a family member experienced trauma? Describe to a classmate prehospital treatment of the trauma. Discuss the effects of the trauma on family members.
- Describe organ donation to family members or friends. Have them describe to you their reasoning either to become or not become organ donors.
- Spend clinical time in the emergency department. Observe how trauma identification is made and the effects of traumatic injury on the client. What immediate medical interventions did you observe? What was the nurse's role in these interventions?

CASE STUDY

A victim experiencing Stage III refractory or irreversible shock is admitted to the emergency department via ambulance. He is carrying an organ donor card. Which law encourages people to carry organ donor cards? Under this act, who can consent for organ donation? How does the process of organ donation begin for this client? Which clients are exceptions to being possible organ donors? What are nursing responsibilities when caring for an organ donor who has been cleared for donation and declared brain dead?

CARE PLAN CRITICAL THINKING ACTIVITY

A 17-year-old female is admitted post elective surgical abortion with possible septic shock. What assessments would you perform immediately to recognize impending septic shock? What nursing interventions would you initiate immediately? What diagnostic laboratory tests can you anticipate?

NCLEX TEST QUESTIONS

1. When administering care to a client in hypovolemic shock, the nurse would expect to observe:
    a. hypertension.
    b. cyanosis.
    c. oliguria.
    d. tachypnea.

2. When a client experiences a severe anaphylactic reaction to a medication, the nurse's initial action is to:
    a. start an IV.
    b. assess vital signs.
    c. place the client in a supine position.
    d. administer oxygen and prepare equipment for intubation.

3. Which of the following is not recommended in the initial treatment of a client experiencing hypovolemia as the result of an accident?
   a. control of bleeding at the source
   b. administration of oxygen
   c. fluid replacement
   d. wound cleansing and dressing

4. An example of a colloid solution used to treat shock is:
   a. Lactated Ringer's solution.
   b. Dextran.
   c. 10% dextrose and water.
   d. Normal saline (0.9% sodium chloride)

5. Clients receiving which of the following types of solutions need their PT (prothrombin time), INR, platelet counts and partial thromboplastin time (PTT) monitored?
   a. crystalloid solutions
   b. TPN (total parenteral nutrition)
   c. colloid solutions
   d. blood products

6. Inotropic drugs (drugs that increase myocardial contractility) are given to trauma clients after fluid restoration to:
   a. decrease cardiac workload and improve renal perfusion.
   b. increase cardiac output and improve tissue perfusion.
   c. cause vasodilatation and increased peripheral resistance.
   d. increase preload and prevent respiratory acidosis.

7. When caring for unconscious clients, the nurse's primary concern must always be:
   a. airway protection and adequate respiratory status.
   b. decreasing intracranial pressure.
   c. fluid balance and cardiac stability.
   d. maintaining range-of-motion and muscle tone.

CHAPTER 7

NURSING CARE OF CLIENTS HAVING SURGERY

LEARNING OUTCOMES

After completing this chapter, you will be able to:

- Describe the various classifications of surgical procedures.
- Identify diagnostic tests used in the perioperative period.
- Describe nursing implications for medications prescribed for the surgical client.
- Provide appropriate nursing care for the client in the perioperative, intraoperative, and postoperative phases of surgery.
- Identify variations in perioperative care for the older adult.
- Describe principles of pain management specific to acute postoperative pain control.
- Discuss the differences and similarities between outpatient and inpatient surgery.
- Use the nursing process as a framework for providing individualized care for the client undergoing surgery.

KEY TOPICS

- The surgical setting
- Surgical risk factors
- Perioperative, intraoperative, and postoperative nursing care
- Managing acute postoperative pain

LECTURE OUTLINE

NURSING CARE OF CLIENTS HAVING SURGERY

- I. Background
  - A. Definitions
    - 1. Surgery: invasive medical procedure

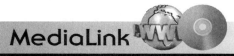

MediaLink

www.prenhall.com/lemone

Additional resources for this chapter can be found on the Student CD-ROM accompanying this textbook, and on the Companion Website at www.prenhall.com/lemone. Click on Chapter 7 to select the activities for this chapter.

CD-ROM
- Audio Glossary
- NCLEX Review

Companion Website
- More NCLEX Review
- Case Study
    The Circulating Nurse
- Care Plan Activity
    Providing Postoperative Care
- MediaLink Application
    Anesthesia and Outpatient
    Surgery

  - 2. Nurse: collaborative and independent role in providing care during all phases of surgical experience
  - B. Phases
    - 1. Preoperative Phase: time from when client and surgeon make decision to

have surgery until client enters operating room

2. Intraoperative Phase: time from entry of operating room until client is admitted to postanesthesia unit

3. Postoperative Phase: time from admittance to postanesthesia unit to time when client is completely recovered from surgery

C. Types of surgery (classified according to purpose)

1. Diagnostic: determine seriousness of alteration in health

2. Curative: cure a health problem

3. Palliative: relief of symptoms

4. Cosmetic: improve physical appearance

5. Preventative: prevent a more serious condition from developing

6. Elective surgery: surgery that can be done at a time convenient for client and surgeon

7. Emergency surgery: must be done as soon as possible to save client's life or ability to function

8. Inpatient surgery: client has been in hospital prior to having surgery done, begins recovery as inpatient client

9. Outpatient surgery: client enters hospital or free standing surgical facility to have surgery done and then is discharged after recovering and stable from anesthesia and surgical procedure
(Many variations of in and outpatient surgery with clients being admitted the morning of surgery and then being inpatients; 23-hour stays post op, etc., in attempt to control costs)

II. Preoperative Phase

A. Diagnostic Testing

1. Purpose: determine client's present health status and ability to tolerate surgical procedure and anesthesia

2. Generally the more involved the surgery, the more involved the diagnostic testing

3. More involved testing with clients who are elderly and/or have multiple pre-existing health problems

4. Nursing advocacy role to make sure physician is aware of any significant abnormalities and follow-up is done

B. Common diagnostic tests prior to surgery

1. Complete Blood Count: hemoglobin and hematocrit: client's ability to tolerate blood loss involved with surgery; white

blood count: general assessment of immune system and healing potential

2. Electrolyte studies: normal range for proper heart and neuromuscular functioning

3. Coagulation studies: ability to clot normally post-surgery

4. Urinalysis: general screening for disease such as renal problems or diabetes

5. Chest x-ray and electrocardiogram: gives basic information about lungs and heart; determine whether client's cardiac and respiratory systems are healthy enough for client to tolerate surgery and anesthesia

6. Blood type and cross match: done if blood transfusion anticipated (For some elective surgeries clients may opt for **autologous blood transfusion:** client donates own blood ahead of time; blood prepared for transfusion during surgery)

7. Other diagnostic tests may be ordered if indicated

8. Preop History and Physical exam is done by surgeon or medical physician; medical specialists may also be consulted

C. Informed Consent

1. Surgeon performing procedure is responsible for obtaining client's informed consent (operative permit)

2. Legal document that includes description and purpose of procedure with possible benefits and risks, right to refuse treatment and withdraw consent, document placed on chart after signed

3. Nurse has advocate role to assist client in getting questions answered and concerns addressed

4. Nurse acts as witness to client's signature on consent; indicates correct person signed consent and was aware of what was signed (not sedated or coerced)

D. Other preoperative interventions

1. Physicians, including surgeon and consultants, give orders to prepare client night before or day of surgery

2. Inpatient clients receive care from nurse; outpatient clients need to understand instructions to prepare for surgery independently

3. Teaching about surgical and postsurgical routines; interventions for pain control and for decreasing the risk of postoperative complications

4. Planning for recovery needs post discharge

5. Common orders
    a. Client's routine medications
        1. Specific instructions regarding medications routinely taken (i.e., diabetic meds, antihypertensives, anticoagulants)
        2. Nurse needs to clarify in advance
        3. Clients often bring meds from home, or a list if outpatient case
    b. Specific preparations ordered by physician (e.g., showering or scrubbing the surgical area with a bacteriostatic cleaner; taking an enema)
    c. NPO status (nothing by mouth): decreases the likelihood of vomiting and decreases the risk of aspiration (serious complication)
        1. Often 6–8 hours depending on time surgery is scheduled
        2. If NPO for several hours, client usually has intravenous fluids ordered to maintain client fluid balance
        3. May be allowed liquids depending on time and type of surgery
    d. Preoperative medications
        1. Ordered at specific time, or "on call," or in surgical holding area
        2. Used to sedate, reduce anxiety, reduce gastric acidity and volume, decrease nausea and vomiting, reduce incidence of aspiration by drying oral and respiratory secretions, or prevent incidence of infection
6. "Preop" Checklist
    a. Nurse completes for inpatient and outpatient surgery clients
    b. Nurse signs that client is fully prepared for surgery
    c. Nurse places documentation on chart and includes
        1. Client has identification and allergy bracelet on
        2. Informed Consent form is signed and witnessed
        3. Diagnostic tests have results documented
        4. History and Physical (H & P) including current height and weight
        5. Preoperative interventions completed as ordered
        6. Preoperative medications administered as ordered
        7. Vital signs documented within 2 hours
        8. Client voided
        9. Family members present with client
        10. Disposition of dentures, glasses, hearing aids per institution policy
        11. Proper attire according to institution policy (jewelry off, nail polish and makeup removed)

III. Intraoperative Nursing Phase
    A. Anesthesia
        1. Medications given to produce unconsciousness, analgesia, reflex loss and muscle relaxation, amnesia
        2. Type determined by condition and type of surgery
        3. Types
            a. General
                1. Given by inhalation and intravenous
                2. CNS depressed: client loses consciousness
                3. Risks for cardiac and respiratory systems
                4. Phases
                    a. Induction: tracheal intubation for airway patency
                    b. Maintenance: positioned, surgery performed
                    c. Emergence: anesthesia reversed; extubation
            b. Regional
            c. Conscious sedation
    B. Surgical team members
        1. Surgeon
        2. Surgical assistant
        3. Anesthesiologist or CRNA
        4. Nursing roles
            a. Circulating nurse: surgery coordinator; assists other team members; documentation; ensures counts of sponges and instruments are correct; client advocate
            b. Scrub nurse: scrubbed in and assists surgeon in surgical procedure
            c. Certified registered nurse anesthetist (CRNA): works with anesthesiologist to maintain anesthesia, and to monitor and maintain physiological status with medications, fluids, blood
            d. Specialty team: nurses specialize for complex surgeries, e.g., open heart surgical team, transplant team
    C. Care of client (especially elderly)
        1. Positioning: minimize risk for pressure sores

2. Communication: client may have sensory impairment being without hearing aids or glasses
   D. Operating room protocols: scrubbing, maintaining sterile fields
IV. Postoperative Phase
   A. Admittance to post-anesthesia recovery unit
      1. Immediate and continuous assessment per protocol; initially every 15 minutes
      2. Monitor patency of airway, vital signs, surgical site, recovery from anesthesia, fluid status, pain control, other postoperative orders, e.g., lab tests, intravenous fluids, etc.
      3. When stable, discharge to hospital room or home
   B. Care focus: prevention of postoperative complications
      1. Cardiovascular
         a. Hemorrhage, shock (hypovolemic most common)
            1. Client restless or less responsive
            2. Monitor postoperative hematocrit/hemoglobin
            3. Hypotension, tachycardia
            4. Pressure for obvious bleeding
            5. Notify surgeon
         b. Deep venous thrombosis (DVT)
            1. Thrombus in deep veins of leg
            2. Client has pain, edema usually in one leg
            3. Bedrest
            4. Contact physician immediately
            5. After diagnosis: anticoagulation
            6. Prevention
               a. Support stockings
               b. Use of intermittent pressure devices on lower legs (e.g., external pneumatic compression machine)
               c. Early ambulation
               d. Adequate hydration
         c. Pulmonary embolism
            1. DVT dislodges, moves, and lodges in pulmonary circulation
            2. Client has chest pain, dyspnea, tachycardia
            3. Bedrest
            4. Contact physician immediately
            5. Prevention includes adequately treating DVT
      2. Respiratory
         a. Atelectasis, pneumonia
         b. Prevention: cough and deep breathe, instruction in incentive spirometry
      3. Elimination
         a. Problems associated with effects of anesthesia, lack of activity, pain medications
         b. Urine elimination
            1. Should urinate within 7 to 8 hours post surgery
            2. Methods to assist people to void
            3. Obtain catheterization order from physician, if indicated
         c. Bowel elimination
            1. Promote activity
            2. Adequate fluid intake
      4. Wound
         a. Healing
            1. Primary Intention: incision edges well-approximated
            2. Secondary Intention: wound gaping, irregular; granulation tissue fills in, some scarring
            3. Tertiary Intention: not sutured, tissue heals by granulation process, wide scar
         b. Wound drainage
            1. Serous: clear or slightly yellow, serum (plasma) of blood
            2. Sanguineous: thick, reddish, contains red blood cells and serum
            3. Purulent: result of infection; contains white blood cells, tissue debris, and bacteria; thick, color varies with causative organism
         c. Wound disruptions
            1. Dehiscence: separation of layers of incision wound
            2. Evisceration: protrusion of body organs through area where incision came apart (with abdominal wounds, may see intestines); cover with sterile dressings soaked in sterile saline; notify physician for surgical close
         d. Suture ("stitches") or staple removal
            1. Some sutures need to be removed; some dissolve
            2. Removed 5 to 10 days post surgery if wound is healing
            3. Often removed at time of client's visit to physician office or removal ordered if inpatient
      5. Acute Pain
         a. Adequate pain control allows client to participate in recovery and avoid complications

b. Client participation in pain assessment and relief
   1. Use of pain scale, administer and evaluate medication effectiveness
   2. Obtain alternate medications or routes if pain control ineffective
   3. Teach client how to splint (brace) incision with movement
   4. Ways of changing position that lessen pull on incision

C. Promotion of recovery from surgery
   1. Discharge instructions
   2. Follow-up plans
   3. Home care, outpatient physical therapy
   4. Wound care; activity restrictions
   5. Prescriptions for medications, lab tests
   6. Supply contact source if client has questions
   7. Follow up appointment with surgeon

FOCUSED STUDY TIPS

- Care for one client in each phase of the surgical experience. Observe how the client's needs differ during each phase. Identify one nursing intervention that meets a client need during each phase.
- Identify baseline testing utilized for all clients scheduled for surgery in your clinical setting. Describe rationales for each test.
- Accompany a family member or friend to outpatient surgery. Observe the nurse's role during each phase of the surgical experience. Compare and contrast this role to inpatient surgical nursing.

CASE STUDY

Ms. Conner has been told that she will be admitted for ambulatory cataract surgery. She is unaware of what that means and what ambulatory or outpatient surgery entails. What explanations can you give Ms. Conner? Describe to Ms. Conner what will most likely happen to her preoperatively and postoperatively.

CARE PLAN CRITICAL THINKING ACTIVITY

The older adult is at risk for increased postoperative complications. How would a postoperative care plan be modified to accommodate age-related changes? How might the nursing care plan differ from one for a younger adult?

NCLEX TEST QUESTIONS

1. The nurse obtains preoperative baseline vital signs for her clients in order to:
   a. establish a baseline postoperatively.
   b. prevent operative hypotension.
   c. provide the anesthetist information necessary for the efficient administration of anesthesia.
   d. judge the client's recovery from the effects of surgery and anesthesia when taking postoperative vital signs

2. Early manifestations of the postoperative complication of atelectasis include:
   a. no urinary output 8 hours postoperatively.
   b. absent bowel sounds.
   c. anorexia.
   d. tachycardia.

3. Management of moderate to severe postoperative pain involves the use of:
   a. NSAIDs (nonsteroidal anti-inflammatory drugs) administered orally, parenterally, or rectally.
   b. opioids.
   c. PCA (patient controlled analgesia administration).
   d. PRN (as needed) oral or intramuscular pain medication.

4. Criteria for discharge from an outpatient surgical center includes:
   a. client is able to eat and drink without vomiting.
   b. client is able to demonstrate postoperative teaching instructions.
   c. client has urinated at least once since surgery.
   d. client has signed a release-of-liability form.

5. A client has not been able to void for 8 hours after surgery. What is the best nursing intervention?
   a. straight catheterization
   b. notify the physician of client's difficulty
   c. apply pressure over the bladder area (Crede's maneuver)
   d. help the client stand at the bedside to void

6. Evaluating the effectiveness of preoperative teaching before colostomy surgery, the nurse expects that the client will be able to:
   a. describe how the procedure will be done.
   b. exhibit acceptance of the surgery.
   c. explain the function of the colostomy.
   d. demonstrate proper application of the colostomy appliance.

7. The nurse can encourage the client to use the incentive spirometer to:
   a. reduce the number of microorganisms in the lungs.
   b. as an alternative to turning, coughing, and deep breathing.
   c. to prevent respiratory complications.
   d. to clear the bronchi of secretions.

CHAPTER 8

NURSING CARE OF CLIENTS WITH INFECTIONS

LEARNING OUTCOMES

After completing this chapter, you will be able to:

- Discuss the components and functions of the immune system and the immune response.
- Compare antibody-mediated and cell-mediated immune response.
- Describe the pathophysiology of wound healing, inflammation, and infection.
- Compare natural and acquired immunity and active and passive immunity.
- Identify factors responsible for nosocomial infections.
- Provide teaching for clients with inflammation or an infection and their families.
- Use the nursing process as a framework to provide individualized care to clients with inflammation and infection.

KEY TOPICS

- Components of the immune system
- Normal immune responses
- Nursing care of the client experiencing infection

LECTURE OUTLINE

NURSING CARE OF CLIENTS WITH INFECTION

I. Immune System
   A. Composition
      Specialized cells, tissues, and organs located throughout body including
      1. White blood cells

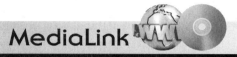

MediaLink

www.prenhall.com/lemone

Additional resources for this chapter can be found on the Student CD-ROM accompanying this textbook, and on the Companion Website at www.prenhall.com/lemone. Click on Chapter 8 to select the activities for this chapter.

CD-ROM
- Audio Glossary
- NCLEX Review

Animations
- Inflammatory Response
- White Blood Cells
- Penicillin

Companion Website
- More NCLEX Review
- Case Study
     Bioterrorism Preparedness
- Care Plan Activity
     Postoperative Infection
- MediaLink Application
     Antibiotic-Resistant Organisms

2. Thymus and bone marrow
3. Spleen, lymphoid tissues and lymph nodes, tonsils
   B. Key functions
      1. Defends against pathogens: bacteria, viruses, fungi, parasites

2. Removes and destroys dead or damaged cells
3. Identifies and removes malignant cells (prevention of tumors)
C. Activation: Response to some type of minor or major injury
   1. Nonspecific: inflammation that prevents or limits entry of invader/injury (local)
   2. Specific: immune response acts when inflammation unable to destroy organisms (systemic)
D. White Blood Cells (WBC) or Leukocytes
   1. Produced in bone marrow
   2. Move through body via blood stream and through tissue spaces
   3. General function: able to distinguish body's own cells from foreign cells and attach and remove foreign cells or own body's damaged cells
   4. Measurement of total WBC
     a. Part of Complete Blood Count (CBC)
     b. Normal WBC count: 4500–10,000/mm^3
     c. Leukocytosis: WBC > 10,000
     d. Leucopenia: WBC < 4500
   5. Types of WBC
     a. Major groups are granulocytes, monocytes, lymphocytes
     b. Measurement: WBC Differential
       1. Short name: "diff"
       2. Count of 100 WBC sorted into the different types
       3. Translates into percentage per type
       4. Significance
         a. Identifies portion of total WBC made up of each specific type
         b. Gives assessment data as to status of immune system and its response to an injury; clues as to infection, inflammation
     c. Types of WBC listed in differential
       1. Neutrophils (also knows as polymorphonuclear leukocytes (PMNs) or polys)
         a. 55–70% total circulating leukocytes
         b. Life span is hours to days
         c. Protect against pathogens, specifically bacteria
         d. Types of neutrophils
           1. Segmented ("segs"): mature, normally 55% of WBC
           2. Bands: immature neutrophils, normally 5% of WBC
         e. Increased level: acute inflammation or infection (bacterial)

2. Eosinophils (EOS)
     a. 1–4% total circulating leukocytes
     b. Found in large amounts in respiratory and GI tract
     c. Protect against parasitic worms and involved in hypersensitivity
3. Basophils
     a. 0.5–1% total circulating leukocytes
     b. Contain protein and chemicals including heparin, histamine, that are released during hypersensitivity reactions, stress
4. Monoctyes: largest of WBC
     a. 2–3% total circulating leukocytes
     b. Migrate to tissues and can live for years
     c. Mature into macrophages in tissue, lungs, connective, liver, etc.
     d. Phagocytic against large foreign particles and cell debris
     e. Defense against chronic infections such as tuberculosis, viral infections
5. Lymphocytes
     a. 20–40% of total circulating leukocytes
     b. Effectors and regulators of specific immune responses
     c. Immune surveillance: monitor for and destroy cancerous cells
     d. Circulate constantly, but concentrate in lymphoid tissues including lymph nodes
     e. Differential only looks at total lymphocyte percentage
     f. 3 different types of lymphocytes which work together:
       1. T Lymphocytes (mature in thymus gland)
       2. B Lymphocytes (mature in bone marrow)
       3. NK cells (natural killer cells): immune surveillance
II. Nonspecific Inflammatory Response
  A. Barrier protection: body's first line defense against infection includes
     1. Intact skin
     2. Mucus of mucous membranes
     3. Bactericidal action of body fluids
  B. Inflammation: nonspecific immune response
     1. Nonspecific: localized, generally same with all types of injury

2. Stages of inflammatory response:
   a. Vascular response: vasodilatation leading to redness, warmth, swelling; three types of exudate: fluid from capillaries into tissue
      1. Serous (plasma)
      2. Sanguineous (mainly red blood cells)
      3. Serosanguineous (mixture)
   b. Cellular response and phagocytosis: margination and WBC's to area
   c. Tissue repair healing: overlap of inflammation and healing
3. Cardinal signs of inflammation: erythema (redness), warmth, swelling, pain, loss of function
4. Acute or Chronic
   a. Acute
      1. Short term, 1–2 weeks
      2. Injurious agent removed
      3. Healing occurs with tissue repair or scarring
   b. Chronic
      1. Slower onset, months–years
      2. Debilitating with severe tissue damage
C. Wound Healing
   1. Phases
      a. Inflammation: debridement occurs, wound prepared for healing
      b. Reconstruction: damaged tissue regenerates
         1. Resolution: original structure and function result
         2. Repair: replacement of destroyed tissue by collagen scar tissue
   2. Requirements
      a. Adequate nutrition
      b. Adequate blood supply
      c. Adequate oxygenation
   3. Other Interfering Factors
      a. Chronic diseases, e.g., diabetes
      b. Drug therapies, e.g., corticosteroids
      c. Infection
III. Immune Response
   A. Definition of Immunocompetent: client has immune system that identifies antigen and destroys or removes it; healthy immune response
   B. Characteristics of healthy immune response
      1. Self-recognition
      2. Specific
      3. Systemic
      4. Has memory (with first exposure, change in host occurs; repeated exposures produces more rapid response)

C. Types of Immune Responses
   1. Antibody-Mediated Immune Response (Humoral Response)
      a. Antigen is bacteria, bacterial toxin, or free virus
      b. B-lymphocyte produces antibody to specific antigen
      c. Antibody (immunoglobulin) binds with antigen to inactivate it
      d. 5 classes of immunoglobulins are IgG, IgA, IgM, IgD, IgE
      e. Antibody—medicated response occurs in 2 phases
         1. Initial exposure: primary response develops
            a. Lag time from exposure to antibody development
            b. Antibodies develop, peak and person recovers
         2. Secondary exposure: with repeat exposure to antigen, memory cells cause immediate rise in antibodies and prevent disease from occurring again
   2. Cell-Mediated Immune Response (Cellular Response)
      a. Antigen is a viral-infected cell, cancer cell, some bacteria, or foreign tissue
      b. T-lymphocytes inactivate antigen without antibody formation
         1. Effector T cell: cytotoxic cell binds with surface antigen on foreign cell or virus-infected cell and destroys it
         2. Regulator T cells include:
            a. Helper T cell: activates B cells for antibodies; assists T cells
            b. Suppressor T cell: provides negative feedback and stops immune process
      c. Cell-mediated response has memory: T cells respond to repeat exposure to antigen
IV. Immunity: Protection of body from disease
   A. Types
      1. Active: body produces antibodies or develops immune lymphocytes against specific antigens
      2. Passive: antibodies are administered to the client; effect temporary
      3. Natural: client contacts antigen, develops the disease, recovers, and is immune
      4. Acquired: antigen introduced into client to stimulate immune system to form antibodies and memory cells but not the actual disease

5. Examples:
   a. Natural Active: client had chicken pox, developed antibodies, is immune
   b. Acquired Active: Tetanus Toxoid given to client; client forms antibodies against tetanus
   c. Natural Passive: maternal antibodies passed to infant through breast milk
   d. Acquired Passive: Tetanus Immune Globulin (Hypertet): antibodies given to client who has not received prior immunizations against tetanus

B. Collaborative Care
   1. Teaching and administration of immunizations, vaccines
   2. Adherence with recommended schedules for immunization (Recommendations subject to change, keep current)
   3. Recommendations for specific groups, e.g., health care workers at risk, Hepatitis B vaccine; elderly, chronically ill, influenza vaccine; travelers to foreign countries, specific disease (typhoid fever) vaccine
   4. Administration of immunizations:
      a. Check client allergies, no upper respiratory infection
      b. No live virus vaccines to immunosuppressed or those who are immunosuppressed in the household
   5. Follow directions regarding administration (routes, sites), use unexpired vaccines (label vials when opened, document lot numbers)

V. Management of Client with Inflammation
A. Diagnostic Testing
   1. White Blood Cell Count with Differential
      a. Total WBC count: increase (acute inflammation or infection) or decrease (consider immunosuppression)
      b. Differential: consider increases or decreases with specific cell type
   2. Erythrocyte Sedimentation Rate (ESR)
      a. Nonspecific
      b. Elevated with inflammation
   3. C-reactive Protein (CRP) Test
      a. Normal is negative
      b. Tests for presence of protein from liver
      c. Indicative of acute or chronic inflammation
   4. Serum Protein
      a. Normal values
         1. Total protein: 6–8 g/dL
         2. Albumin: 3.2–4.5 g/dL
         3. Globulin: 2.3–3.4 g/dL

      b. Determine whether there is adequate protein intake and liver functioning for healing, immune system functioning
      c. Globulin decreased with immunologic deficiencies
   5. Protein electrophoresis: Measurement of immunoglobulins IgG, IgA, IgM, IgD, IgE (antibodies)
   6. Antibody testing: Titer levels measured to determine whether client has developed antibodies to an infection or with an immunization
   7. Skin testing: assesses cell-mediated immunity
      a. Known antigen injected intradermally, e.g., tuberculin test
      b. Note induration indicating previous exposure and sensitization to antigen
      c. If no reaction, depressed cellular immunity (anergy)

B. Medications
   1. Purpose: to provide comfort or decrease inflammatory response and damage
   2. Types
      a. Acetaminophen
         1. Comfort only
         2. Reduces pain and fever
         3. No anti-inflammatory effect
      b. Aspirin and salicylates
         1. Higher doses required (650–1000 mg QID—4 times a day) for anti-inflammatory effect
         2. Inhibits prostaglandin synthesis; anti-pyretic; anti-platelet effect
         3. Irritates gastrointestinal tract
      c. Nonsteroidal anti-inflammatory drugs (NSAIDs)
         1. Multiple types of NSAID medications; all have potential cross-sensitivity to aspirin, irritate gastrointestinal tract
         2. Ketorolac (Toradol), only NSAID that can be given parenterally
         3. Indomethacin and phenylbutazone most toxic
      d. Corticosteroids: hormones produced by adrenal cortex
         1. Inhibit inflammation; do not cure underlying condition, but palliative
         2. Have serious side effects, can mask infections
         3. Guidelines for use of glucocorticoids
            a. Prefer local acting such as topical or intra-articular injection if effective

b. Give smallest possible dose that will be effective

c. If oral, alternate-day dosing schedule to maintain adrenal gland functioning

d. With high-dose therapy, must taper dose; do not stop abruptly to allow adrenal glands to resume normal functioning

C. Proper nutrition: essential for healing
   1. Definitions
      a. Inflammation: catabolic state (tissue breakdown)
      b. Healing: anabolic process (tissue build up)
   2. Diet requirements
      a. Adequate protein, calories, fat
      b. Vitamins: A, B-complex, K^+; mineral: zinc
      c. Adequate fluids 2500/ 24 hr
      d. Prevent weight loss, protein depletion
D. Nursing Diagnoses
   1. Pain
   2. Impaired Tissue Integrity
   3. Risk for Infection

VI. Infection
A. Occurrence: when pathogen colonizes and multiplies within host and host experiences injury, inflammation or organ dysfunction in response to infection or toxin
B. Pathogen Factors
   1. Virulence: disease-causing potential
   2. Chain of infection (reservoir, transmission, vector)
   3. Organism resistance
   4. Damage caused through toxin production
C. Host Factors: ability to resist infection
   1. Physical barrier: intact skin and mucous membranes
   2. Internal environment (body secretions, respiratory defenses)
   3. Specific and nonspecific immune responses
D. Stages of infectious process
   1. Incubation
      a. Pathogen active replication
      b. No symptoms
   2. Prodromal
      a. Symptoms begin to appear
      b. Non-specific
   3. Acute
      a. Pathogen proliferates, maximum symptoms
      b. Fever and chills; may be confined to specific organ/system

c. Stress to body
   1. Catabolic effects
   2. Inflammatory process in response to toxins
   3. Possible trigger of autoimmune disease process
   4. Convalescent
      a. Tissues repair
      b. Symptoms resolve
E. Possible complications: Septicemia, septic shock
F. Nosocomial infections: Infections acquired in health care setting (5% infection rate)
   1. Risk factors for hospitalized clients
      a. Compromised immune systems
      b. Medications including antibiotics, steroids
      c. Treatments including invasive procedures
      d. Increased incidence among elderly
   2. Prevention
      a. Effective handwashing
      b. Enforcement of policies for invasive procedures
G. Antibiotic-resistant microorganisms
   1. Increasing due to inappropriate or prolonged antibiotic therapy
   2. Current resistant strains
      a. Methicillin-resistant Staphylococcus aureus (MRSA)
      b. Multi-drug resistant tuberculosis (MDR-TB)
      c. Penicillin-resistant Streptococcus pneumoniae (PRSP)
      d. Vancomycin-resistant Enterococci (VRE)
      e. Vancomycin Intermediate-resistant Staphylococcus aureus (VISA)
   3. Follow recommended contact precautions/isolation techniques
H. Collaborative Care
   1. Diagnostic Tests
      a. WBC Count with Differential
         1. Leukocytosis with infections
         2. Neutrophilia increased segs; also shift to left (increased band count)
      b. Culture of wound, blood, and/or other body fluids
         1. Obtain specimen prior to starting antibiotic, if not, note antibiotic received on culture request form
         2. Gram stain: to identify probable pathogen
         3. Culture: organism incubated and grown; takes 24–48 hours

4. Sensitivity: cultured organism subjected to different antibiotics to determine whether sensitive (antibiotic will kill organism) or resistant (antibiotic will not kill organism)
   c. Serology: detect antibodies to suspected organism
   d. Direct antigen: detect antigens in body specimens
   e. Antibiotic Peaks and Troughs: monitor therapeutic levels of antibiotics to ensure proper dose for optimum treatment while avoiding toxic levels
      1. Peak: highest level of antibiotic
      2. Trough: lowest level of antibiotic
   f. X-rays, ultrasound examination of organs
   g. Lumbar puncture (LP) to obtain cerebrospinal fluid (CSF) for examination and culture
I. Administration of anti-infective therapy
   1. Check for allergies, risk to fetus in child-bearing aged women
   2. Know client renal, hepatic function; if medication metabolized through this system, monitor lab tests
   3. Best route to effectively treat microorganism in infection site
   4. Antibiotics
      a. Bacteriostatic (inhibit growth) or bactericidal (kill organism)
      b. Specific against different categories of microorganisms that have cell wall
         1. Gram positive
         2. Gram negative
         3. Both (broad spectrum)
      c. Known toxicities to specific organ systems
      d. Superinfection
         1. Major concern
         2. Antibiotics change normal bacterial flora in GI tract, mouth, vagina
         3. Overgrowth of fungus or bacteria
         4. May be treated with antifungal medications or eating yogurt with live cultures
   5. Antiviral: selective since virus is parasite within host's cells
   6. Antifungal: treat fungal infections
   7. Antiparasitic: treat parasitic infections including protozoans
J. Antibiotic categories/specifics
   1. Penicillins: "cillins"
      a. Stop immediately if any sign of hypersensitivity and be ready to treat reaction
      b. Cross sensitivity with cephalosporins
   2. Cephalosporins
      a. 4 generations
      b. Cross sensitivity with penicillins
      c. Monitor for kidney and liver toxicity
   3. Aminoglycosides: "mycins"
      a. Ototoxic, nephrotoxic
      b. Monitor weight, BUN, creatinine
   4. Fluoroquinolones
      a. Fluid intake 2–3 L daily to prevent crystalluria
      b. Monitor for hepatotoxicity
   5. Tetracyclines
      a. Take 1 hour before or 2 hours after meals
      b. Can interfere with anticoagulants
   6. Macrolides (Erythromycin)
      a. For clients allergic to penicillin
      b. GI distress; take on empty stomach or just before meals
   7. Sulfonamides and Trimethoprim
      a. Used for urinary tract infections (UTI), otitis media, Pneumocystis carinii pneumonia
      b. Check for any sulfa allergy
      c. Protect from photosensitivity
      d. Take on empty stomach
      e. Fluid intake 2 L per day
   8. Metronidazole (Flagyl)
      a. No alcohol intake (causes illness—Antabuse effect)
      b. May make urine reddish brown
      c. Need adequate fluid intake 2.5 L daily
K. Isolation techniques
   According to Centers for Disease Control and Prevention (CDC) Guidelines
   1. Standard Precautions
      a. Barrier precautions with body fluids, especially blood
      b. Guidelines for needles, sharp objects disposal
   2. Category-specific Precautions
      a. Airborne precautions
      b. Droplet precautions
      c. Contact precautions
L. Nursing Diagnoses
   1. Risk for infections
   2. Anxiety
   3. Hyperthermia
      a. Chills indicate rising temperature; monitor
      b. Lower temperature cautiously to avoid shivering which raises temperature
      c. Restore fluid balance; increased loss with fever

FOCUSED STUDY TIPS

- Reflect on your clinical practice. Identify three behaviors demonstrated that prevent the development of nosocomial infection.
- Review your personal immunization record. Identify vaccines that provide active and passive immunity.
- Describe to a family member or friend the pathophysiology of wound healing, inflammation, and infection. Evaluate understanding. Ask him/her to identify the usefulness of this information.

CASE STUDY

A friend who is also a nursing student always wears gloves when doing anything for ill clients. You are more selective in your use of gloves. She tells you that you are a fool for "taking chances" and that you are putting your family at risk for "who knows what." Should this be a matter of personal preference? Whose position is more consistent with good nursing practice? Are your instructors consistent in how they address these questions?

CARE PLAN CRITICAL THINKING ACTIVITY

An elderly neighbor keeps complaining about getting respiratory infections and small infected wounds. He asks for your help in preventing this. When developing a teaching plan for him, what assessments are necessary? What nursing interventions would you implement? How would you evaluate whether or not your teaching plan was effective?

NCLEX TEST QUESTIONS

1. A left shift in a WBC (white blood cell count) differential seen in acute infection is a result of:
   a. production of more erythrocytes by the bone marrow.
   b. passive immunity to the infecting agent.
   c. increased immature neutrophils in the circulation.
   d. poor bone marrow functioning.

2. The classification of antibiotics especially effective against gram-negative organisms is:
   a. penicillins.
   b. cephalosporins.
   c. aminoglycosides.
   d. sulfonamides.

3. Which statement best defines interferon?
   a. antiviral substance produced by the spleen
   b. protein substance produced by WBCs (white blood cells) and other body cells
   c. a by-product of protein metabolism
   d. a carbohydrate produced by the liver

4. The nurse knows to minimize local reactions to the vaccines that should be administered:
   a. one at a time, preferably 24 hours apart.
   b. IM (intramuscularly) in the deltoid or gluteus.
   c. ID (intradermally).
   d. in the client's dominant arm.

5. The laboratory result that should be monitored regularly in a client who is receiving gentamicin (Garamycin) is:
   a. serum creatinine.
   b. serum calcium.
   c. platelet count.
   d. white blood cell (WBC) count.

6. Social isolation is a problem when a client is in strict isolation. To reduce or eliminate social isolation the nurse can:
   a. keep the door of the room open so the client can visualize others.
   b. provide a radio or television for diversional activity.
   c. encourage family to visit as often as possible.
   d. take paperwork into the room and sit with the client as much as possible.

7. A nursing student asks the purpose of sensitivity studies. The correct answer is these studies determine:
   a. which antibiotic will inhibit the growth of a microorganism.
   b. the type of microorganism causing the infection.
   c. viral resistance to an antibiotic.
   d. the pathogenicity of the microorganism.

CHAPTER 9

NURSING CARE OF CLIENTS WITH ALTERED IMMUNITY

LEARNING OUTCOMES

After completing this chapter, you will be able to:

- Review normal anatomy and physiology of the immune system and the immune response (see Chapter 8).
- Describe the four types of hypersensitivity reactions.
- Discuss the pathophysiology of autoimmune disorders and tissue transplant rejection.
- Discuss the characteristics of immunodeficiencies.
- Identify laboratory and diagnostic tests used to diagnose and monitor immune response.
- Describe pharmacologic and other collaborative therapies used in treating clients with altered immunity.
- Provide teaching for clients with altered immune responses and their families.
- Correlate the pathophysiological alterations with the manifestations of HIV/AIDS infection.
- Use the nursing process as a framework to provide individualized care to clients with altered immune responses.

KEY TOPICS

- Altered immune responses
- Nursing care of clients with altered immune responses

LECTURE OUTLINE

I. Background
  A. A healthy immune system identifies antigens and effectively destroys or removes them

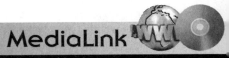

MediaLink

www.prenhall.com/lemone

Additional resources for this chapter can be found on the Student CD-ROM accompanying this textbook, and on the Companion Website at www. prenhall.com/lemone. Click on Chapter 9 to select the activities for this chapter.

CD-ROM
- Audio Glossary
- NCLEX Review

Animations
- Histamine
- T-Cell Destruction of HIV

Companion Website
- More NCLEX Review
- Case Study
    HIV Prevention
- Care Plan Activity
    A Clients with AIDS
- MediaLink Application
    At Risk for HIV/AIDS

B. Alterations that occur within immune system and result in illness
  1. Overreaction: hypersensitivity, as with allergic reactions

2. Incompetency: Immune deficiency or malignancy as with Acquired Immune Deficiency Disorder (AIDS)
    3. Autoimmune disorder: Loss of ability to recognize self
C. Immune responses
    1. Antibody-mediated immune response: action of B lymphocytes (B-cells); acquired immunity
    2. Cell-mediated immune response: T lymphocytes (T-cells) attack antigens directly and activate B-cells
    3. Types of T-cells
        a. Effector cells: Cytotoxic (Killer T)
            1. Carry CD8 antigen
            2. Attack malignant cells
            3. Responsible for transplanted organ rejection and grafted tissues
        b. Regulator cells
            1. Helper T cells
                a. Carry CD4 antigen
                b. Initiate immune response
            2. Suppressor T cells
                a. Carry CD8 antigen
                b. Stop immune response
    4. Immune function declines with age
II. Hypersensitivity Reaction
A. Definition: Altered immune response to antigen resulting in harm to client, e.g., allergy
B. Categories
    1. Range from irritating to life threatening (as with laryngospasm)
    2. Immediate (e.g., anaphylaxis) vs. delayed (e.g., contact dermatitis)
C. Pathophysiology
    1. Antigen-antibody interaction:
        a. Causes tissue damage
        b. Involves immediate reaction after a prior sensitization
        c. Includes systemic reactions: Types I, II, III
            1. Type I
                a. From allergic reaction with IgE
                b. Mast cells and basophils factors released, which causes serious reaction
                c. Most serious reaction: Anaphylaxis
                    1. Signs and symptoms: hives, swelling, difficulty breathing, anaphylactic shock

2. Client needs: Air way protection; prompt reversal (parenteral epinephrine)
            2. Type II
                a. IgG or IgM
                b. Antibodies formed
                c. Complement cascade activated and destroys cells, e.g., hemolytic transfusion blood reaction (ABO, Rh)
            3. Type III
                a. IgG or IgM
                b. Antibody-antigen immune complexes in circulation and block tissues, e.g., reaction to toxin post strep infection, glomerulonephritis
    2. Antigen-lymphocyte reaction
        a. Type IV
        b. Delayed 24–48 hours; contact dermatitis (e.g., latex allergy, positive tuberculin test)
D. Collaborative Care
    1. Overall Focus
        a. Minimize exposure to allergen
        b. Prevent hypersensitivity response
        c. Perform prompt, effective interventions for allergic responses
    2. Nursing history and status before any procedure/medication
        a. Document allergies and reaction(s) that occurred with event
        b. Maintain record; allergy bracelet for in-patient
        c. Ask about anesthesia allergy for local and general preoperative clients
    3. Diagnostic tests
        a. WBC count with differential: Type I allergy: eosinophilia
        b. Radioallergosorbent test (RAST): detects IgE toward specific antigens
        c. Blood type and crossmatch: prevents ABO and Rh reactions
        d. Indirect Coombs: detects circulating antibodies (normal: negative)
        e. Direct Coombs: detects antibodies on client's red blood cells (RBC's) (normal: negative)
        f. Immune complex assays: detects Antibodies Type III reactions
        g. Complement assays: detects amount of available complement; determines amount used
        h. Skin tests: detects allergens, includes intradermal testing

4. Medications
   a. Antihistamines
      1. Blocks histamine receptors
      2. Relieves symptoms of urticaria and angioedema
      3. Diphenhydramine (Benadryl): can be given parenterally or orally
   b. Epinephrine
      1. Immediate treatment for anaphylaxis
      2. Relieves the vasodilatation and bronchoconstriction
      3. Given subcutaneously (SQ) or intravenously (IV)
      4. "Bee sting kit": carried by clients with known serious allergies
   c. Cromolyn (Intal)
      1. Blocks histamine release
      2. Given by inhaler or nasal spray
   d. Glucocorticoids
      1. Both topical and systemic effects
      2. Anti-inflammatory
5. Plasmapheresis
   a. Non-medication treatment
   b. Removal of harmful components in plasma by passing blood through blood cell separator to remove immune complexes
6. Nursing Diagnoses
   a. Ineffective Airway Clearance (as with anaphylaxis)
   b. Decreased Cardiac Output (as with anaphylactic shock)
   c. Risk for Injury (as with blood transfusion reaction)

III. Autoimmune Disorders
   A. Definition: Immune system's ability to recognize self is impaired, and immune defenses are directed against person's own tissues
   B. Common autoimmune disorders
      1. Tissue/organ specific (Hashimoto's thyroiditis)
      2. Systemic (rheumatoid arthritis, systemic lupus erythematosis (SLE))
   C. Pathophysiology (not entirely certain but possibly the following:)
      1. Hidden antigens elicit immune response, development of autoantibodies
      2. Body has changes from bacterial or viral infections, defective immune system
   D. Characteristics of autoimmune disorders
      1. Genetic predisposition
      2. Occur in females more than males

3. Onset associated with stress
4. Frequently are progressive, with periods of exacerbation and remission
   E. Collaborative Care
      1. Diagnostic Tests:
         a. Serologic assays
            1. Tests used to identify autoantibodies, measured in titers, i.e., levels in circulation
            2. Occur with autoimmune state
            3. Not specific for certain disease
         b. Antinuclear antibody (ANA)
         c. Lupus erythematosus (LE) prep
         d. Rheumatoid Factor (RF)
         e. Complement assay: detects amount of available complement; determines amount used
      2. Medications
         a. Anti-inflammatory drugs: aspirin, NSAIDs, corticosteroids
         b. Antirheumatic drugs: gold salts, hydroxychloroquine (Plaquenil)
         c. Cytotoxic drugs
      3. Plasmapheresis may be used
      4. Nursing Care according to signs and symptoms of specific disorder
      5. Common Nursing Diagnoses
         a. Activity Intolerance
         b. Ineffective Coping (with chronic disease)
         c. Ineffective Protection
         d. Risk for Ineffective Therapeutic Regimen Management
         e. Interrupted Family Processes

IV. Tissue transplants
   A. Background
      1. Human Leukocyte Antigens (HLA)
         a. Specific cell surface markers unique to each individual person
         b. Transplant success tied to obtaining organs with HLA close to those of recipient
      2. Types of transplants
         a. Autograft: transplant of client's own tissue
         b. Allograft: most common, grafts between member of same species, but different genotypes and HLA antigens; cadaver donors are most common
         c. Xenograft: transplant from animal species to human, e.g., pig valves
      3. Preparation for allograft: tissue typing

a. Determine histocompatibility, i.e., identify recipient's HLA type, blood type (ABO, Rh), and pre-formed antibodies

b. Match as closely as possible with the donor

4. Types of rejections: typically begin after first 24 hours post transplant

a. Hyperacute tissue rejection

1. Occurs 2–3 days post transplant

2. Due to pre-formed antibodies

3. More common with previous transplant or blood transfusion

b. Acute tissue rejection

1. Most common and treatable

2. Occurs between 3 days and 4 months post transplant

3. Due to cellular immune response

4. Signs and symptoms: fever, redness, swelling and tenderness over graft site; signs of organ failure (reflected by lab values)

c. Chronic tissue rejection

1. Occurs 4 months to years post transplant

2. Due to antibody-mediated immune response

3. Leads to ischemia and to eventual organ deterioration

4. Graft-versus-Host Disease (GvHD): frequent and potentially fatal complication of bone marrow transplant; grafted tissue recognizes host tissue as foreign and mounts a cell-mediated response; primarily affects skin, liver, gastrointestinal tract

B. Collaborative Care

1. Overall goal of pre and post transplant care is to reduce the risk of tissue rejection or GvHD

2. Diagnostic testing—prior to transplant

a. Blood type, Rh factor, crossmatch

b. HLA histocompatibility: used primarily with living donors for kidney or bone marrow transplants

c. Mixed lymphocyte culture (MLC) assay test: histocompatibility between donor and recipient

3. Diagnostic testing—post transplant

a. Ultrasound or magnetic resonance imaging (MRI) of transplanted organ

b. Tissue biopsies of transplanted organ; done routinely to assess evidence of rejection

4. Medications

a. Antibiotics and antiviral medications

1. *Trimethoprim-sulfamethoxazole (Septra, Bactrim):* protects against gram-negative bacteria infection

2. *Acyclovir (Zovirax):* protects from herpes simplex virus (HSV) infection

3. *Ganciclovir (Cytovene):* protects from development of cytomegalovirus (CMV) infection

b. Immunosuppressive agents: Corticosteroids, also anti-inflammatory

1. *Azathioprine (Imuran)*

a. Mainstay, inhibits both cell-mediated and antibody-mediated immunity

b. Metabolized by liver; safe for renal transplant clients

c. Major adverse effect: bone marrow depression (monitor CBC)

2. *Cyclosporine*

a. Inhibits T-cell function and cell-mediated immune responses

b. Monitor blood levels closely to check for toxicity; nephrotoxic and hepatotoxic

c. Signs of toxicity: hypertension, CNS symptoms

3. *Muromonab-CD3 (OKT3, Orthoclone)*

a. Monoclonal antibody, blocks T cell generation and function

b. Used with steroid-resistant organ rejections

4. *Antilymphocyte globulin (ALG), antithymocyte globulin (ATG):* Polyclonal antilymphoctye antibodies

5. Nursing Care involves acute and chronic care for client and family

6. Common Nursing Diagnoses

a. Ineffective Protection

b. Risk for Impaired Tissue Integrity

c. Dealing with psychological consequences of chronic illness

1. Powerlessness

2. Ineffective Coping

3. Anxiety

7. Common nursing interventions

a. Assessment for signs of infection, organ rejection, adverse effects of medications, frequent laboratory testing

b. Medications, handwashing and protective isolation in hospital and post discharge for client and family

c. Stress-reduction, counseling, support group referral

V. Impaired Immune Response

A. Two types

1. Congenital: rare
2. Acquired: acquired immune deficiency syndrome (AIDS)

B. Background

1. Cases recognized in male homosexual population in 1981
2. Human immunodeficiency virus (HIV) isolated in 1984
3. Retrovirus transmitted by
   a. Direct contact with infected blood and body fluids
   b. Contaminated needles
   c. Infants born to HIV positive mothers (15–30%)

C. Risks: Behavorial

1. Unprotected anal sex
2. Injection drug use (sharing needles)
3. Heterosexual intercourse with infected persons
4. Receiving blood transfusions, blood products
5. Occupational risk to health care workers, especially through needle sticks

D. Pathophysiology

1. Retrovirus
   a. Carries genetic code in RNA
   b. Infects cells with CD4 antigen
   c. Takes over cell's DNA and then duplicates
   d. May remain dormant or become active
   e. Active: forms virions which destroy host cell
2. Seroconversion
   a. 6 weeks to 6 months post initial infection, antibodies to HIV are produced and will test positive
   b. Actual virus may remain inactive in cells for years
   c. Antibodies are ineffective against the virus
3. Cells affected by HIV
   a. Helper T (CD4) cells
   b. Macrophages
   c. Cells of CNS
4. Loss of helper T cells leads to typical immunodeficiencies that result in multiple opportunistic infections and cancers

E. Typical Course of HIV Infection

1. Contraction of virus

a. Acute mononucleosis-type illness within days to weeks
b. Symptoms include: fever, sore throat, joint and muscle achiness, rash, lymphadenopathy
c. Asymptomatic period
   1. Mean period 8 to 10 years
   2. Virus can be transmitted to others through blood and body fluids, even though client seems well
   3. Some clients experience persistent lymphadenopathy

2. Development into AIDS

a. Manifestations include: general malaise, fever, fatigue, night sweats, involuntary weight loss, often diarrhea, rash, oral lesions and candidiasis
b. Multiple opportunistic infections, cancers
c. 40–60% develop neurological symptoms

F. Post-infection Related Issues

1. AIDS Dementia Complex

a. Direct effect of virus on brain
b. Starts with fluctuating memory loss; confusion to apathy, to severe dementia; tremor; spasticity; incontinence
c. CNS infections and lesions including toxoplasmosis, non-Hodgkin's lymphoma as space-occupying lesions, cryptococcal meningitis, cytomegalovirus (CMV) infections

2. Opportunistic Infections

a. Occur when CD4 count is less than 200 (normal greater than 1000/mm^3)
b. Pneumonia (*Pneumocystis carinii*)
   1. Most common opportunistic infection (75–80%)
   2. Nonspecific manifestations: fever, cough, shortness of breath, tachypnea, tachycardia
c. Tuberculosis
   1. Often multidrug-resistant strains
   2. Rapid progressive, diffuse pulmonary and disseminated (other body organs)
d. Candidiasis (*Candida albicans*)
   1. Very common
   2. Oral thrush, esophagitis, or vaginitis in women
e. *Mycobacterium avium:* Complex (MAC)
   1. 25% of AIDS cases

2. Major cause of "wasting syndrome"
3. Signs and symptoms include: chills, fever, weakness, night sweats, abdominal pain, diarrhea, weight loss

   f. Other Infections
     1. Viral: Herpes simplex or herpes zoster virus, CMV of retina, GI tract, lungs
     2. Parasitic: Toxoplasma gondii, Cryptococcus neoformans, Cryptosporidium

  3. Secondary cancers
    a. Kaposi's Sarcoma
      1. Often presenting symptom
      2. Skin lesions with vascular macules, papules, violet lesions on skin and viscera; often on face, gastrointestinal tract, lungs
      3. Initially painless, but become painful
      4. Indicator of late-stage disease
    b. Lymphomas
      1. Non-Hodgkin's lymphoma and primary lymphoma of brain
      2. Aggressive and rapid spread
    c. Invasive cervical carcinoma: Women with HIV usually die of cervical cancer, not AIDS

G. Collaborative Care
  1. Treatment
    a. No cure for HIV infection and AIDS
    b. Current research for treatment and cure
    c. Still universally fatal nature of disease
    d. Prevention is vital strategy
  2. Goals of care
    a. Early identification of infection
    b. Promote health-maintenance activities
    c. Prevent opportunistic infections
    d. Treatment of disease complications (cancers)
    e. Provide emotional and psychosocial support
  3. Diagnostic Testing
    a. Enzyme-linked immunosorbent assay (ELISA)
      1. Widely used as screening test for HIV infection; detects HIV antibodies, not virus
      2. Could be negative in early course of infection before detectable antibodies develop
      3. Results 99.5% positive
        a. False positives can occur

        b. If positive, always repeat test and confirm by another method, such as Western blot
    b. Western blot antibody testing: combined with ELISA greater specificity (> 99.9%)
    c. HIV viral load tests: measure amount of activity replicating HIV virus
    d. CBC: detect anemia, leucopenia, thrombocytopenia
    e. CD4 cell count: used to monitor progress of disease and guide therapy
    f. Tests to detect secondary cancers and opportunistic infections
      1. Tuberculin skin testing
      2. Magnetic resonance imaging (MRI) of the brain
      3. Specific cultures and serology for infections
      4. Pap smears every 6 months to detect cervical cancer

  4. Medications
    a. Purposes
      1. Suppress the HIV infection and prolong client's life
      2. Treat opportunistic infections and cancers
    b. Effectiveness measured by
      1. Viral load and CD4 cell counts (above 500 mm^3)
      2. Often used in combinations according to effectiveness
    c. Classes of medications used to suppress HIV infection
      1. Nucleoside Reverse Transcriptase Inhibitors (NRTIs)
        a. Works at level of DNA
        b. Zidovudine (Retrovir, AZT) widespread use; also used prophylactically post parenteral exposure to HIV
      2. Protease Inhibitors: Blocks viral enzymes
      3. Nonnucleoside Reverse Transcriptase Inhibitors
      4. Other agents: Interferons
    d. Medications against opportunistic infections/cancers
      1. Antibiotics, antivirals, anti-cancer agents
      2. Vaccines for pneumococcal, influenza, hepatitis B, haemophilus influenzae serotype b

3. Isoniazid (INH) prophylactically for positive tuberculin test
4. Prophylactic trimethoprim-sulfamethoxazole (Bactrim) if CD4 cell count is below 200 to prevent *Pneumocystis carinii* Pneumonia (PCP)

5. Nursing Care
   a. Prevention of infection
      1. Safe sexual practices
      2. No sharing of needles and drug paraphernalia (drug users)
      3. Screening of donated blood and use of autologous
      4. Use of standard precautions by health care workers

b. Care of the client with HIV
   1. Maintain health and prevent development of opportunistic infections, cancers; physical needs change over course of illness
   2. Still a stigma associated with illness; assist client, family to cope
   3. Intense medical care, client development of support systems, use of psychosocial support

c. Nursing Diagnoses (many and change with course of illness)
   1. Ineffective Coping: Dealing with stigma, contagious disease, chronic illness, terminal illness

FOCUSED STUDY TIPS

- Identify a classmate, family member, or friend with a hypersensitivity reaction. Evaluate which of the four types it is. Discuss the medical management of the reaction.
- Develop a care plan for a client with HIV infection undergoing surgery. Compare and contrast postoperative care for this client to clients without HIV infection.

CASE STUDY

A friend shares with you that she thinks she may be infected with the AIDS virus and asks, "What are the early signs and symptoms I might have if I do have AIDS? What tests can be done to show if I do have AIDS? What should I do?" Answer your friend's questions. Detail what assessment questions you will need to ask her. How does your support of her differ as a nurse and as a friend?

CARE PLAN CRITICAL THINKING ACTIVITY

A client receiving an intravenous antibiotic by IV piggyback over a period of 30 minutes suddenly complains of chest pain and difficulty breathing. What immediate assessments and interventions would you make while another nurse is contacting the physician?

NCLEX TEST QUESTIONS

1. When caring for a client experiencing a Type I hypersensitivity reaction, the nurse's first priority is:
   a. supportive care to relieve the client's discomfort.
   b. administration of antihistamines or anti-inflammatory medications.
   c. managing the client's airway.
   d. maintaining cardiac output.

2. A client is receiving a blood transfusion. The client begins to complain of itching. The nurse observes a red rash beginning on the client's arm above the IV (intravenous) site. The best action by the nurse is:
   a. stop the blood transfusion and call the doctor.
   b. slow the blood transfusion and call the doctor.
   c. smooth Benadryl cream over the area and monitor the client closely.
   d. report the incident to the charge nurse ASAP.

3. The most successful type of tissue transplant is an:
   a. isograft.
   b. allograft.
   c. xenograft.
   ___ d. autograft.
4. Plaquenil and penicillamine are slow-acting antirheumatic drugs used in the treatment of:
   a. tissue rejection.
   b. Type III hypersensitivity reactions.
   ___ c. autoimmune disorders.
   d. lymphomas.
5. The most common cancer associated with AIDs (acquired immune deficiency syndrome) is:
   a. pneumocystis carinii.
   b. Hodgkin's lymphoma.
   c. lymphoma.
   ___ d. Kaposi's sarcoma.

6. An effective means of preventing anaphylactic responses to insect venom is:
   ___ a. immunotherapy.
   b. allergy testing.
   ___ c. prophylactic administration of antihistamines.
   d. topical administration of corticosteroids.
7. Potential complications of plasmapheresis include:
   ___ a. development of Goodpasture's syndrome.
   b. pyelonephritis.
   ___ c. alterations of blood clotting.
   d. tissue rejection.

CHAPTER 10

NURSING CARE OF CLIENTS WITH CANCER

LEARNING OUTCOMES

After completing this chapter, you will be able to:

- Define cancer and differentiate benign from malignant neoplasms.
- Discuss the theories of carcinogenesis, known carcinogens, and risk factors for cancer.
- Compare the mechanisms and characteristics of normal cells with those of malignant cells.
- Describe the effects of cancer on the body.
- Describe the laboratory and diagnostic tests used to diagnose cancer.
- Discuss the role of chemotherapy in cancer treatment.
- Discuss the use of surgery, radiation therapy, and biotherapy in the treatment of cancer.
- Describe the nursing interventions required for selected oncologic emergencies.
- Provide teaching to the client and family experiencing cancer.
- Use the nursing process as a framework for providing individualized care to the client with cancer.

KEY TOPICS

- Cancer risk factors
- Pathophysiology of cancer
- Physiological and psychological effects of cancer
- Chemotherapy
- Nursing care of clients with cancer
- Nursing interventions for oncologic emergencies

MediaLink

www.prenhall.com/lemone

Additional resources for this chapter can be found on the Student CD-ROM accompanying this textbook, and on the Companion Website at www.prenhall.com/lemone. Click on Chapter 10 to select the activities for this chapter.

CD-ROM
- Audio Glossary
- NCLEX Review

Companion Website
- More NCLEX Review
- Case Study
   Pain Management
- Care Plan Activity
   Weight Loss and Chemotherapy
- MediaLink Application
   Terminal Cancer Support Groups

LECTURE OUTLINE

I. Cancer Background
   A. Definition
      1. Family of complex diseases
      2. Affect different organs and organ systems
      3. Normal cells mutate into abnormal cells that take over tissue
      4. Eventually harm and destroy host
      5. Historically, cancer is a dreaded disease
   B. Oncology
      1. Study of cancers
      2. Oncology nurses specialize in the care, treatment of clients with cancer
   C. Incidence and Prevalence
      1. Cancer accounts for about 25% of death on yearly basis
      2. Males: 3 most common types of cancer are prostate, lung and bronchial, colorectal
      3. Females: 3 most common types of cancer are breast, lung and bronchial, and colorectal
   D. Risk factors for cancer: (some are controllable; some are not)
      1. Heredity: 5–10% of cancers; documented with some breast and colon cancers
      2. Age: 70% of all cancers occur in persons > 65
      3. Lower socio-economic status
      4. Stress
         a. Leads to greater wear and tear on body in general
         b. Type C personality ("cancer personality") persons who tend to others' needs to exclusion of their own
      5. Diet: certain preservatives in pickled, salted foods; fried foods; high-fat, low fiber foods; charred foods
      6. Occupational risk: exposure to know carcinogens, radiation, high stress
      7. Infections, especially specific organisms and organ (e.g., human papillomavirus (HPV) causing genital warts and leading to cervical cancer)
      8. Tobacco Use: lung, oral and laryngeal, esophageal, gastric, pancreatic, bladder cancers
      9. Alcohol Use: also tied with tobacco use
      10. Sun exposure (radiation) e.g., skin cancer
   E. Nursing role includes health promotion to lower the controllable risks
      1. Routine medical check up and screenings
      2. Client awareness to act if symptoms of cancer occur
      3. Screening examination recommendations by American Cancer Society; specifics are made according to age and frequencies
         a. Breast Cancer: breast self exam (BSE), breast examination by health care professionals, screening mammogram
         b. Colon and Rectal Cancer: fecal occult blood, flexible sigmoidoscopy, colonoscopy
         c. Cervical, Uterine Cancer: Papanicolaou (Pap) test
         d. Prostate Cancer: digital rectal exam, Prostate-specific antigen (PSA) test

II. Physiology of Cancer
   A. Background
      1. Normal Cell Growth includes two events
         a. Replication of cellular DNA (deoxyribonucleic acid)
         b. Mitosis (cell division)
      2. Five Phases of cell cycle
         a. G1: Gap 1 Phase; cell enlarges, synthesizes proteins to prepare for DNA replication
         b. Synthesis (S) Phase: DNA replicates and chromosomes duplicate
         c. G2: Gap 2 Phase: cell prepares for mitosis
         d. Mitosis M Phase: mitosis occurs with 2 copies of cell (daughter cells)
         e. G1 or G0 phase: resting phase
      3. Cell cycle is under control of cyclins which control process by working with enzymes; some cyclins "brake" (stop) the cellular division
      4. Forms the basis of how some chemotherapeutic agents work against cancers
      5. Differentiation: normal process occurring over many cell cycles for special tasks
         a. Some unproductive differentiations occur (seen on biopsy reports)
            1. Hyperplasia: increase in number or density of normal cells
            2. Metaplasia: protective response to adverse conditions
            3. Dysplasia: loss of DNA control over differentiation (e.g., changes in cervical cells in response to continued irritation)
            4. Anaplasia: regression of cell to immature or undifferentiated cell type
         b. Hyperplasia, metaplasia, and dysplasia are all reversible

B. Theories of carcinogenesis (what causes cancer to occur)
  1. Cellular mutation
     a. Cells begin to mutate (change the DNA to unnatural cell reproduction)
     b. Three stages: initiation, promotion, progression
     c. Example: cells mutate after years of smoking: lung cancer
  2. Oncogenes/tumor suppressor genes Abnormalities
     a. Oncogenes are genes that promote cell proliferation and can trigger cancer
     b. Tumor suppressor genes normally suppress oncogenes
  3. Exposure to known carcinogens
     a. Act by directly altering the cellular DNA (genotoxic)
     b. Act by affecting the immune system (promotional)
  4. Viruses (weaken immune system or cause malignancies)
  5. Drugs and Hormones
     a. Sex hormones often affect cancers of the reproductive systems (estrogen in some breast cancers; testosterone in prostate cancer)
     b. Glucocorticoids and steroids alter immune system
  6. Chemical Agents
     a. Industrial and chemical
     b. Examples: hydrocarbons in soot; arsenic in pesticides; chemicals in tobacco
  7. Physical Agents
     a. Exposure to radiation
     b. Example: nuclear power plant accidents
C. Neoplasms: also called tumors (mass of new tissue that grows independently of surrounding organs)
  1. Types of neoplasms
     a. Benign
        1. Localized growths respond to body's homeostatic controls
        2. Encapsulated
        3. Stop growing when they meet a boundary of another tissue
        4. Can be destructive
     b. Malignant
        1. Have aggressive growth, rapid cell division outside the normal cell cycle
        2. Not under body's homeostatic controls

  3. Cut through surrounding tissues causing bleeding, inflammation, necrosis (death) of tissue
  2. Malignant tumors can metastasize
     a. Tumor cells travel through blood or lymph circulation to other body areas and invade tissues and organs there
        1. Primary tumor: the original site of the malignancy
        2. Secondary tumor (sites): areas where malignancy has spread, i.e., metastasis (metastatic tumor)
        3. Common sites of metastasis are lymph nodes, liver, lungs, bones, brain
        4. 50–60% of tumors have metastasized by time primary tumor identified
     b. Cancerous cells must avoid detection by immune system
  3. Malignant neoplasms can recur after surgical removal of primary and secondary tumors and other treatments
  4. Malignant neoplasms vary in differentiation
     a. Highly differentiated resemble the originating tissue
     b. Undifferentiated neoplasms consist of immature cells with no resemblance to originating tissue
  5. Malignant cells progress in deviation with each generation and do not stop growing and die, as do normal cells
  6. Malignant cells are irreversible, i.e., do not revert to normal
  7. Malignant cells promote their own survival by hormone production, cause vascular permeability; angiogenesis; divert nutrition from host cells
D. Effects of cancer
  1. Disturbed or loss of physiological functioning, from pressure or obstruction
     a. Anoxia and necrosis of organs
     b. Loss of function: bowel or bladder obstruction
     c. Increased intracranial pressure (ICP)
     d. Interrupted vascular/venous blockage
     e. Ascites
     f. Disturbed liver functioning
  2. Hematologic Alterations: impaired function of blood cells
     a. Abnormal WBC's: impaired immunity
     b. Diminished RBC's and platelets: anemia and clotting disorders

3. Infections: fistula development and tumors may become necrotic; erode skin surface
4. Hemorrhage: tumor erosion, bleeding, severe anemia
5. Anorexia-Cachexia Syndrome: wasting away of client
   a. Unexplained rapid weight loss, anorexia with altered smell and taste
   b. Catabolic state: use of body's tissues and muscle proteins to support cancer cell growth
6. Paraneoplastic Syndromes: ectopic sites with excess hormone production
   a. Parathyroid hormone (hypercalcemia)
   b. Ectopic secretion of insulin (hypoglycemia)
   c. Antidiuretic hormone (ADH: fluid retention)
   d. Adrenocorticotropic hormone (ACTH)
7. Pain: major concern of clients and families associated with cancer
   a. Types of cancer pain
      1. Acute: symptom that led to diagnosis
      2. Chronic: may be related to treatment or to progression of disease
   b. Causes of pain
      1. Direct tumor involvement including metastatic pain
      2. Nerve compression
      3. Involvement of visceral organs
8. Physical Stress: body tries to respond and destroy neoplasm
   a. Fatigue
   b. Weight loss
   c. Anemia
   d. Dehydration
   e. Electrolyte imbalances
9. Psychological Stress
   a. Cancer equals death sentence
   b. Guilt from poor health habits
   c. Fear of pain, suffering, death
   d. Stigmatized

III. Collaborative Care
   A. Diagnostic tests used to diagnose cancer
      1. Determine location of cancer
         a. X-rays
         b. Computed tomography (CT)
         c. Ultrasounds (US)
         d. Magnetic resonance imaging (MRI)
         e. Nuclear imaging
         f. Angiography
      2. Diagnosis of cellular type can be done through tissue samples from biopsies,

shedded cells (e.g., Papanicolaou smear) washings
      a. Cytologic examination: tissue examined under microscope
      b. Identification system of tumors: Classification–Grading—Staging
         1. Classification: according to the tissue or cell of origin, e.g., sarcoma, from supportive
         2. Grading:
            a. Evaluates degree of differentiation and rate of growth
            b. Grade 1 (least aggressive) to Grade 4 (most aggressive)
         3. Staging
            a. Relative tumor size and extent of disease
            b. TNM (Tumor size; Nodes: lymph node involvement; metastases)
      3. Tumor markers: specific proteins which indicate malignancy
         a. PSA (Prostatic-specific antigen): prostate cancer
         b. CEA (Carcinoembryonic antigen): colon cancer
         c. Alkaline Phosphatase: bone metastasis
      4. Direct visualization
         a. Sigmoidoscopy
         b. Cystoscopy
         c. Endoscopy
         d. Bronchoscopy
         e. Exploratory surgery; lymph node biopsies to determine metastases
      5. Other non-specific tests
         a. CBC with diff (differential or CBC with differential)
         b. Electrolytes
         c. Blood Chemistries: (liver enzymes: alanine aminotransferase (ALT); aspartate aminotransferase (AST) lactic dehydrogenase (LDH)

IV. Treatment Goals: depending on type and stage of cancer
   A. Cure
      1. Recover from specific cancer with treatment
      2. Alert for reoccurrence
      3. May involve rehabilitation with physical and occupational therapy
      4. Three Seasons of survival
         a. Diagnosis/treatment
         b. Extended survival: treatment completed and watchful waiting
         c. Permanent survival: risk of recurrence is small

B. Control: of symptoms and progression of
cancer
   1. Continued surveillance
   2. Treatment when indicated (e.g., some
   bladder cancer, prostate cancer)
C. Palliation of symptoms: may involve
terminal care if client's cancer is not
responding to treatment
V. Treatment Options (depend on type of cancer)
alone or with combination
A. Chemotherapy
   1. Chemotherapy
      a. Includes phase-specific and non-phase
      specific drugs for specific cancer types
      b. Often combinations of drugs in specific
      protocols over varying time periods
      c. Cell-kill hypothesis: with each cell cycle
      a percentage of cancerous cells are killed
      but some remain; repeating chemo kills
      more cells until those left can be handled
      by body's immune system
   2. Classes of Chemotherapy Drugs
      a. Alkylating agents
         1. Action: create defects in tumor DNA
         2. Examples: Nitrogen mustard,
         Cisplatin
      b. Antimetabolites
         1. Action: specific for S phase
         2. Examples: Methotrexate;
         5 fluorouracil
         3. Toxic Effects: nausea, vomiting,
         stomatitis, diarrhea, alopecia,
         leukopenia
      c. Antitumor Antibiotics
         1. Action: non-phase specific;
         interfere with DNA
         2. Examples: Actinomycin D,
         Bleomycin
         3. Toxic Effect: damage to cardiac
         muscle
      d. Miotic inhibitors
         1. Action: Prevent cell division during
         M phase
         2. Examples: Vincristine, Vinblastine
         3. Toxic Effects: affects
         neurotransmission, alopecia, bone
         marrow depression
      e. Hormones
         1. Action: stage specific G1
         2. Example: Corticosteroids
      f. Hormone Antagonist
         1. Action: block hormones on
         hormone-binding tumors (breast,
         prostate, endometrium); cause
         tumor regression

   2. Examples: Tamoxifen (breast);
   Flutamide (prostate)
   3. Toxic Effects: altered secondary sex
   characteristics
3. Effects of chemotherapy
   a. Tissues (fast growing) frequently
   affected
   b. Examples: mucous membranes, hair
   cells, bone marrow, specific organs
   with specific agents, reproductive
   organs (all fetal toxic, impair ability to
   reproduce)
4. Administration of chemotherapeutic
agents
   a. Trained and certified personnel,
   according to established guidelines
   b. Preparation
      1. Protect personnel from toxic effects
      2. Extreme care for correct dosage;
      double check with physician orders,
      pharmacist's preparation
   c. Proper management clients'
   excrement
   d. Routes of administration
      1. Oral
      2. Body cavity (intraperitoneal or
      intrapleural)
      3. Intravenous (IV)
         a. Use of vascular access devices
         because of threat of
         extravasation (leakage into
         tissues) and long-term therapy
         b. Types of vascular access devices
            1. PICC lines (peripherally
            inserted central catheters)
            2. Tunneled catheters (Hickman,
            Groshong)
            3. Surgically implanted ports
            (accessed with 90-degree
            angle needle)
   e. Nursing care of clients receiving
   chemotherapy
      1. Assess and manage
         a. Toxic effects of drugs (report to
         physician)
         b. Side effects of drugs: manage
         nausea and vomiting,
         inflammation and ulceration of
         mucous membranes, hair loss,
         anorexia, nausea and vomiting
         with specific nursing and
         medical interventions
      2. Monitor lab results (drugs withheld
      if blood counts seriously low); blood
      and blood product administration

3. Assess for dehydration, oncologic emergencies
4. Teach regarding fatigue, immunosuppression precautions
5. Provide emotional and spiritual support to clients and families

B. Surgery
1. Diagnosis, staging, and sometimes treatment of cancer
2. Involves removal of body part, organ, sometimes with altered functioning (e.g., colostomy)
3. Debulking (decrease size of) tumors in advanced cases
4. Reconstruction and rehabilitation (e.g., breast implant post mastectomy)
5. Psychological support to deal with surgery as well as cancer diagnosis

C. Radiation Therapy
1. Treatment of choice for some tumors to kill or reduce tumor, relieve pain or obstruction
2. Delivery
   a. Teletherapy (external): radiation delivered in uniform dose to tumor
   b. Brachytherapy: delivers high dose to tumor and less to other tissues; radiation source is placed in tumor or next to it
   c. Combination
3. Goals
   a. Maximum tumor control with minimal damage to normal tissues
   b. Caregivers must protect selves by using shields, distancing and limiting time with client, following safety protocols
4. Treatment schedules
   a. Planned according to radiosensitivity of tumor, tolerance of client
   b. Monitor blood cell counts
5. Side effects
   a. Skin (external radiation): blanching, erythema, sloughing
   b. Ulcerated mucous membranes: pain, lack of saliva
   c. Gastrointestinal: nausea and vomiting, diarrhea, bleeding, sometimes fistula formation
   d. Radiation pneumonia

D. Biotherapy
1. Modification of biologic processes that result in malignancies; based on immune surveillance hypothesis
2. Used for hematological malignancies, renal and melanoma
3. Monoclonal antibodies (inoculate animal with tumor antigen and retrieve antibodies against tumor for human)

E. Photodynamic Therapy
1. Client giving photosensitizing compound which concentrates in malignant tissue
2. Later given laser treatment to destroy tumor

F. Bone Marrow Transplantation (BMT) and Peripheral Blood Stem Cell Transplantation (PBSCT)
1. Stimulation of nonfunctioning marrow or replace bone marrow
2. Common treatment for leukemias

G. Pain Control
1. Includes pain directly from cancer, treatment, or unrelated
2. Necessary for continuing function or comfort in terminally ill clients
3. Goal is maximum relief with minimal side effects
4. Multiple combinations of analgesics (narcotic and non-narcotic) and adjuvants such as steroids or antidepressants; includes around the clock (ATC) schedule with additional medications for break-through pain
5. Multiple routes of medications
6. May involve injections of anesthetics into nerve, surgical severing of nerves, radiation
7. May need to progress to stronger pain medications as pain increases and client develops tolerance to pain medication

VI. Nursing Diagnoses for clients with cancer
A. Anxiety
1. Therapeutic interactions with client and family; community resources such as American Cancer Society, "I Can Cope"
2. Availability of community resources for terminally ill (Hospice care in-patient, home care)

B. Disturbed Body Image
1. Includes loss of body parts (e.g., amputations); appearance changes (skin, hair); altered functions (e.g., colostomy); cachexic appearance, loss of energy, ability to be productive
2. Fear of rejection, stigma

C. Anticipatory grieving
1. Facing death and making preparations for death
2. Offer realistic hope that cancer treatment may be successful

D. Risk for Infection

E. Risk for Injury
1. Organ obstruction
2. Pathological fractures

F. Altered Nutrition: less than body requirements
1. Consultation with dietician, lab evaluation of nutritional status
2. Managing problems with eating: anorexia, nausea and vomiting
3. May involve use of parenteral nutrition
G. Impaired Tissue Integrity
1. Oral, pharyngeal, esophageal tissues (due to chemotherapy, bleeding due to low platelet counts, fungal infections such as thrush)
2. Teach inspection, frequent oral hygiene, specific non-irritating products, thrush control
VII. Oncologic Emergencies
A. Pericaridal effusion and neoplastic cardiac Tamponade
1. Concern: compression of heart by fluid in pericardial sac, compromised cardiac output
2. Treatment: pericardiocentesis
B. Superior vena cava Syndrome
1. Concern: obstruction of venous system with increased venous pressure and stasis; facial and neck edema with slow progression to respiration distress
2. Treatment: respiratory support; decrease tumor size with radiation or chemotherapy
C. Sepsis and Septic Shock
1. Concern: Early recognition of infection
2. Treatment: prompt

D. Spinal cord compression
1. Concern: pressure from expanding tumor can cause irreversible paraplegia; back pain initial symptom with progressive paresthesia and leg pain and weakness
2. Treatment: early detection and radiation or surgical decompression
E. Obstructive uropathy
1. Concern: blockage of urine flow; undiagnosed can result in renal failure
2. Treatment: restore urine flow
F. Hypercalcemia
1. Concern: high calcium from ectopic parathyroid hormone or metastases
2. Behaviors: fatigue, muscle weakness, polyuria, constipation progressing to coma, seizures
3. Treatment: restore fluids with intravenous saline; loop diuretics; more definitive treatments
G. Hyperuricemia
1. Concern: occurs with rapid necrosis of tumor cells as with chemotherapy; can result in renal damage and failure
2. Prevention and treatment with fluids and alopurinol (Zyloprim)
H. SIADH (Syndrome of Inappropriate Antidiuretic Hormone Secretion)
1. Concern: ectopic ADH production from tumor leads to excessive hyponatremia
2. Treatment: restore sodium level

FOCUSED STUDY TIPS

- Interview a client with cancer. Ask him/her to share with you how the cancer was diagnosed and the initial impact the diagnosis had on the family.
- Contact the local cancer society. Identify actions they take to promote the early detection of cancer. What information is available to health professionals and to community members?
- Visit a local pharmacy. Ask the pharmacist for a package insert for any frequently prescribed chemotherapeutic agent. Read the literature. Become familiar with the drug and its side effects.

CASE STUDY

Your client is a 60-year-old male dying of liver cancer. He is being discharged from the hospital to home with hospice services. His family includes his wife and two adult daughters who live close by. His physician has recommended radiation therapy as a palliative measure. The family agrees, but the client voices reluctance to follow his physician's recommendations. The family has solicited your help in convincing the client to move forward with treatment. What interview questions are necessary to ask at this point? What physical assessments should be made? List three client goals or outcomes for this client and his family.

CARE PLAN CRITICAL THINKING ACTIVITY

A client you are working with has just been diagnosed with metastatic breast cancer. She is scheduled to undergo chemotherapy. Her husband asks why these drugs are used in his wife's treatment and what they will do for her. How do you answer his question?

NCLEX TEST QUESTIONS

1. Cancer is the second major cause of death in the United States. What is the first step toward cancer control?
   a. increasing government control of carcinogens
   b. changing habits and customs that predispose individuals to cancer
   c. create mass screening programs
   d. educating of the public about cancer

2. Alkylating drugs utilized in cancer therapy stop cancer growth by:
   a. destroying messenger RNA.
   b. creating systemic hormonal imbalances.
   c. interrupting the production of necessary cellular metabolites.
   d. damaging DNA in the cell nucleus.

3. A client is experiencing severe side effects from chemotherapy. She is nauseated and she is vomiting. In addition to antiemetic medications, the nurse might suggest:
   a. increasing salt in the diet.
   b. drinking fluids between meals, not with meals.
   c. low-protein meals.
   d. high-calorie, high-protein dietary supplements.

4. The nurse understands that the most common site of cancer for a female is the:
   a. uterine cervix.
   b. Fallopian tubes.
   c. vagina.
   d. uterine body.

5. Of the following screening methods for cancer prevention, the most important one for the client to be aware of is:
   a. sigmoidoscopy.
   b. magnetic resonance imaging (MRI).
   c. colonoscopy.
   d. breast self-examination (BSE).

6. When teaching a class on cancer prevention and treatment, which of the following symptoms does the nurse identify as an early warning sign of cancer?
   a. persistent headache
   b. fever, chills, and cough
   c. muscle cramping and exercise intolerance
   d. changes in bowel or bladder habits

7. When the nurse is counseling clients about preventive measures for cancer, one of the most important behaviors to emphasize is to:
   a. decrease fat intake and avoid obesity.
   b. avoid exposure to the sun.
   c. avoid tobacco use.
   d. avoid stress and obtain adequate exercise.

CHAPTER 11

NURSING CARE OF CLIENTS EXPERIENCING LOSS, GRIEF, AND DEATH

LEARNING OUTCOMES

After completing this chapter, you will be able to:

- Describe theories of loss and grief.
- Discuss factors affecting responses to loss.
- Begin to assess own feelings and values related to loss, grief, and death.
- Discuss legal and ethical issues in end-of-life care.
- Describe the philosophy and activities of hospice.
- Identify physiological changes in the dying client.
- Provide nursing interventions to promote a comfortable death.
- Use the nursing process as a framework for providing individualized care for clients and families experiencing loss, grief, or death.

KEY TOPICS

- Theories of loss, grief, and dying
- Factors affecting responses to loss
- End-of-life considerations
- Nursing care of the client experiencing loss and grief
- Nursing care of the dying client

LECTURE OUTLINE

I. Background
   A. Definitions
      1. Grief: internal process a person works through due to a loss
      2. Loss: actual or potential situation in which someone or something is no longer present or available to a person
      3. Bereavement: form of depression accompanied by anxiety in response to loss of loved one
      4. Mourning: actions and expressions of bereavement including rituals, symbols, actions
   B. Nurses deal with clients experiencing many different types of losses, and expressing grief in various ways; in various stages of grief
   C. Multiple Theories of Grief
      1. Helps nurses make sense of how people grieve

MediaLink

www.prenhall.com/lemone

Additional resources for this chapter can be found on the Student CD-ROM accompanying this textbook, and on the Companion Website at www.prenhall.com/lemone. Click on Chapter 11 to select the activities for this chapter.

CD-ROM
- Audio Glossary
- NCLEX Review

Companion Website
- More NCLEX Review
- Case Study
   Dysfunctional Grieving
- Care Plan Activity
   Anticipatory Grieving
- MediaLink Application
   Grief and Unexpected Death

2. Allows nurses to develop insight into the grief process and empathy for those grieving
3. Develop nurses' awareness of own feelings and experiences regarding grief
4. Common Theories
   a. Engel: Three main stages of grief
      1. Shock and disbelief
      2. Awareness
      3. Restitution
   b. Lindemann
      1. Anticipatory grief: cluster of predictable responses to anticipated loss
      2. Morbid grief: delayed and dysfunctional reaction to loss including debilitating health problems
   c. Caplan: Factors that affect how people deal with a loss
      1. Psychic pain of broken bond
      2. Living without the assets and guidance of lost person or resource
      3. Reduced cognitive and problem-solving ability that occurs with distress
   d. Kuebler-Ross: stages of coping with loss (not all mandatory, or sequential)
      1. Denial: "I can't believe it"; serves as buffer to mobilize defenses
      2. Anger: resisting the loss; directed toward family, health care providers
      3. Bargaining: attempt to postpone reality of loss
      4. Depression: realization of full impact of loss
      5. Acceptance: coming to terms
   e. Carter: Themes of bereavement
      1. Grief's changing character: "waves of intense pain"
      2. Holding: process of preserving fact and meaning of loss
      3. Expectations: norms of how the grieving should act
      4. Role of personal history in grief process
D. Factors affecting how people respond to loss
   1. Age
   2. Social support
   3. Families
   4. Spirituality
   5. Rituals of mourning
   6. Personal experience

II. End of Life issues
   A. Background
      1. State laws dictate specifics; laws vary from state to state
      2. Clients are requested to submit specific documents when they enter the health care system; nurses participate in process
      3. Patient Self-Determination Act requires that all facilities receiving Medicare or Medicaid funds provide clients written information and counseling about advance directives and the institution's policies; nurses participate in process
   B. Legal documents
      1. Advance Directives: legal documents allowing person to plan for health care and/or financial affairs in the event of incapacity
      2. Durable Power of Attorney for Health Care: legal document issued by a mentally competent person to give another mentally competent adult the right to make health care decisions on that person's behalf if the person is unable to do so
      3. Living Will: legal document formally expressing person's wishes regarding life-sustaining treatment in the event of terminal illness or permanent unconsciousness
   C. Common Practices
      1. Do-Not-Resuscitate Orders (DNR) or "no code"
         a. Order written by a physician stating no cardiopulmonary resuscitation to be performed if client quits breathing or heart stops
         b. The person may be near death or may be someone who has significant chronic disease and/or advanced age and does not wish extraordinary measures
         c. Specific implementation details vary from state to state
      2. Comfort measures only
         a. Indicates no further life-sustaining interventions will be done
         b. Measures will be taken to allow the person a dignified comfortable death
   D. Ethical Issues: Euthanasia—mercy killing
      1. Controversial and illegal in all states except Oregon
      2. Involves efforts and actions to end a person's life
      3. Can be voluntary (desired by client) or involuntary (done without client's consent)

4. Legally may be considered murder with the person involved subject to prosecution

E. Hospice
1. Model of care for clients with limited life expectancy and their families
2. Dying is normal part of life and supports dignified and peaceful death
3. 1986 Medicare Hospice Benefit Act provides hospice benefits
4. Time frame: begins when client has 6 months or less until death and ends for family one year post death
5. Interdisciplinary care team
6. Nurses are skilled in pain and symptom management
7. Can be delivered in freestanding hospice, care facility such as nursing home, or client's home

F. End of Life Care standards to ensure peaceful death (American Association of Colleges of Nursing—AACN)
1. Comfort care standards
2. Respect for client wishes
3. Symptom assessment and relief, especially pain
4. Assist client and family through grief process

III. Death
A. Physiological Changes: no set speed or with exact sequence of signs and symptoms
1. Fatigue
2. Loss of interest in eating, anorexia
3. Fluid and electrolyte imbalances including dehydration (lack of intake)
4. Hypotension and renal shutdown
5. Neurological dysfunction
   a. Decreased level of consciousness, confusion, agitation
   b. Hearing thought to be last remaining sense; those around need to be careful of conversations near client
6. Altered respirations
   a. irregular, dyspnea, episodes of apnea
   b. "Death Rattle": common term for noisy respirations (fluid accumulation)
7. Bowel and/or bladder incontinence

B. Pronouncement of death
1. Legal declaration that person has died by physician or other designated health care personnel
2. Information obtained for death certificate

C. Postmortem Care
1. Depending on situation, client's body made presentable and family notified
2. Family encouraged to view and touch body

3. Discussion with family regarding autopsy (may be required if legal matter with death; if autopsy, do not remove any of tubes or lines in body)
4. Family signs paper and designates funeral home for care; body taken to morgue
5. Client belongings given to family members
6. Documentation of all activities
7. Nurse expression of sympathy to family, deal with grief

IV. Collaborative care with clients in grief process
A. Nurses encounter clients in grief process before, during, post loss
1. Assist clients to resolve through process to avoid health, mental problems in future
2. Length of grief is individual process and time frame varies with individual

B. Signs and symptoms commonly experienced in relation to the grief process
1. Gastrointestinal Behaviors
   a. Difficulties with eating
   b. Weight loss or gain
   c. Bowel disturbances
2. Distress behaviors
   a. Crying and overwhelming sadness
   b. Extreme weakness
   c. Hyperventilation
   d. Choking sensation
   e. Shortness of breath
3. Energy and sleep behaviors
   a. Changes in activity level
   b. Insomnia
   c. Preoccupation with sleep

C. Spiritual assessment/promoting coping behaviors
1. Client and family faith impact on how client deals with loss
   a. Belief in God or supreme being
   b. Belief in afterlife
2. Nurse being open to client and family communication regarding spirituality
3. Assist with contact and communication with religious personnel according to client's wishes

D. Psychosocial assessment/interventions
1. Assist client and family in dealing with anxiety
2. Acknowledgement of loss is beginning point
3. Teaching client and family: grief is natural reaction, common reactions to grief, takes time
4. Persons frequently need to grieve/resolve past loss before dealing with present loss
5. Resources available in community

6. Teaching about ways to decrease and deal with stress
E. Nursing Diagnoses

1. Anticipatory grieving
2. Chronic sorrow
3. Death Anxiety

FOCUSED STUDY TIPS

- Assess the level of understanding within your family regarding the physiological process of dying. Describe to them the normal changes that occur during the dying process. Identify and clarify knowledge deficits. How will this information be used?
- What are your personal preferences for your own end-of-life care? Share these thoughts with a classmate. Compare and contrast your classmate's preferences to your own. How will your end-of-life care differ?
- Contact a local hospice agency. Learn what services it provides for clients. How do clients access these services?

CASE STUDY

A terminally ill client you are caring for dies. You are present at the moment of death. He is surrounded by family and friends. Although his death has been anticipated, the family is very distraught. They have requested an autopsy. Detail all necessary nursing interventions for postmortem care for this client. How do you interact with the family while at the same time delivering your care?

CARE PLAN CRITICAL THINKING ACTIVITY

Compare and contrast the care that a man dying of cancer would receive in a critical care unit or at home with hospice care. Identify the advantages and disadvantages of each. Use your analysis to help you describe these options to future clients.

NCLEX TEST QUESTIONS

1. Which of the following would be considered the most therapeutic nursing intervention for encouraging communication with a dying client?
   a. talking about current events and orienting the client frequently
   b. explaining the care for the shift
   c. asking the client frequent yes or no questions
   d. sitting silently at the bedside

2. During a home nursing visit, the nurse observes that a terminally ill client's husband appears pale, tired, and depressed. Which of the following will the nurse suggest?
   a. getting an appointment with a physician to follow up on symptoms
   b. hospitalizing the client for a few days to allow the husband to rest
   c. finding someone to relieve the husband on a regular basis
   d. getting a prescription for an antidepressant

3. Palliative treatment refers to:
   a. providing aggressive forms of current treatment of disease.
   b. encouraging clients to participate in cancer research.
   c. using measures that make clients feel more comfortable.
   d. use of experimental drugs and procedures to prolong life.

4. Nursing care of the client nearing death includes:
   a. gentle ROM (range-of-motion) exercises.
   b. hourly urinary output monitoring.
   c. every 1 hour vital signs.
   d. gentle massage to improve circulation and shift edema.

5. Kubler-Ross defines the second stage of responding to loss as:
   a. anger.
   b. bargaining.
   c. denial.
   d. acceptance.

6. The nurse can pronounce death in some states of the United States. Where would the nurse find this parameter of practice?
   a. state nursing practice acts
   b. state ethics boards
   c. community councils
   d. physicians for whom the nurse works

CHAPTER 12

NURSING CARE OF CLIENTS WITH PROBLEMS OF SUBSTANCE ABUSE

LEARNING OUTCOMES

After completing this chapter, you will be able to:

- Discuss risk factors associated with substance abuse.
- Describe common characteristics of substance abusers.
- Identify major addictive substances.
- Explain the effects of addictive substances on physiological, cognitive, psychological, and social well-being.
- Discuss collaborative care for the client with substance abuse problems, including diagnostic tests, emergency care for overdose, and treatment of withdrawal.
- Use the nursing process as a framework for providing individualized nursing care for clients experiencing problems with substance abuse.

KEY TOPICS

- Major addictive substances
- Risk factors associated with substance abuse
- Nursing care of clients experiencing substance abuse problems

LECTURE OUTLINE

  I. Background/Definitions
    A. Substance abuse
      1. Use of any chemical in any fashion inconsistent with medical or culturally defined social norms
      2. Estimated 9% of U.S. have substance abuse disorder
      3. Alcohol is most commonly used and abused substance in U.S.

    B. Substance dependence: Severe condition in which use of chemical substance no longer under person's control for at least 3 months
    C. Tolerance: Cumulative state in which particular dose of the chemical elicits a smaller response than previously

D. Withdrawal
1. Uncomfortable state occurring when a person stops taking a chemical substance they are addicted to
2. Lasts several days
3. Signs and symptoms: tremors, diaphoresis, anxiety, elevated blood pressure and pulse, possible convulsions
E. Dual diagnosis or disorder
1. Coexistence of substance abuse and psychiatric disorder in one person
2. Examples: cannibis abuse with psychoses; heroin and/or alcohol with depression
II. Risk factors: why one person develops addiction and another does not
A. Biological factors
1. Heredity, especially with alcohol
2. Early onset
a. Increased incidence with males
b. Inability to abstain
c. Antisocial personality
3. Later onset (post age 25)
a. Inability to stop after one drink
b. Passive-dependent personality
B. Psychological factors according to different theories
1. Fixation at oral stage of development (psychoanalytic)
2. Learned, maladaptive behavior (behavioral)
3. Pattern of family relationships (family systems)
4. Positive link with history of sexual or physical abuse as children; low self-esteem, difficulty expressing emotions
C. Sociocultural factors
1. Cultural
2. Religious
III. Common personality characteristics of persons who have substance abuse
A. Tendency to be impulsive and prone to take risks
B. Low tolerance for frustration and pain
C. Seek pleasure and avoid stress
D. Rebellious against social norms, antisocial behaviors
E. Prone to anxiety, anger, low self-esteem
IV. Common addictive substances
A. Nicotine (source: tobacco)
1. Physiology
a. Stimulant on CNS
b. Activates pleasure center of brain
2. Symptoms of withdrawal after chronic use: craving, restlessness, irritability, insomnia, impaired concentration, increased appetite, weight gain

B. Tetrahydrocannabinol (THC) (source: Cannabis/marijuana)
1. Physiology
a. Acts as opioids or cocaine
b. Produces pleasurable sensation
2. Dose-related, prolonged use results
a. Airway constriction
b. Decreased fertility in both sexes
c. Lack of motivation, apathy
C. Alcohol (alcoholic beverages) (ETOH)
1. Physiology: CNS depressant
2. Chronic use results
a. Neurologic and psychiatric disorders
1. Wernicke's encephalopathy: nystagmus, ptosis, ataxia, confusion, coma, possible death (thiamine deficiency)
2. Korsakoff's psychosis: secondary dementia with progressive cognitive deterioration, confabulation, peripheral neuropathy and myopathy (thiamine deficiency)
b. Malnutrition: thiamine depletion leading to Wernicke-Korsakoff syndrome
c. Liver damage including fatty liver and cirrhosis
d. Sleep disturbances including worsening of sleep apnea
e. Increased incidence of accidents: 0.10% is legal level of intoxication in most states
3. Symptoms of withdrawal: Tachycardia, hypertension, diaphoresis, nausea, vomiting, tremors, irritability, delirium tremens (DTs), seizures
D. Central Nervous System Depressants: barbiturates, benzodiazepines
1. May develop cross-tolerance to alcohol and general anesthetics
2. Depressant behaviors are dose dependent
3. Combination of alcohol and barbiturates increase risk for death
E. Psychostimulants (cocaine, amphetamines)
1. High potential for abuse
2. Produces euphoria, highly addictive
3. Routes include smoking, snorting, injecting intravenously
4. Physiologic effects of cocaine
a. Mild overdose: agitation, tremor
b. Severe overdose: anxiety, hyperpyrexia, convulsions, ventricular dysrhythmias, possible hemorrhagic stroke, myocardial infarction
c. Use during pregnancy causes fetal addiction

        d. Long term snorting causes nasal mucosal atrophy and perforation of the nasal septum

    5. Physiologic effects of amphetamines

        a. State of arousal

        b. Sense of increased strength and mental capacity

        c. Decreased need for food and sleep

        d. Long-term use results in hallucinations and paranoia

        e. Causes increase in pulse and blood pressure

    6. Dependence is more psychological than physical

  F. Opiates (morphine, heroin)

    1. Abused by persons of all socioeconomic statures

    2. Taken intravenously

    3. Initial withdrawal symptoms

        a. Drug craving

        b. Lacrimation

        c. Rhinorrhea

        d. Diaphoresis lasting 10 days

    4. Later withdrawal behaviors

        a. Insomnia

        b. Fatigue

        c. GI hyperactivity lasting for months

  G. Hallucinogens (psychedelics, LSD; Ecstasy, PCP (animal anesthetic))

    1. Taken orally, smoked, or by injection

    2. Simulates psychosis: dream-like thoughts, perceptions

    3. Persons experience flashbacks

  H. Inhalants

    1. Types

        a. Anesthetics (e.g., nitrous oxide, laughing gas)

        b. Volatile nitrates (e.g., amyl nitrate)

        c. Organic solvents (e.g., inhaling lighter fluid, paint thinner)

    2. Physiology: stimulants, may result in sudden death

V. Collaborative Care

  A. Clients enter health system for care under different ways

    1. Overdose: life-threatening requiring emergency hospitalization

    2. Client or family seeking help; legal requirement

  B. Interdisciplinary team approach with different therapies

    1. Detoxification

    2. Aversion therapy

    3. Group or individual psychotherapy

    4. Psychotropic medications

    5. Cognitive-behavioral strategies

    6. Family counseling

    7. Self-help groups

  C. Diagnostic Testing

    1. Most commonly used tests include

        a. Urine Drug Screen (UDS)

        b. Blood Alcohol Level (BAL)

            1. Legal intoxication is 0.10%

                a. Clumsiness

                b. Impaired reaction time

            2. 0.20% level: brain is depressed, ataxia

            3. May experience withdrawal symptoms if BAL is high

    2. Length of time drugs can be found in urine and blood varies with dosage and metabolic properties of drug

D. Treatments

    1. Emergency care for overdose Respiratory status is most important; may need mechanical ventilation At risk for seizures Possibly intentional act for suicide, institute precautions Be alert for symptoms of withdrawal

    2. Treatment of withdrawal

        a. Dangerous progression with withdrawal from alcohol, benzodiazepines, and barbiturates

        b. Course

            1. Signs after few hours

            2. Peak in 24–48 hours

            3. Disappear until delirium tremens occurring 2–5 days post withdrawal, lasting 2–3 days

            4. Monitor vital signs (rise in temperature, pulse rate, and blood pressure)

        c. Severe withdrawal (delirium tremens)

            1. Medical emergency

            2. Symptoms: disorientation, paranoid delusions, visual hallucinations, possible seizures

        d. Treatment

            1. Symptomatic care with acetaminophen, vitamins, tranquilizers (benzodiazepines minimize discomfort of withdrawal)

            2. Supportive care

            3. Protection from harming self

            4. Limit sensory input, quiet and dimly lit room

            5. Emphasize safe environment

            6. Understand that hallucinations seem real to client but are not present

            7. Do not argue about delusions or hallucinations

8. Reinforce real events
   e. Clients withdrawing from opiates are mostly sick with gastrointestinal symptoms; clients withdrawing from cocaine may become suicidal
E. Nursing Care
   1. Assessment
      a. Style: comprehensive; open ended questioning, non-threatening, professional manner
      b. Includes
         1. History of past substance abuse
            a. Substances used
            b. Starting
            c. History of withdrawal or overdoses
            d. Attempts to quit
            e. Criminal offenses or driving arrests related to drug or alcohol use
         2. Medical and psychiatric history for:
            a. Cirrhosis
            b. Pancreatitis
            c. Gastritis
            d. Depression
            e. Wernicke-Korsakoff syndrome
            f. Suicide or homicidal ideation
            g. History of abuse with acts of violence towards self or others
         3. Psychosocial concerns
            a. Living style and stress
            b. Ability to hold job
            c. Substance abuse effect on relationships with family and others
            d. Support system
      c. Assessment tools: brief screening tests that detail severity of dependency or abuse and give self-assessment feedback to client
      d. Results of blood and urine screening tests
   2. Nursing Diagnoses
      a. Risk for Injury
         1. Determine disorientation, level of agitation, risk for suicide or harm to self or others

2. Protective environment, frequent observation
3. Vital signs q15 minutes: feedback for symptoms of withdrawal
      b. Ineffective Denial
         1. Establish non-judgmental therapeutic relationship
         2. Assist to recognize maladaptive behaviors; non acceptance of manipulative and blaming behaviors, caring confrontation
         3. Therapeutic group activities for peer feedback
      c. Ineffective Individual Coping
         1. Limit setting; encourage expression of feelings, fears
         2. Teach alternative ways of dealing with stress
      d. Altered Nutrition: Less than Body Requirements
         1. Referral to dietician; nutritional assessment including blood work
         2. Client modification of diet, goal setting for weight according to need
      e. Self-Esteem Disturbance
         1. Acceptance of person
         2. Focus on strength and accomplishments
      f. Altered Sensory Perceptions
      g. Altered Thought Processes
   3. Client Teaching
      a. Negative effects of substance abuse on client physically and psychosocially
      b. Prevention of relapse
         1. After-care programs, self-help groups, community resources (Alcoholics Anonymous, Narcotics Anonymous, National Alliance for Mentally Ill, Employee Assistance Programs)
         2. Medication, such as Naltrexone (ReVia) reduces craving for alcohol; disulfiram (Antabuse) maintains abstinence since client becomes ill with alcohol use

FOCUSED STUDY TIPS

■ Contact the public health department in your community. Identify the major substances abused in your community. Describe to classmates preventative measures utilized to discourage substance abuse in the community.

- Identify alcohol treatment options in your community. Compare and contrast access to these services.
- Ask to care for a client with a history of substance abuse. Read the complete history and physical exam for the client and determine the effects the addiction has had on the client's cognitive, psychosocial, social, and physical well-being.

CASE STUDY

Brian is seen in the emergency department as a suspected substance abuser. Describe the importance of respiratory assessment while caring for Brian. How frequently is it needed? Why? Detail one psycho-social nursing intervention necessary when developing Brian's plan of care. Describe how your intervention will impact Brian's long term rehabilitation.

CARE PLAN CRITICAL THINKING ACTIVITY

Ms. Becker has a long history of multiple substance abuse. She requires hospitalization for a gynecological surgery. Her anticipated stay is 5 days. What problems might occur? What information is necessary to obtain before her surgery? How will this information affect her plan of care? How will her pain management differ, if at all?

NCLEX TEST QUESTIONS

1. An acronym that assists the client in recognizing behaviors that lead to relapse is:
   a. STOP.
   b. HELP.
   c. HALT.
   d. CARE.
2. Severe cognitive impairment seen in chronic alcoholics is a feature of:
   a. GABA.
   b. Wernicke-Korsakoff syndrome.
   c. B_{12} vitamin deficiency.
   d. polysubstance abuse.
3. Recreational use of which of the following drugs can cause decreased testosterone levels in males and decreased levels of follicle-stimulating, luteinizing, and prolactin hormones in females?
   a. alcohol
   b. opioids
   c. marijuana
   d. amphetamines
4. Which of the following groups of individuals has the highest risk for opiate abuse?
   a. lawyers
   b. young middle-class adults
   c. surgical clients
   d. health care professionals

5. Airway constriction leading to bronchitis, sinusitis, and asthma can occur with the chronic use of:
   a. inhalants.
   b. alcohol.
   c. hallucinogens.
   d. marijuana.
6. Smoking during pregnancy leads to such increased risks for infants as:
   a. prolonged labor resulting in complications from hypoxia.
   b. increased risk for lung cancer.
   c. hyperbilirubinemia.
   d. sudden infant death syndrome.
7. Which of the following nursing interventions help the client to develop insight?
   a. discussions that focus on the client's perception of reality
   b. giving negative reinforcement when thinking and behavior are inappropriate
   c. allowing the client to verbalize feelings in a nonthreatening environment
   d. stress management techniques

CHAPTER 13

ASSESSING CLIENTS WITH INTEGUMENTARY DISORDERS

LEARNING OUTCOMES

After completing this chapter, you will be able to:

- Review the anatomy and physiology of the skin, hair, and nails.
- Discuss factors that influence skin color.
- Identify specific topics for consideration during a health history interview of the client with problems involving the skin, hair, and nails.
- Describe techniques for assessing the skin, hair, and nails.
- Describe normal variations in assessment findings for the client with dark skin.
- Identify abnormal findings that may indicate impairment of the integumentary system.

KEY TOPICS

- Review of anatomy and physiology of the integumentary system
- Assessing the integumentary system

LECTURE OUTLINE

I. Assessment Background
   A. Integumentary system is composed of skin, hair, nails
   B. Skin has many major functions
      1. Protection from external environment
      2. Protection from pathogenic invasion
      3. Barrier to loss of fluid and heat
      4. Sensory organ touch and temperature
      5. Wound repair

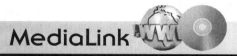

MediaLink

www.prenhall.com/lemone

Additional resources for this chapter can be found on the Student CD-ROM accompanying this textbook, and on the Companion Website at www.prenhall.com/lemone. Click on Chapter 13 to select the activities for this chapter.

CD-ROM
- Audio Glossary
- NCLEX Review

Animation
- Integumentary Repair

Companion Website
- More NCLEX Review
- Functional Health Pattern Assessment
- Case Study
   Assessing a Rash

C. Layers
   1. Epidermis: outermost, made up of epithelial cells
      a. Contains melanocytes: produce *melanin,* a pigment that protects against ultraviolet light

      b. Contains keratinocytes: produce *keratin,* which is fibrous, water repellent

  2. Dermis: second deeper layer

      a. Composed of connective tissue and richly supplied with blood and lymphatic vessels, nerve fibers, hair follicles, sebaceous (oil) and sweat glands

      b. Under the skin is layer of subcutaneous tissue called superficial fascia

  D. Terminology

    1. Melanin: color pigment yellow to brown, darkening or tanning in light skin

    2. Carotene: color pigment yellow to orange, in palms of hands

    3. Erythema: reddening of skin due to blushing, fever, hypertension, inflammation

    4. Cyanosis: bluish discoloration due to poor oxygenation of hemoglobin

    5. Pallor: paleness that can occur with shock, fear, anger, anemia, hypoxia

    6. Jaundice: yellow to orange coloration due to bilirubin deposits as with hepatic disorders

    7. Vitiligo: abnormal loss of melanin in patches, usually over face, hands, groin

II. Health Assessment Interview

  A. Facts about skin problem

    1. Determine onset

    2. Characteristics and course

    3. Precipitating and relieving factors

    4. Associated symptoms

  B. Factors associated with skin problem

    1. Determine associated allergies

    2. Other disorders such as cardiovascular endocrine, hepatic, hematologic conditions

    3. Occupational and social history including travel

    4. Exposure to environmental substances

    5. Stress

  C. Risk factors for skin cancer: malignant melanoma, such as sunburn history

III. Physical Assessment of Skin

  A. Skin Color: Abnormal findings

    1. Pallor or cyanosis

      a. Occurs with exposure to cold and with decreased perfusion and oxygenation

      b. Dark skinned persons: loss of glow and ashen appearance of skin; cyanosis visible in mucous membranes and nail beds

    2. Jaundice

      a. Occurs with deposits of bilirubin due to hepatic malfunction

      b. Dark skinned clients: most apparent in nail beds

    3. Erythema

      a. Occurs with various rashes, inflammations, infections, burns

      b. Appears as redness, swelling, pain

    4. Vitiligo

      a. Loss of melanin in patches, mostly occurring over face, hands, groin

      b. Thought to be autoimmune disorder

  B. Skin lesions

    1. Pearly-edged nodules with a central ulcer, e.g., basal cell carcinoma

    2. Scaly red, fast-growing papules, e.g., squamous cell carcinoma

    3. Dark, asymmetric multicolored patches or moles with irregular edges, e.g., malignant melanoma

    4. Circular lesions, e.g., ringworm and tinea versicolor

    5. Grouped vesicles, e.g., contact dermatitis

    6. Linear lesions, e.g., poison ivy and herpes zoster

    7. Patches of pale, itchy wheals in erythematous area, e.g., hives

    8. Scaly, red patches on scalp, knees, back, and genitals, e.g., psoriasis

    9. Vesicles along sensory nerve paths, turning into pustules and then crusting over, e.g., herpes zoster

    10. Raised bluish or yellowish vascular lesions, e.g., bruises

  C. Determine skin temperature by palpation

    1. Warm, red skin, e.g., inflammation, elevated body temperature

    2. Cool skin, e.g., decreased blood flow as in shock (generalized condition) or arteriosclerosis (localized)

  D. Determine skin texture by palpation

    1. Changes may indicate irritation, trauma

    2. Soft and smooth skin, e.g., hyperthyroidism

    3. Coarse skin, e.g., hypothyroidism

  E. Determine skin moisture by palpation

    1. Dry skin, common with age and may indicate hypothyroidism

    2. Oily skin, common with adolescents and young adults; may be normal or indicative of acne vulgaris

    3. Excessive perspiration may be indicative of shock, fever, increased activity, anxiety

  F. Determine skin turgor by palpation

    1. Tenting occurs in thin elderly clients

    2. Decreased in dehydration

    3. Increased in edema and scleroderma

G. Presence of edema
1. Findings are described
a. 1+ Slight pitting with no obvious distortion
b. 2+ Deeper pitting with no obvious distortion
c. 3+ Pitting is obvious; extremities are swollen
d. 4+ Pitting remains with obvious distortion
2. Edema common with cardiovascular disorders, renal failure, cirrhosis
3. Always compare both sides of body for symmetry; existence of edema in only one extremity may indicate injury or some type of pathology
H. Hair
1. Hair quality and distribution
a. Deviation from normal hair distribution in genital area of males or females may indicate endocrine disorder
b. Hirsutism: as in Cushing's syndrome, acromegaly and ovarian dysfunction
c. Alopecia: may indicate hormonal changes or occurs with chemical or drug treatment
d. Male pattern baldness is usually genetic
2. Hair texture: may be affected by systemic disease
a. Hypothyroidism: hair becomes coarse
b. Hyperthyroidism: hair becomes fine
3. Scalp condition, presence of lesions
a. Mild dandruff may be normal, greasy flakes indicate seborrhea
b. Hair loss, pustules, scales indicate tinea capitis (ringworm of scalp)
c. Red swollen pustules around infected hair follicles are called furuncles
d. Oval whitish pearly particles that will not flake off at the base of the hair shaft are seen with head lice; the skin around the area may be reddened due to pruritis secondary to lice

IV. Fingernails
A. Curvature of nail
1. Clubbing in which angle of nail base > 180°
2. Nail becomes thick, hard, shiny and curved at end
3. Occurs with respiratory and cardiovascular disorders, cirrhosis, colitis, and thyroid disease
B. Surface of the nails
1. Nail folds are inflamed and swollen, may be loose: occurs with paronychia, infection of nails
2. Inflammation and transverse rippling of nail: occurs with chronic paronychia and eczema
3. Nail plate separation from bed (oncolysis): occurs with trauma, psoriasis, Pseudomonas and Candida infections
4. Nail grooves occurs with inflammation, planus, nail biting
5. Nail pitting: occurs with psoriasis
6. Transverse groove (Beau's line): occurs with trachoma and/or acute diseases
7. Spoon-shaped nails: occurs with anemia
C. Color
1. Pigmented band: normal finding in 90% African Americans; sudden appearance may indicate melanoma
2. Yellowish nails: occurs with psoriasis and fungal infections
3. Dark nails: occurs with trauma, Candida infections and hyperbilirubinemia
4. Blackish-green nails: occurs with injury and Pseudomonas infection
5. Red splinter longitudinal hemorrhages: may occur with injury or psoriasis
D. Nail thickness
1. Thickened nails occurs with trauma, psoriasis, fungal infections, and ischemia
2. Thinning nails occurs with nutritional deficiencies

FOCUSED STUDY TIPS

- Teach a family member or friend how to perform a complete physical assessment of the skin. How might this skill contribute to optimal health of an individual?
- Compare skin assessments of clients in the clinical setting. List factors that contribute to the difference in assessment findings.

CASE STUDY

Mr. Barnett is seen in the outpatient clinic for diagnosis of a skin disorder. What questions would you ask Mr. Barnett when taking an initial history?

CARE PLAN CRITICAL THINKING ACTIVITY

Conduct the physical assessment and examination of the integumentary systems of the following clients:

An older woman recovering from a broken leg at home

A 23-year-old male hospitalized with paralysis from a skateboarding accident

A dark-skinned child with a body cast

What seven physical characteristics are you checking for in all four clients? Compare the differences in how the assessments are implemented.

NCLEX TEST QUESTIONS

1. Risk factors for skin cancer include:
   a. chronic skin disorders such as eczema, freckles, and an easy ability to tan.
   b. daily exposure to sunlight, female gender, age under 50.
   c. extended exposure to sunlight, male gender, age over 50.
   d. light-colored hair or eyes, residence in northern latitudes, exposure to smoke.

2. The substance responsible for pigmentation or coloring of the skin is:
   a. keratin.
   b. lunula.
   c. vitiligo.
   d. melanin.

3. Equipment necessary for skin assessment includes:
   a. ruler, flashlight, and gloves.
   b. gloves, slides for samples, and pen for marking lesions.
   c. magnifying glass, gloves, and alcohol swabs.
   d. gloves, diagram for documenting location of lesions, and camera.

4. Nursing interventions during a skin assessment should include providing for:
   a. frequent rest periods during the exam.
   b. modesty and privacy.
   c. signed, informed consent.
   d. videotaping of the assessment.

5. While performing a skin assessment, the nurse identifies multiple bruises in various stages of healing. The nurse knows that this finding suggests:
   a. autoimmune disorder.
   b. nutritional disorder.
   c. abuse.
   d. decreased peripheral vascular blood supply.

6. When assessing dark-skinned clients for jaundice, the nurse knows jaundice in these clients is most apparent:
   a. on the palms of the hands and soles of the feet.
   b. in the sclera of the eyes.
   c. in the mucous membranes.
   d. when skin is visualized with a flashlight.

7. While reading a client's chart regarding care given during the night, the nurse identifies documentation for edema described as "3+." The nurse knows this documentation means:
   a. the client has slight pitting with no obvious distortion.
   b. pitting occurs and remains with obvious distortion of the extremity.
   c. pitting is obvious with swollen extremities.
   d. moderate pitting is observable with no obvious distortion of the extremity.

CHAPTER 14

NURSING CARE OF CLIENTS WITH INTEGUMENTARY DISORDERS

LEARNING OUTCOMES

After completing this chapter, you will be able to:

- Apply knowledge of normal anatomy, physiology, and assessments of the integumentary system when providing nursing care for clients with disorders of the skin, hair, and nails (see Chapter 13).
- Describe the manifestations and nursing care of common skin problems and lesions.
- Compare and contrast the pathophysiology and collaborative care of clients with infections and infestations of the skin.
- Discuss the etiology, pathophysiology, and collaborative care of inflammatory disorders of the skin.
- Describe the pathophysiology and collaborative care of clients with malignant skin neoplasms.
- Explain the risk factors for, pathophysiology of, and nursing interventions to prevent and care for pressure ulcers.
- Discuss surgical options for excision of neoplasms, reconstruction of facial or body structures, and cosmetic procedures.
- Explain the pathophysiology of selected disorders of the hair and nails.
- Discuss nursing implications for pharmacologic agents used to treat disorders of the skin.
- Provide teaching appropriate for prevention and self-care of disorders of the integumentary system.
- Use the nursing process as a framework for providing individualized care to clients with disorders of the integumentary system.

KEY TOPICS

- Common skin problems and lesions
- Infections and infestations of the skin
- Inflammatory disorders of the skin

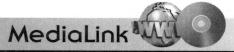

MediaLink

www.prenhall.com/lemone

Additional resources for this chapter can be found on the Student CD-ROM accompanying this textbook, and on the Companion Website at www.prenhall.com/lemone. Click on Chapter 14 to select the activities for this chapter.

CD-ROM
- Audio Glossary
- NCLEX Review

Companion Website
- More NCLEX Review
- Case Study
    Lesions and Pruritis
- Care Plan Activity
    Pressure Ulcers

- Malignant skin disorders
- Skin trauma
- Hair and nail disorders
- Nursing care of clients with integumentary disorders

LECTURE OUTLINE

I. Client with pruritis (itching sensation with urge to scratch)
   A. Cause due to stimulation of itch receptors in skin
      1. Internal or external environment
      2. Secondary to systemic disorders, such as some cancers, diabetes mellitus, hepatic disease, renal failure
      3. Heat, prostaglandins, histamine, morphine
   B. Itch-scratch-itch cycle leads to
      1. Excoriation
      2. Erythema
      3. Pigmentation changes
      4. Infections
      5. Loss of sleep
   C. Management
      1. Identify and eliminate dry skin as a precipitating cause
      2. Medications for itch control
         a. Antihistamines (oral, topical)
         b. Tranquilizers
         c. Corticosteroid (oral, topical)
   D. Often associated with dry skin (xerosis) due to
      1. Aging with less functioning of sebaceous and sweat glands
      2. Low humidity
      3. High heat environment, sunlight
      4. Excessive bathing
      5. Dehydration
   E. Nursing care focus (includes client/family teaching)
      1. Limit baths as necessary with tepid water and mild soaps
      2. Apply skin lubricants after baths
      3. Increase fluid intake, humidify air
      4. Prevent itching and scratching
II. Clients with benign skin lesions
   A. Types of lesions
      1. Cysts: closed sacs, in or under skin
      2. Keloids
         a. Elevated, irregularly shaped progressively enlarging scars
         b. Occur more often in families, with persons of African or Asian descent, with skin trauma
      3. Nevi (moles): macules or papules
         a. Arise from melanocytes
         b. Color from flesh to black

      c. Require observation for changes in size, thickness, color, bleeding, itch
      4. Angiomas (hemangiomas): benign vascular tumors
         a. Includes nevus flammeus (port-wine stain)
         b. Cherry angiomas (red to purple color)
         c. Spider angiomas (dilated superficial arteries)
         d. Telangiectases (single dilated capillaries on cheeks or nose)
         e. Venous lakes (small flat blue blood vessels)
      5. Skin tags: soft papules on a pedicle
      6. Seborrheic keratoses: overgrown, thickened cornified epithelium
   B. Collaborative care:
      1. Usually do not require treatment
      2. May be removed due to irritation or appearance change
III. Clients with psoriasis
   A. Definition
      1. Chronic skin disorder
      2. Raised, reddened, round circumscribed plaques covered with white/silver scales (purple in persons with dark skin) on scalp, arms and legs, elbows, knees, sacrum
      3. Symptoms disappear and recur
   B. Pathophysiology
      1. Epidermal cells (keratinocyte) have shorter than normal growth cycle and produce abnormal keratin forming thick flaky scales: hyperkeratosis
      2. Cause: unknown but familial history and post skin trauma are factors
   C. Manifestations
      1. Psoratic lesions
         a. Associated with pruritis
         b. Lesions where skin touches skin develop into painful fissures
         c. Nails thicken, become infected
      2. Exacerbations appear to be associated with sunlight, stress, hormone, steroid withdrawal, and some drugs
   D. Collaborative Care
      1. Diagnosis
         a. Usually by manifestations
         b. Skin biopsy, ultrasound

2. Treatment
   a. No cure available
   b. Goal: lesion and symptom control
   c. Medications
      1. Corticosteroids, topical and oral
      2. Topical retinoids
      3. Topical tar preparations
      4. Topical anthralin (dithranol)
   d. Photochemotherapy: used with severe psoriasis
      1. Methoxsalen
         a. Antimetabolite acting against hyperkeratosis
         b. Administered orally; then activated by ultraviolet-A (UVA) light in a treatment given two hours later
         c. Treatments usually are 2–3 per week for 10–20 treatments
         d. Clients need eye protection and must avoid sunlight for 8–12 hours after each treatment
         e. Treatments achieve remission but age skin, alter immune function
      2. Ultraviolet-B (UVB) light treatment
         a. Light therapy with gradual increase for exposure time to cause mild erythema and decrease hyperkeratosis
         b. Used along with tar preparations
         c. Clients need eye protection
3. Nursing Care
   a. Clients with psoriasis face self-treatment with time-consuming and "messy" topical preparations
   b. Affects appearance and ability to wear clothes they wish
4. Nursing Diagnoses
   a. Impaired Skin Integrity
      1. Teaching about topical medication application
      2. Teaching about avoiding skin infection
   b. Disturbed Body Image
      1. Clients may isolate themselves from social contacts, normal roles
      2. Clients may feel powerless

IV. Clients with Infections and Infestations
   A. Bacterial Infections
      1. Commonly caused by gram-positive Staphyloccus aureus and beta-hemolytic streptococci
      2. Specific names of infections involving skin
         a. Folliculitis: infected hair follicle
         b. Furuncle: a boil, infected hair follicle
         c. Carbuncle: group of boils
         d. Cellulitis
            1. Localized infections of dermis and subcutaneous tissue
            2. Skin develops red, swollen, painful streaks, which spread along surface of skin, sometimes vesicles
            3. Clients may feel ill with malaise
            4. Clients often treated with short term intravenous antibiotics to stop progression
         e. Erysipelas: similar to a severe cellulitis
            1. Caused by group A streptococci
            2. Client has prodromal symptoms of chills, fever, malaise before rash develops
         f. Impetigo: Infection has vesicles and pustules, which have yellow drainage often forming crusts around mouth
            1. Caused by Staphylococcus aureus or beta-hemolytic streptococci
            2. Contagious and usually found with children (not allowed in school)
      3. Collaborative Care
         a. Diagnosis
            1. Usually by sign and symptoms
            2. May have blood culture, if client is ill systemically
         b. Treatment: Antibiotics, orally and topically
         c. Nursing Care
            1. Teaching with prescribed care
            2. Proper hand washing
            3. Containing drainage
            4. Observing for worsening or expanding local to systemic infection (contact medical provider)
            5. Maintaining proper hygiene, nutrition, and fluid balance
   B. Fungal (mycoses) infections
      1. Background
         a. Plantlike organisms
         b. Spread by direct or indirect contact
         c. Need moisture
      2. Risk Factors
         a. Antibiotic therapy, which disturbs normal flora inside body
         b. Immunodeficiencies
         c. Diabetes mellitus (hyperglycemia)
         d. Pregnancy
         e. Age
      3. Types of fungal infections
         a. Superficial
            1. Dermatophytoses or ringworm

2. Named for affected area of body e.g., tinea pedis (athlete's foot); tinea capitis (scalp); tinea cruris ("jock itch")

   b. Candidiasis caused by *Candida albicans*, "yeast infection"

     1. Occurs in moist areas: outer layers of skin and mucous membranes of mouth, vagina, deep skinfolds

     2. Lesions include different appearances: pustule with burning and itching; areas white to yellow curdlike drainage, reddened areas with clearly demarcated borders (may have internally, e.g., esophagus)

4. Collaborative Care

   a. Diagnosis

     1. Usually by observation

     2. Skin scrapings, observation of skin under ultraviolet light

   b. Treatment

     1. Control contact, contagious

     2. Keep skin clean, dry

     3. Wear cotton underwear

     4. Medications: antifungal agents

       a. Topical, oral, or vaginal suppositories, e.g., Nystatin (Mycostatin)

       b. Fluconazole (Diflucan) oral antifungal agent

     5. Re-establish normal flora with live culture yogurt

C. Parasitic Infestations

  1. Pediculosis (Lice)

   a. Parasites that live on blood and lay eggs on client

   b. Types

     1. Pediculosis corporis (body lice)

     2. Pediculosis pubis (pubic lice or "crabs")

     3. Pediculosis capitis (head lice) found in school children

   c. Intense itching eggs are laid and appear on hair shafts

  2. Scabies

   a. Caused by parasitic mite, *Sarcoptes scabiei*

   b. Mites burrow in skin and lay eggs, which develop into larvae

   c. Causes intense itching and excoriation

   d. Rash appears in warm areas of body, e.g., finger webs, inner wrists, axillae, belt line

  3. Collaborative Care

   a. Diagnosis

     1. Appearance

     2. Microscopic examination of skin scrapings with scabies

   b. Treatment

     1. Examine contacts of infected clients (roommates in a facility, families of children, schoolmates) and treat all if infected

     2. Apply topical medications after nits (lice eggs) removed with fine-toothed comb or lice comb

     3. Must follow exact directions for medication, such as permethrin (NIX) or lindane (Kwell); repeated use, more than the recommendations, could result in toxicities

     4. Must wash or clean clothing, linens

     5. Take care in hospital not to contaminate self from linens

     6. Notify or observe contacts (family members, school mates, sexual partners) for infestations

D. Viral infections: caused by viruses, which depend on live cells for reproduction

  1. Warts

   a. Caused by human papillomavirus (HPV)

   b. Nongenital are benign; genital may be precancerous

   c. Types

     1. Common warts (verruca vulgaris) often on fingers

     2. Plantar warts: soles of feet

     3. Venereal warts (condylomata acuminate) cauliflowerlike in appearance

   d. Resolve spontaneously when immunity develops (5 years)

   e. Treatment for non-genital warts includes topical acid therapy, cryotherapy (freezing), electrodesiccation and curettage

  2. Herpes Simplex (fever blister, cold sore)

   a. Caused by herpes virus Type I (HSV I) (most above the waist); Type II (HSV II) often cause of genital herpes

   b. Course

     1. Begins with burning or tingling sensation

     2. Followed by development of erythema, then vesicle with pustule, ulcer, crusting and then healing in 10–14 days

     3. Initial infection has systemic signs: fever, sore throat

     4. Remains in nerve ganglia and recurs in response to sun, menstruation, stress

c. Treatment: Acyclovir (Zovirax) shortens symptoms, speeds healing
3. Herpes Zoster (shingles)
   a. Caused by *Varicella zoster*
   b. Initial infection causes chickenpox; virus remains in sensory dorsal ganglia
   c. Virus travels to dermatome section of skin supplied by ganglia
   d. Affects persons over 50; clients with Hodgkins, some leukemias, lymphomas; and immunocompromised (clients with HIV, radiation or transplant clients receiving chemotherapy)
   e. Manifestations
      1. Lesions are vesicles with reddened base
      2. On skin, follows pattern of dermatome: usually unilaterally on face, trunk, thorax
      3. New lesions erupt for 3–5 days and then crust over
      4. Recovery usually occurs in 2–3 weeks
      5. Severe pain occurs prior and during eruption and may continue after healing
   f. Complications
      1. Post-herpetic neuralgia: sharp spasmodic pain along nerves
      2. Vision loss if lesion includes ophthalmic nerve
      3. Encephalitis/death, if becomes disseminated in immunocompromised clients
   g. Collaborative care
      1. Diagnosis: usually manifestations, but can have more defined tests
      2. Treatment
         a. Anti-viral Agents
            1. Acyclovir (Zovirax) topical, oral, parenteral
            2. Administer within 1–2 days of lesion appearance for improved effectiveness, less severe symptoms and may prevent post-herpetic neuralgia
            3. Other antiviral agents available
         b. Pain relief
            1. Limit all contact to involved area
            2. Non-narcotic and narcotic medications
            3. Antihistamines for pruritis

4. Ophthalmic topical medications, if eye is involved
   c. Infection control
      1. Fluid in lesions contains virus
      2. Caregivers wear gloves
      3. Prevent contact for those immunocompromised or susceptible to chicken pox
   3. Nursing Diagnoses
      a. Acute Pain
      b. Disturbed Sleep Pattern
      c. Risk for Infection (scratching and excoriation can lead to bacterial infection)
V. Clients with Inflammatory Conditions
   A. Dermatitis
      1. Inflammation of skin with erythema, pain, and/or pruritis
      2. Lichenification: thickening and darkening of skin occurs with chronic dermatitis
      3. Types
         a. Contact: hypersensitivity response to contact chemical, plants
         b. Atopic (eczema): altered immune responses, erythema, scaling, intense pruritis
         c. Seborrheic: yellow or white plaques with scales and crusts
            1. Occurs in scalp (dandruff), eyebrows, ear canals
            2. Young (cradle cap) to very old
         d. Exfoliative: excessive peeling or shedding of skin with other dermatitis or psoriasis
      4. Collaborative Care
         a. Diagnosis usually by manifestations
         b. Medications: antihistamines, corticosteroids, topical and oral, dressings
         c. Nursing care includes teaching for self-care
   B. Acne
      1. Disorder involving the hair and sebaceous glands in which lesions called comedones appear
      2. May be open (pimples, whiteheads, blackheads), pustules (if close to surface of skin), or cysts (if in the deeper areas of the skin)
      3. Inflammation results from irritation from fatty acid (part of sebum) and products from *Propionibacterium acnes* bacteria when comedones rupture
      4. Types
         a. Acne Vulgaris: common in adolescents and young to middle adults

b. Acne Rosacea: facial acne in middle and older adults
   1. Redness over cheeks and nose with enlargement of pores
   2. Nose may develop bullous irregular thickening (rhinophyma)
c. Acne Conglobata: begins in middle age; commonly on back, buttocks, chest
5. Collaborative Care
   a. Treatment with medications
      1. Use of topical medications, which are keratolytic and loosen the comedones
      2. Topical antibiotics
      3. Oral isotretinoin (Accutane), which is tetragenic to fetus if client becomes pregnant and is controversial (associated with suicide with some clients)
   b. Treatment with dermabrasion and laser
   c. Teaching regarding skin care, diet, exposure to sunlight but not sunburn, keeping hands from face and not squeezing pimples
C. Pemphigus Vulgaris
   1. Chronic disorder of skin and oral mucous membranes with vesicle formation
   2. Auto-immune in origin and, if untreated, can be fatal
   3. Associated with IgG antibodies and acantholysis (separation of epidermal cells from one another)
   4. Manifestations
      a. Blisters that eventually ulcerate; first in mouth and scalp and then spread to body areas (face, back, chest, groin)
      b. Eventually there is denuded skin, crusting, and oozing of fluid with musty odor and pain
      c. Fluid loss from blisters can lead to fluid and electrolyte imbalance and risk for secondary bacterial infection, which can be fatal
   5. Collaborative Care
      a. Diagnosis
         1. Immunofluorescence microcopy to identify IgG antibodies in epidermis and serum
         2. Skin biopsy
      b. Treatment
         1. Medications: topical corticosteroids; systemic corticosteroids, immunosuppressive agents
         2. Antibiotic therapy for secondary infections

3. Plasmapheresis
   c. Nursing Care
      1. Includes skin assessment, monitoring for signs of infection
      2. Application of dressings to denuded areas
      3. Pain control
      4. Bathing and oral care
      5. Assistance with fluid and nutritional needs
      6. Precautions for immunocompromised clients
      7. Teaching for home care with referral
D. Lichen Planus
   1. Inflammatory condition of skin and mucous membranes with violet colored papules that are intensely pruritic; becoming hypertrophic and thickened
   2. Condition is self-limiting; lasts 12–18 months
   3. Treatment with corticosteroids and antihistamines for itching
E. Toxic Epidermal Necrolysis (TEN)
   1. Rare life-threatening disease in which epidermis peels off dermis in sheets leaving large areas of denuded skin, conjunctivitis, mucositis
   2. Mortality range 25–100%
   3. Cause can be drug reaction, result of cancer or AIDS
   4. Thought to be due to hypersensitivity or immune response
   5. Needs critical care since multiple body systems are affected
VI. Clients with Malignant Skin Disorders
   A. Background
      1. Most common of all cancers
      2. Arises from epithelial cells
   B. Actinic keratosis
      1. Premalignant; related to chronic sun exposure and photodamage
      2. May progress to squamous cell carcinoma
      3. Appearance: reddened rough macules that are shiny or scaly; skin bleeds underneath if scales removed
   C. Nonmelanoma Skin Cancer
      1. Most common malignant neoplasm in fair-skinned Americans
      2. High cure rate if detected and treated early
      3. Increased incidence with age; in males
   D. Types of Nonmelanoma Skin Cancer
      1. Basal Cell Cancer
         a. Most common, least aggressive, rarely metastasizes (except keratotis found on outer ear)

b. 4 different types, one type is pigmented
c. Starts as papules and develops into nodules
d. Tends to recur
e. If untreated, nodules enlarge and may destroy body parts, like eyelid or nose

2. Squamous cell carcinoma
   a. Occurs on areas of skin exposed to ultraviolet rays and weather; arise on skin that was burned or chronically inflamed
   b. More aggressive and more apt to metastasize than basal cell
   c. Begins as small firm red nodule; crusted with keratin, may ulcerate, bleed and become painful
   d. Recurring cancers may become invasive and metastasize
   e. Risk factors
      1. Environmental: ultraviolet light exposure, pollutants, treatments for psoriasis including UVA light, tar medications, radiation treatment for malignancies, skin that has been burned, human papillomavirus
      2. Host factors: persons with light skin (low levels of melanin), persons with premalignant lesions, persons undergoing immunosuppression therapy, such as transplant clients
   f. Collaborative Care
      1. Diagnostic Tests: various types of skin biopsies
      2. Treatments
         a. Surgical excision, Mohs micrographic surgery, curettage and electrodesiccation
         b. Radiation for inoperable cancers
      3. Nursing care
         a. Teach prevention and early detection
         b. Minimize sun exposure from 10 am–3 pm
         c. Use of sun screens, protective clothing and hats
         d. Avoid tanning booths
         e. Teach self-examination and seek medical attention for skin lesions and changes in moles, freckles

E. Malignant Melanoma
   1. Serious skin cancers, malignancies arise from melanocytes
   2. Increasing incidence; more common in fair-skinned persons, those with history of blistering sunburn as children, those who sun tan or use tanning booths
   3. May arise in skin not exposed to sun
   4. Worse prognosis for lesions on hands, feet, scalp
   5. Most melanomas develop initially in epidermis over a long period of time; once it advances through to dermis prone to metastasis
   6. Pathophysiology/Manifestations
      a. Precursor lesions
         1. Congenital nevi (moles)
         2. Dysplastic nevi, which appear during childhood
         3. Lentigo Maligna (Hutchinson's freckle) tan or black patch on skin often on face of older adult with excessive sun exposure
      b. Characterized by radial and/or vertical growth phases
         1. Radial growth phase: spreads horizontally and highly curable by surgical excision
         2. Vertical growth phase; spreads down into dermis and subcutaneous tissue leading to metastasis and fatal outcome
   7. Collaborative Care
      a. Identification: most common sites (male: trunk; women: lower extremities)
         1. Visual examination of skin surfaces with skin assessment (70% persons with malignant melanoma report change in nevi)
         2. ABCD Rule used to assess suspicious lesions
            A: Asymmetrical
            B: Border irregularity
            C: Color variation or dark black color
            D: Diameter greater than 6 mm. (pencil erasure)
      b. Diagnosis
         1. Biopsy
         2. Also test for metastasis (liver function tests, CT scan of liver, chest x-ray, bone scan, CT scan of brain)
      c. Staging: Determine level of malignant melanoma invasion and tumor thickness
      d. Treatment
         1. Surgical excision: with wide excision to include full thickness of skin and subcutaneous tissue around melanoma and involved or elective lymph node dissection
         2. Surgery may also be done for palliative management of isolated

metastasis (areas include brain, liver, lung, GI tract, subcutaneous tissue)
3. Immunotherapies including interferons, interleukins, monoclonal antibodies, BCG; still under investigation
4. Radiation especially with metastasis to brain, bone, GI tract
8. Nursing Care
a. Observe skin lesions
b. Teach clients prevention and early detection
c. Clients at risk should conduct monthly self-examination to detect any changes in lesions
9. Nursing Diagnoses
a. Impaired skin integrity and risk for infection
b. Hopelessness (response to diagnosis of cancer)
c. Anxiety (response to diagnosis of cancer; assist with coping skills)
VII. Clients with Skin Trauma
A. Pressure Ulcers (bedsores, decubitus ulcers)
1. Due to ischemia from external pressure
2. Develop frequently over bony prominences: heels, greater trochanter, sacrum, ischia
3. Also any part of body exposed to pressure, friction, or shearing forces
4. Pathophysiology
a. External pressure greater than capillary pressure for 2 hours causes tissue ischemia and hypoxia
b. Shearing forces result when one tissue layer slides over another, damaging blood vessels causing injury and thrombosis
5. Classifications of pressure sores
a. Stage I: skin intact, redness remains, no blanching
b. Stage II: Partial thickness skin loss, involving epidermis or dermis; superficial abrasion, blister, or shallow crater
c. Stage III: full thickness with damage or necrosis of subcutaneous tissue; damage not through to fascia
d. Stage IV: full thickness skin loss with extensive tissue destruction or necrosis, may involve muscle, bone, supporting structures
6. Risk Factors
a. Limited mobility as with aged, critically ill, paralyzed, large fractures, spinal cord injuries
b. Incontinence
c. Nutritional deficits
7. Collaborative Care
a. Identify clients at risk; initiate preventative measures
1. Systematic risk assessment with validated tool (e.g., Braden scale) daily
2. Documentation of any skin lesion or ulcer
a. Location
b. Stage estimation
c. Measurement of ulcer
d. Presence of any abnormal pathways
1. Sinus tract (channel under skin)
2. Tunneling (opening at skin level)
3. Undermining (tissue destruction under skin)
4. Visible necrotic tissue
5. Presence of exudates
6. Evidence of granulation tissue
b. Institute skin care and preventative interventions
1. Restore hydration to skin
2. Cleansing and protection of skin from incontinent urine or stool and wound exudate
3. Use proper positioning and correct methods of turning and transferring
4. Pressure relieving protocols (turning schedules, air mattresses, pillows, etc)
5. Assess nutritional status and restore nutritional deficits
6. Maintain client's current level of activity
7. Treatments to promote healing and restore skin integrity, including topical creams, antibiotics, wound care protocols, special dressings
c. Nursing care includes teaching client and/or family; home care referrals
B. Frostbite
1. Injury to skin from freezing; less severe if only skin and subcutaneous tissues
2. Most common sites are exposed and peripheral areas (nose, hands, feet, ears)
3. Manifestations
a. Skin appears cyanotic, reddened, or white
b. Client experiences numbness, itching, prickling; stiffness and paresthesia with deeper frostbite

c. As skin thaws, skin becomes yellow or white with loss of elasticity; burning pain
d. May go on to develop edema, blisters, necrosis, gangrene
4. Treatment
   a. Outdoors
      1. Apply firm pressure with warm hand, or place in axillae
      2. Remove wet footwear, dry feet, apply dry footwear; do not rub with snow
   b. In hospital
      1. Rewarm affected areas in circulating water; do not rub or massage areas
      2. Supportive care and treatment according to level of tissue damage; some frostbite results in amputation
C. Cutaneous Surgery and Procedures: Treatments for conditions of skin, to restore function, change appearance
1. Fusiform Excision
   a. Removal of full thickness of epidermis and dermis and thin layer of subcutaneous tissue
   b. Often for biopsies or removal of malignant skin lesions under local anesthesia
2. Electrosurgery
   a. Destruction of tissue with high-frequency alternating electrical current
   b. Removal of skin lesions, excision of tissues
3. Cryosurgery
   a. Destruction of tissue with freezing agents or cold
   b. Treat many skin lesions; post-operatively prevent infection
4. Curettage
   a. Remove lesions with curette (semisharp surgical instrument)
   b. Obtain biopsies
5. Laser Surgery
   a. Uses intense light to excise, coagulate, vaporize a lesion
   b. Sometimes local anesthesia is used
6. Chemical Destruction: Application of chemical to destroy benign or premalignant skin lesions
7. Sclerotherapy
   a. Removal of benign skin lesion with sclerosing agent
   b. Treatment for spider veins; sclerosing agents include hypertonic saline.

D. Plastic Surgery
1. Surgery which alters, replaces, or restores visible portion of the body
2. Includes correction of disfiguring conditions, restore parts of body removed as treatment or with trauma, enhance attractiveness of natural features
3. Types
   a. Skin graft
      1. Surgical method of detaching skin from donor site and placing it on recipient site
      2. Method of covering wounds which have good blood supply, would otherwise take a long time to granulate in
      3. Split-thickness graft: contains epidermis and part of dermis; thin thickness often taken from anterior thigh
      4. Full-thickness graft: contains epidermis and dermis; able to withstand trauma
   b. Flap
      1. Piece of tissue in which free end moved from donor site to a recipient site while maintaining blood supply through connection at base (pedicle)
      2. Used to cover large wound or cover area with poor circulation; used with reconstruction surgery as with repair after excision of skin cancer from face, burn injury
      3. Nursing care, includes monitoring circulation to graft area or flap post-operatively
      4. Donor sites may be covered with gauze dressings or transparent dressings
      5. Donor sites often more painful than skin graft itself
   c. Chemical peeling
      1. Application of chemical to produce controlled and predictable injury to alter skin
      2. Cosmetic surgery that removes fine wrinkles
   d. Liposuction
      1. Aspiration of fat from subcutaneous tissue layer to change the contours of body
      2. Pressure dressing applied afterward to help skin conform to new tissue size

e. Dermabrasion
1. Face is sprayed with chemical to cause light freezing
2. Abraded with sandpaper or brush to remove facial scars, severe acne, pigments
f. Facial Reconstructive Surgery
1. Surgeries done to correct deformities or improve cosmetic appearance
2. Rhinoplasty: improve appearance of nose; usually also submucous resection of nasal septum (SMR) to improve nasal airway
3. Blepharoplasty: cosmetic surgery to remove skin from drooping eyelids
4. Rhytidectomy: facelift to remove facial wrinkles and tighten facial tissues
4. Nursing Care
a. Some procedures are done as outpatient; others, like skin grafts and flaps, are in-patient
b. Promotion of healing and prevention of infection is key to good response to surgery
5. Common Nursing Diagnoses
a. Impaired Skin Integrity
b. Risk for Infection
c. Acute Pain
d. Altered Body Image
VIII. Clients with Disorders of Hair
A. Hirsutism (hypertrichosis)
1. Excessive hair in normal/abnormal areas in women

2. May be due to increase in androgen levels in women
3. Diagnostic tests to determine if systemic condition: serum testosterone level, CT scan of adrenal glands
4. Treatment: according to underlying cause
B. Alopecia: loss of hair, baldness
1. Common types
a. Male pattern baldness: genetically predetermined
b. Female pattern alopecia: starting in 20–30's, progressive thinning
2. Treatment
a. Male pattern baldness treated with topical minoxidil (Rogaine)
b. Surgical treatment: movement of tissue containing hair to restore hair or limit areas of alopecia
IX. Clients with Disorder of Nails
A. May be due to systemic disease, trauma, irritants or allergies
B. Types
1. Onycholoysis: separation of distal nail plate from nail bed
2. Paronychia: infection on cuticle of finger or toenails
3. Onychomcosis: fungal infection of nail plate
4. Unguis incarnatus: ingrown toenail
C. Treatment of nail problems: Surgical removal or pharmacologic treatment

FOCUSED STUDY TIPS

- Locate a common skin lesion on a family member or friend. Identify the type of lesion. Describe treatment for the lesion.
- Care for a client with a pressure ulcer. Research how the ulcer developed. Develop a teaching plan for the client or the caregiver to prevent the development of other pressure ulcers.
- Review a medical text of skin disorders. Look at the pictures and read captions. Identify pictures of disorders that have been reviewed in this chapter.

CASE STUDY

Mrs. Smith is admitted to the critical care unit with bacterial pneumonia. She was diagnosed 10 years ago with multiple sclerosis. She has utilized a wheelchair for the past year. On initial assessment, the nurse finds a Stage III decubitus to her coccyx. Mrs. Smith is unaware of this pressure ulcer. What do you tell Mrs. Smith about her pressure ulcer? What are the factors contributing to the development of this decubitus? When developing a plan of care for Mrs. Smith, what do you include in your teaching plan to prevent this ulcer from progressing to Stage IV? How does her current illness affect the health of her pressure ulcer? How can Mrs. Smith manage the care of her pressure ulcer when she is discharged from the hospital?

CARE PLAN CRITICAL THINKING ACTIVITY

You are caring for a client with severe pruritus due to jaundice secondary to cirrhosis of the liver. What nursing interventions can be utilized to relieve the client's discomfort?

NCLEX TEST QUESTIONS

1. During physical assessment, the nurse identifies a sacral decubitus that appears blistered and cracked. The lesion is correctly identified as a decubitus in which stage?
   a. Stage III
   b. Stage II
   c. Stage I
   d. Stage IV

2. To promote healing of a decubitus ulcer, the proper nursing intervention would involve:
   a. maintaining proper body alignment with the bed in the low position.
   b. placing the client in a wheelchair for 4 hours every shift.
   c. preventing friction when moving the client and decreasing fluid intake to prevent incontinence.
   d. frequent position changes and gentle massaging of the affected area.

3. If the client experiencing psoriasis complains about pruritus, the nurse should suggest using:
   a. drying soaps or astringents.
   b. hot water when bathing.
   c. emollient lubricants.
   d. vigorous drying with cotton towels after bathing.

4. Herpes zoster, or shingles, manifests as a cluster of small vesicles usually occurring on the back, face, or scalp. One major problem with this condition is:
   a. pain.
   b. reverse isolation is necessary.
   c. it is not curable.
   d. requires months of antibiotic therapy.

5. Immunotherapy is a relatively new treatment for:
   a. nonmelanoma skin cancer.
   b. squamous cell carcinoma.
   c. malignant melanoma.
   d. pemphigus vulgaris.

6. For the client at risk for pressure ulcers, the goal of care is:
   a. collaborative treatment to promote healing.
   b. restoration of skin integrity.
   c. prevention.
   d. increased mobility.

7. Any client with impaired skin integrity is at risk for:
   a. pressure ulcers.
   b. secondary bacterial infections.
   c. immunosuppression.
   d. excoriation.

CHAPTER 15

NURSING CARE OF CLIENTS WITH BURNS

LEARNING OUTCOMES

After completing this chapter, you will be able to:

- Apply knowledge of normal integumentary anatomy, physiology, and assessments when providing nursing care for clients with burns (see Chapter 13).
- Discuss types and causative agents of burns.
- Explain burn classification by depth and extent of injury.
- Describe the stages of burn wound healing.
- Explain the pathophysiology, collaborative care, and nursing care for the client with a minor burn.
- Discuss the systemic pathophysiologic effects of a major burn.
- Identify the collaborative care necessary during the emergent/resuscitative stage, the acute stage, and the rehabilitative stage of a major burn.
- Discuss the nursing implications of medications administered to the client with a major burn.
- Discuss the nursing implications for burn wound management.
- Use the nursing process as a framework for providing individualized care to clients with a burn.

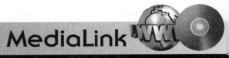

MediaLink

www.prenhall.com/lemone

Additional resources for this chapter can be found on the Student CD-ROM accompanying this textbook, and on the Companion Website at www.prenhall.com/lemone. Click on Chapter 15 to select the activities for this chapter.

CD-ROM
- Audio Glossary
- NCLEX Review

Companion Website
- More NCLEX Review
- Case Study
    Full-Thickness Burns
- Care Plan Activity
    Inhalation Injury
- MediaLink Applications
    Teaching Plan: Fire Prevention

KEY TOPICS

- Types and classifications of burn injuries
- Stages of burn wound healing
- Medical management of burns
- Nursing care of clients experiencing burn injury

LECTURE OUTLINE

I. Background
  A. Definition
    1. A burn is an injury resulting from heat, chemicals, radiation, electrical current
    2. The transfer of energy from source of heat causes physiologic changes and damage to tissues
    3. Systemic infection is the leading cause of death in major burn clients
  B. Factors associated with burns
    1. Age (children and older adults)
    2. Careless smoking
    3. Alcohol or drug intoxication
    4. Physical and/or mental disabilities
    5. Certain occupations
  C. Types of burns
    1. Thermal
      a. Results from exposure to dry heat, as with flame; or moist heat, as with steam or hot fluids
      b. Most common type of burn injuries
    2. Chemical
      a. Direct skin contact with acid or alkaline agents and agent destroys tissue protein
      b. Alkali burns are deeper and more severe than acid burns
      c. Organic compound burns, as from petroleum distillates, cause cutaneous damage through fat solvent action; also cause liver and kidney damage
    3. Electrical
      a. Severity dependent on type and duration of current, and amount of voltage
      b. Destructive process from electrical burn is concealed, persists for weeks post
      c. Electricity follows path of least resistance: along muscles, bones, blood vessels, nerves
      d. Blood coagulation at site of injury leads to impaired blood flow and necrosis of tissue
      e. Alternating current from manufactured electricity burns results in sustained muscles contractions and respiratory arrest
      f. Direct current, as with a lightning strike, is high voltage for an instant; have entry and exit wounds and flash over the skin, which can mean less internal damage

    4. Radiation
      a. Often from sunburn or radiation treatments as with treatment for cancer
      b. Functions of skin are left intact
  D. Classification of burns: Determined by Tissue Damage
    1. Depth of burn (layers of underlying tissues affected)
      a. Superficial: First degree
        1. Involvement: only epidermal layer
        2. Causes: sunburn, ultraviolet light, minor flash injuries, mild radiation burns
        3. Appearance of burn
          a. Skin color pink to bright red, slight edema
          b. Mildly painful
        4. Usual treatment: mild analgesia, application water-soluble lotions
      b. Partial-thickness burns: Second degree
        1. Involvement: superficial partial-thickness burn or deep partial-thickness burn depending on the depth of burn through the layers of the dermis
        2. Causes
          a. Superficial: Brief exposure to flash flame, dilute chemical agents, hot surface
          b. Deep: Hot liquids, solids; flash or direct flame, radiant energy, chemical agents
        3. Appearance of burn
          a. Blisters
            1. Superficial: bright red, moist glistening appearance
            2. Deep: pale and waxy, moist or dry
          b. Severe pain in response to air or heat
        4. Usual treatment: analgesia, skin substitutes, grafting may be necessary
      c. Full-thickness burns: Third degree
        1. Involvement: all layers of skin, may extend into subcutaneous fat, connective tissue, muscle, bone
        2. Causes: prolonged contact with flames, steam, chemicals, high-voltage electrical current
        3. Appearance of burn
          a. Pale, waxy, yellow, brown, mottled, charred, or nonblanching red

b. No sensation of pain or light touch since receptors were destroyed

4. Usual treatment: requires skin grafting

2. Methods of determining extent of burn (percentage of body surface)

a. Rule of 9's: involvement of parts of body

b. Lund and Browder: surface area for body parts according to client age

c. American Burn Assn: extent and depth of burn (minor, moderate, major)

E. Process of healing with burn occurs more slowly than with other types of injuries

1. Physiologic events

a. Hemostasis: platelets aggregate, thrombus formation, wound walled off

b. Inflammation: local vasodilatation; increased capillary permeability

c. Proliferation: Granulation tissue begins to form (epithelialization) (peak 14 days post burn)

d. Remodeling: Collagen fibers reorganized, scars contract

2. Two types of excessive scarring, if burn injury extended into dermal layer

a. Hypertrophic scar: overgrowth of dermal tissue but remains within boundaries of wound

b. Keloid: scar extends beyond boundaries of wound

II. Prehospital Client Management: First Aid at scene

A. Stop the burning process to limit severity

1. Thermal burns

a. "Stop, drop, and roll" to control fire

b. Remove clothing and lavage area with cool water, no ice

c. Cover to prevent hypothermia

2. Chemical burns

a. Remove clothes and shower or lavage with water

b. Contact poison control center if necessary

3. Electrical burns: disconnect electrical current to protect rescuers

4. Radiation burns: shield, distance, and limit time exposure to radioactive source

B. Support vital functions

1. CPR, if indicated

2. Note any other injuries

3. Initiate fluid replacement

4. Cover client

III. Care of Clients with Burns

A. Minor burns

1. Not extensive, superficial split-thickness < 15%, full thickness < 2%

2. Not associated with immunosuppression, hypermetabolism, increased susceptibility to infection

3. Pathophysiology

a. Skin remains intact

b. Includes sunburns, minor scald burns

4. Collaborative Care: Treatment

a. Wash with mild soap and water

b. Tetanus toxoid, if needed

c. Prescribed wound care topical agents, dressings

d. Controlling pain: analgesics

e. Range of motion to affected joints

f. Teaching about home care

g. Follow up appointments

B. Major burns

1. Serious injury to underlying layers or skin and cover large body surface area

2. Criteria include

a. > 25% total body surface area if client < 40

b. > 20% total body surface area if client > 40

c. > 10% total body surface area full thickness burn

d. Injuries involving face, eyes, ears, feet, hands, perineum

e. High-voltage electrical burns

f. All burns involving inhalation injury or major trauma

3. Pathophysiology: involves all body systems

a. Integumentary

1. Bull's eye appearance: most severe burn located centrally, lesser burns at peripheral edge of wound (like 3 concentric circles)

a. Outer zone of hyperemia: blanches, heals 2–7 days

b. Middle zone of stasis: moist, red blisters, blanches on pressure; pale and necrotic 3–7 days post burn

c. Inner zone of coagulation: leathery, coagulated and merges with middle zone days 3–7 days

2. Eschar: hard crust that forms over necrotic skin and tissue

b. Cardiovascular

1. Hypovolemic Shock (Burn Shock)

a. Fluid shift from intracellular and intravascular to interstitial area

b. Occurs due to increased cell permeability, intracellular edema, and osmosis

c. Initially, hypotension, vasoconcentration reflected in CBC

d. Usually lasts 24 hours, followed by fluid shift back and diuresis

2. Cardiac rhythm alterations: burns > 40% total body surface area cause myocardial dysfunction, cardiac dysrhythmias

3. Peripheral vascular compromise: blood vessel damage, compartment syndrome

c. Respiratory: direct inhalation injury or systemic response to injury

1. Inflammation: cilia stop functioning causing bronchial congestion and infection

2. Interstitial Pulmonary Edema: fluid from pulmonary vasculature, sloughed burned lung tissue

3. Upper airway thermal injury: soot, charring, blisters, edema in oropharynx

4. Smoke poisoning: irritant gases, particulate matter, direct cytotoxic effect

5. Carbon monoxide: impairs oxygen delivery and cellular use

d. Gastrointestinal: dysfunction related to size of burn wound

1. Paralytic ileus (gastric distention, absent bowel sounds)

2. Stress (Curling's) ulcers: acute ulceration of stomach or duodenum (hematemesis)

3. Ischemic bowel leads to bacterial translocation and sepsis and multiple organ dysfunction

e. Urinary

1. Early stages: decreased renal blood flow and glomerular filtration rate

2. Myoglobinuria: dark brown concentrated urine due to damaged erythroctyes from burn injury

3. May result in renal failure

f. Immune System

1. Cell-mediated and humoral immune system impaired

2. High risk for infection

g. Metabolism

1. Two phases of metabolic response to burn injury

a. Ebb stage (first 3 days) decreased oxygen consumption

b. Flow stage after burn resuscitation accomplished

2. Hypermetabolism: basal metabolic rate significantly increased

3. Protein catabolism, lipolysis, gluconeogenesis

4. Collaborative Care/Burn Team: Three Stages of Treatment

a. Emergent/resuscitative stage

1. Scope: Onset of injury through successful fluid resuscitation

2. Includes

a. Estimate of depth and extent of burn injury

b. First aid measures

1. Limit severity of burns

2. Ventilation maintenance including intubation for all clients with burns of chest, face, or neck

c. Fluid resuscitation

1. Restore circulating blood volume; counteract burn shock, replace fluid and electrolyte losses

2. 2 large bore IV's for venous access

3. Fluid of choice: Crystalloids, i.e., warmed Lactated Ringers Parkland formula or Modified Brooke formula which individualize amounts and rates (most in first 8 hours post burn)

4. Enough fluid to maintain urinary output 30–50 ml per hour and pulse rate < 120 (adult)

3. Emergency department staff obtains history of burn injury

a. Time of injury

b. Causative agents

c. Early treatment of burn

d. Client's past medical history

e. Client age and body weight

4. May include transfer to burn center if client has significant burn

b. Acute stage

1. Scope: Starts at beginning of diuresis and ends with closure of burn wound

2. Includes
   a. Wound care management: hydrotherapy, excision, grafting
   b. Nutritional therapies: Enteral and parenteral nutritional interventions
   c. Measures to control infections: Topical and systemic antimicrobials
   d. Pain management, physical therapy
   e. Observation for complications
3. Specific treatment of burn may include surgeries as indicated by client healing
   a. Escharotomy
      1. Circumferentially eschar acts as a tourniquet
      2. Incision made into eschar to restore circulation
   b. Surgical debridement to achieve
      1. Excision of wound to level of fascia
      2. Removal of thin slices of burn wound to level of viable tissue
   c. Autografting: Skin removed from healthy tissue and applied to burn wound
4. Dressings
   a. Biologic and biosynthetic dressings used to promote healing and prepare wound for skin grafting in future
   b. Includes
      1. Allograft (human skin)
      2. Heterograft/xenograft from animal (usually pig), amniotic membranes, synthetic materials
   c. Rehabilitative stage
      1. Scope: Starts with wound closure and ends when client reaches high level of health restoration; may take years
      2. Biopsychosocial adjustment by client
         a. Prevention of contractures and scars
         b. Client returns to work, family, and social roles
         c. May include vocational, occupational, physical and psychosocial rehabilitation

IV. Nursing Care for Clients with Burns
   A. Monitoring of vital signs/changes in stability
      1. Critical care nursing
      2. Cardiac and hemodynamic monitoring
      3. Pulse oximetry
   B. Diagnostic Tests
      1. Urinalysis: adequacy renal perfusion, myoglobinuria
      2. Regular monitoring of CBC, electrolytes, serial Arterial Blood Gases (ABG's)
      3. Creatine phosphokinase (CPK) for muscle damage with electrical burns
      4. Renal function tests (BUN, Creatinine) closely monitored
      5. Blood glucose, elevated transiently post burn and with parenteral nutrition
      6. Nutritional assessment (most reliable in rehabilitative stage): Total protein, albumin, transferrin, prealbumin
      7. Monitor cardiovascular/respiratory status as needed: chest x-rays, electrocardiograms
   C. Medications
      1. Pain control
         a. Intravenous morphine is drug of choice in early stages of care
         b. Pain medications are often administered prior to hydrotherapy and physical therapy
         c. Alternative therapies added to plan of care for pain control
      2. Antimicrobial agents
         a. Topical antimicrobial therapy used to eliminate infection of surface of burn wound
         b. Most widely used topical agents
            1. Mafenide acetate (Sulfamylon) cream
            2. Sulfadiazine (Silvadene) cream
            3. Silver nitrate 0.5% soaks
         c. Systemic antibiotics preoperatively and postoperatively with excisions and autograftings
      3. Tetanus prophylaxis: During acute phase to prevent Clostridium tetani infection
      4. Control gastric hyperacidity
         a. Goal to maintain gastric pH above 5.0
         b. Clients have nasogastric tube in place in emergent phase of care
         c. Intravenous Histamine H_2 blockers, e.g., famotidine (Pepsid), ranitidine (Zantac)
      5. Respiratory management: Bronchodilators and mucolytic agents
   D. Wound Management
      1. Goals
         a. Remove nonviable tissues

b. Control microbial colonization

c. Promote tissue granulation

d. Achieve wound coverage as soon as possible

2. Debridement of wounds

a. Process of removing loose tissue, wound debris, eschar from wounds

b. Types of debridement

1. Mechanical: wet to dry or wet to moist dressings; hydrotherapy and/or irrigation; scissors and tweezers

2. Enzymatic: use of topical enzyme agents to dissolve and remove necrotic tissue, i.e., collagenase (Santyl), fibrinolysis-deoxyribonuclease (Elase)

3. Surgical (in operating room)

c. Dressing of wounds

1. Open: burn wound open to air with topical agent applied

2. Closed

a. Topical agent applied

b. Burn wound covered with gauze or nonadherent dressing

c. Wrapped with roller gauze bandages

d. Distal to proximal circumferentially, wrap fingers and toes separately

E. Prevention of contractures and scarring/maintain function

1. Physical therapy with correct positioning

a. Use of splints to maintain in flexion except when exercising

b. Early ambulation

c. Range of motion (ROM), passive or active every two hours

2. Support garments

a. Uniform pressure reduces hypertrophic scarring

b. Tubular support bandages

c. Later, custom-made elastic pressure garments

F. Nutritional Support

1. Resting energy need increases as much as 100% of normal

2. 4000–6000 kcal per day; reverse negative nitrogen balance; adequate protein to build new tissues

3. Enteral feedings, plus oral feedings if feasible

4. Total Parenteral Nutrition (TPN) via central venous catheter in case of Curling's ulcer, septic ileus, bowel obstruction, pancreatitis

G. Psychosocial Support

1. Psychiatric consultation, social worker consultation

2. Support group for burn clients and families

3. Client's religious support and/or hospital chaplain

H. Nursing Diagnoses

1. Altered skin integrity

2. Altered fluid volume (deficit, then excess)

3. Acute pain

4. Risk for infection

5. Impaired physical mobility

6. Imbalanced nutrition, less than body requirements

7. Powerlessness

I. Health Promotion

1. Primary goals

a. Prevention

b. Reduction in incidence of burns

2. Strategies

a. Smoke alarms, sprinkler systems

b. No smoking in bed

c. Care and observation with candle use

d. Teaching regarding control of fire, first aid for burns

FOCUSED STUDY TIPS

- Visit a local pharmacy. What OTC (over-the-counter) pharmaceuticals are available for treatment of minor burns?
- Develop a first-aid treatment plan for burns occurring in the home. Familiarize family members with the plan. Assess their level of understanding of burn treatment and potential complications. Identify and clarify any knowledge deficits.
- Care for a client in the clinical setting experiencing burn injury. Identify burn management for this client. Discuss short-term and long-term goals for the client with your instructor.

CASE STUDY

Ms. Hanson was severely burned around her head, neck, chest, and arms. She has three small children at home. Her care is anticipated to be intense while in the hospital, and a lengthy rehabilitation is anticipated. While hospitalized, what major complications does the nurse anticipate with her burn injury? What diagnostic tests might be helpful in determining Mrs. Hanson's health status? When developing a plan of care for Mrs. Hanson, what are her priority nursing diagnoses? What priority nursing interventions will be implemented? Describe how her priority nursing diagnoses will change as she approaches discharge. What will her focus of care become? How will her plan of care differ from her initial admission plan of care? What major issues will she be facing?

CARE PLAN CRITICAL THINKING ACTIVITY

Develop a care plan for a 65 kg burn victim undergoing fluid resuscitation. What nursing diagnoses are utilized? What are the goals for fluid resuscitation for this client? What nursing interventions will be implemented? How are evaluations made?

NCLEX TEST QUESTIONS

1. Which of the following types of burns will not require skin grafting?
   a. small, partial thickness
   b. large, partial thickness
   c. small, full thickness
   d. large, full thickness

2. The preferred diet for severely burned clients is:
   a. high fat, low carbohydrate.
   b. low fat, high carbohydrate.
   c. high protein, high calorie.
   d. low protein, high calorie.

3. Anti-deformity positioning prevents scar contracture across joints by placing them in:
   a. flexion.
   b. extension.
   c. hyperextension.
   d. abduction.

4. A method of permanent burn wound closure is:
   a. xenograft.
   b. allograft.
   c. autograft.
   d. homograft.

5. Clients who are critically burned are at high risk for which complication during the resuscitative phase?
   a. neurogenic shock
   b. cardiogenic shock
   c. burn shock
   d. myocardial infarction

6. Fluid resuscitation is necessary in all burn wounds that involve _____ percent total body surface area burned. Total Body Surface Area (TBSA)
   a. 10
   b. 20
   c. 25
   d. 15

7. Inhalation injury is a frequent burn complication resulting in upper-airway edema during which time period?
   a. 1 to 2 hours
   b. 8 to 12 hours
   c. 24 to 48 hours
   d. 12 to 24 hours

CHAPTER 16

ASSESSING CLIENTS WITH ENDOCRINE DISORDERS

LEARNING OUTCOMES

After completing this chapter, you will be able to:

- Review the anatomy and physiology of the endocrine glands.
- Explain the functions of the hormones secreted by the endocrine glands.
- Identify specific topics to consider during a health history interview of the client with health problems involving endocrine function.
- Describe techniques for physical assessment of endocrine structure and function.
- Identify abnormal findings that may indicate malfunction of the endocrine system.

KEY TOPICS

- Review of anatomy and physiology of the endocrine system
- Overview of hormones
- Assessing endocrine function

LECTURE OUTLINE

I. Background: Organs of Endocrine System
   A. Pituitary gland (hypophysis, master gland)
      1. Anterior portion: adenohypophysis
         Hormones produced:
         a. Growth Hormone (GH), somatotrophin:
            Function: stimulates growth of body (epiphyseal plates of long bones)
         b. Prolactin (PRL)
            Function: stimulates production of breast milk

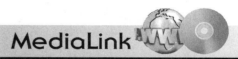

   c. Thyroid-stimulating hormone (TSH)
      Function: stimulates synthesis and release of thyroid hormones by thyroid
   d. Adrenocorticotropic hormone (ACTH)
      Function: stimulates production of hormones from adrenal cortex especially glucocorticoids

97

e. Gonadotropin hormone
Function: stimulates gonads
f. Follicle-stimulating hormone (FSH)
Function: stimulates gonads
FSH: female, development of ovarian follicles, estrogenic sex hormones; male, development and maturation of sperm
g. Luteinizing hormone (LH)
Function: stimulates gonads
LH: female, ovulation and formation of corpus luteum; male, called Interstial cell-stimulating hormone (ICSH), stimulates testes to produce male sex hormones
2. Posterior portion: neurohypophysis
Releases hormones produced by hypothalamus:
a. Antidiuretic hormone (ADH), vasopressin: inhibits urine production by causing reabsorption of water by renal tubules
b. Oxytocin: induces contraction of smooth muscle during labor; ejection of milk from breasts
B. Thyroid gland
Produces Thyroid hormone (TH) composed of:
1. Thyroxine (T4)
2. Triiodothyronine (T3)
Function: increase metabolism, growth and development in children
3. Calcitonin
Function: decreases excessive calcium by slowing calcium release by bone cells
C. Parathyroid gland: produces parathyroid hormone (PTH), parathormone
Function: phosphate metabolism (increases renal excretion of phosphate, decreases excretion of calcium, releases calcium from bone)
D. Adrenal Gland
2 parts:
1. Adrenal Medulla
Hormones: catecholamines
a. Epinephrine
Functions:
1. Increases blood glucose, stimulating ACTH, glucocorticoids
2. Increases rate and force of cardiac contractions
3. Constricts blood vessels in skin, mucous membranes, kidneys
4. Dilates blood vessels in skeletal muscles, coronary and pulmonary arteries

b. Norepinephrine
1. Increases heart rate and force of contractions
2. Constricts blood vessels throughout body
2. Adrenal Cortex
Hormones: corticoids
a. Mineralocorticoids
Aldosterone: retains sodium and water to increase blood volume and pressure
b. Glucocorticoids: cortisol, cortisone
Functions:
1. Carbohydrate metabolism by regulating glucose use in body tissue, mobilizing fat, shifting energy source for muscle cells from glucose to fat
2. Responds to stress
3. Depresses inflammatory response, inhibits immune system
E. Pancreas (endocrine portion)
1. Glucagon (alpha cells) increases blood glucose
2. Insulin (beta cells) decreases blood glucose
3. Somatostatin (delta cells) inhibits secretion of glucagons and insulin
F. Gonads
1. Androgens: (mainly testosterone) male sex hormones
2. Estrogen and progesterone: female sex hormones (there are several types of estrogens)
II. Physiology of Endocrine System
A. Hormones are chemical messengers that exert action on target organs by binding to specific receptor sites on target organs
B. Hormones cause effect by regulating tissue responses
C. Hormone levels are controlled by pituitary gland, feedback mechanisms
D. Negative feedback: sensors detect changes in hormone level and respond, e.g., if level decreases, action made to increase level; when level rises, action made to decrease level
E. Positive feedback: increased level on one hormone causes another gland to release a hormone
III. Assessment of Endocrine Function
Signs and symptoms of dysfunction, often nonspecific
A. Health assessment interview
1. Client medical history
2. Family history

3. Changes in size or functioning of organs, skin, hair
4. Changes in thirst, appetite, weight, energy, sleep
5. Use of medications that may affect hormones
6. Changes in reproductive functioning, secondary sex characteristics

B. Physical Assessment
1. Palpation of thyroid: technique
2. Inspection of skin, hair, nails, facial appearance
3. Reflexes, musculoskeletal system
4. Height, weight, vital signs
5. Assessment for hypocalcemia

C. Abnormal findings
1. Skin assessment
   a. Pigmentation: "hyper" or "hypo" with adrenocortical dysfunction
   b. Rough, dry skin, yellow cast with hypothyroidism
   c. Smooth, flushed skin with hyperthyroidism
   d. Purple striae (stretch marks)
   e. Skin lesions on extremities: diabetes mellitus
2. Hair and nails
   a. Pigmentation with hypoadrenocorticofunction
   b. Dry, thick, brittle nails and hair with hypothyroidism

c. Thin, brittle nails, thin soft hair with hyperthyroidism
d. Excessive hair growth with hyperadrenocortical function

3. Facial Assessment
   a. Abnormal growth, symmetry with excess growth hormone
   b. Exophthalmos (protruding eyes) with hyperthyroidism
4. Thyroid assessment
   a. Enlargment of thyroid gland or goiter
   b. One or multiple palpable nodules
5. Motor function assessment
   a. Increased deep tendon reflexes with hyperthyroidism
   b. Decreased deep tendon reflexes with hypothyroidism
6. Sensory function assessment
   Peripheral neuropathy or paresthesias with diabetes, hypothyroidism, excess growth hormone
7. Musculoskeletal assessment
   Size and proportion, insufficient or excess growth hormone
8. Hypocalcemic tetany (possible thyroid, parathyroid abnormalities)
   a. Trousseau's sign (carpal spasm with inflation of blood pressure cuff)
   b. Chvostek's sign (tap front of client's ear in angle of jaw to elicit facial muscle contraction)

FOCUSED STUDY TIPS

- Practice a health assessment interview assessing endocrine functioning with a classmate. Take notes and determine normal and abnormal assessment findings.
- Identify three laboratory tests utilized in the clinical setting to diagnose endocrine disorders.

CASE STUDY

When caring for a client with an endocrine dysfunction, the physician suspects hypocalcemic tetany. To determine its presence, the physician asks you to check two signs of the disorder. What are the signs' names? What is the assessment technique for each sign? What would be a positive finding for each sign? Practice identifying each sign on a classmate, friend, or family member. What laboratory test would collaborate your findings if the disorder were present and both signs were positive?

CARE PLAN CRITICAL THINKING ACTIVITY

Assessing the endocrine system is difficult because hormones affect all body tissues and organs. Manifestations of dysfunction are often nonspecific. When doing a physical assessment of the endocrine system, describe five different areas to assess and describe one abnormal finding for each area. What possible medical diagnosis may exist for each of your abnormal findings?

NCLEX TEST QUESTIONS

1. An excess of glucocorticoids in the body:
   a. depresses the inflammatory response and inhibits effectiveness of the immune system.
   b. stimulates the release of aldosterone from the adrenal cortex.
   c. increases stress.
   d. stimulates the secretion of somatotropin.

2. When planning care for a client with hyperthyroidism, the nurse knows hyperthyroidism exists when:
   a. amount of circulating thyroid hormone is unchanged.
   b. the client is lethargic and symptomatic.
   c. thyroxin blood level is high.
   d. thyroxin blood level is low.

3. Another name for ADH (antidiuretic hormone) is:
   a. vasopressor.
   b. calcitonin.
   c. somatostatin.
   d. vasopressin.

4. Trousseau's sign and Chvostek's sign are assessment techniques utilized to assess the client for the presence of:
   a. hypercalcemic tetany.
   b. thyroid toxicity.
   c. hypoparathyroidism.
   d. hypocalcemic tetany.

5. The adrenal glands are located:
   a. behind the stomach and between the spleen and duodenum.
   b. on top of the kidneys.
   c. on the ovaries in women and the testicles in men.
   d. at the base of the skull near the top of the cervical spine.

6. The hormones responsible for growth and development in children are:
   a. parathyroid hormone (PTH).
   b. cortisol and cortisone.
   c. thyroid hormones.
   d. estrogens and androgens.

7. Which gland is responsible for the secretion of all corticosteroids?
   a. pancreas
   b. adrenal cortex
   c. adrenal medulla
   d. pituitary

CHAPTER 17

NURSING CARE OF CLIENTS WITH ENDOCRINE DISORDERS

LEARNING OUTCOMES

After completing this chapter, you will be able to:

- Apply knowledge of normal anatomy, physiology, and assessments of the thyroid, parathyroid, adrenal, and pituitary glands when providing nursing for clients with endocrine disorders (see Chapter 16).
- Identify diagnostic tests used to diagnose disorders of the thyroid, parathyroid, adrenal, and pituitary glands.
- Compare and contrast the manifestations of disorders that result from hyperfunction and hypofunction of the thyroid, parathyroid, adrenal, and pituitary glands.
- Explain the nursing implications for medications prescribed to treat disorders of the thyroid and adrenal glands.
- Provide appropriate nursing care for the client before and after a subtotal thyroidectomy and an adrenalectomy.
- Use the nursing process as a framework for providing individualized care to clients with disorders of the thyroid, parathyroid, adrenal, and pituitary glands.

KEY TOPICS

- Disorders of the thyroid gland
- Disorders of the parathyroid glands
- Disorders of the pituitary gland
- Nursing care of clients with endocrine dysfunction

LECTURE OUTLINE

I. Multiple problems when caring for clients with endocrine disorders
  A. Multiple diagnostic tests that can be exhausting

B. Changing physical appearance and emotional responses
C. Permanent lifestyle changes

101

II. Disorders of the Thyroid Gland
  A. Systems affected
    1. Metabolism
    2. Cardiovascular
    3. Gastrointestinal
    4. Neuromuscular
  B. Clients with Hyperthyroidism (Thyrotoxicosis)
    1. Definition: excessive delivery of thyroid hormone to peripheral tissues
    2. Pathophysiology
      a. Autoimmune reactions (Grave's disease)
      b. Excess secretion of TSH from pituitary gland
      c. Neoplasms (toxic multinodular goiter)
      d. Thyroiditis
      e. Excessive intake of thyroid medications
    3. Signs and symptoms
      a. Metabolism
        1. Hypermetabolism
        2. Increased appetite with weight loss
        3. Heat intolerance, increased sweating
      b. Cardiovascular
        1. Systolic hypertension
        2. Tachycardia, atrial fibrillation
        3. Dysrhythmias, palpitations
        4. Possibly angina, congestive heart failure
      c. Gastrointestinal
        1. Increased peristalsis with diarrhea
        2. Hyperactive bowel sounds
      d. Neuromuscular
        1. Nervousness, restlessness
        2. Insomnia
        3. Fine tremor
        4. Emotional lability (mood swings)
      e. Other
        1. Fine hair
        2. Smooth and warm skin
    4. Specific conditions
      a. Graves' disease
        1. Most common cause of hyperthyroidism
        2. Antibody against TSH receptor site
        3. Cause unknown, but hereditary link
        4. More common in females aged 20–40
        5. Signs and symptoms
          a. Signs of hyperthyroidism plus
          b. Enlarged thyroid gland (goiter)
          c. Proptosis (forward displacement of eyes) causing blurred vision, diplopia, lacrimation, photophobia
          d. Exophthalmos (forward protrusion of eyes) causing corneal dryness, irritation, ulceration
          e. Changes in menstruation
      b. Toxic Multinodular Goiter
        1. Nodules in thyroid tissue secrete excessive thyroid hormone
        2. Usually female in 60–70's, has had goiter for a number of years
      c. Thyroiditis
        1. Viral infection of thyroid
        2. May become chronic and lead to hypothyroidism
      d. Thyroid crisis (Thyroid Storm)
        1. Extreme state of hyperthyroidism; rare now
        2. Occurs with untreated hyperthyroidism or hyperthyroid person with stressor like infection, trauma; manipulation of thyroid during surgery
        3. Life-threatening condition with excess metabolic symptoms such as temperature elevation to 102–106, hypertension, tachycardia, and agitation advancing to seizures, psychosis, delirium
        4. Treatment includes reducing thyroid secretion, stabilizing cardiovascular system, and managing respiratory distress
    5. Diagnostic tests
      a. Serum thyroid antibodies (TA): antibodies in Graves' disease
      b. TSH test: (from pituitary) suppressed with primary hyperthyroidism
      c. T3 and T4: elevated for diagnosis of hyperthyroidism, thyroiditis
      d. T3 uptake test; elevated with hyperthyroidism
      e. RAI uptake test
        1. Oral or intravenous dose of radioactive iodine (131I) given to client
        2. Thyroid scan after 24 hours
        3. Size and shape of gland revealed
        4. Uptake is increased with Grave's disease
      f. Thyroid suppression test
        1. RAI and T4 measured and then remeasured after client takes thyroid hormone
        2. No suppression with hyperthyroid

6. Treatment of hyperthyroidism
    a. Medications
        1. Antithyroid medications: block synthesis of thyroid hormones
            a. Propylthiouracil (PTU)
            b. Methimazole (Tapazole)
        2. Beta-adrenergic blockers: control symptoms (tachycardia, tremor, etc.)
            a. Propanolol (Inderal)
            b. Atenolol (Tenormin); for those with cardiac or asthma problems
    b. Radioactive Iodine Therapy
        1. Process:
            a. Iodine is taken up by thyroid
            b. Concentrates in the thyroid gland and destroys cells
            c. Less hormone is produced
            d. Dose given orally
            e. Results occur in 6 to 8 weeks
        2. Not to be given to pregnant women
        3. Client often hypothyroid after treatment
    c. Surgery
        1. Subtotal thyroidectomy: only part of thyroid removed
        2. Total thyroidectomy to treat cancer of thyroid: client will need life-long thyroid replacement
        3. Prior to surgery: get client into euthyroid state
        4. Iodine (Potassium Iodide) given prior to surgery to decrease size and vascularity of thyroid
        5. Post-op concerns
            a. Airway: maintain airway; oxygen, suction, tracheostomy set available
            b. Hemorrhage: check neck dressing including posteriorly; could compress trachea
            c. Hypocalcemia: parathyroid glands may be removed or damaged; resulting in low calcium; have calcium chloride or calcium gluconate available
7. Nursing Diagnoses
    a. Risk for Decreased Cardiac Output
    b. Disturbed Sensory Perception: Visual
        1. Interventions to protect eye from corneal irritation and to maintain moisture
        2. Lubricants and taping eyes shut at night
    c. Imbalanced Nutrition—Less than body requirements: Diet high in protein and calories
    d. Disturbed Body Image: Exophthalmos may continue post treatment
8. Nursing Care: Client teaching regarding
    a. Medications
    b. Signs and symptoms of altered thyroid function
    c. Hyperthyroid client at risk for hypothyroid post treatment
C. Clients with Hypothyroidism
    1. Definition
        a. Thyroid gland produces insufficient amount of thyroid hormone
        b. Myxedema: characteristic accumulation of nonpitting edema in connective tissues throughout body; water retention in mucoprotein deposits in interstitial spaces
        c. More common females aged 30–60
    2. Pathophysiology
        a. Primary (more common)
            1. Defect in thyroid gland
            2. Congenital defects
            3. Post treatment of hyperthyroidism
            4. Thyroiditis
            5. Iodine deficiency
        b. Secondary
            1. Deficiency in TSH (pituitary gland)
            2. Peripheral resistance to thyroid hormones
    3. Signs and Symptoms: Slow onset over months to years
        a. Metabolism: slowed
            1. Intolerance to cold
            2. Sleepiness
            3. Fatigue, weakness
        b. Cardiovascular
            1. Bradycardia, alterations in blood pressure
            2. Tendency for development of congestive heart failure, myocardial infarction
        c. Gastrointestinal
            1. Enlarged tongue, anorexia, vomiting
            2. Constipation
        d. Neuromuscular: Apathy, slow movement and thinking
        e. Other
            1. Goiter: thyroid gland enlarges in attempt to produce more hormone
            2. Edema in hands, feet, face; dry skin and hair

4. Specific Conditions
   a. Iodine Deficiency
      1. Dietary foods grown in iodine poor soil
      2. Use of non-iodized salt
      3. Medications, such as lithium carbonate, amiodarone (Cordarone)
   b. Hashimoto's Thyroiditis
      1. Autoimmune disorder
      2. Antibodies produced against thyroid tissue
   c. Myxedematous coma
      1. Life-threatening complication of long-standing and untreated hypothyroidism
      2. Hyponatremia, hypoglycemia, acidosis
      3. Precipitated by stressors, failure to take thyroid replacement meds
      4. Treatment includes restoring balance throughout systems and increasing thyroid hormone levels
5. Diagnostic Tests
   a. Serum thyroid antibodies (TA): antibodies in Hashimoto's Thyroiditis
   b. TSH test: (from pituitary) elevated with primary hypothyroidism
   c. T3 and T4: decreased for diagnosis of hypothyroidism
   d. T3 uptake test; decreased with hypothyroidism
   e. RAI (radioactive iodine) uptake test
      1. Oral or intravenous dose of radioactive iodine (131I or 123I) given to client
      2. Thyroid scanned after 24 hours
      3. Uptake decreased with hypothyroidism
      4. Size and shape of gland revealed
   f. Serum cholesterol is elevated
6. Treatment of hypothyroidism
   a. Medication
      1. Thyroid hormone replacement life long
      2. Synthroid, Levothroid
   b. Surgery: partial thyroidectomy, if goiter large enough to interfere with breathing or swallowing
7. Nursing Diagnoses
   a. Decreased Cardiac Output
   b. Constipation
   c. Risk for Impaired Skin Integrity: due to over all edema high risk for skin breakdown: preventative interventions

D. Client with Cancer of Thyroid (relatively rare)
   1. Types
      a. Papillary thyroid carcinoma
         1. More common in female in 40's
         2. Usually single nodule
         3. Risks: exposure of area to x-ray, nuclear fallout, family history
      b. Follicular thyroid cancer: more common in female in 50's
   2. Diagnosis
      a. Palpable firm nontender nodule in thyroid
      b. Usually no elevation in thyroid hormones
      c. Thyroid scans, needle biopsy of nodule
   3. Treatment
      a. Subtotal or total thyroidectomy
      b. Radioactive iodine therapy with 131I
      c. Client will need continued medical followup; thyroid replacement
      d. 95% survival rate without metastasis
III. Disorders of Parathyroid
   A. Clients with hyperparathyroidism
      1. Definition
         a. Increased secretion of parathyroid hormone (PTH) affecting kidneys, bones
         b. Occurs rarely and results in increased serum calcium
      2. Pathophysiology: may be due to tumor or hyperplasia of parathyroid, resulting in hypercalcemia, hypophosphatemia
      3. Signs and Symptoms
         a. Usually clients are asymptomatic
         b. Behaviors result from hypercalcemia: "bones, stones, abdominal groans"
            1. Bone decalcification (increased of bone fractures)
            2. Renal calculi
            3. Abdominal pain, constipation
         c. Clients may also have metabolic acidosis, hypokalemia, dysrhythmias, muscle weakness
      4. Collaborative care
         a. Diagnostic tests
            1. Exclude other causes of hypercalcemia
            2. Serum calcium, phosphorus, magnesium, electrolytes, bone x-rays and scans
         b. Treatment
            1. Focus on decreasing calcium levels
            2. Increase fluid intake, remain active
            3. Avoid calcium supplements, thiazide diuretics

4. Medications to inhibit bone reabsorption: Alendronate (Fosamax), Pamidronate (Aredia)
5. Removal of parathyroid gland, if tumor exists
6. Severe hypercalcemia involves hospitalization and intravenous saline

B. Clients with hypoparathyroidism
   1. Definition
      a. Abnormal low parathyroid hormone levels
      b. Occurs rarely and results in decreased serum calcium
   2. Pathophysiology
      a. Often due to damage or removal of parathyroid glands during thyroidectomy
      b. Hypocalcemia, elevated blood phosphate levels, decreased activation of Vitamin D in intestines
   3. Signs and Symptoms of Hypocalcemia
      a. Numbness
      b. Tingling around mouth, fingertips
      c. Muscle spasms of hands and feet
      d. Tetany
      e. Laryngospasms
   4. Collaborative Care
      a. Diagnostic tests
         1. Calcium and phosphorus levels, assess for Chvostek and Trousseau's signs
         2. Rule out other causes of hypocalcemia (renal failure, absorption or nutritional disorders)
      b. Treatment
         1. Treat hypocalcemia
         2. Intravenous calcium gluconate in severe cases
         3. Long-term therapy with supplemental calcium
         4. Dietary teaching
         5. Vitamin D therapy

IV. Disorders of Adrenal Glands
   A. Client with Hypercortisolism (Cushing's Syndrome)
      1. Definition
         a. Chronic disorder hyperfunction of adrenal cortex producing excessive amounts of ACTH or cortisol
         b. More common in females between the ages of 30 and 50

c. Occurs in persons on high-dose steroids for long periods of time
      2. Pathophysiology
         a. Tumors in pituitary cause hypersecretion of ACTH; some cancerous tumors secrete ACTH (e.g., small-cell lung cancer)
         b. Tumors, either benign or malignant, in adrenal cortex cause excessive production of cortisol and suppress ACTH production, causing atrophy of other uninvolved adrenal cortex
         c. Iantrogenic form, clients who are on long-term glucocorticoid therapy
      3. Signs and Symptoms
         a. Pattern related to adrenal cortex functions
            1. Effect functions of adrenal cortex "sugar, sex, and salt"
            2. Glucose metabolism, secondary sex characteristics, and mineralcorticoid levels
         b. Obesity and redistribution of body fat: central obesity, fat pads under clavicles, upper back ("buffalo hump"), rounded face
         c. Glucose and electrolyte abnormalities
            1. Hyperglycemia
            2. Sodium retention
            3. Hypokalemia causing hypertension
         d. Thinning of skin, bruises easily, abdominal striae
         e. Altered immunity, delayed healing, prone to infection
         f. Altered calcium absorption increasing osteoporosis and risk for fractures
         g. Increased gastric acid secretion increasing risk for ulcers
         h. Emotional changes from depression to psychosis
         i. Changes in secondary sexual characteristics, e.g., hirsuitism in females, gynecomastia in males
         j. Menstrual irregularities
      4. Collaborative Care
         a. Long-term steroid therapy
            1. Clients with iatrogenic Cushing's syndrome due to long-term steroid therapy for another condition must be aware of potential problems and remain under medical treatment
            2. Clients are maintained at lowest level of steroids needed for adequate treatment and efforts are made to minimize untoward effects

b. Diagnostic tests
  1. Measurement of plasma cortisol, ACTH: Alterations in normal diurinal alteration: higher in mornings, lower in afternoons and evenings
  2. 24-hour urine collections for measurements of hormones
    a. 17-ketosteroids and 17-hydroxycorticosteroids, which are elevated
    b. Important that collections are done properly with correct additives in specimens
  3. Electrolytes, calcium, and glucose levels (elevated Na^+, glucose; decreased K^+, Ca^2)
  4. ACTH suppression: synthetic cortisol (dexamethasone) given and plasma cortisol levels measured
c. Treatment: tumors may be treated with surgery, radiation, medications, or a combination
  1. Surgery
    a. Adrenalectomy: removal of adrenal gland if tumor is in the adrenal gland; if both glands are removed, client will need to be on lifelong hormone replacement
    b. Hypophysectomy (removal of pituitary gland): removal of pituitary gland through transphenoidal (through nostril) route or craniotomy
  2. Medications: for clients whose pituitary or adrenal tumors are inoperable
    a. Suppress adrenal cortex, decrease cortisol synthesis
    b. Examples: Mitotane, Metyrapone, Ketoconazole
d. Nursing Diagnoses for clients with Cushing's syndrome
  1. Fluid Volume Excess
  2. Risk for Injury: potential for falls, fractures
  3. Risk for Infection
  4. Disturbed Body Image (changes revert when Cushing's syndrome is treated)
e. Nursing Care
  1. Post-operatively, clients being treated for adrenal or pituitary surgery need intensive care and are usually in large medical centers

  2. Clients who have undergone treatment often need to be on life-long hormone replacement; must wear medical identification bracelet
  3. Clients must not abruptly stop hormone replacement or could develop Addisonian crisis
B. Client with Chronic Adrenocortical Insufficiency (Addison's Syndrome)
  1. Definition
    a. Dysfunction of adrenal cortex
    b. Chronic deficiency of cortisol, aldosterone, adrenal androgens
    c. More common in women and those adults under 60
  2. Pathophysiology
    a. Autoimmune destruction of adrenal, accounts for 80% of spontaneous cases; occurs alone or with polyglandular autoimmune syndrome
    b. Untoward effect from anticoagulant, trauma in which client has bilateral adrenal hemorrhage
    c. Pituitary dysfunction from tumors, surgery, radiation, exogenous steroid
    d. Abrupt withdrawal from long-term, high-dose corticosteroid therapy
  3. Signs and Symptoms
    a. Slow onset; relate to decreased levels of cortisol and aldosterone
    b. Relate to lack of functions of adrenal cortex or decrease in "sugar, salt and sex"
    c. Hyponatremia, hyperkalemia, low circulating blood volume
    d. Postural hypotension, syncope, and possibly hypovolemic shock
    e. Dizziness, confusion, cardiac dysrhythmias
    f. Hypoglycemia, nausea, vomiting, weakness, lethargy, diarrhea
    g. Hyperpigmentation due to increased ACTH levels (bronzed appearance in Caucasians)
  4. Specific condition: Addisonian Crisis
    a. Life-threatening response to acute adrenal insufficiency
    b. Occurs in clients with Addison's disease in response to major stressors
    c. Major symptoms are high fever, weakness, abdominal pain, severe hypotension, circulatory collapse, shock, coma

      d. Treatment is rapid intravenous replacement of fluids and glucocorticoids

  5. Collaborative Care

    a. Diagnostic tests

      1. Serum cortisol and urine 17-ketosteroids and 17-hydroxycorticosteroids are decreased

      2. Plasma ACTH is increased, if cause is from adrenal dysfunction

      3. ACTH stimulation test

      4. Electrolytes show hyponatremia, hyperkalemia

      5. Serum glucose is decreased

      6. Hematocrit and hemoglobin are elevated; BUN is elevated as with dehydration

      7. CT scan of head may be done to determine if intracranial lesion affecting pituitary

    b. Medications

      1. Hydrocortisone

      2. Fludrocortisone (Florinef), a mineralcorticoid replacement

    c. Diet with increased sodium

    d. Nursing Care

      1. Clients must continue under medical care and should wear medical identification bracelet

      2. Client and family must be aware of need to continue medications and signs and symptoms of insufficient hormone levels

      3. Care must be taken whenever client will face stressor such as surgery, serious illness

      4. Any client on long-term, high-dose corticosteroid therapy must be gradually tapered from cortisone to allow adrenals to regain functioning

    e. Nursing Diagnoses

      1. Fluid Volume Deficit

      2. Risk for Ineffective Therapeutic Regime Management

C. Clients with tumors of Adrenal Medulla (Pheochromocytoma)

  1. Definition

    a. Adrenal medulla produces catecholamines (epinephrine, norephinephrine)

    b. Tumors of adrenal medulla produce excessive levels of catecholamines

  2. Signs and Symptoms

    a. Paroxysmal severe hypertension (systolic: 200–300; diastolic 150–175) with tachycardia

    b. Can be life threatening and stressor induced

  3. Diagnostic tests: Catecholamine levels (serum and urine) are elevated

  4. Treatment: Adrenalectomy to remove tumor

V. Disorders of Pituitary Gland

  A. Disorders of anterior pituitary gland

    1. Hyperfunction of anterior pituitary gland

    2. Pathophysiology: Most often benign adenoma producing excess hormones; growth hormone (GH), Prolactin (PRL), or ACTH

    3. Specific Conditions

      a. Gigantism: Growth hormone hypersecretion occurs prior to puberty resulting in person becoming excessively tall (over 7 feet tall)

      b. Acromegaly: Growth hormone hypersecretion occurs after puberty resulting in bone and connective tissue continuing to grow, resulting in enlargement of face, hands, and feet

      c. Overproduction of Prolactin secretion: Results in decreased reproductive and sexual function

      d. Cushing's Syndrome

    4. Treatment: Surgical removal or irradiation of pituitary tumor

  B. Disorders of Posterior Pituitary Gland

    1. Excessive or deficiency in antidiuretic hormone (ADH)

    2. ADH is secreted in response to changes in serum osmolality (hypothalamus)

    3. Specific Conditions

      a. Syndrome of Inappropriate ADH Secretion (SIADH)

        1. Definition

          a. High levels of ADH is absence of hypoosmolality

          b. Results in hyponatremia and water intoxication

        2. Pathophysiology

          a. Malignant tumors (e.g., oat cell or small cell lung cancer) which secret ADH,

          b. Post head injury, side effect of some medications including diuretics and anesthetics

        3. Signs and Symptoms: neurologic symptoms including decreased

level of consciousness, confusion, muscle twitches, seizures
4. Treatment: correction of Na^+ deficit, restriction of fluids, treat underlying cause
b. Diabetes Insipidus
1. Definition: ADH insufficiency from neurogenic or nephrogenic origin
2. Pathophysiology: brain tumors, closed head trauma, other brain conditions, renal failure
3. Signs and Symptoms: excretes large amounts of dilute urine; client at risk for dehydration and hypernatremia
4. Treatment: administer intravenous hypotonic fluids, oral fluids and replace ADH hormone (Desmopressin acetate)

FOCUSED STUDY TIPS

■ Identify a medication used to treat an endocrine disorder. Describe to classmates how it affects the disorder it treats. Describe routes of administration, normal adult dosages, side effects, and contraindications. Share laboratory tests and values needed to determine efficacy. Make a drug card for this medication for each classmate.

■ Care for a client utilizing hormones. Identify the drug and the condition it is being used for. What symptoms will the client experience if overdosed or underdosed with this drug?

■ Practice physical assessment of the thyroid gland on a family member, friend, or classmate. Describe normal and abnormal findings.

CASE STUDY

Mrs. Jones has just been diagnosed with hyperparathyroidism. What symptoms and laboratory values may have contributed to her diagnosis? How is her disease treated if hospitalization is required? How will it be treated when she is discharged? Develop a preoperative and postoperative teaching plan for this client if surgical correction of this disorder is necessary.

CARE PLAN CRITICAL THINKING ACTIVITY

Home care is an integral part of treating the client with adrenal insufficiency. What are the priorities of a teaching plan for a client being discharged with adrenal insufficiency? How would you measure the client's understanding of these priorities?

NCLEX TEST QUESTIONS

1. When teaching a client about hyperthyroidism, the nurse tells the client that this disorder is most often referenced or identified by the following term?
   a. Cretinism
   b. Colloid goiter
   c. Myxedema
   d. Grave's disease

2. The medical term for hypersecretion of growth hormone in adults is:
   a. Grave's disease.
   b. gigantism.
   c. acromegaly.
   d. Simmond's disease.

3. Cushing's syndrome is a chronic disorder resulting in:
   a. increased serum levels of ADH (antidiuretic hormone).
   b. increased circulating cortisol or ACTH (adrenocorticotropic hormone).
   c. lifelong need of steroid replacement therapy
   d. adrenal insufficiency

4. When reviewing bloodwork for a client with Addison's disease, the nurse expects to find:
   a. increased serum cortisol levels.
   b. low BUN (blood urea nitrogen).
   c. decreased serum cortisol levels.
   d. elevated blood glucose levels.

5. While caring for a client with hypothyroidism, the nurse assesses the client for hypocalcemia. If present, the nurse would expect to observe:

    a. a negative Chvostek's sign.

    b. hyperventilation.

    c. pitting edema of the lower extremities.

    d. spasms of the hands and feet.

6. Diabetes insipidus is the result of:

    a. insulin insufficiency.

    b. ADH (anti-diuretic hormone) insufficiency.

    c. excessive production of ACTH (adrenocorticotropic hormone).

    d. high serum levels of ADH (anti-diuretic hormone).

7. Manifestations of SIADH (syndrome of inappropriate ADH secretion) occur as a result of:

    a. water retention, hyponatremia, and serum hypoosmolality.

    b. water retention, hypernatremia, and serum hyperosmolality.

    c. dehydration, seizures, and hypernatremia.

    d. fever, dehydration, and polyuria.

CHAPTER 18

NURSING CARE OF CLIENTS WITH DIABETES MELLITUS

LEARNING OUTCOMES

After completing this chapter, you will be able to:

- Apply knowledge of normal endocrine anatomy, physiology, and assessments when providing nursing care for clients with diabetes mellitus (see Chapter 16).
- Describe the prevalence and incidence of diabetes mellitus.
- Explain the pathophysiology, risk factors, manifestations, and complications of Type 1 and Type 2 Diabetes Mellitus.
- Compare and contrast the manifestations and collaborative care of hypoglycemia, diabetic ketoacidosis (DKA), and hyperosmolar hyperglycemic state (HHS).
- Identify the diagnostic tests used for screening, diagnosis, and monitoring of diabetes mellitus.
- Discuss the nursing implications for insulin and oral hypoglycemic agents used to treat clients with diabetes mellitus.
- Provide accurate information to clients with diabetes mellitus to facilitate self-management of medications, diet planning, exercise, and self-assessment, including foot care.
- Use the nursing process as a framework for providing individualized care to clients with Diabetes Mellitus.

KEY TOPICS

- Pathophysiology of diabetes mellitus
- Complications of diabetes mellitus
- Medical management of diabetes mellitus, including glucose monitoring, medications, diet, and exercise
- Nursing care of clients with diabetes mellitus

MediaLink

www.prenhall.com/lemone

Additional resources for this chapter can be found on the Student CD-ROM accompanying this textbook, and on the Companion Website at www.prenhall.com/lemone. Click on Chapter 18 to select the activities for this chapter.

CD-ROM
- Audio Glossary
- NCLEX Review

Animation
- Glipizide

Companion Website
- More NCLEX Review
- Case Study
   Diabetes Mellitus Type 1
- Care Plan Activity
   Diabetes Mellitus Type 2
- MediaLink Applications
   Diabetes Foot Care

LECTURE OUTLINE

I. Diabetes Mellitus: Overview
  A. Definition: metabolic disorder characterized by hyperglycemia due to an absolute or relative lack of insulin or to a cellular resistance to insulin
  B. Major classifications
    1. Type 1 Diabetes
    2. Type 2 Diabetes
  C. Impact on health of American population
    1. Sixth leading cause of death due to cardiovascular effects resulting in atherosclerosis, coronary artery disease, and stroke
    2. Leading cause of end stage renal failure
    3. Major cause of blindness
    4. Most frequent cause of non-traumatic amputations
    5. Diabetes affects estimated 15.7 million people (10.3 million are diagnosed; 5.4 million are undiagnosed)
    6. Increasing prevalence of Type 2 Diabetes in older adults and minority groups (African American, American Indian and Hispanic populations)
    7. Estimated 11% of older U.S. population (65–74) have diabetes
II. Diabetes Type 1
  A. Definition
    1. Metabolic condition in which the beta cells of pancreas no longer produce insulin; characterized by hyperglycemia, breakdown of body fats and protein and development of ketosis
    2. Accounts for 5–10% of cases of diabetes; most often occurs in childhood or adolescence
    3. Formerly called juvenile onset diabetes or insulin-dependent diabetes (IDDM)
  B. Pathophysiology
    1. Autoimmune reaction in which the beta cells that produce insulin are destroyed
    2. Alpha cells produce excess glucagons causing hyperglycemia
  C. Risk Factors
    1. Genetic predisposition for increased susceptibility; Human Leukocyte Antigens (HLA) linkage
    2. Environmental triggers stimulate an autoimmune response
      a. Viral infections (mumps, rubella, coxsackievirus B4)
      b. Chemical toxins
  D. Manifestations
    1. Process of beta cell destruction occurs slowly; hyperglycemia occurs when

80–90% is destroyed; often trigger stressor event (e.g., illness)
    2. Hyperglycemia leads to
      a. Polyuria (hyperglycemia acts as osmotic diuretic)
      b. Glycosuria (renal threshold for glucose: 180 mg/dL)
      c. Polydipsia (thirst from dehydration from polyuria)
      d. Polyphagia (hunger and eats more since cell cannot utilize glucose)
      e. Weight loss (body breaking down fat and protein to restore energy source
      f. Malaise and fatigue (from decrease in energy)
      g. Blurred vision (swelling of lenses from osmotic effects)
    3. Without treatment (exogenous source of insulin) person will develop diabetic ketoacidosis
  E. Diabetic Ketoacidosis (DKA)
    1. Results from breakdown of fat and overproduction of ketones by the liver and loss of bicarbonate
    2. Occurs when Diabetes Type 1 is undiagnosed or known diabetic has increased energy needs, when under physical or emotional stress or fails to take insulin
    3. Pathophysiology
      a. Hypersomolarity (hyperglycemia, dehydration)
      b. Metabolic acidosis (accumulation of ketones)
      c. Fluid and electrolyte imbalance (from osmotic diuresis)
    4. Diagnostic tests
      a. Blood glucose greater than 250 mg/dL
      b. Blood pH less than 7.3
      c. Blood bicarbonate less than 15 mEq/L
      d. Ketones present in blood
      e. Ketones and glucose present in urine
      f. Electrolyte abnormalities (Na^+, K^+, Cl^-)
    5. Treatment
      a. Requires immediate medical attention and usually admission to hospital
      b. Frequent measurement of blood glucose and treat according to glucose levels with regular insulin (mild ketosis, subcutaneous route; severe ketosis with intravenous insulin administration)
      c. Restore fluid balance: initially 0.9% saline at 500–1000 mL/hr.; regulate fluids according to client status; when

blood glucose is 250 mg/dL add dextrose to intravenous solutions

   d. Correct electrolyte imbalance: client often is hypokalemic and potassium is added to intravenous fluids and levels monitored frequently

   e. Monitor cardiac rhythm since hypokalemia puts client at risk for dysrhythmias

   f. Treat underlying condition precipitating DKA

III. Diabetes Type 2

  A. Definition: condition of fasting hyperglycemia occurring despite availability of body's own insulin

  B. Pathophysiology

    1. Sufficient insulin production to prevent DKA; but insufficient to lower blood glucose through uptake of glucose by muscle and fat cells

    2. Cellular resistance to insulin increased by obesity, inactivity, illness, age, some medications

  C. Risk Factors

    1. History of diabetes in parents or siblings; no HLA

    2. Obesity (especially of upper body)

    3. Physical inactivity

    4. Race/ethnicity: African American, Hispanic, or American Indian origin

    5. Women: history of gestational diabetes, polycystic ovary syndrome, delivered baby with birth weight > 9 pounds

    6. Clients with hypertension; HDL cholesterol < 35 mg/dL, and/or triglyceride level > 250 mg/dL.

  D. Manifestations

    1. Client usually unaware of diabetes

     a. Discovers diabetes when seeking health care for another concern

     b. Usually does not experience weight loss

    2. Possible symptoms or concerns

     a. Hyperglycemia (not as severe as with Type 1)

     b. Polyuria

     c. Polydipsia

     d. Blurred vision

     e. Fatigue

     f. Paresthesias (numbness in extremities)

     g. Skin Infections

  E. Hypersomolar Hyperglycemic State (HHS)

    1. Potential complication of Diabetes Type 2

    2. Life threatening medical emergency, high mortality rate

    3. Characterized by

     a. Plasma osmolarity 340 mOsm/L or greater (normal: 280–300)

     b. Blood glucose severely elevated, 600–2000 (normal 70–110)

     c. Altered level of consciousness

    4. Precipitating factors

     a. Infection (most common)

     b. Therapeutic agent or procedure

     c. Acute or chronic illness

    5. Slow onset 1–14 days

    6. Pathophysiology

     a. Hyperglycemia leads to increased urine output and dehydration

     b. Kidneys retain glucose; glucose and sodium rise

     c. Severe hyperosmolar state develops leading to brain cell shrinkage

    7. Manifestations

     a. Altered level of consciousness (lethargy to coma)

     b. Neurological deficits: hyperthermia, motor and sensory impairment, seizures

     c. Dehydration: dry skin and mucous membranes, extreme thirst

    8. Treatment

     a. Usually admitted to intensive care unit of hospital for care since client is in life-threatening condition: unresponsive, may be on ventilator, has nasogastric suction

     b. Correct fluid and electrolyte imbalances giving isotonic or colloid solutions and correct potassium deficits

     c. Lower glucose with regular insulin until glucose level drops to 250 mg/dL

     d. Treat underlying condition

IV. Complications of Diabetes

  A. Alterations in blood sugars: hyperglycemia and hypoglycemia

  B. Macrocirculation (large blood vessels)

    1. Atherosclerosis occurs more frequently, earlier in diabetics

    2. Involves coronary, peripheral, and cerebral arteries

  C. Microcirculation (small blood vessels)

    1. Affects basement membrane of small blood vessels and capillaries

    2. Involves tissues affecting eyes and kidneys

  D. Prevention of complications

    1. Managing diabetes

    2. Lowering risk factors for conditions

3. Routine screening for complications
4. Implementing early treatment
V. Complications of Diabetes: Alterations in blood sugars
  A. Hyperglycemia: high blood sugar
    1. DKA (mainly associated with Diabetes Type 1)
    2. HHS (mainly associated with Diabetes Type 2)
    3. Dawn phenomenon: rise in blood sugar between 4 A.M. and 8 A.M., not associated with hypoglycemia (associated with Diabetes Type 1 and 2)
    4. Somogyi effect: combination of hypoglycemia during night with a rebound morning hyperglycemia that may lead to insulin resistance for 12 to 48 hours
  B. Hypoglycemia (insulin reaction, insulin shock, "the lows"): low blood sugar
    1. Mismatch between insulin dose, carbohydrate availability and exercise
    2. May be affected by intake of alcohol, certain medications
    3. Manifestations
      a. Result of compensatory response by autonomic nervous system and impaired cerebral function (brain cells need near continuous glucose to function properly)
      b. Vary with individuals
      c. Often client or family recognize early signs or symptoms
      d. Blood glucose < 45–60 mg/dL
    4. Specific manifestations
      a. Cool, clammy skin
      b. Rapid heartbeat
      c. Hunger
      d. Nervousness, tremor
      e. Faintness, dizziness
      f. Unsteady gait, slurred and/or incoherent speech
      g. Vision changes
      h. Seizures, coma
    5. Severe hypoglycemia can result in death
    6. Clients taking medications, such as beta-adrenergic blockers may not experience manifestations associated with autonomic nervous system
    7. Hypoglycemia unawareness: clients with Diabetes Type 1 for 4 or 5 years or more may develop severe hypoglycemia without symptoms which can delay treatment
    8. Treatment for mild hypoglycemia
      a. Immediate treatment: client should take 15 gm of rapid-acting sugar (half cup of fruit juice; 8 oz of skim milk, 3 glucose tablets, 3 life savers)
      b. 15/15 rule: wait 15 minutes and monitor blood glucose; if still low, client should eat another 15 gm of sugar
      c. Continue until blood glucose level has returned to normal
      d. Client should contact medical care provider if hypoglycemia occurs more that 2 or 3 times per week
    9. Treatment for severe hypoglycemia is often hospitalization
      a. Client is unresponsive, has seizures, or has altered behavior; blood glucose level is less than 50 mg/dL
      b. If client is conscious and alert, administer 15 gm of sugar
      c. If client is not alert, administer
        1. 25%–50% solution of glucose intravenously, followed by infusion of 5% dextrose in water
        2. Glucagon 1 mg by subcutaneous, intramuscular, or intravenous route; follow with oral or intravenous carbohydrate
      d. Monitor client response physically and also blood glucose level
VI. Complications Affecting Cardiovascular System, Vision, and Kidney Function
  A. Coronary Artery Disease
    1. Major risk of myocardial infarction in Type 2 diabetics
    2. Most common cause of death for diabetics (40–60%)
    3. Diabetics more likely to develop Congestive Heart Failure
  B. Hypertension
    1. Affects 20–60% of all diabetics
    2. Increases risk for retinopathy, nephropathy
  C. Stroke: Type 2 diabetics are 2–6 times more likely to have stroke
  D. Peripheral Vascular Disease (PVD)
    1. Increased risk for Types 1 and 2 diabetics
    2. Development of arterial occlusion and thrombosis resulting in gangrene
    3. Gangrene from diabetes most common cause of non-traumatic lower limb amputation
  E. Diabetic Retinopathy
    1. Definition
      a. Retinal changes related to diabetes
      b. Leads to retinal ischemia and breakdown of blood-retinal barrier
      c. Involves 3 stages

2. Leading cause of blindness ages 25–74
   a. Affects almost all Type 1 diabetics after 20 years
   b. Affects 60% of Type 2 diabetics
3. Diabetics should be screened for retinopathy and receive treatment (laser photocoagulation surgery) to prevent vision loss
4. Diabetics also have increased risk for cataract development

F. Diabetic Nephropathy
   1. Definition: glomerular changes in kidneys of diabetics leading to impaired renal function
   2. First indicator: microalbuminuria
   3. Diabetics without treatment go on to develop hypertension, edema, progressive renal insufficiency
      a. In Type 1 diabetics, 10–15 years
      b. May occur soon after diagnosis with Type 2 Diabetes since many are undiagnosed for years
   4. Most common cause of end-stage renal failure in U.S.
   5. Kimmelstiel-Wilson syndrome: glomerulosclerosis associated with diabetes

VII. Complications Affecting Peripheral and Autonomic Nervous System
A. Diabetic neuropathies are disorders involving changes in blood vessels that supply nerves and result in impaired nerve conduction
B. Types of diabetic neuropathies
   1. Peripheral (Somatic) Neuropathies
      a. Polyneuropathy: bilateral sensory disorders most common to affect diabetics; begins in toes and feet and may include:
         1. Distal paresthesias (change in sensation like numbness or tingling)
         2. Pain including aching, burning, feelings of cold
         3. Altered or impaired sensation
      b. Mononeuropathy: affects single nerve, e.g., diabetic femoral neuropathy
   2. Visceral (Autonomic) Neuropathies
      a. Includes the actual functioning of a particular area of autonomic nervous system
      b. Examples include sweating, gastrointestinal, sexual dysfunction

VIII. Other Complications from Diabetes
A. Increased susceptibility to infection
   1. Predisposition is combined effect of other complications

2. Normal inflammatory response is diminished
3. Slower than normal healing
B. Periodontal disease
C. Foot ulcers and infections: predisposition is combined effect of other complications

IX. Collaborative Care
A. Based on research from 10-year study of Type 1 diabetics conducted by NIH focus is on keeping blood glucose levels as close to normal by active management interventions; complications were reduced by 60%
B. Treatment interventions are maintained through
   1. Medications
   2. Dietary management
   3. Exercise
C. Management of diabetes with pancreatic transplant, pancreatic cell or Beta cell transplant is in investigative stage

X. Diagnostic Tests
A. To diagnose Diabetes Mellitus, one of the three following tests must be positive and must be confirmed on another day with one of the three tests
   1. Client has symptoms of diabetes and casual plasma glucose > 200 mg/dL (Casual plasma glucose is drawn at any time of day without regard to time of last meal)
   2. Fasting plasma glucose level > 126 mg/dL
   3. During a oral glucose tolerance test (OGTT), the 2 hour plasma glucose > 200 mg/dL
B. Diagnostic tests to monitor diabetes management
   1. Fasting Blood Glucose (normal: 70–110 mg/dL)
   2. Glycosylated hemoglobin (c) (Hemoglobin A1C)
      a. Considered elevated if values above 7–9%
      b. Blood test analyzes glucose attached to hemoglobin. Since rbc lives about 120 days gives an average of the blood glucose over previous 2 to 3 months
   3. Urine glucose and ketone levels (part of routine urinalysis)
      a. Glucose in urine indicates hyperglycemia (renal threshold is usually 180 mg/dL)
      b. Presence of ketones indicates fat breakdown, indicator of DKA; ketones may be present if person not eating
   4. Urine albumin (part of routine urinalysis)
      a. If albumin present, indicates need for workup for nephropathy

 b. Typical order is creatinine clearance testing
 5. Cholesterol and Triglyceride levels
  a. Recommendations
   1. LDL < 100 mg/dL
   2. HDL > 45 mg/dL
   3. Triglycerides < 150 mg/dL
  b. Monitor risk for atherosclerosis and cardiovascular complications
 6. Serum electrolytes in clients with DKA or HHS
C. Client monitoring of blood glucose levels
 1. Goals: Diabetic can monitor glucose control and avoid episodes of hypoglycemia
 2. Recommendations by American Diabetic Association
  a. Type 1 diabetics: at least 3 times a day
  b. Type 2 diabetics: enough to reach glucose goals
  c. More often when treatment is being modified, client is ill or pregnant, or experiencing hyperglycemia or hypoglycemia
 3. Equipment includes blood glucose monitor, test strips which react to blood, lancet device to perform finger-stick and obtain specimen
 4. Client needs to be aware of and follow specific instructions of monitor to insure obtaining accurate results
 5. Health care personnel must be verified competent in utilizing blood glucose monitoring devices used in hospital or nursing home; equipment must be maintained and verified
XI. Medications
 A. Insulin
  1. Sources: standard practice is use of human insulin prepared by alteration of pork insulin or recombinant DNA therapy
  2. Clients who need insulin as therapy:
   a. All Type 1 diabetics since their bodies essentially no longer produce insulin
   b. Some Type 2 diabetics, if oral medications are not adequate for control (both oral medications and insulin may be needed)
   c. Diabetics enduring stressor situations such as surgery, corticosteroid therapy, infections, treatment for DKA, HHS
   d. Women with gestational diabetes who are not adequately controlled with diet
   e. Some clients receiving high caloric feedings including tube feedings or parenteral nutrition

 3. Terms describing time and effect of insulin
  a. Onset: the time span after administration when insulin will begin to affect the blood glucose level
  b. Peak: the time span after administration when insulin will have the greatest effect on the blood glucose level
  c. Duration: the time span after administration when insulin will continue to affect the blood glucose level
 4. Types of preparations/specifics: differ regarding timed effects
  a. Rapid acting (ultra-short): insulin lispro (Humalog)
  b. Short-acting: Regular insulin (only insulin for intravenous administration)
  c. Intermediate-acting: NPH, Lente insulin
  d. Long-acting: Ultralente, Lantus (no defined onset or peak)
  e. Combination insulins: specific manufactured combinations of intermediate and rapid or short acting insulins
 5. Insulin Administration
  a. Equipment
   1. Insulin syringes are specific for insulin administration; needle is thin, short (25–27 gauge, 0.5 inch long) specific for subcutaneous administration
   2. Calibrated for U 100 insulin; standard concentration is 100 units in 1 mL; (U 500 insulin rarely used; clients are severely insulin resistant.)
   3. Some diabetics may use an insulin pump
    a. CSII device with small pump that holds syringe of insulin connected with tubing to needle placed subcutaneously in skin in abdomen
    b. Delivers a constant amount of programmed insulin round the clock; client can administer bolus to cover blood glucose elevation
  b. Route
   1. Insulin is only given parenterally; current research for nasal or oral forms
   2. All insulins can be given subcutaneously; only regular insulin can be given intravenously.

c. Preparation
1. Insulin can be kept at room temperature for 4 weeks
2. Insulin should be stored in refrigerator; brought to room temperature prior to administration
3. Regular insulin is clear; other insulins are cloudy and vials need to be gently rolled to mix adequately prior to withdrawal of insulin into syringe
4. Care taken to withdraw insulin without air bubbles to obtain correct dose
5. If mixing insulins, draw clear (regular) first, then cloudy intermediate insulin
d. Administration
1. Designated areas of body with subcutaneous tissue but sites differ in absorption rates: abdomen fastest and recommended
2. Usually given at 90-degree angle; do not massage site after injection but can apply pressure
3. Distance injection sites an inch and avoid scars, incisions
4. Lipodystrophy and lipostrophy (hardening of tissues) are not seen much since use of human insulin, room temperature insulin
B. Oral Hypoglycemic Agents
1. Used to treat Diabetes Type 2
2. Client must also maintain prescribed diet and exercise program; monitor blood glucose levels
3. Not used with pregnant or lactating women
4. Several different oral hypoglycemic agents and insulin may be prescribed for the client
5. Specific drug interactions may affect the blood glucose levels
6. Classifications and action
a. Sulfonylureas
1. Action: Stimulates pancreatic cells to secrete more insulin and increases sensitivity of peripheral tissues to insulin
2. Used: to treat non-obese Type 2 diabetics
3. Example: Glipizide (Glucotrol)
b. Meglitinides
1. Action: stimulates pancreatic cells to secret more insulin
2. Example: Repaglinide (Prandin)

c. Biguanides
1. Action: decreases overproduction of glucose by liver and makes insulin more effective in peripheral tissues
2. Example: Metformin (Glucophage)
d. Alpha-glucoside Inhibitors
1. Action: Slow carbohydrate digestion and delay glucose absorption
2. Example: Acarbose (Precose)
e. Thizaolidinediones
1. Action: Sensitizes peripheral tissues to insulin
2. Example: Rosiglitazone (Avandia)
f. D-pheylalanine (Amino Acid) Derivative
1. Action: Stimulates very rapid and short insulin secretion to decrease spikes in glucose following meals; reduces overall glucose level
2. Example: Nateglinide (Starlix)
C. Aspirin Therapy: daily dose recommended to decrease risk of cardiovascular complications
XII. Role of Diet in Diabetic Management
A. Goals for diabetic therapy include
1. Maintain as near-normal blood glucose levels as possible with balance of food with medications
2. Obtain optimal serum lipid levels
3. Provide adequate calories to attain or maintain reasonable weight
B. Diet Composition
1. Carbohydrates: 60–70% of daily diet
2. Protein: 15–20% of daily diet
3. Fats: No more than 10% of total calories from saturated fats
4. Fiber: 20 to 35 grams/day; promotes intestinal motility and gives feeling of fullness
5. Sodium: recommended intake 1000 mg per 1000 kcal
6. Sweeteners approved by FDA instead of refined sugars
7. Limited use of alcohol: potential hypoglycemic effect of insulin and oral hypoglycemics
C. Meal planning
1. Different methods to achieve adequate nutrition and maintain adequate diabetic control yet consider the diabetic individual
2. Consistent-Carbohydrate Diabetes Meal Plan
a. Clients count carbohydrate content
b. Based on individual diet prescription and Food Guide Pyramid

3. Exchange Lists: Diet consists of specific number of exchanges (servings) of specific food groups per meals or snacks

D. Diet specifics for Type 1 diabetics
1. Correlation of eating patterns with insulin onset and peak of action
2. Meals, snacks, insulin regimens take into account individual's life-style (exercise, occupation, ethnicity, religion, and finances)
3. Self-monitoring of blood glucose allows clients to adjust insulin and diet

E. Diet specifics for Type 2 diabetics
1. Often includes plan for weight loss, which will improve glucose control
2. Three meals spaced at 4–5 hour intervals with one or two snacks
3. Includes decrease of fat intake

F. Diet guidelines when client is ill, i.e., "sick day management"
1. Monitor blood glucose at least 4 times per day
2. Test urine for ketones, if blood glucose level > 240 mg/dL
3. Continue insulin or oral hypoglycemic agent
4. Sip 8–12 ounces of fluid hourly
5. Substitute easily digested foods or liquids that are carbohydrate equivalents, if unable to tolerate solid foods
6. Contact healthcare provider if unable to eat for 24 hours or vomiting and diarrhea lasts more than 6 hours

XIII. Exercise
A. Effects in the diabetic client
1. Increases uptake of glucose by muscle cells, possibly reducing need for insulin
2. Decreases cholesterol and triglyceride levels, thus reducing risk for cardiovascular complications
3. Clients should consult with health care provider before beginning or changing exercise program; may recommend cardiac and other risk screenings first

B. Recommendations while exercising for all diabetics by American Diabetic Association
1. Proper footware; inspecting feet before and after exercise
2. Avoid exercise in temperature extremes
3. Avoid exercise during times of poor glucose control

C. Specific concerns for Type 1 diabetics
1. Increases risk for hypoglycemia and hyperglycemia
2. Exercise should be moderate and regular
3. Self-monitoring of blood glucose levels needed before and after exercise

4. Fluid intake (such as water) must be increased; food intake may need to be increased (should have snack available after exercise)

D. Specific concerns for Type 2 diabetics
1. Very important since promotes weight loss and thus glycemic control, decreases risks for cardiovascular complications
2. Clients may experience decrease need for hypoglycemic agents with compliance with prescribed diet, exercise program, and weight loss
3. Regular exercise may delay the onset of Type 2 Diabetes in individuals at high risk

XIV. Care of diabetic surgical clients
A. Clients face increased risks for
1. Postoperative infection
2. Delayed wound healing
3. Fluid and electrolyte imbalances
4. Hypoglycemia
5. DKA

B. Preoperative care: general guidelines
1. Clients should be in best possible metabolic state
2. Usual diabetic medication or insulin changed the day of surgery:
a. Clients may receive regular insulin according to blood glucose levels as client is given intravenous glucose therapy
b. Clients may receive half dose of intermediate- or long-acting insulin dose prior to surgery
3. Surgery should be scheduled early in morning to minimize fasting
4. Postoperative glucose affected by ability to eat, gastric suctioning
5. Blood glucose usually monitored at set intervals with orders for regular insulin coverage

XV. Care of diabetic older clients
A. 40% of all clients with diabetes are over age of 65
B. Need to include spouse, members of family in teaching who may assist with client meeting medical needs
C. Diet changes may be difficult to implement since client has established eating habits
D. Exercise programs may need adjustment to meet individual's abilities (such as physical limitations from other chronic illnesses)
E. Individual reluctance to accept assistance to deal with chronic illness, assist with hygiene
F. Limited assets for medications, supplies, dietary

G. Visual deficits or learning challenges to learn insulin administration, blood glucose monitoring

XVI. Nursing Care
  A. Assessment, planning, implementation with client according to type and stage of diabetes
  B. Prevention, assessment and treatment of complications through client self-management and keeping appointments for medical care
  C. Client and family teaching for diabetes management
  D. Health promotion includes education of healthy lifestyle, lowering risks for developing diabetes for all clients
  E. Blood glucose screening at 3 year intervals starting at age 45 for persons in high-risk groups

XVII. Common Nursing Diagnoses and Specific Teaching Interventions
  A. Risk for impaired skin integrity: Proper foot care
    1. Daily inspection of feet
    2. Checking temperature of any water before washing feet
    3. Need for lubricating cream after drying but not between toes
  B. Risk for infection
    1. Frequent hand washing
    2. Early recognition of signs of infection and seeking treatment
    3. Meticulous skin care
    4. Regular dental examinations and consistent oral hygiene care
  C. Risk for injury: Prevention of accidents, falls and burns
  D. Sexual dysfunction
    1. Effects of high blood sugar on sexual functioning,
    2. Resources for treatment of impotence, sexual dysfunction
  E. Ineffective coping
    1. Assisting clients with problem-solving strategies for specific concerns
    2. Providing information about diabetic resources, community education programs, and support groups
    3. Utilizing any client contact as opportunity to review coping status and reinforce proper diabetes management and complication prevention

FOCUSED STUDY TIPS

- Determine your risk factors for diabetes mellitus. Instruct a family member or friend on how to do the same.
- Plan a health fair with classmates. What suggestions would you make for screening participants for diabetes mellitus?
- Compare and contrast management of a juvenile or adolescent diabetic with management of an elderly diabetic. What will they have in common with the management of their disease in terms of diet, exercise, drug therapy, and glucose monitoring? What will their differences be in these areas? How will lifestyle impact their disease?

CASE STUDY

Martin Bailey has had Type I diabetes since childhood; he is now 42 years old. He comes to the outpatient client for routine follow-up and asks you about continuous subcutaneous insulin infusion (CSII). What do you tell him? Describe the physical characteristics of the pump, how it functions, and how it is programmed. He asks you what the advantages and disadvantages of CSII are. Answer in detail.

CARE PLAN CRITICAL THINKING ACTIVITY

Ms. Anderson has been treated for diabetes for 9 years. She is seen in an oupatient clinic. Her most recent glycosylated hemoglobin is 9.2%. What influence will this test result have in planning a teaching session for Ms. Anderson? What questions will you include in your health assessment? What physical assessments will you make? What goals will you make with the client? Is further evaluation necessary? Why or why not?

NCLEX TEST QUESTIONS

1. When teaching a self-care plan to diabetics with flu, cold, or minor gastrointestinal upsets, the nurse makes the following recommendation:
   a. "Notify your physician immediately to avoid diabetic complications."
   b. "Hold insulin and eat or drink whatever you are able to keep in your stomach."
   c. "Self-care interventions are necessary only if vomiting and diarrhea are present."
   d. "If unable to eat usual foods, replace these items with soft foods or liquids that are considered to be complex carbohydrates."

2. While preparing regular insulin for administration, the nurse knows:
   a. the client must eat approximately 1/2 hour after the injection.
   b. regular insulin is administered after meals only.
   c. the client must eat 3 to 4 hours after the injection.
   d. regular insulin peaks 4 hours after administration; food is necessary before the injection.

3. The nurse assesses the client experiencing diabetic ketoacidosis for:
   a. tachycardia.
   b. lethargy.
   c. tremors.
   d. profuse diaphoresis.

4. Which of the following factors would most likely decrease the client's need for insulin?
   a. steroid therapy
   b. acute illness
   c. nutritional support
   d. oral antidiabetic agents

5. Clinical manifestations of diabetic ketoacidosis include:
   a. fluid overload.
   b. progressive dehydration.
   c. absence of ketonuria.
   d. loss of consciousness.

6. Peripheral neuropathies affect:
   a. motor functions.
   b. optic functions.
   c. vascular functions.
   d. sensory functions.

7. Diabetic retinopathy causes blindness by:
   a. deposit of glucose on the retinal surface.
   b. thickening of the retina.
   c. scarring of the optic nerve.
   d. infarction of the retinal tissue.

CHAPTER 19

ASSESSING CLIENTS WITH NUTRITIONAL AND GASTROINTESTINAL DISORDERS

LEARNING OUTCOMES

After completing this chapter, you will be able to:

- Review the anatomy and physiology of the gastrointestinal system.
- Describe the processes of carbohydrate, fat, and protein metabolism.
- Describe the sources of nutrients and vitamins and their functions in the human body.
- Identify specific topics to consider during a health history assessment interview of the client with nutritional and gastrointestinal disorders.
- Describe physical assessment techniques used to evaluate nutritional and gastrointestinal status.
- Identify abnormal findings that may indicate impairment in gastrointestinal function.

KEY TOPICS

- Review of anatomy and physiology of the gastrointestinal system
- Assessment of nutritional status and the gastrointestinal system

LECTURE OUTLINE

 I. Background Anatomy and Physiology
   A. Digestive organs
      1. Mouth (oral, buccal cavity)
         a. Structures: lips, cheeks, tongue, teeth
         b. Processes:
            1. Food is chewed and mixed with saliva to form a mass or *bolus*
            2. Saliva from salivary glands facilitates taste and provides enzymes which initiate chemical breakdown of starches

      2. Pharynx
         a. Structures: oropharynx, laryngopharynx
         b. Processes
            1. Provide passageways for food, fluids, air

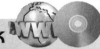

MediaLink

www.prenhall.com/lemone

Additional resources for this chapter can be found on the Student CD-ROM accompanying this textbook, and on the Companion Website at www.prenhall.com/lemone. Click on Chapter 19 to select the activities for this chapter.

CD-ROM
- Audio Glossary
- NCLEX Review

Animations
- Digestive System
- Carbohydrates
- Lipids
- Proteins

Companion Website
- More NCLEX Review
- Functional Health Pattern Assessment
- Case Study
   Weight Loss

2. Pharyngeal mucosa produces fluid to facilitate passage of bolus as it is swallowed
3. Muscles of pharynx move bolus to esophagus through peristalsis
3. Esophagus: passageway for food from pharynx to stomach
  a. Structures:
    1. Epiglottis: flap of cartilage over top of larynx that prevents food from entering larynx during swallowing
    2. Gastroesophageal sphincter: closure of esophagus at cardiac orifice of stomach
  b. Process: Food passes from pharynx to stomach
4. Stomach
  a. Regions of stomach: cardiac, fundus, body, pylorus
  b. Structures: Stomach lining
    1. Gastric glands produce gastric juice
    2. Mucous cells: produce alkaline mucus to protect stomach lining
    3. Zymogenic cells: produce pepsinogen (inactive form of pepsin)
    4. Parietal cells: secrete 2 substances:
      a. Hydrochloric acid: bactericidal; acts in protein digestion
      b. Intrinsic factor: needed for absorption of vitamin B_{12} in small intestine
    5. Enteroendocrine cells: secrete gastrin (regulates secretion and motility), histamine, endorphins, serotonin, somatostatin
  c. Innervation
    1. Secretory activity regulation
      a. Vagus nerve (parasympathetic) increases secretory activity
      b. Stimulation of sympathetic nerves decreases secretory activity
    2. Secretory activity has 3 phases
      a. Cephalic phase: preparation for digestion; triggered by sight, odor, taste, or thought of food
      b. Gastric phase: begins when food enters stomach; more gastric juice and hydrochloric acid secreted
      c. Intestinal phase: initiated by partially digested food entering small intestine; continued gastric secretion
  d. Processes:
    1. Acts as storage reservoir for food

2. Continues mechanical breakdown of food
3. Begins process of protein digestion
4. Mixes food with gastric juices into thick fluid: chyme
5. Connects esophagus and small intestine
6. Pyloric sphincter controls emptying of stomach into duodenum
7. Empties completely in 4–6 hours post normal meal
  a. Large volumes speed process
  b. Solid and fats slow process
5. Small Intestine
  a. Regions of small intestine:
    1. Duodenum (pancreatic enzymes and bile enter)
    2. Jejunum
    3. Ileum
  b. Structures
    1. Circular folds of mucosa and submucosa
    2. Villi
    3. Microvilli provide large surface area
  c. Processes
    1. Connects stomach (at pyloric sphincter) to large intestine (at ileocecal junction)
    2. Peristalsis moves contents
    3. Production of secretin and cholecystokinin when chyme enters stimulating
    4. Pancreatic enzymes and bile to enter at duodenum
    5. Chemical digestion of foods by enzymes
      a. Amylase acts on starches
      b. Trypsin and chymotrypsin act on proteins
      c. Lipases act on lipids
      d. Bile salts emulsify triglycerides
      e. Intestinal enzymes continue to further break down starches and proteins
    6. Absorption of almost all food products, water, vitamins and most electrolytes; (i.e., 10 L of fluid enters small intestine; < 1L reaches large intestine daily)
B. Accessory Digestive Organs
  1. Liver
    a. Structure:
      1. Four lobes: right, left, caudate, quadrate
      2. Encased in fibroelastic capsule

3. Tissue as lobules, plates of hepatocytes
4. Each lobule communicates with branch of hepatic artery, branch of hepatic portal vein, bile duct
5. Sinusoids, blood-filled spaces are within lobules
6. Kupffer cell line sinusoids and remove debris from blood

b. Processes
1. Synthesis of
    a. Plasma proteins and clotting factors
    b. Fats from carbohydrates and proteins for energy or as adipose tissue
    c. Phospholipids and cholesterol for production of bile salts, steroids, plasma membranes
2. Responds to glucose levels in blood
    a. Releases glucose in response to hypoglycemia
    b. Stores glucose as glycogen or fat in response to hyperglycemia
3. Stores
    a. Blood and releases stored blood during hemorrhage
    b. Iron as ferritin (needed in production of red blood cells)
    c. Fat soluble vitamins
4. Converts amino acids to carbohydrates
5. Metabolizes bilirubin
6. Lessens toxicity of chemicals, foreign molecules, hormones
7. Secretes bile: needed for emulsification and absorption of fats

2. Gallbladder
a. Structure
    1. Small sac on inferior surface of liver
    2. Connected to cystic duct which is joined to hepatic duct forming common bile duct: pathway for bile from liver to small intestine
b. Processes
    1. Concentration and storage of bile
    2. Secretion of bile into cystic duct to enter duodenum at sphincter of Oddi when fatty food enters duodenum

3. Pancreas (exocrine portion)
a. Structure: Acini, i.e., secretory cells drain into pancreatic duct, which joins the common bile duct

b. Processes
1. Secretion of pancreatic juice containing enzymes amylase, lipase, trypsin, chymotrypsin
2. Alkaline pancreatic juice neutralizes acidic chyme to optimum pH for digestion and absorption of food

C. Metabolism
1. Biochemical reaction occurring at cellular level, which produces and provides energy to maintain life
2. Metabolic reactions are either anabolic or catabolic
    a. Anabolic processes involve simple molecules combining to build more complex structures, i.e., amino acids bind to form proteins
    b. Catabolic processes involve the breakdown of complex structures to simpler forms, i.e., breakdown of carbohydrates releasing ATP, energy molecule necessary for cellular activity
3. Kilocalorie
    a. Measurement of energy value of food
    b. Amount of heat energy needed to raise temperature of 1 kilogram of water 1 degree centigrade

D. Categories of nutrients
1. Carbohydrates
    a. Primary Sources: plant foods: sugars (milk, fruits) and starches (grains, root vegetables)
    b. Energy value: 4 kcal per gram; excess converted to glycogen or fat
    c. Recommended daily intake: 125–175 gm (mostly complex)
    d. Body function: converted to glucose for cellular function
    e. Deficiency: over time tissue wasting since protein and fats are broken down and metabolic acidosis could result
2. Proteins
    a. Primary Sources
        1. Complete (all essential amino acids): animal products
        2. Incomplete (lack some amino acids): plant sources: legumes, nuts
    b. Energy value: 4 kcal per gram
    c. Recommended daily intake
        1. Male: 56 gm
        2. Female: 45 gm
        3. Additional needed with growth, pregnancy, tissue repair and healing

  d. Body function: building body tissues, enzymes, hormones, hemoglobin
3. Fats
  a. Source
    1. Saturated fats: animal products, coconuts
    2. Unsaturated fats: seeds, nuts, vegetable oil; cholesterol: meats, milk products, egg yolks
  b. Energy value: 9 kcal per gram
  c. Recommended daily intake
    1. 30% or less of daily caloric intake
    2. < 10% saturated fat
    3. Cholesterol no more than 250 mg
  d. Body function
    1. Fatty acids are essential for body cell membranes for some substances, including hormones
    2. Concentrated source of cell fuel
  e. Deficiency: excessive weight loss and skin lesions
4. Vitamins
  a. Essential organic compounds facilitate body's use of nutrients
  b. Categories:
    1. Fat Soluble: A, D, E, K which are produced or stored in body and can reach toxic levels
      a. Vitamin A: needed for vision, skin and mucous membrane integrity
      b. Vitamin D
        1. Needed for calcium homeostasis
        2. Body produces: formed by sunlight action in skin
        3. Additive to milk
      c. Vitamin E: antioxidant
      d. Vitamin K
        1. Needed for clotting proteins by the liver
        2. Body produces: synthesized by bacteria in large bowel
    2. Water Soluble: B vitamins and C which are excreted and seldom reach toxic levels
      a. Vitamin B_1 (Thiamin) needed for function of heart, muscles, nerves
      b. Vitamin B_2 (riboflavin) needed to utilize other nutrients
      c. Vitamin B_6 (pyridoxine) needed for protein metabolism
      d. Vitamin B_{12} (cyanocobalamin)
        1. Essential for red blood cell formation

    2. Not found in any plant foods
      e. Vitamin C (ascorbic acid)
        1. Antioxidant
        2. Needed for healing wounds
        3. Found in citrus fruits, vegetables
      f. Niacin (nicotinamide) needed for carbohydrate and fat metabolism
      g. Biotin needed for catabolism of fatty acids and carbohydrates
      h. Pantothenic acid needed for steroid, heme synthesis
      i. Folic acid (folacin) needed for formation of red blood cells, health of nervous system
5. Minerals
  a. Necessary for maintenance of body's structures and functioning
  b. Major minerals needed include: calcium, phosphorus, potassium, sulfur, sodium, chloride, magnesium
  c. Trace elements (necessary in small amounts) include: iron, iodine, copper, zinc, selenium
II. Health Assessment Interview: Subjective Data
  A. Record presence of any problems client relates to nutrition, digestion, discomfort in eating, bowel function
  B. Follow with specific questions related to anorexia, nausea, vomiting, diarrhea, or constipation
  C. Address specifically any changes in weight or appetite, or changes in functioning
  D. Ask client to describe typical dietary intake over 24-hour period; include beverages and water
  E. Ask client if taking any vitamins, herbal supplements
  F. Address alcohol intake
  G. Address intake of fluids especially those with sugar and/or caffeine
  H. Record presence of any food allergies of intolerance to foods
  I. Ask client to describe a healthy diet and assess the individual's diet
  J. Ask about health history including surgeries or diseases of gastrointestinal system or metabolism (diabetes mellitus), dental history
III. Physical Assessment
  A. Includes techniques of inspection, auscultation, percussion, and palpation
  B. Palpation is performed last to avoid problems with assessment of bowel sounds or causing pain

C. Parts
  1. Anthropometric assessment: obtain measurement and compare to standards
     a. Weigh client and compare to ideal body weight (IBW)
        1. 10–20% < IBW: malnutrition
        2. 10% > IBW: overweight
        3. 20% > IBW: obese
     b. Triceps Skinfold Thickness (TST) measurement
        1. Readings 10% or more below standards: malnutrition
        2. Readings 10% or more above standards: obesity
     c. Midarm circumference (MAC) measurement
        1. Decreased with malnutrition
        2. Increased with obesity
     d. Midarm Muscle Circumference (MAMC) calculation
        1. MAMC < 90% standard: mild malnutrition
        2. MAMC 60–90% standard: moderate malnutrition
        3. MAMC < 60% standard: severe malnutrition
  2. Oral assessment: examiner must wear gloves
     a. Abnormal findings of the lips
        1. Cheliosis: painful lesions at corners of mouth associated with riboflavin or niacin deficiency
        2. Clear vesicles or cold sore with herpes simplex 1
     b. Abnormal findings of the tongue
        1. Moisture: vertical fissures with dehydration
        2. Color: bright red with folic acid, B_{12}, iron deficiency; Black and hairy with post antibiotic therapy
     c. Abnormal findings of the buccal mucosa
        1. Leukoplakia (small white patches) possibly pre-malignant
        2. Reddened, dry, or swollen as with stomatitis
        3. White cheesy patches that bleed when scraped as with candidiasis
     d. Abnormal findings of the teeth and gums
        1. Excessive cavities, plaque on teeth
        2. Swollen, bleeding gums: periodontal disease, vitamin C deficiency
     e. Abnormal findings of the throat and tonsils: red swollen with white spots as with acute infections
     f. Abnormal findings of the breath
        1. Foul odor: significant for poor hygiene, liver disease, respiratory infections
        2. Fruity, sweet odor: as with ketoacidosis
        3. Acetone odor: uremia
  3. Abdominal assessment
     a. Abnormal findings upon inspection
        1. Generalized abdominal distention: obesity, gas retention
        2. Generalized abdominal distention with eversion of umbilicus: could signify ascites, presence of tumor(s)
        3. Lower abdominal distention: as with pregnancy, ovarian mass, distended bladder
        4. Sunken abdomen: malnutrition or muscle replacing fat
        5. Striae (stretch marks): conditions with rapid weight gain
        6. Spider angiomas: could signify liver disease
        7. Dilated veins: indicate possible hepatic problem
        8. Increased pulsation: could indicate aortic aneurysm
     b. Abnormal findings upon auscultation
        1. Absent bowel sounds: post surgery, late bowel obstruction, peritonitis
        2. Borborygmus (hyperactive or growling bowel sounds): diarrhea, early bowel obstruction
        3. Bruit: restricted blood flow
        4. Venous hum over liver: as with liver cirrhosis
        5. Friction rub: inflammation of spleen or liver
     c. Abnormal findings upon percussion: Dullness is heard where bowel is displaced with fluid, tumors, or filled with fecal mass
     d. Abnormal findings upon palpation
        1. Do not use deep palpation with clients with a pulsatile abdominal mass, risk for hemorrhage, renal transplant, or polycystic kidneys
        2. Findings
           a. Abdominal pain with involuntary muscle spasms could signify peritoneal irritation
           b. Abnormal masses, as with aortic aneurysm, tumors, distended bowel or bladder

    c. Boardlike abdomen: perforated
       bowel
    d. Rebound tenderness: signifies
       peritoneal irritation
  3. Specific areas
    a. Right upper quadrant pain: acute
       cholecystitis
    b. Upper middle abdominal pain:
       acute pancreatitis
    c. Right lower quadrant pain: acute
       appendicitis
    d. Left lower quadrant pain: acute
       diverticulitis

  4. Palpation of liver
    a. Enlargement with smooth tender
       edge: hepatitis, venous
       congestion
    b. Enlargement, nontender:
       malignancy
    c. Sharp pain on inspiration and
       client stops inspiring (Murphy's
       sign): inflammation of
       gallbladder

FOCUSED STUDY TIPS

- Practice physical assessment of the gastrointestinal system Become familiar with different bowel sounds. Teach a child to listen for bowel sounds and describe at his level what he is hearing.
- Evaluate a family member's level of understanding of normal nutritional status. What changes can you help him or her identify and make?

CASE STUDY

Mrs. Post is admitted to the emergency room complaining of severe abdominal pain, nausea, and vomiting. She is 3 days postop appendectomy. Her right lower quadrant abdominal incision is stapled and is clean and dry with no signs of infection. She has not had a bowel movement since surgery. Her abdomen is firm and slightly distended. No bowel sounds are audible. List subjective and objective data. Identify any abnormal assessment findings and their possible etiologies. What questions are relevant when taking Mrs. Post's history? What should be included in Mrs. Post's care plan regarding observations, measurements, and nursing interventions?

CARE PLAN CRITICAL THINKING ACTIVITY

Create a list of medical terms related to gastrointestinal assessment that are utilized when implementing a care plan. Choose terms a client must be familiar with before discharge to home. Include them in a teaching plan.

NCLEX TEST QUESTIONS

1. Which of the following vitamins is water-soluble?
   a. Vitamin C
   b. Vitamin D
   c. Vitamin B
   d. Vitamin A

2. Clients with inflamed gallbladders experience sharp pain on inspiration, then stop inspiring. This manifestation is called:
   a. McBurney's sign.
   b. McMurray's sign.
   c. Trousseau's sign.
   d. Murphy's sign.

3. An adult client tells the nurse that he needs to increase his intake of water-soluble vitamins. The nurse encourages him to increase his dietary intake of:
   a. fortified milk.
   b. wheat germ.
   c. fortified cereals.
   d. orange juice.

4. A vegetarian client asks a nurse how to increase protein intake of a meal consisting of corn tortillas and refried beans. The nurse's best response is:
   a. try to convert to eating only fish as an alternative to being a strict vegetarian.
   b. lettuce and tomato salad.
   c. add cheese and sour cream to the tortilla and beans.
   d. add lentil rice soup to the meal.

5. When doing a health assessment interview, the client states that she has lost 25 pounds in the previous 2 months. The nurse should assess the client for:
   a. positive nitrogen balance.
   b. anabolism.
   c. negative nitrogen balance.
   d. catabolism.

6. When teaching a group of clients about healthy nutrition, the nurse describes linoleic acid as the only essential fatty acid not synthesized by the body. She instructs the clients to obtain this fatty acid by including which of the following in the diet?
   a. sunflower oil
   b. butter
   c. organ meats
   d. margarine

7. The energy value of foods is measured in:
   a. calories.
   b. mg/kg.
   c. k/cal.
   d. % IBW.

CHAPTER 20

NURSING CARE OF CLIENTS WITH NUTRITIONAL DISORDERS

LEARNING OUTCOMES

After completing this chapter, you will be able to:

- Compare and contrast the pathophysiology and manifestations of nutritional disorders.
- Identify diagnostic tests used to find nutritional disorders.
- Discuss nursing implications for collaborative care for clients with nutritional disorders.
- Provide appropriate nursing care for a client receiving enteral or parenteral nutrition.
- Use appropriate techniques to assess clients with nutritional disorders (see Chapter 19).
- Use the nursing process as a framework for providing individualized nursing care for clients with nutritional disorders.

KEY TOPICS

- Obesity
- Malnutrition
- Eating disorders
- Nursing care of clients with nutritional disorders

MediaLink

www.prenhall.com/lemone

Additional resources for this chapter can be found on the Student CD-ROM accompanying this textbook, and on the Companion Website at www.prenhall.com/lemone. Click on Chapter 19 to select the activities for this chapter.

CD-ROM
- Audio Glossary
- NCLEX Review

Companion Website
- More NCLEX Review
- Case Study
  Obesity
- Care Plan Activity
  Malnutrition
- MediaLink Applications
  Establishing a Balanced Diet

LECTURE OUTLINE

I. Impact of Nutritional Disorders
   A. Affect many body systems and organs
   B. Can result in serious and chronic health disorders
   C. Involve multiple issues including developmental, sociocultural, psychologic and physiologic factors

II. Client with Obesity
   A. Incidence and prevalence
      1. One-third of Americans are obese
      2. Increased incidence in women, African Americans, economically disadvantaged
      3. Rising in children and young adults

127

© 2004 by Pearson Education, Inc.

B. Pathophysiology
1. Obesity results from excess energy intake, decreased energy expenditure or combination
2. Appetite affects food intake; regulated by central nervous system (hunger and satiety centers of hypothalamus)
3. Hormonal effects: thyroid, insulin, leptin (produced by fatty tissues)
4. Insulin associated with body fat distribution
   a. Upper body obesity (central obesity)
      1. Waist-hip ratio > 1 males; 0.8 females
      2. More intro-abdominal fat
      3. Higher levels of free fatty acids
      4. Higher risk for cardiovascular complications
   b. Lower body obesity (peripheral obesity)
      1. Waist/hip ratio < 0.8
      2. Common in females
      3. Risk cardiovascular complications
      4. More difficult to treat
C. Risk factors for obesity
1. Heredity
2. Physical inactivity
3. Environmental influences including abundance of food, fast-food restaurants; cultural, family, religious rituals centered around food
4. Psychologic factors: low self-esteem, result of anxiety, depression, "addiction to food"
D. Complications
1. Morbid obesity: weight is >100% over ideal body weight; increased mortality
2. Increased risk of insulin resistance and Diabetes Type 2
3. Altered reproductive function; in women Polycystic ovarian syndrome (PCOS)
4. Increased risk for cardiovascular disease
E. Collaborative Care: Ongoing process and individualized program of
1. Exercise
2. Diet
3. Behavior modification
F. Diagnostic Tests
1. Body Mass Index
   a. Identify percentage of fat in body
   b. Calculated by weight (kg) divided by height in meters squared (m^2)
   c. At ideal body weight: males have 10–20% body fat; females: 20–30%

2. Tests to determine physiologic cause or complication of obesity
   a. Thyroid Profile (T3, T4, TSH): thyroid problem
   b. Serum glucose: Diabetes Type 2
   c. Serum cholesterol
   d. Lipid profile (LDL, HDL levels)
   e. Electrocardiogram (effects on cardiac status)
G. Treatments
1. Exercise
   a. Increases energy consumption, promotes weight loss while preserving lean body mass; theoretically a pound of body fat is equivalent to 3500 kcal
   b. Program is tailored to meet individual needs and likes
   c. Health evaluation by health practitioner prior to starting program
   d. Clients should stop if chest pain or shortness of breath occurs
   e. Sample: 30 minutes of aerobic exercise 3–5 times/week
2. Dietary Management
   a. Low calories and fat with adequate nutrients, minerals and fiber
   b. Regular meals with small servings
   c. Gradual weight loss of no more than 1–2 pounds per week
   d. Usually 1000 to 1500 calories per day
   e. Best diet plan contains modifications without severe restrictions, low fat, well-balanced nutrition and improved eating habits
3. Behavior Modification
   a. Strategies to alter eating habits
   b. May include altering external cues which stimulate eating
   c. Support and group programs, e.g., Weight Watchers
4. Medications
   a. Short-term use
      1. Long-term efficacy questionable
      2. Also possible tolerance, addiction, side effects;
   b. Amphetamines: high potential for abuse
   c. Sibutramine (Meridia): appetite suppressants, acts on CNS, increases metabolic rate
   d. Orlistat (Xenical) inhibits fat absorption from GI tract
   e. Over-the-counter medications
      1. Phenylpropanolamine (Acutrim, Dexatrim) is adrenergic agent suppressing appetite

       2. Bulk-forming products that create sense of fullness

  5. Surgery

    a. Limited to morbidly obese who must be able to tolerate surgery, be addiction free and have had psychologic evaluation

    b. Procedures: vertical banded gastroplasty and roux-en-Y gastric bypass

    c. Reduce stomach capacity; postoperative complications high, mortality rate is low

  6. Maintaining Weight Loss

    a. Majority of dieters regain weight within 2-year period

    b. Long-term weight loss is lifelong commitment

  7. Nursing Care

    a. Promote healthy weight throughout life span; maintain active life style

    b. Adults should reduce consumed calories as energy needs change

  8. Nursing Diagnoses

    a. Imbalanced Nutrition: More than Body Requirements

    b. Activity Intolerance

    c. Ineffective Therapeutic Regimen Management

      1. Develop realistic goals

      2. Develop strategies to deal with stress eating

    d. Chronic Low Self-Esteem: Referral for counseling as appropriate

III. Client with Malnutrition

  A. Definition: inadequate intake of nutrients; major (calories, carbohydrates, proteins, fats) or micronutrients (vitamins, minerals)

  B. Incidence and Prevalence

    1. Groups at risk in U.S. include young, poor, elderly, homeless, low-income women, ethnic minorities

    2. More than half of all hospitalized clients are malnourished from serious illness or surgery

  C. Pathophysiology

    1. Starvation (inadequate dietary intake)

      a. Glycogen used for energy initially for 24 hours

      b. Proteins used to form glucose for energy (gluconeogenesis)

      c. Fats broken down into fatty acids and ketones

      d. Size of all body compartments reduces; energy expenditure decreases

    2. Acute stress: hypermetabolism and catabolism (as with illness or trauma)

      a. Increased energy expenditure and nutrient needs

      b. Lean body mass broken down to meet needs

    3. Protein-Calorie Malnutrition (PCM): condition of many hospitalized clients

      a. Admitted in starvation state and then surgery or illness promote the stress response

      b. Deficient in both calories and protein

    4. Kwashiorkor: chronic protein deficiency with adequate calories for energy

    5. Marasmus: insufficient protein and calories for body's needs

  D. Risk Factors for Malnutrition

    1. Age (older adults)

    2. Poverty, homelessness

    3. Functional health problems limiting mobility and/or vision

    4. Oral or gastrointestinal problems affecting eating, digestion

    5. Chronic illnesses and/or pain

    6. Medications or treatments that affect the appetite

    7. Acute health problems including infection, surgery, trauma

  E. Manifestations

    1. Weight loss (most apparent)

    2. Wasted appearance including dry, brittle hair, pallor

    3. Peripheral or abdominal edema

  F. Complications

    1. Impaired mobility

    2. Skin and tissue breakdown including pressure ulcers

    3. Delayed wound healing, increased risk for infection

    4. Postural hypotension related to decrease in cardiac output

  G. Collaborative Care

    1. Goal

      a. Restore ideal body weight

      b. Replace and restore adequate nutrition

    2. Diagnostic Tests

      a. Calculation of Body Mass Index (BMI) $< 18–20/m^2$

      b. Serum albumin reduced (< 3.0 g/dL)

      c. Total lymphocyte count is reduced

      d. Electrolytes: Potassium is often low with severe malnutrition

      e. Specialized procedures to evaluate malnutrition

        1. Bioelectric impedance analysis

2. Total daily energy expenditure
3. Medications: supplemental vitamin and minerals
4. Fluid and Dietary Management
   a. Correction of imbalances, particularly potassium, magnesium, calcium
   b. Gradual re-introduction of protein and calories; vitamins and minerals
   c. Fat and lactose introduced lastly
   d. Gradual refeeding to prevent further electrolyte imbalances, malabsorption and diarrhea
5. Enteral Nutrition
   a. Tube feedings used to meet caloric and protein requirements in clients unable to consume adequate food
   b. Used for clients with difficulty swallowing, unresponsiveness, oral or neck trauma/surgery, anorexia, serious illness
   c. May be total nutrition or used as a supplement
   d. Tubes
      1. Nasogastric or nasoduodenal (small-caliber soft tubes)
      2. Gastrostomy or jejunostomy tubes
   e. Tube placement checked by monitoring pH
      1. Stomach pH < 4
      2. Jejunum pH > 6
      3. Some institutions also measure length of nasal tubes at set intervals
   f. Feeding solutions
      1. Standard is 1 calorie per mL with 14% protein; 60% carbohydrates, 25–30% fat with added vitamins and minerals to meet recommended daily intake
      2. Different formulas provide more calories, protein, lower fat, fiber
      3. Usually initiated as half strength solution, small volume gradually increased
   g. Tube feedings may be administered as continuous drip feeding regulated with feeding pump or by bolus (gravity) feeding
   h. Most common complications: aspiration and diarrhea
      1. Head of bed elevated at least 30 degrees during feeding and 1 hour after feeding
      2. Tube in jejunum decreases aspiration risk

3. Formulas with fiber added can reduce diarrhea
4. Additional water is administered to prevent dehydration
6. Parenteral Nutrition
   a. Total Parenteral Nutrition (TPN) also called hyperalimentation is intravenous administration of carbohydrates, protein, electrolytes, vitamins, minerals, and fat emulsions
   b. Usually administered through a central vein, sometimes with triple lumen catheter; lesser concentrations may be given through peripheral vein
   c. Used with clients who have undergone major surgery, trauma, or are seriously malnourished
   d. Frequently maintained at home by client and family with monitoring by home health nurses
   e. Client risks associated with TPN therapy
      1. Pneumothorax, malposition with insertion of central venous catheter; correct placement and no pneumothorax is confirmed by post-insertion x-ray prior to initiation of TPN solution
      2. Potential for leakage, clotting off, dislodgement, breakage; frequent observation and infused using locked tube connections and a pump
      3. Infection: high glucose solutions are good media for bacteria and skin is disrupted from line insertion; Meticulous sterile technique with tubing and dressing changes according to protocols
      4. Fluid overload, electrolyte imbalance, hyperglycemia; Frequent monitoring of electrolytes, chemistries to guide solution content; blood glucose levels monitored by fingerstick every 6 hours
7. Nursing Care
   a. Nurses can prevent malnutrition in clients by assessing client needs and ability to meet nutritional needs
   b. NPO status should be used only as necessary
   c. Efforts should be taken to promote normal eating patterns of clients whenever possible

8. Nursing Diagnoses
   a. Imbalanced Nutrition: Less than body requirements
   b. Risk for Infection
   c. Risk for Fluid Volume Deficit: clients with malnutrition need to have intake and output monitored
   d. Risk for Impaired Skin Integrity

IV. Client with an Eating Disorder
   A. Anorexia nervosa
      1. Severely disturbed eating behavior and weight management
         a. Maintains weight loss by restricted calorie intake
         b. Sometimes includes excessive exercise
         c. Have extreme fear of gaining weight
         d. May exhibit binge-purge behavior
      2. More common in females beginning in adolescence
      3. Clients have body weight less than 85% expected for age and
      4. Often show physiological manifestations associated with starvation
      5. May develop serious complications affecting cardiac, electrolyte, acid-base status
      6. Clients tend to be obsessive, perfectionistic
   B. Bulimia nervosa
      1. Severely disturbed eating behavior and weight management
         a. Client performs binge eating followed by purging 5–10 times per week
         b. Foods eaten during binge are usually high in calories and fat
      2. Client induces vomiting by stimulating gag reflex or takes excessive quantities of laxatives or diuretics
      3. Client's weight is usually normal or slightly overweight
      4. Develop complications with fluid, electrolyte imbalance
   C. Collaborative Care
      1. Clients may require hospitalization if weight < 75% normal
      2. Treatment involves nutrition, behavioral and psychologic aspects; anti-depressant therapy
      3. Families support and involvement is essential to treatment
      4. Nursing Care
         a. Nursing role in identifying clients and referring them for treatment
         b. Early intervention may prevent altered growth and development of complications
      5. Nursing Diagnoses
         a. Imbalanced Nutrition: Less than body requirements
            1. Intervention: monitoring caloric intake
            2. Intervention: observing client 1 hour post meals to prevent purging
         b. Altered Patterns of Sexuality
         c. Chronic Low Self-esteem
         d. Disturbed Body Image
         e. Ineffective Family Therapeutic Regimen Management

FOCUSED STUDY TIPS

- Review medical records in the clinical setting to determine various nutritional abnormalities. What laboratory values are of value to determine the presence or absence of nutritional disorders?

- Visit the dietary department of a hospital or long-term care facility. Ask for sample menus for clients with nutritional disorders. Become familiar with the menus. Prepare and practice nursing interactions to convince clients of the role diet will play in achieving optimal health.

- Evaluate your diet for a 24-hour period. What excesses or deficiencies can you identify? What changes can you make to prevent nutritional disorders that may result from these excesses or deficiencies?

CASE STUDY

R.T. is a 34-year-old male admitted to the hospital with a recurrence of symptoms of inflammatory bowel disease. He is placed NPO. His initial laboratory studies in the emergency room indicate a severe electrolyte imbalance, as well as malnutrition. TPN is ordered. What are the indications for the use of total parenteral nutrition (TPN)? What is the composition of TPN? Describe anticipated nursing interventions for the client receiving TPN therapy.

CARE PLAN CRITICAL THINKING ACTIVITY

T. E. is an elderly woman being discharged from the hospital following a stroke. She has a gastrostomy tube in place and will require continuous feeds at home. She will leave with her daughter who will assume her care. What elements must discharge plans include? Prepare a teaching plan for care of the gastrostomy tube. Identify educational interventions that will indicate understanding of information presented.

NCLEX TEST QUESTIONS

1. According to the U.S. guidelines, which of the following would be the correct daily caloric requirement for a sedentary male whose IBW (ideal body weight) is 165 pounds?
   a. 2640
   b. 2740
   c. 2800
   d. 2930

2. VCLD (very low-calorie diets) are reserved for those clients who:
   a. fast.
   b. have 15 to 20% body fat.
   c. are greater than 20% overweight.
   d. are greater than 35% overweight.

3. The most accurate means to identify obesity is:
   a. weight.
   b. measures of body fat.
   c. serum lipid levels.
   d. visual assessment.

4. A client is trying to lose 6 pounds over 3 weeks. Her normal caloric intake is 1800 calories/day. The nurse helps her to plan a diet with a daily caloric intake of:
   a. 1000.
   b. 1200.
   c. 1300.
   d. 1150.

5. A client visits the clinic and tells the nurse that although she has been on a 1200 calorie diet for 3 weeks, she continues to gain weight. She also complains of fatigue, dry skin, and amenorrhea. The nurse suspects the client may be experiencing a deficiency of:
   a. hemoglobin.
   b. pancreatic enzyme.
   c. vitamins.
   d. serum thyroxine.

6. A home health nurse visits an elderly male postoperative client who tells her he has lost a lot of weight since surgery. To obtain anthropometric data from the client, the nurse should:
   a. determine if the client consumes adequate protein.
   b. gather information about medication usage.
   c. ask the client to keep a food diary to be reviewed at her next visit.
   d. measure skin folds from several body sites.

7. Which of the following is an example of aggressive nursing assessment or intervention to help prevent malnutrition associated with hospitalization or long-term care?
   a. monitoring intake and output
   b. weighing the client daily
   c. asking for immediate restoration of diet orders after NPO status
   d. keeping a food log for the client

CHAPTER 21

NURSING CARE OF CLIENTS WITH UPPER GASTROINTESTINAL DISORDERS

LEARNING OUTCOMES

After completing this chapter, you will be able to:

- Describe the pathophysiology of common disorders of the mouth, esophagus, and stomach.
- Relate the manifestations of upper gastrointestinal disorders to the pathophysiologic processes.
- List diagnostic tests used to identify disorders of the upper gastrointestinal tract.
- Discuss the nursing implications for collaborative care measures used to treat clients with upper gastrointestinal disorders.
- Use knowledge of normal anatomy and physiology and assessments to provide nursing care for clients with upper gastrointestinal disorders (see Chapter 19).
- Use the nursing process to assess needs, plan, and implement individualized care for the client with an upper gastrointestinal disorder.

KEY TOPICS

- Disorders of the mouth
- Disorders of the esophagus
- Disorders of the stomach and duodenum
- Cancers of the upper gastrointestinal system
- Nursing care of clients with upper gastrointestinal disorders

MediaLink
www.prenhall.com/lemone

Additional resources for this chapter can be found on the Student CD-ROM accompanying this textbook, and on the Companion Website at www.prenhall.com/lemone. Click on Chapter 21 to select the activities for this chapter.

CD-ROM
- Audio Glossary
- NCLEX Review

Animations
- Mouth and Throat
- Ranitidine

Companion Website
- More NCLEX Review
- Case Study
    Peptic Ulcer Disease
- Care Plan Activity
    Peptic Ulcer Disease and Pain
- MediaLink Applications
    Oral Cancer

LECTURE OUTLINE

I. Care of Clients with Disorder of the Mouth
   A. Disorder includes inflammation, infection, neoplastic lesions

B. Pathophysiology
   1. Causes include mechanical trauma, irritants such as tobacco, chemotherapeutic agents

133

© 2004 by Pearson Education, Inc.

2. Oral mucosa is relatively thin, has rich blood supply, exposed to environment
C. Manifestations
  1. Visible lesions or erosions on lips or oral mucosa
  2. Pain
D. Collaborative Care
  1. Direct observation to investigate any problems; determine underlying cause and any coexisting diseases
  2. Any undiagnosed oral lesion present for > 1 week and not responding to treatment should be evaluated for malignancy
  3. General treatment includes mouthwashes or treatments to cleanse and relieve irritation
    a. Alcohol-based mouthwashes cause pain and burning
    → b. Sodium bicarbonate mouthwashes are effective without pain
  4. Specific treatments according to type of infection
    a. Fungal (candidiasis): nystatin "swish and swallow" or clotrimazole lozenges
    b. Herpetic lesions: topical or oral acyclovir
    c. Bacterial infections: antibiotic based on culture or smear results
E. Nursing Care
  1. Goal: to relieve pain and symptoms, so client can continue food and fluid intake in health care facility and at home
  2. Impaired oral mucous membrane
    a. Assess clients at high risk
    b. Assist with oral hygiene post eating, bedtime
    c. Teach to limit irritants: tobacco, alcohol, spicy foods
  3. Imbalanced nutrition: less than body requirements
    a. Assess nutritional intake; use of straws
    b. High calorie and protein diet according to client preferences
F. Client with Oral Cancer
  1. Background
    a. Uncommon (5% of all cancers) but has high rate of morbidity, mortality
    b. Highest among males over age 40
    c. Risk factors include smoking and using oral tobacco, drinking alcohol, marijuana use, occupational exposure to chemicals, viruses (human papilloma virus)
  2. Pathophysiology
    a. Squamous cell carcinomas

    b. Begin as painless oral ulceration or lesion with irregular, ill-defined borders
    c. Lesions start in mucosa and may advance to involve tongue, oropharynx, mandible, maxilla
    d. Non-healing lesions should be evaluated for malignancy after one week of treatment
  3. Collaborative Care
    a. Elimination of causative agents
    b. Determination of malignancy with biopsy
    c. Determine staging with CT scans and MRI
    d. Based on age, tumor stage, general health and client's preference, treatment may include surgery, chemotherapy, and/or radiation therapy
    e. Advanced carcinomas may necessitate radical neck dissection with temporary or permanent tracheostomy; Surgeries may be disfiguring
    f. Plan early for home care post hospitalization, teaching family and client care involved post surgery, refer to American Cancer Society, support groups
  4. Nursing Care
    a. Health promotion:
      1. Teach risk of oral cancer associated with all tobacco use and excessive alcohol use
      2. Need to seek medical attention for all non-healing oral lesions (may be discovered by dentists); early precancerous oral lesions are very treatable
    b. Nursing Diagnoses
      1. Risk for Ineffective Airway Clearance
      2. Imbalanced Nutrition: less than body requirements
      3. Impaired Verbal Communication: establishment of specific communication plan and method should be done prior to any surgery
      4. Disturbed Body Image
II. Care of Clients with Disorders of Esophagus
  A. Gastroesophageal Reflux Disease (GERD)
    1. Definition
      a. Gastroesophageal reflux is the backward flow of gastric content into the esophagus

b. GERD common, affecting 15–20% of adults

c. 10% of persons experience daily heartburn and indigestion

d. Because of location near other organs, symptoms may mimic other illnesses including heart problems

2. Pathophysiology

 a. Gastroesophageal reflux result from transient relaxation or incompetence of lower esophageal sphincter, sphincter, or increased pressure within stomach

 b. Factors contributing to gastroesophageal reflux include

  1. Increased gastric volume (post meals)

  2. Position pushing gastric contents close to gastroesophageal juncture (such as bending or lying down)

  3. Increased gastric pressure (obesity or tight clothing)

  4. Hiatal hernia

 c. Normally the peristalsis in esophagus and bicarbonate in salivary secretions neutralize any gastric juices (acidic) that contact the esophagus; during sleep and with gastroesophageal reflux esophageal mucosa is damaged and inflamed; prolonged exposure causes ulceration, friable mucosa, and bleeding; untreated there is scarring and stricture

3. Manifestations

 a. Heartburn after meals, while bending over, or recumbent

 b. May be regurgitation of sour materials in mouth, pain with swallowing

 c. Atypical chest pain

 d. Sore throat with hoarseness

4. Complications

 a. Esophageal strictures, which can progress to dysphagia

 b. Barrett's esophagus: changes in cells lining esophagus with increased risk for esophageal cancer

5. Collaborative Care

 a. Diagnosis may be made of history of symptoms and risks

 b. Treatment includes

  1. Lifestyle changes

  2. Diet modifications

  3. Medications

 c. Surgery may be indicated for clients with serious complications

6. Diagnostic Tests

 a. Barium swallow (evaluation of esophagus, stomach, small intestine)

 b. Upper endoscopy: direct visualization; biopsies may be done

 c. 24-hour ambulatory pH monitoring

 d. Esophageal manometry which measure pressures of esophageal sphincter and peristalsis

7. Medications

 a. Antacids for mild to moderate symptoms, e.g., Maalox, Mylanta, Gaviscon

 b. H_2 receptor blockers: decrease acid production; given BID or more often, e.g., cimetidine, ranitidine, famotidine, nizatidine

 c. Proton-pump inhibitors: reduce gastric secretions, promote healing of esophageal erosion and relieve symptoms, e.g., omeprazole (Prilosec); lansoprazole (Prevacid) initially for 8 weeks; or 3 to 6 months

 d. Promotility agent: enhances esophageal clearance and gastric emptying, e.g., metoclopramide (Reglan)

8. Dietary and Lifestyle Management

 a. Elimination of acid foods (tomatoes, spicy, citrus foods, coffee)

 b. Avoiding food which relax esophageal sphincter or delay gastric emptying (fatty foods, chocolate, peppermint, alcohol)

 c. Maintain ideal body weight

 d. Eat small meals and stay right 2 hours post eating; no eating 3 hours prior to going to bed

 e. Elevate head of bed on 6–8" blocks to decrease reflux

 f. No smoking

 g. Avoiding bending and wear loose fitting clothing

9. Surgery indicated for persons not improved by diet and lifestyle changes

 a. Laparoscopic procedures to tighten lower esophageal sphincter

 b. Open surgical procedure: Nissen fundoplication

10. Nursing Care

 a. Pain usually controlled by treatment

 b. Assist client to institute home plan

B. Hiatal Hernia

 1. Definition

  a. Part of stomach protrudes through the esophageal hiatus of the diaphragm into thoracic cavity

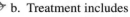

      b. Most cases are asymptomatic; incidence increases with age

      c. Sliding hiatal hernia: gastroesophageal junction and fundus of stomach slide through the esophageal hiatus

      d. Paraesophageal hiatal hernia: the gastroesophageal junction is in normal place but part of stomach herniates through esophageal hiatus; hernia can become strangulated; client may develop gastritis with bleeding

    2. Manifestations: Similar to GERD

    3. Diagnostic Tests

      a. Barium swallow

      b. Upper endoscopy

    4. Treatment

      a. Similar to GERD: diet and lifestyle changes, medications

      b. If medical treatment is not effective or hernia becomes incarcerated, then surgery; usually Nissen fundoplication by thoracic or abdominal approach

C. Impaired Esophageal Motility

    1. Types

      a. Achalasia: characterized by impaired peristalsis of smooth muscle of esophagus and impaired relaxation of lower esophageal sphincter

      b. Diffuse esophageal spasm: nonperistaltic contraction of esophageal smooth muscle

    2. Manifestations: Dysphagia and/or chest pain

    3. Treatment

      a. Endoscopically guided injection of botulinum toxin

      b. Balloon dilation of lower esophageal sphincter

D. Esophageal Cancer

    1. Definition: Relatively uncommon malignancy with high mortality rate, usually diagnosed late

    2. Pathophysiology

      a. Squamous cell carcinoma

        1. Most common affecting middle or distal portion of esophagus

        2. More common in African Americans than Caucasians

        3. Risk factors: cigarette smoking and chronic alcohol use

      b. Adenocarcinoma

        1. Nearly as common as squamous cell affecting distal portion of esophagus

        2. More common in Caucasians

        3. Associated with Barrett's esophagus, complication of chronic GERD and achalasia

    3. Manifestations

      a. Progressive dysphagia with pain while swallowing

      b. Choking, hoarseness, cough

      c. Anorexia, weight loss

    4. Collaborative Care: Treatment goals

      a. Controlling dysphagia

      b. Maintaining nutritional status while treating carcinoma (surgery, radiation therapy, and/or chemotherapy)

    5. Diagnostic Tests

      a. Barium swallow: identify irregular mucosal patterns or narrowing of lumen

      b. Esophagoscopy: allow direct visualization of tumor and biopsy

      c. Chest x-ray, CT scans, MRI: determine tumor metastases

      d. Complete Blood Count: identify anemia

      e. Serum albumin: low levels indicate malnutrition

      f. Liver function tests: elevated with liver metastasis

    6. Treatments: Dependent on stage of disease, client's condition and preference

      a. Early (curable) stage: surgical resection of affected portion with anastomosis of stomach to remaining esophagus; may also include radiation therapy and chemotherapy prior to surgery

      b. More advanced carcinoma, treatment is palliative and may include surgery, radiation, and chemotherapy to control dysphagia and pain

      c. Complications of radiation therapy include perforation, hemorrhage, stricture

    7. Nursing Care: Health promotion; education regarding risk associated with smoking and excessive alcohol intake

    8. Nursing Diagnoses

      a. Imbalanced Nutrition: less than body requirements (may include enteral tube feeding or parenteral nutrition in hospital and home)

      b. Anticipatory Grieving (dealing with cancer diagnosis)

      c. Risk for Ineffective Airway Clearance (especially during postoperative period if surgery was done)

III. Care of Clients with Disorders of Stomach and Duodenum
   A. Gastritis
      1. Definition: Inflammation of stomach lining from irritation of gastric mucosa (normally protected from gastric acid and enzymes by mucosal barrier)
      2. Types
         a. Acute Gastritis
            1. Disruption of mucosal barrier allowing hydrochloric acid and pepsin to have contact with gastric tissue: leads to irritation, inflammation, superficial erosions
            2. Gastric mucosa rapidly regenerates; self-limiting disorder
            3. Causes of acute gastritis
               a. Irritants include aspirin and other NSAIDS, corticosteroids, alcohol, caffeine
               b. Ingestion of corrosive substances: alkali or acid
               c. Effects from radiation therapy, certain chemotherapeutic agents
            4. Erosive Gastritis: form of acute which is stress-induced, complication of life-threatening condition (Curling's ulcer with burns); gastric mucosa becomes ischemic and tissue is then injured by acid of stomach
            5. Manifestations
               a. Mild: anorexia, mild epigastric discomfort, belching
               b. More severe: abdominal pain, nausea, vomiting, hematemesis, melena
               c. Erosive: not associated with pain; bleeding occurs 2 or more days post stress event
               d. If perforation occurs, signs of peritonitis
            6. Treatment
               a. NPO status to rest GI tract for 6–12 hours, reintroduce clear liquids gradually and progress; intravenous fluid and electrolytes if indicated
               b. Medications: proton-pump inhibitor or H_2 receptor blocker; sucralfate (carafate) acts locally; coats and protects gastric mucosa
               c. If gastritis from corrosive substance: immediate dilution and removal of substance by gastric lavage (washing out stomach contents via nasogastric tube), no vomiting
         b. Chronic Gastritis
            1. Progressive disorder beginning with superficial inflammation and leads to atrophy of gastric tissues
            2. Type A: autoimmune component and affecting persons of northern European descent; loss of hydrochloric acid and pepsin secretion; develops pernicious anemia
            3. Type B: more common and occurs with aging; caused by chronic infection of mucosa by *Helicobacter pylori;* associated with risk of peptic ulcer disease and gastric cancer
            4. Manifestations
               a. Vague gastric distress, epigastric heaviness not relieved by antacids
               b. Fatigue associated with anemia; symptoms associated with pernicious anemia: paresthesias
            5. Treatment: Type B: eradicate *H. pylori* infection with combination therapy of two antibiotics (metronidazole and clarithomycin or tetracycline) and proton-pump inhibitor
      3. Collaborative Care
         a. Usually managed in community
         b. Teach food safety measures to prevent acute gastritis from food contaminated with bacteria
         c. Management of acute gastritis with NPO state and then gradual reintroduction of fluids with electrolytes and glucose and advance to solid foods
         d. Teaching regarding use of prescribed medications, smoking cessation, treatment of alcohol abuse
      4. Diagnostic tests
         a. Gastric analysis: assess hydrochloric acid secretion (less with chronic gastritis)
         b. Hemoglobin, hematocrit, red blood cell indices: anemia including pernicious or iron deficiency
         c. Serum vitamin B_{12} levels: determine pernicious anemia

    d. Upper endoscopy: visualize mucosa, identify areas of bleeding, obtain biopsies; may treat areas of bleeding with electro or laser coagulation or sclerosing agent
  5. Nursing Diagnoses
    a. Fluid Volume Deficit
    b. Imbalanced Nutrition: less than body requirements
B. Peptic Ulcer Disease (PUD)
  1. Definition and risk factors
    a. Break in mucous lining of GI tract comes into contact with gastric juice; affects 10% of U.S. population
    b. Duodenal ulcers: most common; affect mostly males ages 30–55; ulcers found near pyloris
    c. Gastric ulcers: affect older persons (ages 55–70); found on lesser curvature and associated with increased incidence of gastric cancer
    d. Common in smokers, users of NSAIDS; familial pattern
  2. Pathophysiology
    a. Ulcers or breaks in mucosa of GI tract occurs with
      1. *H. pylori* infection (spread by oral to oral, fecal-oral routes) damages gastric epithelial cells reducing effectiveness of gastric mucus
      2. Use of NSAIDS: interrupts prostaglandin synthesis which maintains mucous barrier of gastric mucosa
    b. Chronic with spontaneous remissions and exacerbations associated with trauma, infection, physical or psychological stress
  3. Manifestations
    a. Pain is classic symptom: gnawing, burning, aching hungerlike in epigastric region possibly radiating to back; occurs when stomach is empty and relieved by food (pain: food: relief pattern)
    b. Symptoms less clear in older adult; may have poorly localized discomfort, dysphagia, weight loss; presenting symptom may be complication: GI hemorrhage or perforation of stomach or duodenum
  4. Complications
    a. Hemorrhage: frequent in older adult: hematemesis, melena, hematochezia (blood in stool); weakness, fatigue, dizziness, orthostatic hypotension and anemia; with significant blood loss may develop hypovolemic shock
    b. Obstruction: gastric outlet obstruction: edema surrounding ulcer blocks GI tract from muscle spasm or scar tissue
      1. Gradual process
      2. Symptoms: feelings of epigastric fullness, nausea, worsened ulcer symptoms
    c. Perforation: ulcer erodes through mucosal wall and gastric or duodenal contents enter peritoneum leading to peritonitis; chemical at first (inflammatory) and then bacterial in 6 to 12 hours
      1. Time of ulceration: severe upper abdominal pain radiating throughout abdomen and possibly to shoulder
      2. Abdomen becomes rigid, boardlike with absent bowel sounds; symptoms of shock
      3. Older adults may present with mental confusion and non-specific symptoms
  5. Zollinger-Ellison syndrome
    a. Peptic ulcer disease caused by gastrinoma (tumor in pancreas, stomach, or intestine which secretes gastrin)
    b. Excess gastric acid leads to ulceration and often bleeding and perforation
    c. Excess hydrochloric acid production also leads to diarrhea and steatorrhea (excess fat in stools)
  6. Collaborative Care
    a. Elimination of *H. pylori*
    b. Prevention of or treatment of ulcers from NSAIDS use
  7. Diagnostic Tests
    a. Upper GI series detects up to 90% of ulcers
    b. Gastroscopy: visualization of esophageal, gastric, and duodenal mucosa for ulcers, perform biopsies
    c. Tests for *H. pylori*
      1. Biopsy urease test on specimen biopsy
      2. Urea breath test (non-invasive)
      3. Serologic testing
    d. Gastric analysis: analysis of stomach contents aspirated through naso-gastric tube; diagnosis of Zollinger-Ellison syndrome

8. Treatment
   a. Medications
      1. Control of *H. pylori* with combination therapy of two antibiotics and proton-pump inhibitors or bismuth subsalicylate
      2. Stop NSAID use or add twice a day proton-pump inhibitors
   b. Specific medication interventions
      1. Proton-pump inhibitors often heal ulcers in 4 weeks
      2. Histamine$_2$ blockers are used for 8 weeks or longer to heal ulcers and can interact with other medications
      3. Sulcralfate: binds to ulcer base forming protective barrier
      4. Bismuth compounds (including Pepto-Bismol) stimulate mucosal bicarbonate and prostaglandin production to heal ulcers; antibacterial against *H. pylori*
      5. Prostaglandin analogs (misoprostol): prevent NSAID-induced ulcers
      6. Antacids: rapid relief of ulcer symptoms; need to be taken frequently and not with other medications, inexpensive
   c. Dietary Management
      1. Maintain good nutrition: balanced meals at regular intervals
      2. Limited alcohol intake; stop smoking
   d. Surgery no longer part of treatment, but may see clients who have had surgical treatment in past and may have long-term complications
   e. Treatment of complication hemorrhage
      1. Restore and maintain circulation with intravenous fluids and/or blood transfusions
      2. Gastroscopy with interventions to control bleeding (laser, electrocautery, sclerosing agents)
      3. Maintain NPO status with nasogastric tube; antacids per nasogastric tube and intravenous H$_2$ receptor blockers
      4. Surgery may be indicated if medical treatment does not control bleeding
   f. Treatment of complication gastric outlet obstruction
      1. Gastric decompression with nasogastric suction, intravenous and electrolyte replacement

2. Intravenous H$_2$ receptor blockers
      3. Endoscopy for balloon dilation of gastric outlet
      4. Surgery if other methods are not successful
   g. Treatment of complication perforation
      1. Gastric decompression with nasogastric suction, intravenous and electrolyte replacement
      2. Fowler's or semi-Fowler's positioning
      3. Aggressive intravenous antibiotic therapy
      4. Laparoscopic or open laparotomy to close perforation
9. Nursing Diagnoses
   a. Pain: clients should eliminate any food found to precipitate pain
   b. Sleep Pattern Disturbance related to ulcer pain
   c. Imbalanced Nutrition: less than body requirements: Six small meals may be more effective in avoiding symptoms
   d. Deficient Fluid Volume: prevent hypovolemic shock and allow adequate replacement for nasogastric drainage with intravenous fluids and electrolytes
10. Home care involves teaching clients medication regimens and an action plan, including recognition of complications and to seek medical assistance for complications
C. Cancer of Stomach
   1. Incidence
      a. Worldwide common cancer, but less common in U.S.
      b. Incidence highest among Hispanics, African Americans, Asian Americans, males twice as often as females
      c. Older adults of lower socioeconomic groups higher risk
   2. Pathophysiology
      a. Adenocarcinoma most common form involving mucus-producing cells of stomach in distal portion
      b. Begins as localized lesion (in situ) progresses to mucosa; spreads to lymph nodes and metastasizes early in disease to liver, lungs, ovaries, peritoneum
   3. Risk factors
      a. *H. pylori* infection
      b. Genetic predisposition
      c. Chronic gastritis, pernicious anemia, gastric polyps

d. Achlorhydria (lack of hydrochloric acid)
e. Diet high in smoked foods and nitrates
4. Manifestations
   a. Disease often advanced with metastasis when diagnosed
   b. Early symptoms are vague: early satiety, anorexia, indigestion, vomiting, pain after meals not responding to antacids
   c. Later symptoms: weight loss, cachexia (wasted away appearance), abdominal mass, stool positive for occult blood
5. Collaborative Care
   a. Support client through testing
   b. Assist client to maintain adequate nutrition
6. Diagnostic Tests
   a. CBC indicates anemia
   b. Upper GI series, ultrasound identifies a mass
   c. Upper endoscopy: visualization and tissue biopsy of lesion
7. Treatment
   a. Surgery if diagnosis made prior to metastasis
      1. Partial gastrectomy with anastomosis to duodenum: Bilroth I or gastroduodenostomy
      2. Partial gastrectomy with anastomosis to jejunum: Bilroth II or gastrojejunostomy
      3. Total gastrectomy (if cancer diffuse but limited to stomach) with esophagojejunostomy
   b. Complications associated with gastric surgery
      1. Dumping Syndrome
         a. Occurs with partial gastrectomy; hypertonic, undigested chyme bolus rapidly enters small intestine and pulls fluid into intestine causing decrease in circulating blood volume and increased intestinal peristalsis and motility
         b. Manifestations 5–30 minutes after meal: nausea with possible vomiting, epigastric pain and cramping, borborygmi, and diarrhea; client becomes tachycardic, hypotensive, dizzy, flushed, diaphoretic
         c. Manifestations 2–3 hours after meal: symptoms of hypoglycemia in response to excessive release of insulin that occurred from rise in blood glucose when chyme entered intestine
         d. Treatment: dietary pattern to delay gastric emptying and allow smaller amounts of chyme to enter intestine
            1. Liquids and solids taken separately
            2. Increased amounts of fat and protein
            3. Carbohydrates, especially simple sugars, reduced
            4. Client to rest recumbent or semi-recumbent 30–60 minutes after eating
            5. Anticholinergics, sedatives, antispasmodic medications may be added
      2. Anemia: iron deficiency and/or pernicious
      3. Folic acid deficiency
      4. Poor absorption of calcium, vitamin D
   c. Radiation and/or chemotherapy to control metastasic spread
   d. Palliative treatment including surgery, chemotherapy; client may have gastrostomy or jejunostomy tube inserted
8. Nursing Diagnoses
   a. Imbalanced Nutrition: less than body requirement: consult dietician since client at risk for protein-calorie malnutrition
   b. Anticipatory Grieving
9. Home care centers around maintaining nutrition (often enteral or parenteral feedings); pain management, hospice care

FOCUSED STUDY TIPS

- Compare and contrast mouth assessments of clients in the clinical setting. Identify differences in assessment findings. Describe factors that influence the differences in the assessments.
- Reflect on nursing interventions you might implement to keep your client's mouth as clean as you want your own.
- Interview a family member, friend, or client experiencing an upper gastrointestinal disorder. Evaluate the impact the disorder has on nutritional status.

CARE PLAN CRITICAL THINKING ACTIVITY

Proton-Pump Inhibitors (PPIs) are the drugs of choice for severe (GERD). What are PPIs and how do they work? What are the nursing responsibilities related to PPI therapy? For discharge teaching of GERD clients, what four primary instructions must clients and family know when going home with this drug therapy?

CASE STUDY

T. C. is 8 months postop partial gastrectomy with jejunal anastamosis. He has been admitted to the hospital for "dumping syndrome." He asks you to explain exactly what this diagnosis is. What do you tell him? How is his nursing care managed in the hospital? What will be included in his discharge teaching plan?

NCLEX TEST QUESTIONS

1. A 40-year-old client is hospitalized for gastrointestinal (GI) bleeding. Orders include nasogastric tube (NGT) placement with irrigations until the returns are clear. Which fluid should be used for the nasogastric (NG) irrigations?
   a. 3% saline
   b. D_5W
   c. normal saline
   d. plain water

2. A client says to the nurse, "My doctor told me my ulcer may have been caused by bacteria. I didn't know that bacteria could cause an ulcer." Which of the following responses by the nurse is the best?
   a. "If it was caused by bacteria, you would have a fever as a result of the inflammatory process."
   b. "We know that ulcers are communicable. They can be spread easily. Be careful you don't spread it to your children."
   c. "Diet and stress have nothing to do with developing an ulcer."
   d. Even though the bacteria *Helicobacter pylori* causes ulcer formation, we really don't know how it does cause ulcers."

3. The nurse is caring for a female client during recuperation following development of a duodenal ulcer. The client suddenly experiences severe abdominal pain, increased heart rate, increased respiratory rate, and diaphoresis. On palpation, the abdomen is rigid; bowel sounds are faint and diminished. Which of the following nursing actions is appropriate?
   a. Immediately place her in high Fowler's position to facilitate breathing.
   b. Help her walk to the bathroom to get rid of any flatus.
   c. Check to see if she has food allergies and see if she ate anything to which she might be allergic.
   d. Establish IV access and call the physician after obtaining the necessary data.

4. A client with a history of peptic ulcer disease is taking ranitidine (Zantac). He questions the action of this drug. The best answer for the nurse to give is:
   a. "It blocks the secretion of hydrochloric (HCl) acid in the stomach."
   b. "It coats the lining of the stomach."
   c. "The release of gastric acid is increased."
   d. "The histamine receptors become more sensitive and act to protect the stomach."

5. A client with borborygmi, cramping pain, vomiting, and diarrhea has a diagnosis of peptic ulcer disease (PUD) with recent surgical treatment. The client is probably experiencing which of the following?
   a. dumping syndrome
   b. complications of the PUD
   c. perforation of the stomach
   d. peritonitis

6. A female client hospitalized for a broken pelvis from a motor vehicle accident is being sent home on an H₂-antagonist and an antacid as part of her home medications. When the client questions why, the nurse explains that
   a. the medications are a preventive measure only.
   b. she has GERD because of the other medications she is taking.
   c. the stress of the accident and injury caused a stress ulcer.
   d. she probably always had an ulcer and didn't know it.

7. A client is taking cimetidine (Tagamet) for treatment of a peptic ulcer. Which of the following instructions should the nurse give the client about the administration of this drug?
   a. Take the drug on an empty stomach.
   b. Take the drug with an antacid.
   c. Avoid fluids for an hour before and after taking the drug.
   d. Take the drug with meals and at bedtime.

8. A client states, "My doctor told me to quit taking aspirin since I've developed this ulcer. I have to take aspirin to keep my arthritis from hurting. I don't know what to do." Which response on the part of the nurse is best?
   a. "Let's worry about treating your ulcer. Your arthritis will have to wait."
   b. "Aspirin is one of the medications that makes an ulcer worse. Another medicine can be ordered by the doctor for your arthritis."
   c. "Go ahead and take the aspirin if it helps, but watch closely for bleeding."
   d. "The doctor knows what is best for you, and you should follow those instructions."

9. Which of the following results would indicate a problem with the patency of a gastrostomy tube?
   a. The nurse aspirates only 5 mL of stomach contents.
   b. The nurse is unable to inject air into the tube.
   c. Blood is coming from the tube opening.
   d. The return aspirate is full of a green bile-like substance.

10. A client has a nasogastric (NG) tube in place for gastric decompression and complains of increasing nausea. Which action should the nurse take first?
    a. advance the tube 2 cm
    b. place client in a recumbent position
    c. instill 20 ml of saline
    d. obtain abdominal X-ray to assess placement

CHAPTER 22

NURSING CARE OF CLIENTS WITH GALLBLADDER, LIVER, AND PANCREATIC DISORDERS

LEARNING OUTCOMES

After completing this chapter, you will be able to:

- Describe the pathophysiology of commonly occurring disorders of the gallbladder, liver, and exocrine pancreas.
- Relate knowledge of normal anatomy and physiology to the manifestations and effects of biliary, hepatic, and pancreatic disorders.
- Discuss diagnostic tests, including client preparation, used to identify biliary, hepatic, and pancreatic disorders.
- Discuss nursing implications for dietary and pharmacologic interventions used for clients with these disorders.
- Provide appropriate nursing care for the client who has surgery of the gallbladder, liver, or pancreas.
- Relate changes in normal assessment data to the pathophysiology and manifestations of gallbladder, liver, and exocrine pancreatic disorders.
- Use the nursing process to plan and provide individualized care for clients with disorders of the gallbladder, liver, or exocrine pancreas.

KEY TOPICS

- Gallbladder disorders
- Liver disorders
- Exocrine pancreatic disorders
- Nursing care of clients with gallbladder, liver, and pancreatic disorders

LECTURE OUTLINE

I. Gallbladder Disorders
   A. Cholelithiasis and Cholecystitis
      1. Definitions

MediaLink

www.prenhall.com/lemone

Additional resources for this chapter can be found on the Student CD-ROM accompanying this textbook, and on the Companion Website at www.prenhall.com/lemone. Click on Chapter 22 to select the activities for this chapter.

CD-ROM
- Audio Glossary
- NCLEX Review

Animation
- Cirrhosis

Companion Website
- More NCLEX Review
- Case Study
   Hepatitis B
- Care Plan Activity
   Hepatitis A
- MediaLink Applications
   Treatment of Liver Cancer

   a. Cholelithiasis: formation of stones (calculi) within the gallbladder or biliary duct system

143

b. Cholecystitis: inflammation of gall bladder

c. Cholangitis: inflammation of the biliary ducts

2. Pathophysiology

   a. Gallstones form due to

     1. Abnormal bile composition

     2. Biliary stasis

     3. Inflammation of gallbladder

   b. Most gallstones are composed primarily of bile (80%); remainder are composed of a mixture of bile components

   c. Excess cholesterol in bile is associated with obesity, high-cholesterol diet and drugs that lower cholesterol levels

   d. If stones from gallbladder lodge in the cystic duct

     1. There can be reflux of bile into the gallbladder and liver

     2. Gallbladder has increased pressure leading to ischemia and inflammation

     3. Severe ischemia can lead to necrosis of the gall bladder

     4. If the common bile duct is obstructed, pancreatitis can develop

3. Risk factors for cholelithiasis

   a. Age

   b. Family history, also Native Americans and persons of northern European heritage

   c. Obesity, hyperlipidemia

   d. Females, use of oral contraceptives

   e. Conditions which lead to biliary stasis: pregnancy, fasting, prolonged parenteral nutrition

   f. Diseases including cirrhosis, ileal disease or resection, sickle-cell anemia, glucose intolerance

4. Manifestations of cholelithiasis

   a. Many persons are asymptomatic

   b. Early symptoms are epigastic fullness after meals or mild distress after eating a fatty meal

   c. Biliary colic (if stone is blocking cystic or common bile duct): steady pain in epigastric or RUQ (right upper quadrant) of abdomen lasting up to 5 hours with nausea and vomiting

   d. Jaundice may occur if there is obstruction of common bile duct

5. Manifestations of acute cholecystitis

   a. Episode of biliary colic involving RUQ pain radiating to back, right scapula, or shoulder; the pain may be aggravated by movement, or deep breathing and lasting 12–18 hours

   b. Anorexia, nausea, and vomiting

   c. Fever with chills

6. Complications of cholecystitis

   a. Chronic cholecystitis occurs after repeated attacks of acute cholecystitis; often asymptomatic

   b. Empyema: collection of infected fluid within gallbladder

   c. Gangrene of gall bladder with perforation leading to peritonitis, abscess formation

   d. Pancreatitis, liver damage, intestinal obstruction

7. Collaborative Care

   a. Treatment depends on the acuity of symptoms and client's health status

   b. Clients experiencing symptoms are usually treated with surgical removal of the stones and gallbladder

8. Diagnostic Tests

   a. Serum bilirubin: conjugated bilirubin is elevated with bile duct obstruction

   b. CBC reveals elevation in the WBC as with infection and inflammation

   c. Serum amylase and lipase are elevated, if obstruction of the common bile duct has caused pancreatitis

   d. Ultrasound of gallbladder: identifies presence of gallstones

   e. Other tests may include flat plate of the abdomen, oral cholecytogram, gall bladder scan

9. Treatment

   a. Treatment of choice is laparoscopic cholecystectomy

   b. If surgery is inappropriate due to client condition

     1. May attempt to dissolve the gallstones with medications

     2. Medications are costly, long duration

     3. Stones reoccur when treatment is stopped

10. Laparoscopic cholecystectomy

   a. Minimally invasive procedure with low risk of complications; required hospital stay < 24 hours

   b. Learning needs of client and family/caregiver include pain control, deep breathing, mobilization, incisional care and nutritional/fluids needs

c. Client is given phone contact for problems

11. Some clients require a surgical laparotomy (incision inside the abdomen) to remove gall bladder

   a. Client will have nasogastric tube in place post-operatively and require several days of hospitalization

   b. If exploration of the common bile duct is done with the cholecystectomy, the client may have a T-tube inserted which promotes bile passage to the outside as area heals

12. Clients with cholelithiasis and cholecystitis prior to surgery can avoid future attacks by limiting fat intake

13. Nursing Diagnoses

   a. Pain

   b. Imbalanced Nutrition: less than body requirements

   c. Risk for Infection

B. Cancer of the Gallbladder

   1. Relatively rare, affecting females > 65

   2. Usually advanced disease at time of diagnosis and is only treated palliatively

   3. Manifestations include intense pain, palpable mass in RUQ, jaundice, weight loss

   4. Nursing care focuses on comfort and palliative care

II. Liver Disorders

A. Hepatitis

   1. Definition: inflammation of the liver due to virus, exposure to alcohol, drugs, toxins; may be acute or chronic in nature

   2. Pathophysiology: metabolic functions and bile elimination functions of the liver are disrupted by the inflammation of the liver

B. Viral Hepatitis

   1. Types (causative agents)

      a. Hepatitis A virus (HAV) Infectious hepatitis

         1. Transmission: fecal-oral route, often contaminated foods, water or direct contact

         2. Contagious through stool up to 2 weeks before symptoms occur; abrupt onset

         3. Benign, self limited; symptoms last up to 2 months

      b. Hepatitis B virus (HBV)

         1. Transmission: infected blood and body fluids

         2. Liver cells damaged by immune response; increased risk for primary liver cancer; causes acute and chronic hepatitis, fulminant hepatitis and carrier state

         3. High risk to health care workers, injection drug users, men who have sex with men, person with multiple sexual partners, persons exposed to blood products (hemodialysis clients)

      c. Hepatitis C virus (HCV)

         1. Transmission: infected blood and body fluids; injection drug use is primary factor

         2. Initial manifestations are mild, nonspecific

         3. Primary worldwide cause of chronic hepatitis, cirrhosis, liver cancer

      d. Hepatitis B-associated delta virus (HDV)

         1. Transmission: infected blood and body fluids; causes infection in people who are also infected with Hepatitis B

         2. Causes acute or chronic infection

      e. Hepatitis E virus (HEV)

         1. Transmission: fecal-oral route, contaminated water supplies in developing nations; rare in U.S.

         2. Affects young adults; fulminant in pregnant women

   2. Disease Pattern Associated with hepatitis (all types)

      a. Incubation Phase (period after exposure to virus): no symptoms

      b. Prodromal Phase (preicteric—before jaundice)

         1. "Flu" symptoms: general malaise, anorexia, fatigue, muscle and body aches

         2. Nausea, vomiting, diarrhea, constipation, and mild RUQ abdominal pain

         3. Chills and fever

      c. Icteric (jaundiced) Phase

         1. 5–10 days after prodromal symptoms

         2. Jaundice of the sclera, skin and mucous membranes occurs

         3. Elevation of serum bilirubin

         4. Pruritis

         5. Stool become light brown or clay colored

         6. Urine is brownish colored

      d. Convalescent Phase

    1. In uncomplicated cases, symptoms improve and spontaneous recovery occurs within 2 weeks of jaundice

    2. Lasts several weeks; continued improvement and liver enzymes improve

3. Chronic hepatitis

  a. Chronic hepatitis: chronic infection from viruses: HBV, HBC, HBD

    1. Few symptoms (fatigue, malaise, hepatomegaly)

    2. Primary cause of cirrhosis, liver cancer, liver transplants

    3. Liver enzymes are elevated

  b. Fulminant hepatitis: rapidly progressive disease with liver failure developing within 2–3 weeks of onset of symptoms; rare but usually due to HBV with HBD infections

  c. Toxic hepatitis

    1. Hepatocellular damage results from toxic substances

    2. Includes alcoholic hepatitis, acute toxic reaction or chronic use

    3. Toxic substances include medications such as acetaminophen, benzene, carbon tetrachloride, halothane, chloroform, poisonous mushrooms

  d. Hepatobiliary hepatitis

    1. Due to cholestasis, interruption of normal flow of bile

    2. Causes include cholelithiasis, oral contraceptive use

4. Collaborative Care: Focus is on determination of cause, treatment and support, and prevention of future liver damage

5. Diagnostic Tests

  a. Liver function tests

    1. Alanine aminotransferase (ALT): specific to liver

    2. Aspartate aminotransferase (AST): heart and liver cells

    3. Alkaline phosphatase (ALP): liver and bone cells

    4. Gamma-glutamyltransferase (GGT): present in cell membranes; rises with hepatitis and obstructive biliary disease

    5. Lactic dehydrogenase (LDH): present in many body tissues; isoenzyme, LDH5 is specific to the liver

    6. Serum bilirubin levels: total, conjugated, unconjugated

  b. Lab tests for viral antigens and antibodies associated with types of viral hepatitis

  c. Liver biopsy: tissue examined to detect changes and make diagnosis

    1. Preparation: signed consent; NPO 4–6 hours before

    2. Prothrombin time and platelet count results; may need Vitamin K first to correct

    3. Client voids prior to procedure, supine position

    4. Local anesthetic; client instructed to hold breath during needle insertion

    5. Direct pressure applied to site after sample obtained; client placed on right side to maintain site pressure

    6. Vital signs monitored frequently for 2 hours

    7. No coughing, lifting, straining 1–2 weeks afterward

6. Medications for prevention of hepatitis

  a. Vaccines available for Hepatitis A and B

  b. Vaccine for Hepatitis B recommended for high-risk groups

  c. Post exposure prophylaxis recommended for household and sexual contacts of persons with HAV or HBV

  d. Hepatitis A prophylaxis: single dose of immune globulin within 2 weeks of exposure

  e. Hepatitis B prophylaxis: Hepatitis B immune globulin (HBIG) for short-term immunity; HBV vaccine may be given at the same time

7. Treatment

  a. Medications

    1. Medication for acute Hepatitis C: interferon alpha to prevent chronic hepatitis

    2. Chronic Hepatitis B: interferon alpha intramuscular or subcutaneously or lamivudine

    3. Chronic Hepatitis C: interferon alpha with ribavirin (Rebetol) oral antiviral drug

  b. Acute hepatitis treatment

    1. As needed bedrest

    2. Adequate nutrition

    3. Avoid substances toxic to the liver especially alcohol

  c. Complementary therapies: Milk thistle (silymarin)

8. Nursing Care: Teaching about prevention by stressing
   a. Hygiene
   b. Handwashing, especially for food handlers
   c. Blood and body fluids precautions
   d. Vaccines for persons at high risk
9. Nursing Diagnoses
   a. Risk for Infection
      1. Standard precautions, proper hand washing at all times
      2. Reporting of contagious disease to health department to control spread of disease
   b. Fatigue
      1. Scheduling planned rest periods
      2. Gradual increase of activity with improvement
   c. Imbalanced Nutrition: Less than body requirements
      1. High caloric diet with adequate carbohydrates
      2. Small frequent meals; nutritional supplements
   d. Body Image Disturbance
10. Home care must include proper infection control measures; continuing medical care

C. Cirrhosis
1. Definition
   a. End state of chronic liver disease
   b. Progressive and irreversible
   c. Tenth leading cause of death in U.S.
2. Pathophysiology
   a. Functional liver tissue gradually destroyed and replaced with fibrous scar tissue
   b. As hepatocytes are destroyed, metabolic functions are lost
   c. Blood and bile flow within liver is disrupted
   d. Portal hypertension develops
3. Alcoholic cirrhosis (Laennec's cirrhosis)
   a. Alcohol causes metabolic changes in liver leading to fatty infiltration (stage in which abstinence from alcohol could allow liver to heal)
   b. With continued alcohol abuse, inflammatory cells infiltrate liver causing necrosis, fibrosis and destruction of liver tissue
   c. Regenerative nodules form, liver shrinks and is nodular
   d. Malnutrition commonly present
4. Biliary cirrhosis: bile flow is obstructed and is retained within liver causing

inflammation, fibrosis and regenerative nodules to form
5. Posthepatic cirrhosis: Chronic Hepatitis B or C and unknown cause leads to liver shrinkage and nodule formation with extensive liver cell loss and fibrosis
6. Manifestations
   a. Early: liver enlargement and tenderness, dull ache in RUQ, weight loss, weakness, anorexia, diarrhea or constipation
   b. Progresses to impaired metabolism causing bleeding, ascites, gynecomastia in men, infertility in women, jaundice, neurological changes, peripheral edema, anemia, low WBC and platelets
7. Complications
   a. Portal hypertension: shunting of blood to collateral blood vessels leading to engorged veins in esophagus, rectum and abdomen, ascites
   b. Splenomegaly: anemia, leucopenia, thrombocytopenia
   c. Ascites: accumulation of protein rich in protein; hypoalbuminemia, sodium and water retention
   d. Esophageal varices: thin walled dilated veins in esophagus which may rupture leading to massive hemorrhage
   e. Hepatic encephalopathy: from accumulated neurotoxins in blood; ammonia produced in gut is not converted to urea and accumulates in blood; medications may not be metabolized and add to mental changes including personality changes, slowed mentation, asterixis (liver flap); progressing to confusion, disorientation and coma
   f. Hepatorenal syndrome: renal failure with azotemia
8. Collaborative Care: Holistic care to client and family addressing physiologic, psychosocial, spiritual needs
9. Diagnostic Tests
   a. Liver function tests (ALT, AST, alkaline phosphatase, GGT); elevated, but not as high as with acute hepatitis
   b. CBC and platelets: anemia, leucopenia, thrombocytopenia
   c. Prothrombin time: prolonged (impaired coagulation due to lack of Vitamin K)

   d. Serum electrolytes: deficiencies in sodium, potassium, phosphate, magnesium
   e. Bilirubin: elevated
   f. Serum albumin: hypoalbuminemia
   g. Serum ammonia: elevated
   h. Serum glucose and cholesterol
   i. Abdominal ultrasound: evaluation of liver size and nodularity, ascites
   j. Upper endoscopy: diagnose and possibly treat esophageal varices
   k. Liver biopsy: may be done to diagnose cirrhosis; may be deferred if bleeding times are elevated
10. Medications
   a. Medications are used to treat complications and effects of cirrhosis; all liver toxic drugs (sedatives, hypnotics, acetaminophen) and alcohol must be avoided
   b. Diuretics: spironolactone (Aldactone) works against increased aldosterone levels, furosemide (Lasix)
   c. Medications to decrease manifestations of hepatic encephalopathy by reducing number of ammonia forming bacteria in bowel and converts ammonia to ammonium which is excreted in stool; Lactulose, Neomycin
   d. Beta-blocker nadolol (Corgard) with isosorbide mononitrate (Ismo, Imdur) used to prevent esophageal varices from rebleeding
   e. Ferrous sulfate and folic acid to treat anemia
   f. Vitamin K to reduce risk of bleeding
   g. Antacids to decrease risk of acute gastritis
   h. Oxazepam (Serax) benzodiazepine antianxiety/sedative drug not metabolized by liver; used to treat acute agitation
11. Treatment: Dietary and fluid management
   a. Fluid and sodium restrictions based on response to diuretic therapy, urine output, electrolyte values
   b. Protein: 75–100 grams per day; unless client has hepatic encephalopathy (elevated ammonia levels), then 60–80 gm/day
   c. Diet high in carbohydrates, moderate in fats or as total parenteral nutrition (TPN)

   d. Vitamin and mineral supplements; deficiencies often include B vitamins, and A, D, E, magnesium
12. Treatment: Complication management
   a. For ascites and associated respiratory distress: Paracentesis
   b. For bleeding esophageal varices
      1. Restore hemodynamic stability with fluids, blood transfusion and fresh frozen plasma (contains clotting factors)
      2. Control bleeding with vasoconstrictive medications: somatostatin or octreotide, vasopressin
      3. Upper endoscopy to treat varices with banding (variceal ligation or endoscopic sclerosis)
      4. Balloon tamponade, if bleeding not controlled or endoscopy unavailable as short term measure: multiple-lumen naso-gastric tube such as Sengstaken-Blakemore tube or Minnesota tube which have gastric and esophageal balloons to apply tension to control bleeding
   c. Insertion of transjugular intrahepatic portosystemic shunt (TIPS), a short-term measure to control portal hypertension (varices and ascites); using a stent to channel blood between portal and hepatic vein and bypassing liver (increases risk for hepatic encephalopathy)
   d. Surgery: liver transplant; contraindications include malignancy, active alcohol or drug abuse, poor surgical risk
13. Nursing Care
   a. Health promotion includes education about relationship of alcohol and drug abuse with liver disorders; avoidance of viral hepatitis
   b. Home care includes teaching family to participate in disease management, possible hospice care
14. Nursing Diagnoses
   a. Fluid Volume Excess
   b. Disturbed Thought Processes: Early identification of encephalopathy and appropriate interventions, i.e., client safety, avoidance of hepatoxic medications, low-protein diet, medications to treat

c. Ineffective Protection: Risks associated with impaired coagulation, esophageal varices, acute gastritis
d. Impaired Skin Integrity: Bile deposits on skin cause severe pruritis; topical treatments
e. Imbalanced Nutrition: Less than body requirements

D. Cancer of the Liver
1. Background
   a. Primary liver cancer is uncommon in U.S.
   b. Common cancer worldwide
   c. Usually advanced at time of diagnosis with poor prognosis
2. Pathophysiology
   a. Most primary cancers arise from liver parenchymal cells
   b. Incidence is linked to alcoholic cirrhosis and chronic Hepatitis B or C
   c. Tumor interferes with normal hepatic function causing biliary obstruction, portal hypertension, and metabolic disruption
   d. Tumors grow rapidly and metastasize early
3. Manifestations
   a. Insidious at first and masked by chronic hepatitis or cirrhosis
   b. Abdominal pain and mass in RUQ often presenting symptoms
4. Collaborative Care
   a. Diagnostic tests
      1. Tumors identified by CT scan or MRI
      2. Liver biopsy may be done to identify the tumor type
      3. Serum AFP (alpha-fetoprotein) rises with hepatocellular cancer
   b. Treatment
      1. Small, localized tumor may be resected surgically but often cancer has metastasized when diagnosed
      2. Radiation therapy may be used to shrink tumor
      3. Chemotherapy including direct continuous hepatic artery infusion
   c. Nursing Care
      1. Client needs to avoid hepatotoxic drugs and alcohol
      2. Focus of care is on pain control; early referral to hospice

E. Liver Trauma
1. Pathophysiology

a. Blunt or penetrating trauma as with motor vehicle accidents, gunshot or stab wounds can damage liver
b. Bleeding is usually the primary problem but may not be immediately apparent (liver is very vascular)
c. Includes hematoma on surface or within parenchyma, liver laceration or disruption of vessels attached to liver

2. Collaborative Care
   a. Diagnostic Tests: diagnostic peritoneal lavage with CT scan, CBC
   b. Treatment: may include immediate surgery and/or treatment to restore blood volume and promote hemostasis including intravenous fluids, blood and clotting products
3. Nursing Diagnoses
   a. Fluid Volume Deficit related to hemorrhage
   b. Risk for Infection: related to wound or abdominal contamination
   c. Altered Protection: related to impaired coagulation

F. Liver Abscess
1. Pathophysiology
   a. Bacterial or amebic in origin; right lobe most frequently affected
   b. Bacterial (pyogenic) liver abscess may be caused by cholangitis, abdominal infections such as peritonitis or diverticulitis, post trauma or surgery; *Escherichia coli* most common causative organism
   c. Amebic abscess can occur with contaminated drinking water
   d. Abscess destroys healthy tissue leaving area of necrosis, inflammatory exudates, and blood
2. Manifestations
   a. Bacterial: acute onset with fever, vomiting, hyperbilirubinemia, abdominal pain in RUQ
   b. Amebic: insidious onset
3. Collaborative Care
   a. Diagnostic tests include CT and ultrasound studies, liver biopsy or aspirate, blood and fecal cultures
   b. Treatment: antibiotics according to culture results for bacterial infections; amebic abscesses often treated with metronidazole (Flagyl) and iodoquinal (Diquinol)

c. Nursing care: Includes preventive teaching and supportive care to prevent dehydration and control pain

III. Disorder of the Exocrine Pancreas
  A. Pancreatitis
    1. Definition
      a. Inflammation of pancreas characterized by release of pancreatic enzymes into pancreatic tissue itself leading to hemorrhage and necrosis
      b. Mortality rate is 10%
      c. Occurs as acute or chronic in form
    2. Risk factors
      a. Alcoholism
      b. Gallstones
    3. Acute Pancreatitis
      a. Pathophysiology
        1. Interstitial pancreatitis: milder form leading to inflammation and edema of pancreatic tissue; often self-limiting
        2. Necrotizing pancreatitis: inflammation, hemorrhage, and necrosis of pancreatic tissue
        3. Exact cause is unknown; gallstones can cause bile reflux activating pancreatic enzymes; alcohol causes duodenal edema, obstructing pancreatic outflow
        4. Other factors are trauma, surgery, tumors, infectious agents
        5. With pancreatitis, large volume of fluid shifts from circulation into retroperitoneal space, peripancreatic space, abdominal cavity
      b. Manifestations
        1. Abrupt onset of continuous severe epigastric and abdominal pain, radiating to back and relieved somewhat by sitting up and leaning forward; initiated by fatty meal or alcohol intake
        2. Nausea and vomiting
        3. Abdominal distention and rigidity
        4. Decreased bowel sounds
        5. Hypotension
        6. Fever, cold and clammy skin
        7. 24 hours later: jaundice;
        8. 3–6 days: retroperitoneal bleeding, bruising in flanks (Turner sign) or around umbilicus (Cullen's sign)
      c. Complications: intravascular volume depletion which can lead to

        1. Acute tubular necrosis and renal failure: 24 hours post
        2. Acute respiratory distress syndrome (ARDS): 3–7 days post
        3. Local complications of pancreatic necrosis, abscess, pseudocysts, pancreatic ascites
    4. Chronic pancreatitis
      a. Background
        1. Characterized by gradual destruction of functional pancreatic tissue
        2. Irreversible process
        3. Primary risk is alcoholism
        4. 10–20% idiopathic
      b. Pathophysiology: pancreatic ducts and flow of pancreatic juices are blocked leading to recurrent inflammation with fibrosis and loss of exocrine function
      c. Manifestations
        1. Recurrent episodes of epigastric and LUQ (left upper quadrant) abdominal pain radiating to back, pain lasts from days to week with increased frequency
        2. Anorexia, nausea and vomiting, weight loss, flatulence, constipation, and steatorrhea (fatty, frothy, foul-smelling stools)
      d. Complications
        1. Malabsorption, malnutrition, peptic ulcer disease
        2. Pancreatic pseudocyst or abscess, stricture of common bile duct
        3. Diabetes mellitus
        4. Increased risk for pancreatic cancer
        5. Risk of narcotic addiction
    5. Collaborative Care
      a. Acute pancreatitis is usually a mild, self-limiting disease with care focused on eliminating causative factors, reducing pancreatic secretions, supportive care
      b. Severe necrotizing pancreatitis requires intensive care management
      c. Chronic pancreatitis focuses on pain management and treatment of malabsorption and malnutrition
    6. Diagnostic Tests
      a. Laboratory tests
        1. Serum amylase: 2–3 times normal in 2–12 hours with acute; returns to normal in 3–4 days

2. Serum lipase: rises and remains elevated 7–14 days
3. Serum trypsinogen: elevated with acute; decreased with chronic
4. Urine amylase: rises with acute
5. Serum glucose: transient elevation with acute
6. Serum bilirubin and alkaline phosphatase: may be increased with compression of common bile duct with acute
7. Serum calcium: hypocalcemia with acute
8. CBC: elevated white blood cells count
9. BUN, Creatinine: monitor renal function
   b. Ultrasounds to diagnose gallstones, pancreatic mass, pseudocyst
   c. CT scan to identify pancreatic enlargement, fluid collections, areas of necrosis
   d. Endoscopic retrograde cholangiopancreatography (ERCP) diagnose chronic pancreatitis (acute pancreatitis can occur after this procedure)
   e. Endoscopic ultrasound
   f. Percutaneous fine-needle aspiration biopsy to differentiate between chronic pancreatitis and malignancy
7. Treatment
   a. Acute pancreatitis is supportive and includes hydration, pain control, and antibiotics
   b. Chronic pancreatitis includes pain management without causing drug dependence
   c. Medications may include
      1. Pancreatic enzyme supplements to reduce steatorrhea
      2. H_2 blockers or proton pump inhibitors to decrease gastric secretions
      3. Octreotide (sandostatin) to suppress pancreatic secretion
   d. Fluid and dietary management
      1. Initially client is NPO usually with nasogastric suction, intravenous fluids and possibly total parenteral nutrition

2. Oral food and fluids begun as condition resolves
3. Low fat diet and no alcohol
   e. Surgeries include
      1. Blocked gallstones may be removed endoscopically
      2. Cholecystectomy for cholelithiasis
      3. Drainage procedures or resection of pancreas may be needed
8. Nursing Diagnoses
   a. Pain
   b. Impaired Nutrition: less than body requirements
   c. Risk for Fluid Volume Deficit
9. Home Care: Client and family teaching to include prevention of future attacks including abstinence from alcohol and smoking; low fat diet; monitoring for signs of infection (as with abscess formation)
B. Pancreatic Cancer
   1. Definition
      a. Accounts for 2% of cancers; most are adenocarcinoma; most common site is head of the pancreas
      b. Very lethal death within 1–3 years after diagnosis
      c. Incidence increases after age 50; slightly higher in females and African Americans over Caucasians
   2. Risk factors
      a. Smoking
      b. Other factors include chemical or environmental toxins, high fat diet, chronic pancreatitis, diabetes mellitus
   3. Manifestations
      a. Usually nonspecific; up to 85% persons seek health care with advanced case
      b. Slow onset: anorexia, nausea, weight loss, flatulence, dull epigastic pain
      c. Cancer in head of pancreas causes bile obstruction resulting in jaundice, clay colored stools, dark urine, pruritus
      d. Late: palpable mass and ascites
   4. Treatment
      a. Surgery is indicated in early cancers
      b. Pancreatoduodenectomy (Whipple's procedure)
      c. Radiation and chemotherapy

FOCUSED STUDY TIPS

- Review laboratory values of clients in the clinical setting that may be indicative of liver disorders. Identify physical assessment manifestations that would collaborate the abnormal values.
- When administrating medications in the clinical setting, identify drugs that are metabolized in the liver.
- Describe to a family member or friend the pathophysiology of jaundice. Explain the difference between newborn jaundice and jaundice occurring with liver dysfunction.

CASE STUDY

E. W. is admitted to the hospital and scheduled for a liver biopsy. In preparation for the procedure, what paperwork is necessary? What assessments must the nurse make before the procedure begins? In what position will the client be placed? What other information will you share with the client and his family before the procedure begins? After the procedure?

CARE PLAN CRITICAL THINKING ACTIVITY

Develop a health-care teaching plan for a client who is recovering from acute pancreatitis.

NCLEX TEST QUESTIONS

1. A client presenting with ascites secondary to liver failure is being evaluated for fluid balance. Which of the following provides the best indicator of fluid status?
   a. intake and output measurement
   b. liver function tests
   c. caloric intake and serum protein levels.
   d. daily weight

2. When providing discharge teaching to the client with chronic cirrhosis, his wife asks the nurse to explain why there is so much emphasis on bleeding precautions. Which of the following provides the most appropriate response?
   a. "The liver affected by cirrhosis is unable to produce clotting factors."
   b. "The low-protein diet will result in reduced clotting factors."
   c. "The increased production of bile decreases clotting factors."
   d. "The required medications reduce clotting factors."

3. When explaining the rationale for the use of lactulose (Chronulac) syrup to the client with chronic cirrhosis, the nurse would choose which of the following statements?
   a. "Chronulac syrup reduces constipation, which is a frequent complaint with cirrhosis."
   b. "Chronulac syrup suppresses the metabolism of ammonia and aids in its elimination through feces."
   c. "Chronulac syrup helps to reverse cirrhosis of the liver."
   d. "Chronulac syrup can be taken intermittently to reduce side effects."

4. Which of the following laboratory values will the nurse interpret as confirming a client's diagnosis of pancreatitis?
   a. elevated amylase, elevated lipase, elevated serum glucose, and decreased serum calcium levels
   b. elevated amylase, elevated lipase, decreased serum glucose, and decreased serum calcium levels
   c. decreased amylase, decreased lipase, elevated serum glucose, and increased serum calcium levels
   d. decreased amylase, decreased lipase, decreased serum glucose, and increased serum calcium levels
   e. high ammonia level

5. The client has just had a liver biopsy. Which of the following nursing actions would be the priority after the biopsy?
   a. Monitor pulse and blood pressure every 30 minutes until stable and then hourly for up to 24 hours.

b. Ambulate every 4 hours for the first day, as long as client can tolerate this.

c. Measure urine specific gravity every 8 hours for the next 48 hours.

d. Maintain NPO status for 24 hours post-biopsy.

6. A male client is being treated for ruptured esophageal varices with a Sengstaken-Blakemore tube. His vital signs have been stable, and the suction port is draining scant amounts of drainage. He suddenly becomes acutely dyspneic, and oximetry reveals an O_2 sat of 74%. The nurse's immediate action is to

a. release the esophageal balloon. *to preserve airway*

b. release the gastric balloon.

c. increase the suction.

d. irrigate the gastric balloon.

7. A newly admitted client with cirrhosis of the liver has a distended abdomen and the umbilicus is protruding. The nurse knows the pathological basis for this is

a. increased fluid intake resulting from excessive use of alcohol causing overhydration.

b. increased size of the liver resulting in abdominal distension.

c. hypoalbuminemia causing fluid to leave the vascular system and enter the peritoneal cavity.

d. shunting of the blood to the collateral circulation in the esophagus resulting in decreased blood volume and accumulation of fluid.

8. A client with pancreatitis complains of numbness around the mouth and tingling in the hands and feet. The nurse interprets that these symptoms are consistent with which of the following disorders?

a. hypercalcemia

b. enhanced digitalis effect

c. hypophosphatemia

d. hypocalcemia

9. A client with a history of liver disease presents with steatorrhea. What implication would this have on the client's nutritional status?

a. This could mean altered protein metabolism.

b. This could be an indication of increased absorption of fat-soluble vitamins.

c. Fat-soluble vitamins will need to be administered in water-soluble form.

d. Increased fat is needed in the diet to reduce the presence of steatorrhea.

10. A client has a history of gallbladder disease and is admitted for a diagnostic workup to rule out pancreatitis. The nurse knows the relationship between these two diseases is

a. when a stone obstructs the common bile duct, a reflux of bile may cause breakdown of pancreatic tissue.

b. the symptoms are very similar, and it is necessary to differentiate between the two diseases.

c. there is no relationship between gallbladder disease and pancreatitis.

d. pancreatitis is directly related to alcohol intake, and this is intensified by gallbladder disease.

CHAPTER 23

ASSESSING CLIENTS WITH BOWEL ELIMINATION DISORDERS

LEARNING OUTCOMES

After completing this chapter, you will be able to:

- Review the anatomy and physiology of the small and large intestines.
- Explain the physiologic processes involved in bowel elimination.
- Identify specific topics for consideration during a health history interview of the client with problems of bowel elimination.
- Describe physical assessment techniques of bowel function.
- Identify manifestations of impairment of bowel function.

KEY TOPICS

- Review of the anatomy and physiology of the small intestine and the large intestine
- Assessing bowel function

LECTURE OUTLINE

I. Background of Anatomy and Physiology
    A. Small Intestine
        1. 20 feet in length; 1 inch (2.5 cm) in diameter
        2. Begins at pyloric sphincter and ends at ileocecal junction
        3. Composed of 3 regions
            a. Duodenum: 10 inches (25 cm): site where pancreatic enzymes and bile enter
            b. Jejunum: 8 feet (2.4 m)
            c. Ileum: 12 feet (3.6 m) meets large intestine at ileocecal valve
        4. Site of chemical digestion and absorption

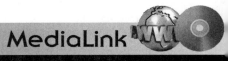

MediaLink

www.prenhall.com/lemone

Additional resources for this chapter can be found on the Student CD-ROM accompanying this textbook, and on the Companion Website at www.prenhall.com/lemone. Click on Chapter 23 to select the activities for this chapter.

CD-ROM
- Audio Glossary
- NCLEX Review

Companion Website
- More NCLEX Review
- Functional Health Pattern Assessment
- Case Study
    Irritable Bowel Syndrome

5. Large amount of surface area for absorption due to circular folds, villi (fingerlike projections of mucous cells) and microvilli (tiny projections of mucous cells); 10 L of intestinal fluid (food, liquids, secretions) enter and less than 1 L reaches large intestine
6. Enzymes which act in small intestine include
    a. Amylase from pancreas which acts on starches
    b. Intestinal enzymes (dextrinase, glucoamylase, maltase, sucrase,

lactase) further break down carbohydrates to monosaccharides

   c. Trypsin and chymotrypsin (from pancreas) and intestinal enzymes break down proteins into peptides

   d. Lipase from pancreas break down lipids

7. Other actions in small intestine

   a. Triglycerides enter as fat globules and are coated and emulsified by bile salts

   b. Nucleic acids are hydrolyzed by pancreatic enzymes; further broken down by intestinal enzymes

8. Enzyme production is initiated by secretion of secretin and cholecystokinin, hormones produced by intestinal mucosal cells when chyme enters small intestine

9. All food products, water, vitamins, most electrolytes are absorbed in small intestine; fibers, water and bacteria enter large intestine

B. Large Intestine (Colon)

1. Begins at ileocecal valve and ends at anus

2. 5 feet in length (1.5 m) and frames small intestine on 3 sides

3. Regions of large intestine include

   a. First section: cecum and appendix (attached to surface as extension)

   b. Colon

   c. Rectum

   d. Anal canal

4. Segments of the colon

   a. Ascending: extends along right side of abdomen to hepatic flexure; where makes right angle turn

   b. Transverse: crosses abdomen to splenic flexure

   c. Descending: descends down left side of abdomen and ends at S-shaped sigmoid colon which terminates at the rectum

5. Rectum is mucosa-lined and is 12 cm in length; has three transverse folds called valves of Houston that retain feces but allow flatus to be passed through anus; ends at anal canal which terminates at anus

6. Anus: has internal involuntary sphincter and external voluntary sphincter; both are usually open only during defecation

7. Anorectal junction separates rectum from anal canal and is site where internal hemorrhoids occur

8. Major function: elimination of indigestible food residue from body

9. Absorption of water, salts, vitamins from food residue and bacteria

10. Chyme enters at ileocecal valve and is moved by peristaltic waves; goblet cells within the lining secrete mucus promotes movement through large intestine

11. Defecation reflex initiated when feces enter rectum and stretches rectal wall: walls of sigmoid colon contract and sphincters relax

12. Valsalva's maneuver: closing glottis and contracting diaphragm and abdominal muscles to increase intra-abdominal pressure to facilitate expulsion of feces

II. Assessment of Bowel Function

A. Health assessment interview: (Subjective data)

1. Analyze any problem with function by analyzing onset, characteristics, course, severity, precipitating factors, associated symptoms

2. Determine if any medical conditions influence bowel elimination pattern, e.g., stroke, spinal cord injury

3. Ask about travel to other countries

4. Determine psychosocial history such as stress and/or depression that may affect bowel elimination pattern (stress: diarrhea; depression; constipation)

5. Address activities of daily living that affect bowel elimination pattern: exercise, sleep-rest patterns, dietary and fluid intake

6. Record presence and characteristics of any pain

   a. Lower abdominal or rectal: distended colon with gas or fluid

   b. Cramping, colicky pain: diarrhea and/or constipation

   c. Sudden lower abdominal cramping: obstruction of colon

   d. LLQ pain: diverticulitis

   e. Rectal pain: stool retention or hemorrhoids

7. Record frequency and characteristics of stools

   a. Diarrhea, constipation, rectal bleeding

   b. Use of laxatives, suppositories, enemas

   c. Use of medication that may affect bowels, e.g., narcotics, antacids

8. For client with an ostomy (stoma), surgical opening into bowel: address stool consistency, functioning, any problems, skin care, appliance usage, feelings regarding ostomy

9. Ask about nutritional status, changes in weight, digestion problems
10. Determine family history of colon cancer, colitis, gallbladder disease, malabsorption syndromes; client risk factors for cancer including history of colon inflammation, polyps; last sigmoidoscopy, colonoscopy
B. Physical Assessment
   1. Abnormal Findings during abdominal assessment including bowel sounds
      a. Generalized abdominal distention: retention of stool or gas
      b. Concave abdomen: malnutrition
      c. High-pitched tinkling, growling bowel sounds: diarrhea or onset of bowel obstruction
      d. Absent bowel sounds: later stages of bowel obstruction, post surgery
   2. Abnormal Findings during perianal examination:
      a. Presence of anal fissures: swollen, painful, longitudinal breaks
      b. Presence of hemorrhoids: dilated anal veins
      c. Prolapsed internal hemorrhoids: reddish mass
      d. Prolapsed rectum: doughnut-shaped red tissue at anal area
      e. Polyps: movable soft masses found upon palpation of anus and rectum
      f. Tumor: hard, irregular embedded masses found upon palpation of anus and rectum
   3. Abnormal Findings during Examination of client's stool
      a. Color: clay colored: lack of bile; black: blood or iron intake
      b. Obvious bleeding: hemorrhoids, fissures
      c. Positive occult blood test: bleeding from within gastrointestinal tract
      d. Foul odor: fat or blood in stool

FOCUSED STUDY TIPS

- Develop a line of questioning to determine problems with bowel elimination for a health history interview. Practice with classmates before utilizing it with clients in the clinical setting.
- Visit a local pharmacy and review OTC (over-the-counter) medications related to bowel elimination disorders. Read the labels. Identify advantages and disadvantages to their use.
- Practice abdominal assessments on classmates or family members. Compare and contrast findings. Practice documenting physical assessment findings.

CASE STUDY

S. R. comes to the clinic complaining of vague abdominal discomfort. When doing her health assessment interview regarding bowel function, she appears uncomfortable and reluctant to speak. What can you do to promote effective rapport? Give seven examples of the type of information for which you will ask.

CARE PLAN CRITICAL THINKING ACTIVITY

Describe the process of physical assessment of the abdomen. What four assessment techniques are utilized? Compare and contrast normal and abnormal findings. What equipment is necessary to perform abdominal assessment?

NCLEX TEST QUESTIONS

1. Paralytic ileus is a frequent complication of postoperative abdominal surgery. According to the physician's orders and the nurse's assessment, a planned intervention would be to
   a. administer PO fluids only.
   b. insert a nasogastric tube.
   c. listen for bowel sounds.
   d. insert a rectal tube
2. When assessing a client's abdomen, the appropriate procedure is
   a. inspection, palpation, percussion, auscultation.

b. inspection, percussion, auscultation, palpation.

c. inspection, auscultation, percussion, palpation.

d. inspection, palpation, auscultation, percussion.

3. Which of the following affects the enzymatic action of protein digestion?

a. pH level

b. presence of food in the oral cavity

c. salivary amylase

d. lingual lipase

4. Which one of the following clinical findings would the nurse associate with malabsorption of fat?

a. steatorrhea

b. increased gastric emptying

c. constipation

d. pallor

5. An elderly client expresses concern about the possibility of constipation, stating "I have not had a bowel movement today at all, and I don't want to get an obstruction." Which response by the nurse is most helpful to the client?

a. "It is better to control your bowel habits with increased fiber and increased fluid intake."

b. "Oh, don't worry about that!"

c. "You probably need to take a laxative."

d. "That's a part of the aging process. It is to be expected."

6. A 39-year-old female complains of right lower-quadrant pain. Prior to performing an abdominal assessment, the nurse determines that she will perform the assessment techniques in the following sequence:

a. inspection, palpation, and auscultation

b. palpation, auscultation, and inspection

c. inspection, auscultation, and palpation

d. auscultation, palpation, and inspection

7. Which of the following statements would be described as a component of a client's past health history?

a. "I had an appendectomy in 1994."

b. "My father died of lung cancer."

c. "I worked in a dry cleaner for 25 years."

d. "I graduated from high school when I was 18."

8. The nurse would use which of the following statements to describe how dietary fiber aids in the processes of digestion, transport, and absorption?

a. "Fiber helps to coat the gastric lining of the stomach in order to decrease the acidic environment."

b. "Soluble fiber adds weight to feces, and insoluble fiber acts as a bulking agent to assist in the elimination process."

c. "A large amount of fiber in the diet has no effect on the digestion of nutrients."

d. "In order for dietary fiber to be effective, it must be taken with mineral oil to facilitate the digestion, transport, and absorption of nutrients."

9. A client, age 60, is admitted to the hospital for a possible acute low-intestinal obstruction. His preoperative workup indicates vital signs of BP 100/70, P 88, R 18, and temperature of 96.4°F. Listening to bowel sounds, the nurse would expect to find

a. absence of bowel sounds.

b. gurgling bowel sounds.

c. hyperactive, high-pitched sounds.

d. tympanic, percussion sounds.

10. For a client who has problems with constipation, which statement would indicate the need for additional teaching?

a. "I need to drink 2500 to 3000 ml of liquid each day."

b. "I should maintain a low-fiber diet."

c. "I will eat three regular meals that include the four basic food groups."

d. "I should exercise several times per week for at least 20 minutes."

CHAPTER 24

NURSING CARE OF CLIENTS WITH BOWEL DISORDERS

LEARNING OUTCOMES

After completing this chapter, you will be able to:

- Relate the effects and manifestations of bowel disorders to normal physiology and assessment findings (Chapter 23).
- Discuss the pathophysiology, manifestations, and management of bowel absorption and elimination disorders.
- List diagnostic tests used to identify disorders of the small and large bowel.
- Discuss the nursing implications of medications used in managing bowel absorption and elimination disorders.
- Discuss care of clients with a colostomy or ileostomy.
- Provide appropriate nursing care for the client before and after intestinal surgery.
- Provide appropriate teaching for clients with bowel absorption and elimination disorders and their families.
- Use the nursing process as a framework for providing individualized care to clients with disorders of bowel absorption and elimination.

KEY TOPICS

- Disorders of intestinal motility
- Fecal incontinence
- Malabsorption syndromes
- Neoplastic disorders
- Structural and obstructional disorders
- Anorectal disorders
- Nursing care of clients with bowel disorders

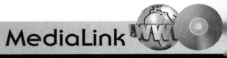

MediaLink

www.prenhall.com/lemone

Additional resources for this chapter can be found on the Student CD-ROM accompanying this textbook, and on the Companion Website at www.prenhall.com/lemone. Click on Chapter 24 to select the activities for this chapter.

CD-ROM
- Audio Glossary
- NCLEX Review

Companion Website
- More NCLEX Review
- Case Study
  Irritable Bowel Syndrome
- Care Plan Activity
  Irritable Bowel Syndrome
- MediaLink Application
  Crohn's Disease

LECTURE OUTLINE

I. Factors affecting bodily function of elimination
  A. GI tract
    1. Food intake
    2. Bacterial flora in bowel
  B. Indirect
    1. Psychologic stress
    2. Voluntary postponement of defecation
  C. Normal bowel elimination pattern
    1. Varies with the individual
    2. 2–3 times daily to 3 stools per week
II. Disorders of intestinal motility
  A. Client with diarrhea
    1. Definition
      a. Increase in frequency, volume, fluid content of stool
      b. Is a symptom rather than primary disorder
      c. Acute: lasts less than a week; often due to infectious agent
      d. Chronic: persists longer that 3–4 weeks; may be caused by inflammatory bowel disorders, malabsorption, endocrine disorders
    2. Pathophysiology
      a. Large volume diarrhea caused by increased water content of stool from osmotic or secretory processes
      b. Small volume diarrhea characterized by small frequent stooling; usually caused by inflammation or disease of colon
    3. Manifestations
      a. Affected by cause, duration, severity, area of bowel affected, client's general health
      b. Varies from several large watery stools daily to very frequent small stools containing mucus, blood, or exudate
    4. Complications
      a. Dehydration, especially in very young or older and/or debilitated adult
      b. Severe diarrhea can lead to vascular collapse, hypovolemic shock; electrolyte imbalances such as hypokalemia, hypomagnesemia; metabolic acidosis
    5. Collaborative Care: management focuses on identifying and treating cause, preventing complications

6. Diagnostic Tests
  a. Stool specimen: gross and microscopic examination to detect WBC's, unabsorbed fat, parasites (if parasitic infection suspected usually get series of 3 specimens at 2–3 day intervals)
  b. Stool culture: enteric pathogen
  c. Serum electrolytes, osmolality, arterial blood gases: assess for complications
  d. Sigmoidoscopy: direct examination of bowel mucosa
  e. Tissue biopsy: identify chronic inflammatory process, infections
7. Medications
  a. Used sparingly or not at all until cause has been identified
  b. Antidiarrheal medications may worsen disease if slows elimination of a toxin from the bowel
  c. Antidiarrheal medications commonly contain opium or derivatives, anticholinergics, absorbants, demulcents
  d. Antibiotics used cautiously since alter normal bowel bacterial flora
  e. Balanced electrolyte solutions, oral or intravenous potassium replacement
8. Dietary Management
  a. Fluid replacement: oral: glucose/balanced electrolyte solution commercially or can be made at home
  b. Solid food withheld first 24 hours to rest bowel; then begin frequent small soft feeding of mild foods
  c. Milk and milk products added last
  d. Foods with roughage, fried and spicy, coffee and alcohol avoided in recovery period
  e. Clients with chronic diarrhea may need to eliminate specific foods found to aggravate and cause diarrhea
9. Nursing Care
  a. Teaching includes safe food handling, measures to take if traveling outside foreign countries or without safe water
  b. Assess information regarding duration and extent of diarrhea, risk factors, abdominal assessment, signs of dehydration

10. Nursing Diagnoses
    a. Diarrhea
    b. Risk for Fluid Volume Deficit: assess for orthostatic hypotension: drop in BP > 10 mm HG and pulse increase of 10 when changing from lying to sitting or standing position
    c. Risk for Impaired Skin Integrity: provide for hygiene, protective ointment for perianal area
11. Home Care: Teaching regarding care including proper hand washing, introduction of food with constipating effect: applesauce, bananas, crackers, rice, potatoes

B. Client with Constipation
1. Definition
    a. Infrequent (2 or <) bowel movements weekly or difficult passage of stools
    b. More frequently affects persons > 65
2. Pathophysiology
    a. May be primary problem or symptom of a disease; acute onset often caused by organic process (tumor or partial bowel obstruction)
    b. Chronic constipation: often functional cause
    c. Overuse of laxatives or enemas can lead to intestinal problems
    d. Fecal impaction: rock-hard or puttylike mass of feces in rectum blocking the passage; client may experience abdominal cramping and rectal fullness and may have diarrhea passed around the impaction
3. Collaborative Care
    a. Determine probable cause by history, physical assessment
    b. Simple or chronic constipation may be treated with education
    c. Acute constipation requires diagnostic testing
4. Diagnostic Testing
    a. Serum electrolytes, thyroid function tests: determine metabolic or endocrine condition
    b. Barium enema: x-ray evaluation of bowel structure and identify tumor or diverticular disease
    c. Sigmoidoscopy or colonoscopy: evaluate acute constipation, identify tumor; suspicious lesions can be biopsied
5. Medications
    a. Laxatives and cathartics: preparations to promote stool evacuation; laxatives are mild; cathartics are stronger

    b. Laxatives appropriate for short term use
    c. Contraindicated if bowel obstruction or impaction suspected or abdominal pain of undetermined origin; could cause mechanical damage or bowel perforation
    d. Bulking agents i.e., psyllium seed, methycellulose, only laxative appropriate for long term use
6. Dietary management
    a. Foods with high fiber which is mostly indigestible: draws water and increases stool bulk which stimulates peristalsis: raw fruit, vegetables, bran
    b. Fluids (6–8 glasses daily) necessary to maintain bowel motility and soft stools
7. Enemas
    a. Generally used only in acute situations, short term basis
    b. Work by
        1. Local irritation to bowel e.g., tap water,
        2. Soap suds; drawing fluid into bowel e.g., phosphate enemas (Fleet)
        3. Softening fecal mass e.g., oil retention
    c. Contraindicated if risk of bowel obstruction, perforation, ulceration; undiagnosed abdominal pain
    d. Repeated use of enemas can lead to electrolyte imbalance, especially tap-water or phosphate enemas
8. Nursing Care and Home Care
    a. Prevention: diet, fluid, exercise
    b. Allowing time and responding to urge
    c. Educate regarding seeking medical attention if change in bowel habits

C. Client with Irritable Bowel Syndrome (IBS) (spastic bowel, functional colitis)
1. Definition
    a. Functional GI tract disorder without identifiable cause characterized by abdominal pain, constipation, diarrhea, or both
    b. Affects up to 20% person in Western civilization; more common in females
2. Pathophysiology
    a. Appears there is altered CNS regulation of motor and sensory functions of bowel
        1. Increased bowel activity in response to food intake, hormones, stress
        2. Increased sensations of chyme movement through gut
        3. Hypersecretion of colonic mucus

b. Lower visceral pain threshold causing abdominal pain and bloating with normal levels of gas
c. Some linkage of depression and anxiety

3. Manifestations
   a. Abdominal pain relieved by defecation; may be colicky, occurring in spasms, dull or continuous
   b. Altered bowel habits including frequency, hard or watery stool, straining or urgency with stooling, incomplete evacuation, passage of mucus; abdominal bloating, excess gas
   c. Nausea, vomiting, anorexia, fatigue, headache, anxiety
   d. Tenderness over sigmoid colon upon palpation

4. Collaborative Care
   a. Management of distressing symptoms
   b. Eliminating precipitating factors, stress reduction

5. Diagnostic Tests: to find a cause for client's abdominal pain, changes in feces elimination
   a. Stool examination for occult blood, ova and parasites, culture
   b. CBC with differential, Erythrocyte Sedimentation Rate (ESR): to determine if anemia, bacterial infection, or inflammatory process
   c. Sigmoidoscopy or colonoscopy
      1. Visualize bowel mucosa, measure intraluminal pressures, obtain biopsies if indicated
      2. Findings with IBS: normal appearance increased mucus, intraluminal pressures, marked spasms, possible hyperemia without lesions
   d. Small bowel series (Upper GI series with small bowel follow through) and barium enema: examination of entire GI tract; used to determine IBS: increased motility

6. Medications
   a. Purpose to manage symptoms
   b. Bulk-forming laxatives: reduce bowel spasm, normalize bowel movement in number and form
   c. Anticholinergic drugs (dicyclomine (Bentyl), hyoscyamine) to inhibit bowel motility; given before meals
   d. Antidiarrheal medications (loperamide (Imodium), diphenoxylate (Lomotil): prevent diarrhea prophylactically

e. Antidepressant medications
f. Research: medications altering serotonin receptors in GI tract

7. Dietary Management
   a. Often benefit from additional dietary fiber: adds bulk and water content to stool reducing diarrhea and constipation
   b. Some benefit from elimination of lactose, fructose, sorbitol
   c. Limiting intake of gas-forming foods, caffeinated beverages

8. Nursing Care
   a. Contact in health environments outside acute care
   b. Home care focus on improving symptoms with changes of diet, stress management, medications; seek medical attention if serious changes occur

9. Nursing Diagnoses
   a. Constipation
   b. Diarrhea
   c. Anxiety
   d. Ineffective Coping

D. Client with Fecal Incontinence
1. Definition
   a. Loss of voluntary control of defecation
   b. More common in older adults

2. Pathophysiology
   a. Interference with sensory or motor control of rectum and anal sphincters
      1. External sphincter paralyzed with spinal cord injury, disease
      2. Sphincter muscles damage or excessive pelvic floor relaxation
   b. Age-related changes in anal sphincter tone and response to rectal distention

3. Collaborative Care
   a. Physical assessment of pelvic floor and anus to evaluate muscle tone; rectal sphincter tone by digital exam, manometry, sigmoidoscopy
   b. Treatment directed toward cause
      1. Medications to control diarrhea, constipation
      2. High fiber, ample fluid, regular exercise
      3. Kegel exercises
      4. Bowel training program: establish set time of day for defecation; may use some type of stimulant
      5. Neurological incontinence may use digital stimulation
      6. Low residue diet if incontinence of solid stool

7. Biofeedback
8. Surgical repair if sphincter damage, rectal prolapse
4. Nursing Diagnoses
    a. Bowel incontinence
    b. Risk for impaired skin integrity
5. Home Care
    a. Teaching regarding not a normal part of aging; seek medical evaluation
    b. Client may become socially isolated, affected with low self-esteem
    c. Support with treatment modalities
III. Acute Inflammatory and Infectious Disorders
    A. Client with Appendicitis
       1. Definition
           a. Appendix is tubelike pouch attached to cecum just below ileocecal valve; appendix becomes inflamed
           b. Common cause of acute abdominal pain; most common reason for emergency abdominal surgery in U.S.
       2. Pathophysiology
           a. Obstruction of proximal lumen of appendix often caused by fecalith (hard mass of feces), foreign body, tumor, inflammation, edema of lymphoid tissue
           b. Appendix becomes distended with fluid secreted by mucosa, impairing blood supply, leading to inflammation, edema, ulceration and infection
           c. Within 24–36 hours tissue necrosis and gangrene results; leading to perforation if untreated and bacterial peritonitis
           d. Pathology depends on timing of surgery i.e., simple, gangrenous, perforated
       3. Manifestations
           a. Initially mild generalized or upper abdominal pain
           b. Over 4 hours, pain intensifies and localizes in RLQ of abdomen; aggravated by moving, walking, coughing
           c. Localizes in right iliac region (McBurney's point) with rebound tenderness (relief of pain with direct pressure; followed by pain on release of pressure)
           d. Client may also have low-grade fever, anorexia, nausea, vomiting
           e. Pain and local tenderness may be less acute in older adults, delaying diagnosis and treatment

4. Complications
    a. Perforation, peritonitis, and abscess
    b. Perforation is manifested by increased pain and high fever
    c. Less common is chronic appendicitis with chronic abdominal pain and recurrent acute attacks at intervals
5. Collaborative Care
    a. Rapid diagnosis and treatment
    b. Admission to hospital, client is NPO with intravenous fluids
    c. Diagnosis is established and appendectomy done
6. Diagnostic Tests: Confirm diagnosis and rule out other causes
    a. WBC count with Differential: WBC elevated with shift to left with appendicitis
    b. Urinalysis: rule out urinary tract infection as source of pain and nausea
    c. Abdominal x-rays (flat and upright): fecalith may be visualized in RUQ or localized ileus noted
    d. Abdominal ultrasound: most effective for diagnosis; quick procedure; useful with older adult clients with atypical symptoms
    e. Pelvic examination: usually done on female clients of child-bearing age to rule out gynecologic disorder or pelvic inflammatory disease
    f. Intravenous pyelogram (IVP): differentiate appendicitis from urinary tract disease
7. Medications
    a. Preoperatively, intravenous fluids with electrolytes
    b. Antibiotic therapy, third-generation cephalosporin to treat gram negative bacteria (bowel flora cause infection if perforation)
8. Surgery
    a. Appendectomy: surgical removal of appendix
    b. 2 approaches:
        1. Laparoscopic approach (endoscopic)
        2. Lapatotomy (open abdominal approach)
    c. Laparoscopic approach advantages
        1. Direct visualization allows definitive diagnosis without laparotomy
        2. Short postop hospitalization with few complications

3. Rapid recovery and return to normalcy
  d. Laparotomy indicated when rupture has occurred; peritoneal cavity irrigated
9. Nursing Care
  a. Prepare client physically and psychologically for emergency surgery; preoperative teaching
  b. No laxatives, enemas, heat applications; risk of perforation
10. Nursing Diagnoses
  a. Risk for Infection
  b. Pain
    1. Analgesia is limited while diagnosis is established; postoperatively pain is controlled adequately
    2. Sudden relief of preoperative pain may signal appendix rupture
11. Home Care
  a. Laparoscopic appendectomy client is discharged on day of or day after surgery
  b. Postop teaching regarding wound care, pain management, telephone contact source
B. Client with Peritonitis
1. Definition
  a. Inflammation of peritoneum, lining that covers wall (parietal peritoneum) and organs (visceral peritoneum) of abdominal cavity
  b. Enteric bacteria enter the peritoneal cavity through a break of intact GI tract (e.g., perforated ulcer, ruptured appendix)
2. Pathophysiology
  a. Peritonitis results from contamination of normal sterile peritoneal cavity with infections or chemical irritant
  b. Release of bile or gastric juices initially causes chemical peritonitis; infection occurs when bacteria enter the space
  c. Bacterial peritonitis usually caused by bacteria (normal bowel flora): *Escherichia coli, Klebsiella, Proteus, Pseudomonas*
  d. Inflammatory process causes fluid shift into peritoneal space (third spacing); leading to hypovolemia; then septicemia
3. Manifestations
  a. Depends on severity and extent of infection, age and health of client
  b. Presents with "acute abdomen"
    1. Abrupt onset of diffuse severe abdominal pain
    2. Pain may localize near site of infection (may have rebound tenderness)
    3. Intensifies with movement
  c. Entire abdomen is tender and boardlike: guarding or rigidity of abdominal muscle
  d. Decreased peristalsis leading to paralytic ileus; bowel sounds are diminished or absent with progressive abdominal distention; pooling of GI secretions lead to nausea and vomiting
  e. Systemically: fever, malaise, tachycardia and tachypnea, restlessness, disorientation; oliguria with dehydration and shock
  f. Older or immunosuppressed client may have
    1. Few of classic signs
    2. Increased confusion and restlessness
    3. Decreased urinary output
    4. Vague abdominal complaints
    5. At risk for delayed diagnosis and higher mortality rates
4. Complications
  a. May be life threatening; mortality rate overall 40%
  b. Abscess
  c. Fibrous adhesions
  d. Septicemia, septic shock; fluid loss into abdominal cavity leads to hypovolemic shock
5. Collaborative Care
  a. Diagnosis, identifying and treating cause
  b. Prevention of complications
6. Diagnostic Tests
  a. WBC with differential: elevated WBC to 20,000; shift to left
  b. Blood cultures: identify bacteria in blood
  c. Liver and renal function studies, serum electrolytes: evaluate effects of peritonitis
  d. Abdominal x-rays: detect intestinal distension, air-fluid levels, free air under diaphragm (sign of GI perforation)
  e. Diagnostic paracentesis
7. Medications
  a. Antibiotics

1. Broad spectrum before definitive culture results identifying specific organism(s) causing infection
2. Specific antibiotic(s) treating causative pathogens
   b. Analgesics
8. Surgery
   a. Laparotomy to treat cause (close perforation, removed inflamed tissue)
   b. Peritoneal lavage: washing out peritoneal cavity with copious amounts of warm isotonic fluid during surgery to dilute residual bacterial and remove gross contaminants
   c. Often have drain in place and/or incision left unsutured to continue drainage of purulent material
9. Treatment
   a. Intravenous fluids and electrolytes to maintain vascular volume and electrolyte balance
   b. Bed rest in Fowler's position to localize infection and promote lung ventilation
   c. Intestinal decompression with nasogastric tube or intestinal tube connected to suction
      1. Relieves abdominal distension secondary to paralytic ileus
      2. NPO with intravenous fluids while having nasogastric suction
10. Nursing Diagnoses
    a. Pain
    b. Fluid Volume Deficit: often on hourly output; nasogastric drainage is considered when ordering intravenous fluids
    c. Ineffective Protection
    d. Anxiety
11. Home Care
    a. Client may have prolonged hospitalization
    b. Home care often includes
       1. Wound care
       2. Home health referral
       3. Home intravenous antibiotics
C. Client with Gastroenteritis
   1. Definition
      a. Inflammation of stomach and small intestine caused by bacteria, viruses, parasites, toxins commonly causing anorexia, nausea, vomiting, and diarrhea
      b. "Food poisoning;" usually self-limited but can be severe for the very young,

old, people with impaired immune function
2. Pathophysiology: infection produces inflammation, tissue damage by 2 primary mechanisms
   a. Production of exotoxins which cause damage and inflammation, impairing intestinal absorption and thus diarrhea and fluid loss
      1. Staphylococcus: causes food poisoning when food is contaminated and left at room temperature (meats, dairy)
         a. Abrupt onset 2–8 hours
         b. Lasts 3–6 hours with abdominal cramping, diarrhea, headache, fever
      2. *Clostridium botulinum:* severe, life threatening from improperly preserved foods (home canned vegetables, smoked meats); spores highly resistant to heat
         a. Toxin blocks acetylcholine causing descending weakness and paralysis
         b. Nausea, vomiting, abdominal cramps may occur
         c. Respiratory muscle paralysis requires ventilatory support or death
         d. Treatment is administration of antitoxin (from horse serum, check allergies); may include gastric lavage and catharsis (GI "washout") or plasmapheresis
      3. Specific strains of *Escherichia coli:* cause hemorrhagic colitis from toxin
         a. Damages bowel mucosa and blood vessels and toxin can damage kidney: hemolytic uremic syndrome and thrombocytopenic purpura
         b. Fecal-oral route from undercooked contaminated beef (hamburger), unpasteurized milk, apple juice
         c. Treatment may include plasmapheresis, renal dialysis if acute tubular necrosis and renal failure occur
      4. *Vibrio cholerae:* causes cholera endemic in parts of Asia, Africa, Middle East from fecal-oral route

a. Often abrupt onset with severe, frequent watery diarrhea "rice water stool"

b. Significant complications are dehydration, hypokalemia, and metabolic acidosis

c. Fatal without supportive treatment

b. Invasion and ulceration of the mucosa directly producing microscopic ulceration, bleeding, fluid exudates and water and electrolyte secretion

1. Shigella (Bacillary dysentery): spread by fecal-oral route through contaminated foods, fomites, vectors (fleas)

   a. Abrupt onset of diarrhea that is watery and contains blood, mucus, exudates; severe abdominal cramping, tenesmus

   b. May develop secondary infection, acute blood loss

2. Salmonella: food poisoning caused from eating raw or improperly cooked meat, poultry, eggs, dairy

   a. Onset is 8 to 48 post bacterial ingestion

   b. Severe diarrhea with abdominal cramping, nausea and vomiting, low-grade fever, chills

3. *Escherichia coli* species

3. Traveler's diarrhea

a. Often persons traveling to other countries develop diarrhea in 2 to 10 days, usually with difference in climate, sanitation, food and drink

b. Causes are most often strains of enterotoxin-producing *Escherichia coli,* shigella, Camylobacter

c. Manifestations include diarrhea (up to 10 stools/day) abdominal cramping resolving in 2–5 days

4. Manifestations (general features)

a. Anorexia, nausea, vomiting

b. Abdominal pain and cramping with *borborygmi* excessively loud and hyperactive bowel sounds

c. Diarrhea, often watery and frequent stools

5. Complications

a. Dehydration and hypovolemia leading to orthostatic hypotension, and hypovolemic shock

b. Electrolyte imbalance:

1. Metabolic alkalosis: from excessive vomiting

2. Metabolic acidosis: from excessive diarrhea

3. Hypokalemia

4. Hyponatremia: if fluids replaced with pure water only

6. Collaborative Care

a. Manage symptoms

b. Prevent complication

c. Identify cause

d. Prevent spread

7. Diagnostic Tests: instituted if symptoms severe or prolonged (48 hours)

a. Stool specimen for culture, ova and parasites, fecal leukocytes; may identify toxin; cultures may take 6 weeks for results

b. Serum toxin levels if botulism suspected

c. Serum osmolality, electrolytes, arterial blood gases: monitor fluid and electrolyte status

d. Sigmoidoscopy may be done to differentiate infectious from inflammatory etiologies

8. Medications

a. Most cases resolve spontaneously and no medications are needed

b. Antibiotics may be prescribed according to culture and for cholera, salmonella, shigella

c. Antidiarrheal medications may be used; not used with botulism

d. Other specific treatments such as antitoxin with botulism

9. Treatment

a. Fluid and electrolyte replacement, orally if feasible

b. Intravenous fluid replacement with balanced electrolyte solutions

c. Specific treatments according to individual client case

10. Health Promotion

a. Proper food handling

1. Thoroughly cooking meet, no pink hamburgers

2. Drinking only pasteurized milk products

3. Prompt refrigeration of meats, eggs, dairy products

4. Proper home canning and boiling home canned foods to destroy potential toxins

5. Discarding foods that appear possibly spoiled
   b. Avoiding contaminated water: using bottled water, water purification tablets as necessary
11. Nursing Diagnoses
    a. Diarrhea
    b. Fluid Volume Deficit
    c. Nausea
    d. Vomiting
    e. Impaired Home Maintenance
12. Home Care
    a. Proper hand washing
    b. Fluid and electrolyte replacement
    c. Medications such as antidiarrheal medications
    d. Symptoms of complications necessitating medical attention

D. Client with protozoan bowel infection: Parasite organism which infects bowel
   1. Giardiasis
      a. Caused by *Giardia lamblia,* affecting children more than adults
      b. Spread by fecal-oral route from contaminated food, water, and direct contact
      c. Manifestations: asymptomatic or mild to severe diarrhea
      d. Malabsorption may occur
   2. Amebiasis (Amebic dysentery)
      a. Caused by protozoan *Entamoeba histolytica*
      b. Oral-fecal route or person to person contact
      c. Usually asymptomatic; may have severe watery, blood, mucus, diarrhea
      d. May have liver enlargement
   3. Cryptosporidiosis (Coccidoisis)
      a. Usually mild diarrhea and traveler's diarrhea
      b. Causes severe diarrhea, malabsorption, weight loss with persons who are immunosuppressed
      c. Transmitted by fecal-oral route, contaminated water is source
   4. Collaborative Care: Identify organism and obtain treatment
   5. Diagnostic Testing
      a. Stool for ova and parasites: obtain 3 times at 3-day intervals
      b. Indirect hemagglutination assay (IHA): detect antibodies
      c. Sigmoidoscopy: examine bowel mucosa, stool specimen; no preparation

   d. Duodenal string test, duodenal aspiration, or biopsy if giardiasis is suspected
   6. Medications: Local and systemic antiparasitic drugs
   7. Nursing Care
      a. Teaching clients about maintaining safe water supplies, proper hand washing and toileting
      b. All members of household should be tested if infectious protozoan identified

E. Client with Helminthic Disorder
   1. Pathophysiology
      a. Helminthic infections are caused by parasitic worms
      b. Different organisms have definitive and intermediate hosts
      c. Most organisms enter body through the GI tract through contaminated and inadequately cooked foods and migrate to other body organs such as liver, lungs
   2. Collaborative Care: Focus is the diagnosis and treatment
   3. Diagnostic Tests
      a. Stool specimen for ova and parasites
      b. Collection of parasite eggs from perianal skin by using cellophane tape over anus
      c. CBC may show anemia
      d. Differential commonly reveals eosoinophilia
      e. Other specific testing for involvement of particular organs and parasites
   4. Treatment
      a. Medication includes single oral dose or 3-day course of antihelminthic drugs such as pyrantel pamoate (Antiminth) or mebendazole (Vermox)
      b. All members of household should be treated
      c. Stool cultures are repeated after treatment
   5. Nursing Care
      a. Preventative teaching including not fertilizing crops with human feces, adequately cooking all meats and fish, maintenance of safe water supplies
      b. Standard precautions need to be followed; linens and beddings need to be properly laundered to prevent re-infection

IV. Chronic Inflammatory Bowel Disease
    A. Client with Inflammatory Bowel Disease

1. Definition
   a. Includes 2 separate but closely related conditions: ulcerative colitis and Crohn's disease; both have similar geographic distribution and genetic component
   b. Etiology is unknown but runs in families; may be related to infectious agent and altered immune responses
   c. Peak incidence occurs between the ages of 15–35; second peak 60–80
   d. Chronic disease with recurrent exacerbations
2. Ulcerative Colitis
   a. Pathophysiology
      1. Inflammatory process usually confined to rectum and sigmoid colon
      2. Inflammation leads to mucosal hemorrhages and abscess formation, which leads to necrosis and sloughing of bowel mucosa
      3. Mucosa becomes red, friable, and ulcerated; bleeding is common
      4. Chronic inflammation leads to atrophy, narrowing, and shortening of colon
   b. Manifestations
      1. Diarrhea with stool containing blood and mucus; 5–10 stools per day leading to anemia, hypovolemia, malnutrition
      2. Fecal urgency, tenesmus, LLQ cramping
      3. Experience fatigue, anorexia, weakness
      4. Severe cases: arthritis, uveitis
   c. Complications
      1. Hemorrhage: can be massive with severe attacks
      2. Toxic megacolon: usually involves transverse colon which dilates and lacks peristalsis (manifestations: fever, tachycardia, hypotension, dehydration, change in stools, abdominal cramping)
      3. Colon perforation: rare but leads to peritonitis and 15% mortality rate
      4. Increased risk for colorectal cancer (20–30 times); need yearly colonoscopies
      5. Sclerosing cholangitis
3. Crohn's Disease (regional enteritis)
   a. Pathophysiology
      1. Can affect any portion of GI tract but terminal ileum and ascending colon are more commonly involved
      2. Inflammatory aphthoid lesion (shallow ulceration) of mucosa and submuscosa develops into ulcers and fissures which involve entire bowel wall
      3. Fibrotic changes occur leading to local obstruction, abscess formation and fistula formation
      4. Fistulas develop between loops of bowel (enteroenteric fistulas); bowel and bladder (enterovesical fistulas); bowel and skin (enterocutaneous fistulas)
      5. Absorption problem develops leading to protein loss and anemia
   b. Manifestations
      1. Often continuous or episodic diarrhea; liquid or semi-formed; abdominal pain and tenderness in RLQ relieved by defecation
      2. Fever, fatigue, malaise, weight loss, anemia
      3. Fissures, fistulas, abscesses
   c. Complications
      1. Intestinal obstruction: caused by repeated inflammation and scarring causing fibrosis and stricture
      2. Fistulas lead to abscess formation; recurrent urinary tract infection if bladder involved
      3. Perforation of bowel may occur with peritonitis
      4. Massive hemorrhage
      5. Increased risk of bowel cancer (5–6 times)
4. Collaborative Care
   a. Establish diagnosis
   b. Supportive treatment
   c. Many clients need surgery
5. Diagnostic Tests
   a. Colonoscopy, sigmoidoscopy: determine area and pattern of involvement, tissue biopsies; small risk of perforation
   b. Upper GI series with small bowel follow-through, barium enema
   c. Stool examination and stool cultures to rule out infections
   d. CBC: shows anemia, leukocytosis from inflammation and abscess formation

e. Serum albumin, folic acid: lower due to malabsorption

f. Liver function tests may show enzyme elevations

6. Medications: goal is to stop acute attacks quickly and reduce incidence of relapse

   a. Sulfasalazine (Azulfidine): sulfonamide antibiotic with topical effect in colon; used with ulcerative colitis

   b. Corticosteroids: reduce inflammation and induce remission; with ulcerative colitis may be given as enema; intravenous steroids are given with severe exacerbations

   c. Immunosuppressive agents (azathioprine (Imuran), cyclosporine) for clients who do not respond to steroid therapy

   d. New therapies including immune response modifiers, anti-inflammatory cyctokines

   e. Antibiotics: metronidazole (Flagyl) or ciprofloxacin (Cipro)

   f. Anti-diarrheal medications

7. Dietary Management

   a. Individualized according to client; eliminate irritating foods

   b. Dietary fiber contraindicated if client has strictures

   c. With acute exacerbations, client may be made NPO and given enteral or total parenteral nutrition (TPN)

8. Surgery: performed when necessitated by complications or failure of other measures

   a. Crohn's disease:

      1. Bowel obstruction leading cause; may have bowel resection and repair for obstruction, perforation, fistula, abscess

      2. Disease process tends to recur in area remaining after resection

   b. Ulcerative Colitis

      1. Total colectomy to treat disease, repair complications (toxic megacolon, perforation, hemorrhage, prophylactic for cancer risk)

      2. Total colectomy with an ileal pouch-anal anastomosis (initially has temporary ileostomy)

   c. Ostomy

      1. Surgically created opening between intestine and abdominal wall that allows passage of fecal material

      2. Stoma is the surface opening which has appliance applied to retain stool and is emptied at intervals

      3. Name of ostomy depends on location of stoma

      4. Ileostomy: opening in ileum; may be permanent with total proctocolectomy or temporary (loop ileostomy)

      5. Ileostomies: always have liquid stool which can be corrosive to skin since contains digestive enzymes

      6. Continent (or Kock's) ileostomy: has intra-abdominal reservoir with nipple valve formation to allow catheter insertion to drain out stool

9. Nursing Care: Focus is effective management of disease with avoidance of complications

10. Nursing Diagnoses

    a. Diarrhea

    b. Disturbed Body Image: diarrhea may become controlling all aspects of life; client has surgery with ostomy

    c. Imbalanced Nutrition: Less than body requirement

    d. Risk for Impaired Tissue Integrity: malnutrition and healing post surgery

    e. Risk for Sexual Dysfunction, related to diarrhea or ostomy

11. Home Care

    a. Inflammatory bowel disease is chronic and day to day care lies with client

    b. Teaching to control symptoms, adequate nutrition; if client has ostomy: care and resources for supplies, support group and home care referral

B. Malabsorption Syndromes

   1. Definition

      a. Condition in which intestinal mucosa ineffectively absorbs nutrients resulting with excretion of nutrients in stool

      b. Common disorders include sprue, lactose intolerance, short bowel syndrome

   2. Pathophysiology

      a. Flattening of intestinal mucosa with loss of villi and microvilli

      b. Loss of absorptive surface and enzyme production

   3. Manifestations

      a. GI: anorexia, abdominal bloating, diarrhea with loose, bulky, foul-smelling stool, steatorrhea

b. Systemic: weight loss, general malaise, weakness, muscle cramps, bone pain, anemia

4. Sprue
   a. Celiac Disease (nontropical sprue)
      1. Chronic malabsorption disorder due to sensitivity to gluten, protein found in wheat, rye, barley, oats; commonly affects Caucasians of European descent
      2. Intestinal mucosa is damaged by immune response; there is loss of the absorptive surface
      3. Manifestations: abdominal bloating and cramps, diarrhea, and steatorrhea; leading to anemia, delayed maturity, symptoms associated with nutritional deficiencies; potential complications are GI malignancies and intestinal lymphoma
      4. Gluten free diet causes manifestations to resolve; treat nutritional deficiencies
   b. Tropical Sprue
      1. Occurs in tropical climates; cause unknown; pathological changes similar to celiac disease but not affected by gluten
      2. Treated with folic acid and tetracycline

5. Diagnostic Tests
   a. Fecal fat: document presence of steatorrhea
   b. Serologic testing for antibodies specific to celiac sprue
   c. Tests to evaluate nutrient deficiencies: serum protein, albumin, cholesterol, electrolytes, iron; evaluate anemia: hemoglobin, hematocrit, RBC indices; vitamin K deficiency: prothrombin time
   d. Enteroscopy: visualize and biopsy upper small bowel
   e. Upper GI series with small bowel follow-through

6. Lactase Deficiency
   a. Lack of enzyme lactase which is needed to absorb lactose, primary carbohydrate in milk and milk products
   b. More common is person of Asian, Native American, African American, Jewish American, and Hispanic heritage
   c. May be asymptomatic with moderate amounts of milk; symptoms include lower abdominal cramping, pain, diarrhea after milk ingestion
   d. May be diagnosed by lactose breath test, lactose tolerance tests
   e. Treatment includes following a lactose-free or reduced lactose diet or milk treated with lactase

7. Short Bowel Syndrome
   a. Condition involving malabsorption in clients who have had surgical resection of significant portions of the small intestine
   b. Absorption of water, nutrients, vitamins, minerals may be affected depending on part of small bowel resected; transit time may be reduced and digestive processes are impaired
   c. Manifestations may include weight loss, diarrhea, and nutritional deficiencies
   d. Diagnostic tests are done to evaluate nutritional deficiencies
   e. Clients often require small frequent feedings with high calories and protein; multivitamin and mineral supplements; proton-pump inhibitor; total parenteral nutrition (TPN) may be required

8. Collaborative Care: Focus on identifying cause; evaluate and treating nutritional deficiencies

9. Nursing Diagnoses
   a. Diarrhea
   b. Imbalanced Nutrition: Less than body requirements

10. Home Care: Focuses on education of treatment, prescribed diet, supplements

V. Neoplastic Disorders
   A. Background
      1. Large intestine and rectum most common GI site affected by cancer
      2. Colon cancer is second leading cause of death from cancer in U.S.
   B. Client with Polyps
      1. Definition
         a. Polyp is mass of tissue arising from bowel wall and protruding into lumen
         b. Most often occur in sigmoid and rectum
         c. 30% of people over 50 have polyps
         d. Most are benign but some have potential to become malignant
      2. Pathophysiology

a. Most polyps are adenomas, benign but considered premalignant; < 1% become malignant but all colorectal cancers arise from these polyps

b. Polyp types include tubular, villous, or tubularvillous

c. Familial polyposis is uncommon autosomal dominant genetic disorder with hundreds of adenomatous polyps throughout large intestine; untreated, near 100% malignancy by age 40

3. Manifestations

a. Most asymptomatic

b. Intermittent painless rectal bleeding is most common presenting symptom

4. Collaborative Care

a. Diagnosis is based on colonoscopy

b. Most reliable since allows inspection of entire colon with biopsy or polypectomy if indicated

c. Repeat every 3 years since polyps recur

5. Nursing Care

a. All clients advised to have screening colonoscopy at age 50 and every 5 years thereafter (polyps need 5 years of growth for significant malignancy)

b. Bowel preparation ordered prior to colonoscopy with cathartics and/or enemas

C. Client with Colorectal Cancer

1. Definition

a. Third most common cancer diagnosed

b. Affects sexes equally

c. Five-year survival rate is 90%, with early diagnosis and treatment

2. Risk Factors

a. Family history

b. Inflammatory bowel disease

c. Diet high in fat, calories, protein

3. Pathophysiology

a. Most malignancies begin as adenomatous polyps and arise in rectum and sigmoid

b. Spread by direct extension to involve entire bowel circumference and adjacent organs

c. Metastasize to regional lymph nodes via lymphatic and circulatory systems to liver, lungs, brain, bones, and kidneys

4. Manifestations

a. Often produces no symptoms until it is advanced

b. Presenting manifestation is bleeding; also change in bowel habits (diarrhea or constipation); pain, anorexia, weight loss, palpable abdominal or rectal mass; anemia

5. Complications

a. Bowel obstruction

b. Perforation of bowel by tumor, peritonitis

c. Direct extension of cancer to adjacent organs; reoccurrences within 4 years

6. Collaborative Care: Focus is on early detection and intervention

7. Screening

a. Digital exam beginning at age 40, annually

b. Fecal occult blood testing at 50, annually

c. Colonoscopies or sigmoidoscopies beginning at age 50, every 3–5 years

8. Diagnostic Tests

a. CBC: anemia from blood loss, tumor growth

b. Fecal occult blood (guiac or Hemoccult testing): all colorectal cancers bleed intermittently

c. Carcinoembryonic antigen (CEA): not used as screening test, but is a tumor marker and used to estimate prognosis, monitor treatment, detect reoccurrence

d. Colonoscopy or sigmoidoscopy; tissue biopsy of suspicious lesions, polyps

e. Chest x-ray, CT scans, MRI, ultrasounds: to determine tumor depth, organ involvement, metastasis

9. Surgery

a. Surgical resection of tumor, adjacent colon, and regional lymph nodes is treatment of choice

b. Whenever possible anal sphincter is preserved and colostomy avoided; anastomosis of remaining bowel is performed

c. Tumors of rectum are treated with abdominoperineal resection (A-P resection) in which sigmoid colon, rectum, and anus are removed through abdominal and perineal incisions and permanent colostomy created

d. Colostomy

1. Ostomy made in colon if obstruction from tumor

a. Temporary measure to promote healing of anastomoses

b. Permanent means for fecal evacuation if distal colon and rectum removed

2. Named for area of colon in which formed
   a. Sigmoid colostomy: used with A-P resection formed on LLQ (left lower quadrant)
   b. Double-barrel colostomy: 2 stomas: proximal for feces diversion; distal is mucous fistula
   c. Transverse loop colostomy: emergency procedure; loop suspended over a bridge; temporary
   d. Hartman procedure: Distal portion is left in place and oversewn; only proximal colostomy is brought to abdomen as stoma; temporary; colon reconnected at later time when client ready for surgical repair

10. Radiation Therapy
    a. Used as adjunct with surgery; rectal cancer has high rate of regional recurrence if tumor outside bowel wall or in regional lymph nodes
    b. Used preoperatively to shrink tumor

11. Chemotherapy: Used postoperatively with radiation therapy to reduce rate of rectal tumor recurrence and prolong survival

12. Nursing Care
    a. Prevention is primary issue
    b. Client teaching
       1. Diet: decrease amount of fat, refined sugar, red meat; increase amount of fiber; diet high in fruits and vegetables, whole grains, legumes
       2. Screening recommendations
       3. Seek medical attention for bleeding and warning signs of cancer
       4. Risk may be lowered by aspirin or NSAID use

13. Nursing Diagnoses for post-operative colorectal client
    a. Pain
    b. Imbalanced Nutrition: Less than body requirements
    c. Anticipatory Grieving
    d. Alteration in Body Image
    e. Risk for Sexual Dysfunction

14. Home Care
    a. Referral for home care

b. Referral to support groups for cancer or ostomy
c. Referral to hospice as needed for advanced disease

VI. Structural and Obstructive Disorders
   A. Client with a Hernia
      1. Definition: Defect in abdominal wall that allows abdominal contents to protrude out of abdominal cavity
      2. Risk Factors
         a. Trauma
         b. Surgery
         c. Increased intra-abdominal pressure from pregnancy, obesity, weight lifting, tumors
      3. Pathophysiology
         a. May be congenital (defect present at birth) or acquired (weakening of normal abdominal musculature)
         b. Reducable hernia
            1. Abdominal contents (peritoneum, bowel, other organs) protrude through abdominal wall to form a sac covered by skin and subcutaneous tissues
            2. Contents move into sac when intra-abdominal pressure increases
            3. Contents returns inside when pressure returns to normal or when manual pressure applied
         c. Incarcerated hernia: contents of hernia cannot be returned to abdominal cavity
         d. Strangulated hernia: blood supply to bowel contents in hernia is compromised leading to necrosis, untreated can result in perforation and peritonitis
         e. Manifestations: abdominal pain and distention, nausea, vomiting, tachycardia, fever
      4. Classification of hernias according to location
         a. Inguinal Hernia: occurs in the groin
            1. Indirect: occurs congenitally; sac of abdominal contents protrude through internal inguinal ring into inguinal canal; may descend into scrotum
            2. Direct: acquired defects from weakness of posterior inguinal wall
            3. Often cause lump in groin while lifting or straining
         b. Femoral Hernia
            1. Peritoneal sac protrudes though femoral ring

  2. Common in pregnant or obese women
  c. Umbilical Hernia: congenital or acquired
    1. More common in females
    2. Risk factors include multiple pregnancies, ascites, abdominal tumors
    3. Prone to strangulation
  d. Incisional or Ventral Hernia
    1. Occur at previous surgical incision or post abdominal tear
    2. Risk factors include poor wound closure or infection, age, debility, obesity, poor nutrition, excessive incisional stress
5. Collaborative Care
  a. Diagnosis made upon physical examination
  b. Felt when client coughs or bears down
6. Surgery
  a. Herniorrhaphy: surgical repair of hernia done electively and prevents incarceration, strangulation, perforation; often done as out-patient surgery
  b. Abdominal wall defect closed by suture and may have mesh inserted over defect
  c. Incarcerated or painful hernia necessitates emergency surgical repair; if infarcted bowel involved may necessitate bowel resection
  d. Post-operatively heavy lifting and manual work restricted 3 weeks
  e. For hernias not surgically repaired: client may be taught to reduce by lying down and pushing gently against mass, or by wearing truss or binder to control protrusion of hernia
7. Nursing Care
  a. Focus for clients with hernias not surgically repaired
    1. Teaching to prevent complications
    2. Seeking medical attention if strangulation occurs
  b. Postoperative care for clients who have had hernia repair
    1. No activities to increase intra-abdominal pressure while healing
    2. Usual care including pain management, asepsis, optimal nutrition
B. Client with Intestinal Obstruction
  1. Definition
    a. May be partial or complete obstruction
    b. Failure of intestinal contents to move through the bowel lumen; most common site is small intestine
    c. With obstruction, gas and fluid accumulate proximal to and within obstructed segment causing bowel distention
    d. Bowel distention, vomiting, third-spacing leads to hypovolemia, hypokalemia, renal insufficiency, shock
  2. Pathophysiology
    a. Mechanical
      1. Problems outside intestines: adhesions (bands of scar tissue), hernias
      2. Problems within intestines: tumors, IBD
      3. Obstruction of intestinal lumen (partial or complete)
        a. Intussusception: telescoping bowel
        b. Volvulus: twisted bowel
        c. Foreign bodies
        d. Strictures
    b. Functional
      1. Failure of peristalsis to move intestinal contents: adynamic ileus (paralytic ileus, ileus) due to neurologic or muscular impairment
      2. Accounts for most bowel obstructions
      3. Causes include
        a. Post gastrointestinal surgery
        b. Tissue anoxia or peritoneal irritation from hemorrhage, peritonitis, or perforation
        c. Hypokalemia
        d. Medications: narcotics, anticholinergic drugs, antidiarrheal medications
        e. Renal colic, spinal cord injuries, uremia
  3. Manifestations small bowel obstruction
    a. Vary and depend on level of obstruction and speed of development
    b. Cramping or colicky abdominal pain, intermittent, intensifying
    c. Vomiting
      1. Proximal intestinal distention stimulates vomiting center
      2. Distal obstruction vomiting may become feculent
    d. Bowel sounds

1. Early in course of mechanical obstruction: borborygmi and high-pitched tinkling, may have visible peristaltic waves
2. Later silent; with paralytic ileus, diminished or absent bowel sounds throughout
   e. Signs of dehydration
4. Complications
   a. Hypovolemia and hypovolemic shock can result in multiple organ dysfunction (acute renal failure, impaired ventilation, death)
   b. Strangulated bowel can result in gangrene, perforation, peritonitis, possible septic shock
   c. Delay in surgical intervention leads to higher mortality rate
5. Large Bowel Obstruction
   a. Only accounts for 15% of obstructions
   b. Causes include cancer of bowel, volvulus, diverticular disease, inflammatory disorders, fecal impaction
   c. Closed-loop obstruction: competent ileocecal valve causes massive colon dilation
   d. Manifestations: deep, cramping pain; severe, continuous pain signals bowel ischemia and possible perforation; localized tenderness or palpable mass may be noted
6. Collaborative Care
   a. Relieving pressure and obstruction
   b. Supportive care
7. Diagnostic Tests
   a. Abdominal x-rays and CT scans with contrast media
      1. Show distended loops of intestine with fluid and/or gas in small intestine, confirm mechanical obstruction; indicates free air under diaphragm
      2. If CT with contrast media meglumine diatrizoate (Gastrografin): check for allergy to iodine, need BUN and Creatinine to determine renal function
   b. Laboratory testing to evaluate for presence of infection and electrolyte imbalance: WBC, Serum amylase, osmolality, electrolytes, arterial blood gases
   c. Barium enema or colonoscopy/sigmoidoscopy to identify large bowel obstruction

8. Gastrointestinal Decompression
   a. Treatment with nasogastric or long intestinal tube provides bowel rest and removal of air and fluid
   b. Successfully relieves many partial small bowel obstructions
9. Surgery
   a. Treatment for complete mechanical obstructions, strangulated or incarcerated obstructions of small bowel, persistent incomplete mechanical obstructions
   b. Preoperative care
      1. Insertion of nasogastric tube to relieve vomiting, abdominal distention, and to prevent aspiration of intestinal contents
      2. Restore fluid and electrolyte balance; correct acid and alkaline imbalances
      3. Laparotomy: inspection of intestine and removal of infarcted or gangrenous tissue
      4. Removal of cause of obstruction: adhesions, tumors, foreign bodies, gangrenous portion of intestines and anastomosis or creation of colostomy depending on individual case
10. Nursing Care
    a. Prevention includes healthy diet, fluid intake
    b. Exercise, especially in clients with recurrent small bowel obstructions
11. Nursing Diagnoses
    a. Fluid Volume Deficit
    b. Ineffective Tissue Perfusion, gastrointestinal
    c. Ineffective Breathing Pattern
12. Home Care
    a. Home care referral as indicated
    b. Teaching about signs of recurrent obstruction and seeking medical attention
C. Client with Diverticular Disease
   1. Definition
      a. Diverticula are saclike projections of mucosa through muscular layer of colon mainly in sigmoid colon
      b. Incidence increases with age; less than a third of persons with diverticulosis develop symptoms
   2. Risk factors
      a. Cultural changes in western world with diet of highly refined and fiber-deficient foods

b. Decreased activity levels

c. Postponement of defecation

3. Pathophysiology

a. Diverticulosis is the presence of diverticula which form due to increased pressure within bowel lumen causes bowel mucosa to herniate through defects in colon wall, causing outpouchings

b. Muscle in bowel wall thickens narrowing bowel lumen and increasing intraluminal pressure

c. Complications of diverticulosis include hemorrhage and diverticulitis, the inflammation of the diverticular sac

d. Diverticulitis: diverticulum in sigmoid colon irritated with undigested food and bacteria forming a hard mass (fecalith) that impairs blood supply leading to perforation

e. With microscopic perforation, inflammation is localized; more extensive perforation may lead to peritonitis or abscess formation

4. Manifestations

a. Pain, left-sided, mild to moderate and cramping or steady

b. Constipation or frequency of defecation

c. May also have nausea, vomiting, low-grade fever, abdominal distention, tenderness and palpable LLQ mass

d. Older adult may have vague abdominal pain

5. Complications

a. Peritonitis

b. Abscess formation

c. Bowel obstruction

d. Fistula formation

e. Hemorrhage

6. Collaborative Care: Focus is on management of symptoms and complications

7. Diagnostic Tests

a. Abdominal x-ray: detection of free air with perforation, location of abscess, fistula

b. Barium enema contraindicated in early diverticulitis due to risk of barium leakage into peritoneal cavity but will confirm diverticulosis

c. Abdominal CT scan, sigmoidoscopy or colonscopy used in diagnosis of diverticulosis

d. WBC count with differential: leukocytosis with shift to left in diverticulitis

e. Hemocult or guiac testing: determine presence of occult blood

8. Medications

a. Broad spectrum antibiotics against gram negative and anaerobic bacteria to treat acute diverticulitis, oral or intravenous route depending on severity of symptoms

b. Analgesics for pain (non-narcotic)

c. Stool softener but not cathartic may be prescribed (nothing to increase pressure within bowel)

9. Dietary Management

a. Diet modification may decrease risk of complications

b. High-fiber diet (bran, commercial bulk-forming products such as psyllium seed (Metamucil) or methycelluose)

c. Some clients advised against foods with small seeds which could obstruct diverticula

10. Treatment for acute episode of diverticulitis

a. Client initially NPO with intravenous fluids (possibly TPN)

b. As symptoms subside reintroduce food: clear liquid diet, to soft, low-roughage diet, psyillium seed products to soften stool and increase bulk

c. High-fiber diet is resumed after full recovery

11. Surgery

a. Surgical intervention indicated for clients with generalized peritonitis or abscess that does not respond to treatment

b. With acute infection, 2 stage Hartman procedure done with temporary colostomy; re-anastomosis performed 2–3 months later

12. Nursing Care: Health promotion includes teaching high-fiber foods in diet generally, may be contraindicated for persons with known conditions

13. Nursing Diagnoses

a. Impaired Tissue Integrity, gastrointestinal

b. Pain

c. Anxiety, related to unknown outcome of treatment, possible surgery

14. Home Care
    a. Teaching regarding prescribed diet, fluid intake, medications
    b. Referral for home health care agency, if new colostomy client

VII. Anorectal Disorders
  A. Client with Hemorrhoids (Piles)
    1. Definition: Varicose veins, varices, or varicosities of veins in anus, anal canal region
    2. Risk Factors
       a. Straining to defecate in sitting or squatting position
       b. Pregnancy (increased intra-abdominal pressure)
       c. Prolonged sitting
       d. Obesity
       e. Chronic constipation
       f. Low-fiber diet
    3. Pathophysiology
       a. Hemorrhoids develop when venous return from anal canal is impaired
       b. Internal hemorrhoids affect venous plexus above mucocutaneous junction of anus
          1. Rarely cause pain but present with bleeding
          2. May vary in severity but recurrent can cause anemia
          3. Associated with portal hypertension
       c. External hemorrhoids affect venous plexus below the mucocutaneous junction
          1. Manifestations include anal irritation, feeling of pressure
          2. As hemorrhoids enlarge may prolapse and protrude through anus (may be manually replaced post defecation or become permanently prolapsed)
       d. Prolapsed hemorrhoid becomes painful when strangulated from edema and thrombosed
    4. Collaborative Care: Focus is on conservative care unless permanent prolapsed or thrombosis occurs
    5. Diagnosis
       a. Client history and examination of anorectal area
       b. Anoscopic exam used to detect and evaluate internal hemorrhoids
    6. Conservative Treatment
       a. High-fiber diet, increased water intake
       b. Bulk-forming products such as psyllium seed (Metamucil) or stool

softeners to prevent constipation and straining
    c. Comfort measures such as suppositories or ointments with anesthetic or astringent effects
    d. Warm sitz baths, bed rest, astringent compresses
    7. Treatment beyond conservative treatment
       a. Sclerotherapy: injecting chemical irritant into tissue surrounding hemorrhoid to cause inflammation and fibrosis and scarring
       b. Rubber band ligation: induce necrosis and slough of hemorrhoid
       c. Cryosurgery, infared photocoagulation, electrocoagulation
    8. Surgery: Hemorrhoidectomy
       a. Surgical excision of hemorrhoids
       b. Anal packing in for 24 hours
       c. Pain management with analgesics and sitz baths, stool softeners, cleansing agents post defecation to prevent infection
  B. Client with Anorectal Lesion
    1. Anal fissures
       a. Definition: Ulcerations occur in the epithelium of anal canal over internal sphincter become abraded
       b. Contributing factors
          1. Irritating diarrheal stools
          2. Tightening of the anal canal with increased sphincter tension
          3. Childbirth trauma
          4. Habitual cathartic use
          5. Laceration by a foreign body
          6. Anal Intercourse
       c. Manifestations
          1. Have periods of exacerbation and remission
          2. Pain that tears or burns occurring with defecation
          3. Bright red bleeding
          4. Constipation due to fear of defecation
       d. Diagnosis: Digital examination and anoscopy
       e. Treatment
          1. Dietary and fluid changes
          2. Bulk-forming laxative
          3. Topical hydrocortisone cream
          4. Internal sphincterotomy if not healed from medical intervention
    2. Anorectal Abscess
       a. Abscess in pararectal space often from multiple pathogens: *Escherichia coli*,

Proteus, streptococci, staphylococci; from infected hair follicle, sebaceous or sweat gland, fissures, or anal trauma
b. Manifestation is pain aggravated by sitting or walking with external swelling, redness, heat, tenderness
c. Usually involves incision and drainage (I and D) for drainage of large amount of pus and antibiotic therapy
d. May lead to fistula which may be surgically closed after infection has cleared

3. Anorectal Fistula
   a. Tract from anal canal to perianal skin
   b. Occur spontaneously from anorectal abscess drainage or Crohn's disease
   c. Treatment is fistulotomy; allowed to heal by secondary intention: from inside outward

4. Pilonidal Disease
   a. Acute abscess or chronic draining sinus in sacrococcygeal area
   b. May be due to hair entrapment or congenital defect
   c. Manifestations include pain, tenderness, redness, warmth, swelling, purulent drainage
   d. Treatment is incision and drainage (I and D); close by primary or secondary intention

5. Nursing Care
   a. Education of preventing constipation
   b. If surgical treatment has occurred emphasis on keeping area clean and dry, pain control

FOCUSED STUDY TIPS

- While caring for a client in the clinical setting, identify a bowel disorder for which the client may be at risk. List nursing interventions to prevent the disorder.
- Care for a client who has experienced bowel surgery. Describe the impact the surgery has had on the client's nutritional status. Describe how the client's eating pattern has been disrupted. Describe how nutritional needs are being met in the immediate postoperative period.
- Compare and contrast colostomy and ileostomy. Care for a client with an ileostomy or colostomy. Interview the client and identify lifestyle changes and changes in dietary patterns that have occurred since the surgery.

CASE STUDY

L. T. has had a stroke and has been incontinent of feces. Her condition is gradually improving. She is regaining muscle tone in her right arm and leg. Her caregivers and physician have asked you to develop a bowel-training program for home use to manage her fecal incontinence. List your topics of instruction for the client and family.

CARE PLAN CRITICAL THINKING ACTIVITY

R. B. is scheduled to have a knee replacement. He also has a colostomy. Create a care plan for his nursing diagnosis of "Alteration in elimination related to intestinal diversion." What extra precautions might need to be taken in the early postoperative period for this client?

NCLEX TEST QUESTIONS

1. Which of the following foods would present a problem for a client diagnosed with celiac disease?
   a. Butter
   b. Oats or barley cereal
   c. Fresh vegetables
   d. Coffee or tea
2. A client with a colostomy has been experiencing increased flatus for the past 3 days. Which client

information provided during assessment would lead the nurse to suspect an etiology for this occurrence?
   a. The client has been eating pasta for the past 3 days.
   b. The client has been eating cereal and milk for breakfast each morning.
   c. The client has been eating at a salad bar for lunch for the past 3 days.

d. The client has been taking more fluids for the past 3 days.

3. A nurse is discussing the home maintenance regimen with a client who has irritable bowel syndrome. Which of the following statements indicates client understanding?
   a. "I'll take a walk after dinner each evening."
   b. "I'll have a cigarette after meals to relax."
   c. "I'll chew gum between meals to curb my appetite."
   d. "I'll eat more fresh vegetables and fruits."

4. A client who has Crohn's disease complains of feeling very tired and extremely thirsty and has experienced excessive diarrhea the last few days. The client has sunken eyeballs and, upon examination, poor skin turgor. The nurse should recommend immediate treatment for
   a. malabsorption syndrome.
   b. electrolyte imbalance.
   c. dehydration.
   d. peritonitis.

5. Which of the following describes the best practice in an attempt to control diverticulosis?
   a. daily intake of vitamins A, C, and E
   b. high intake of dietary fiber
   c. high intake of carbohydrates
   d. increasing intake of fluids

6. A client is admitted to the unit with a large, distended bowel, acute tenderness upon palpation of the abdomen, fever, rigidity, and absent bowel sounds. After being on the unit, the client's level of consciousness decreases, and he begins to have feculent vomit. The priority therapeutic intervention would be to
   a. reduce the fever through antipyretics.
   b. insert an NG tube-to-wall suction and monitor the output.
   c. administer pain medications to relax the client.
   d. listen to bowel sounds.

7. When teaching the elderly client who is taking psyllium (Metamucil) for constipation, the nurse would instruct the client to
   a. expect results the evening of the first day the medicine is taken.

   b. mix the powder in applesauce to mask the taste.
   c. take each dose with 8 ounces of water and increase fluid intake.
   d. expect that the stools will become black in color.

8. Following a gunshot wound to the abdomen, a 27-year-old male has a complete colectomy with creation of an ileostomy. Nursing measures that will be necessary for the client, considering the fact that the function of the large intestine has been eliminated, will include
   a. administration of proteolytic enzymes via tube feedings.
   b. observation of intake and output, since reabsorption of water will be diminished.
   c. administration of proteolytic enzymes via tube feedings and administration of emulsifying agents.
   d. observation of intake and output and administration of emulsifying agents.

9. A client being admitted to a hospital unit is complaining of severe pain in the lower abdomen and is lying on the bed with his knees flexed. Admission vital signs reveal an oral temperature of 101.2°F. Which of the following would suggest a diagnosis of appendicitis?
   a. The pain is localized at a position halfway between the umbilicus and the right iliac crest.
   b. The client describes the pain as occurring 2 hours after eating.
   c. The pain subsides after eating.
   d. The pain is in the left lower quadrant.

10. A child with a confirmed diagnosis of appendicitis has been scheduled for an emergency appendectomy. Suddenly, the child states his pain is much less. The best interpretation of this is that
    a. he is tolerating the pain much better.
    b. there is a possibility the appendix has ruptured.
    c. his level of consciousness has decreased.
    d. perhaps the problem has been resolved.

CHAPTER 25

ASSESSING CLIENTS WITH URINARY SYSTEM DISORDERS

LEARNING OUTCOMES

After completing this chapter, you will be able to:

- Review the anatomy and physiology of the urinary system.
- Explain the role of the urinary system in maintaining homeostasis.
- Identify specific topics for consideration during a health history interview of the client with health problems involving the urinary system.
- Describe techniques for assessing the integrity and function of the urinary system.
- Identify abnormal findings that may indicate impairment of the urinary system.

KEY TOPICS

- Review of anatomy and physiology of the urinary system
- Formation of urine
- Maintaining normal composition and volume of urine
- Renal hormones
- Assessing urinary system functioning

LECTURE OUTLINE

   I. Background of Anatomy and Physiology
      A. Kidneys
         1. Outside of peritoneal cavity on either side of vertebral column at levels of T12–L3
         2. Supported by 3 layers of connective tissue
            a. Outer renal fascia: surrounds kidney and adrenal gland
            b. Middle adipose capsule: cushions and holds kidney in place

            c. Inner renal capsule: barrier against infection; protects kidneys from trauma
         3. Functions
            a. Balance solute and water transport
            b. Excrete metabolic waste products
            c. Conserve nutrients

d. Regulate acid-base balance
e. Secrete hormones to help regulate blood pressure, erythrocyte production, calcium metabolism
f. Form urine

4. Internal regions of each kidney:
   a. Cortex: outer region; contains glomeruli
   b. Medulla: contains renal pyramids (formed from bundles of collecting tubules); renal columns (extensions of cortex)
   c. Pelvis: innermost region continuous with ureter as leaves hilum
      1. Major and minor calyces, branches of pelvis, extend toward medulla and collect urine and empty into pelvis
      2. Urine channeled through ureter into bladder for storage
      3. Walls of calyces, renal pelvis, and ureter contain smooth muscle and move urine by peristalsis

5. Each kidney contain about 1 million nephrons
   a. Nephron: contains tuft of capillaries called glomerulus, which is surrounded by glomerular capsule (Bowman's space)
   b. Renal corpuscle: glomerulus and capsule
   c. Endothelium of capillaries of glomerulus are very porous
   d. Solute-rich fluid (filtrate) pass from capillaries into capsule; then channeled into Proximal Convoluted Tubule (PCT) of nephron
   e. Peritubular capillaries reabsorb substances into plasma from filtrate
      1. Active transport: glucose, sodium, potassium, amino acids, proteins, vitamins
      2. Passive transport: 70% water, chloride, bicarbonate
   f. Filtrate moves into loop of Henle and is concentrated
   g. Filtrate moves to Distal Convoluted Tubule (DCT) where solutes are secreted into filtrate
   h. Collecting duct receives newly formed urine from many nephrons and channels urine through calyces of renal pelvis into ureter

B. Ureters
   1. Bilateral tubes 10–12 inches long (25–30 cm)
   2. Transport urine from kidney to bladder through peristalsis
   3. Wall of ureter has 3 layers
      a. Inner is epithelial mucosa
      b. Middle is smooth muscle
      c. Outer is fibrous connective tissue

C. Urinary Bladder
   1. Posterior to symphysis pubis
      a. Males: immediately in front of rectum
      b. Females: next to vagina and uterus
   2. Storage of urine
   3. Trigone is smooth triangular portion of base of bladder outlined by openings for ureters and urethra
   4. Layers
      a. Epithelial mucosa lining (internal)
      b. Connective tissue submucosa
      c. Smooth muscle layer: detrusor muscle made up of fibers arranged to allow bladder to expand or contract according to amount of urine in it
      d. Fibrous outer layer
   5. Size of healthy adults holds 300–500 ml before internal pressure rises and signals need to empty
   6. Sphincters
      a. Internal: relaxes in response to full bladder and signals need to urinate
      b. External: formed by skeletal muscle, under voluntary control

D. Urethra
   1. Thin-walled muscular tube that channels urine to outside of body
   2. Extends from base of bladder to external urinary meatus
      a. Males: 8 inches long (20 cm) channels for semen and urine; prostate gland encircles urethra at base of bladder; urinary meatus located at end of the glans penis
      b. Females: 1.5 inches long (3–5 cm) anterior to vaginal orifice

E. Formation of Urine
   1. Kidneys process 180 liters (47 gallons) of blood-derived fluid each day; 1% excreted as urine; rest is returned to circulation
   2. Done by nephron through 3 processes:
      a. Glomerular filtration
      b. Tubular reabsorption
      c. Tubular secretion

F. Glomerular filtration
   1. Definition: passive, nonselective process in which hydrostatic pressure forces fluid and solutes through a membrane

2. Glomerular filtration fate (GFR): amount of fluid filtered from blood into capsule per minute
3. GFR is influenced by 3 factors
   a. Total surface area available for filtration
   b. Permeability of filtration membrane
   c. Net filtration pressure (proportional to GFR)
4. Net filtration pressure responsible for formation of filtrate
5. Net filtration pressure determined by 2 forces
   a. Hydrostatic pressure ("push")
   b. Osmotic pressure ("pull")
6. Normal GFR in both kidneys is 120–125 ml/min in adults; held constant under normal conditions by
   a. Renal autoregulation: Diameter of afferent arterioles responds to pressure changes in renal blood vessels:
      1. Increase in systemic blood pressure: renal vessels constrict
      2. Decline in blood pressure: afferent arterioles dilate
   b. Renin-angiotensin mechanism
      1. Juxtaglomerular apparatus located in distal tubules respond to slow filtrate flow by releasing chemical that causes intense vasodilation of afferent arterioles
      2. Increase in flow of filtrate promotes vasoconstriction, decreasing GFR
      3. Drop in systemic blood pressure triggers juxtaglomerular cells to release renin; acts on angiotensinogen to release angiotensin I which is converted to angiotensin II causing systemic vaso-constriction and causes systemic blood pressure to rise
   c. Extrinsic control through sympathetic nervous system
      1. Under extreme stress causes strong constriction of afferent arterioles and inhibits filtrate formation
      2. Causes release of renin, increasing systemic blood pressure
G. Tubular reabsorption: Proximal tubules constantly regulate and adjust rate and degree of water and solute reabsorption according to hormonal signals
H. Tubular secretion
   1. Substances (hydrogen and potassium ions, creatinine, ammonia, organic acids) move from blood into tubules as filtrate
   2. Mechanism for disposal of substance such as medications
   3. Rids body of undesirable substances that had been reabsorbed and rids body of excess potassium ions (regulation of pH)
I. Normal Composition and Volume of Urine
   1. Result of countercurrent exchange of fluid through tubes of loop of Henle and vasa recta (tiny capillaries)
   2. Dilution or concentration of urine largely determined by action of antidiuretic hormone (ADH)
   3. Urine by volume is 95% water; 5% solutes; most of weight from urea
J. Clearance of waste products
   1. Renal plasma clearance: ability of kidney to clear a given amount of plasma of particular substance in a given time
   2. Waste products cleared by kidneys
      a. Urea: nitrogenous waste product from breakdown of amino acids by liver; 25–30 gram daily
      b. Creatinine: end product of creatine phosphate, found in skeletal muscle
      c. Uric acid: metabolite of nucleic acid metabolism
      d. Ammonia
      e. Bacterial toxins
      f. Water-soluble drugs
   3. Tests of renal clearance used to determine GFR and glomerular damage
K. Renal hormones
   1. Activation of Vitamin D: absorption of calcium and phosphate
      a. Vitamin D enters body though dietary intake of action of ultraviolet rays on cholesterol in skin
      b. Activated first in liver and then kidneys under stimulation by parathyroid hormone
   2. Erythropoietin
      a. Produced by kidneys in response to decreased levels of oxygen to kidney
      b. Hormone stimulates bone marrow to produce red blood cells
   3. Natriuretic hormone
      a. Released by right atrium of heart in response to increased volume and stretch
      b. Inhibits ADH secretion which makes collecting tubules less porous, producing large amount of dilute urine
II. Assessment of Urinary System Function
   A. Health assessment interview to collect subjective data

1. Obtain information about current urinary status including
   a. Urine: color, odor, amount
   b. Any difficulty starting stream
   c. Frequency or urgency in urinating
   d. Dysuria: painful urination
   e. Nocturia: excessive urination at night
   f. Hematuria: blood in the urine
   g. Oliguria: voiding small amounts of urine
   h. Polyuria: voiding large amounts of urine
   i. Presence of any discharge
   j. Presence of flank pain
2. For any problem identified
   a. Analyze onset
   b. Characteristics and course
   c. Severity
   d. Factors that precipitate or relieve problem
   e. Associated symptoms
   f. Timing and circumstances
3. Additional information regarding urinary status
   a. Hematuria:
      1. Determine use of medications
      2. Presence of bleeding problems
      3. In females, whether menstruating
   b. Pyuria (cloudy, foul-smelling urine):
      1. Indicative of infection, determine whether client has temperature elevations, chills, malaise
      2. In males, retrograde ejaculation
   c. Pain
      1. Location, duration, intensity
      2. Kidney pain: present in back and costovertebral angle and may spread toward umbilicus
      3. Renal colic: severe, sharp, stabbing, excruciating in flank, bladder, urethra, testes, ovaries
      4. Bladder and urethral pain: dull, continuous or spasmodic
      5. Distended bladder: constant pain increased by any pressure over bladder
4. History: Family history of altered structure or function
   a. End-stage renal disease
   b. Renal calculi
   c. Frequent infections
   d. Hypertension
   e. Diabetes Mellitus

5. Life-style, diet, work history
   a. Cigarette smoking
   b. Exposure to toxic chemicals
   c. Usual amount and type of fluid intake
   d. Usual voiding habits
   e. Self-care measures
B. Physical assessment to collect objective data
   1. Skin assessment with abnormal findings
      a. Pallor of skin and mucous membranes: anemia
      b. Decreased skin turgor: dehydration
      c. Edema: fluid volume excess
      d. Uremic frost (uric acid crystals): untreated renal failure
   2. Abdominal assessment with abnormal findings
      a. Enlargement or asymmetry: hernia or superficial mass
      b. Prominent veins: renal dysfunction
      c. Distended, glistening, tight skin: fluid retention
      d. Fluid accumulation in peritoneal cavity: ascites
   3. Urinary meatus assessment with abnormal findings
      a. Redness, swelling, discharge: could be indicative of infection or sexually transmitted disease
      b. Ulceration: sexually transmitted disease
      c. In males, deviation from midline of meatus: congenital defect
   4. Kidney assessment with abnormal findings
      a. Systolic bruits: renal artery stenosis
      b. Tenderness and pain on percussion in costovertebral angle: glomerulonephritis or glomerulonephrosis
      c. Palpation of kidney:
         1. Mass or lump: tumor or cyst
         2. Pain or tenderness: inflammatory process
         3. Soft or sponginess: chronic renal failure
         4. Bilaterally enlarged kidneys: polycystic kidney disease
         5. Unequally sized kidneys: sign of hydronephrosis
   5. Bladder assessment with abnormal findings
      a. Dull percussion tone over bladder after voiding: urinary retention
      b. Palpation of bladder as firm, rounded organ: distended bladder

FOCUSED STUDY TIPS

- Memorize normal serum BUN (blood urea nitrogen) and serum creatinine levels. Always review and evaluate these values when caring for clients in the clinical setting.
- Keep track of your I & O (intake and output) for a 24-hour period. Evaluate your results. Are you close to normal values necessary to maintain homeostasis? If not, develop a plan to correct the imbalance.
- Practice palpating bladders. Palpate bladders when full. Palpate bladders immediately after voiding. Compare and contrast differences in assessment findings. Practice documenting assessments.

CASE STUDY

You are asked to give an inservice on urinary elimination to nursing assistants. One nursing assistant asks you, "How is urine made?" Write out your answer.

CARE PLAN CRITICAL THINKING ACTIVITY

What assessment data would you need to determine whether or not a client has a UTI (urinary tract infection)?

NCLEX TEST QUESTIONS

1. The creatinine level is a valuable indicator of glomerular filtration rate because
   a. creatinine levels are directly proportional to renal excretory function.
   b. creatinine only enters the glomerulus when glomerular filtration pressures exceed 60 mm Hg.
   c. creatinine filtration is unaffected by renal disease.
   d. creatinine is formed in the glomerulus.

2. What is the dominant effect of ADH (antidiuretic hormone) on the kidneys?
   a. Increased excretion of water and sodium
   b. Increased water reabsorption and more concentrated urine
   c. Greater reabsorption of sodium and potassium excretion
   d. Greater potassium reabsorption and sodium excretion

3. The reason females are more prone to urinary tract infections (UTI's) than males is attributed to the length of their
   a. ureters.
   b. urethra.
   c. pelvic bones.
   d. renal arteries.

4. If a urine specimen is needed for a client with signs and symptoms of acute renal failure (ARF), the nurse should instruct the client to collect a urine specimen

   a. midstream.
   b. at the beginning of urination.
   c. at the end of urination.
   d. first morning void.

5. When the nurse is evaluating the postoperative kidney function of a client, how much urine output will indicate normal renal perfusion?
   a. 10 mL per hour
   b. 30 mL per hour
   c. 50 mL per hour
   d. 90 mL per hour

6. As part of an annual physical exam, a 60-year-old adult male has had lab work done. Which of the following serum creatinine levels would indicate that the client has a mild degree of renal insufficiency?
   a. 5.0 mg/dL
   b. 4.3 mg/dL
   c. 1.7 mg/dL
   d. 0.8 mg/dL

7. The nurse is collecting a 24-hour urine specimen from a client. After collecting the first specimen, the nurse should
   a. save it as part of the collection.
   b. discard the specimen, and then begin collecting.
   c. test the specimen, and then discard it.
   d. collect 100 mL of the specimen, then discard the rest.

8. Which of the following statements by a student nurse reflects correct understanding about the body's attempt to restore homeostasis during periods of acidosis?
   a. "The kidneys start to work within seconds after an imbalance occurs and are very effective in restoring the body to a correct acid-base balance."
   b. "The kidneys may not start to function immediately but are very effective as a buffer system to restore the acid-base balance."
   c. "The kidneys are not as effective as the lungs in restoring the acid-base balance because the bicarbonate ion is not a good buffer."
   d. "The kidneys are very slow to respond to any acid-base imbalance but are very effective in ridding the body of carbonic acid."

9. Which of the following findings in the urinalysis report would the nurse consider abnormal?
   a. Straw-colored urine
   b. Glucose negative
   c. Blood negative
   d. Specific gravity of 1.10

10. The nurse evaluating for tenderness in the area of the kidneys would plan to use which of the following assessment techniques?
   a. Percussion
   b. Auscultation
   c. Inspection
   d. Light palpation

CHAPTER 26

NURSING CARE OF CLIENTS WITH URINARY TRACT DISORDERS

LEARNING OUTCOMES

After completing this chapter, you will be able to:

- Apply knowledge of the structure and function of the urinary tract to caring for clients with urinary tract disorders.
- Describe the pathophysiology of commonly occurring urinary tract disorders.
- Identify laboratory and diagnostic tests used to diagnose disorders affecting the urinary tract.
- Compare and contrast the manifestations of common urinary tract disorders.
- Discuss the nursing implications of medications prescribed for clients with urinary tract disorders.
- Provide appropriate nursing care for clients having surgery of the urinary tract.
- Use the nursing process as a framework for providing individualized care to clients with urinary tract disorders.

KEY TOPICS

- Urinary tract infection (UTI)
- Cancer of the urinary tract
- Trauma to the urinary tract
- Urinary obstructions
- Neurological conditions affecting the urinary tract

LECTURE OUTLINE

I. Client with a Urinary Tract Infection (UTI)
   A. Background
      1. Bacterial infections of urinary tract are very common reason to seek health services
      2. Common in young females and uncommon in males under age 50

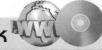

MediaLink
www.prenhall.com/lemone

Additional resources for this chapter can be found on the Student CD-ROM accompanying this textbook, and on the Companion Website at www.prenhall.com/lemone. Click on Chapter 26 to select the activities for this chapter.

CD-ROM
- Audio Glossary
- NCLEX Review

Companion Website
- More NCLEX Review
- Case Study
   Urinary Tract Infection
- Care Plan Activity
   Urinary Tract Infection
- MediaLink Application
   Urinary Tract Disorders

3. Common causative organisms
   a. *Escherichia coli* (gram-negative enteral bacteria) causes most community acquired infections
   b. *Staphylococcus saprophyticus*, gram-positive organism causes 10–15%

c. Catheter-associated UTI's caused by gram-negative bacteria: Proteus, Klebsiella, Seratia, Pseudomonas

4. Normal mechanisms that maintain sterility of urine
   a. Adequate urine volume
   b. Free-flow from kidneys through urinary meatus
   c. Complete bladder emptying
   d. Normal acidity of urine
   e. Peristaltic activity of ureters and competent ureterovesical junction
   f. Increased intravesicular pressure preventing reflux
   g. In males, antibacterial effect of zinc in prostatic fluid

B. Pathophysiology
   1. Pathogens which have colonized urethra, vagina, or perineal area enter urinary tract by ascending mucous membranes of perineal area into lower urinary tract
   2. Bacteria can ascend from bladder to infect the kidneys
   3. Classifications of infections
      a. Lower urinary tract infections: urethritis, prostatitis, cystitis
      b. Upper urinary tract infection: pyelonephritis (inflammation of kidney and renal pelvis)

C. Risk Factors
   1. Aging:
      a. Increased incidence of diabetes mellitus
      b. Increased risk of urinary stasis
      c. Impaired immune response
   2. Females: short urethra, having sexual intercourse, use of contraceptives that alter normal bacteria flora of vagina and perineal tissues; with age increased incidence of cystocele, rectocele (incomplete emptying)
   3. Males: prostatic hypertrophy, bacterial prostatitis, anal intercourse
   4. Urinary tract obstruction: tumor or calculi, strictures
   5. Impaired bladder innervation
   6. Bowel incontinence
   7. Diabetes mellitus
   8. Instrumentation of urinary tract

D. Cystitis
   1. Most common UTI
   2. Remains superficial, involving bladder mucosa which becomes hyperemic and may hemorrhage
   3. General manifestations of cystitis:
      a. Dysuria
      b. Frequency and urgency

c. Nocturia
d. Urine has foul odor, cloudy (pyuria), bloody (hematuria)
e. Suprapubic pain and tenderness

4. Older clients may present with different manifestations
   a. Nocturia, incontinence
   b. Confusion
   c. Behavioral changes
   d. Lethargy
   e. Anorexia
   f. Fever or hypothermia

5. Readily responds to treatment
6. Untreated, may involve kidneys
7. Severe or prolonged may cause sloughing of bladder mucosa with ulcer formation
8. Chronic cystitis may lead to bladder stone formation

E. Catheter-Associated UTI
   1. Longer a catheter is in place, greater risk for infection
   2. Bacteria may enter catheter system at connection between catheter and drainage system or through emptying tube of drainage bag
   3. UTI's may be asymptomatic
   4. Most infections resolve with removal of catheter and short course of antibiotic
   5. Most significant complication is gram-negative bacteremia

F. Pyelonephritis
   1. Inflammation of renal pelvis and parenchyma (functional kidney tissue)
   2. Acute pyelonephritis
      a. Results from infection that ascends to kidney from lower urinary tract
      b. Risk factors
         1. Pregnancy
         2. Urinary tract obstruction and congenital malformation
         3. Urinary tract trauma, scarring
         4. Renal calculi
         5. Polycystic or hypertensive renal disease
         6. Chronic diseases i.e., diabetes mellitus
         7. Vesicourethral reflux
      c. Pathophysiology
         1. Infection spreads from renal pelvis to renal cortex
         2. Kidney grossly edematous; localized abscesses in cortex surface
         3. *E. coli* responsible organism for 85% of acute pyelonephritis; also *Proteus, Klebisella*

  d. Manifestations
     1. Rapid onset with chills and fever
     2. Malaise
     3. Vomiting
     4. Flank pain
     5. Costovertebral tenderness
     6. Urinary frequency, dysuria
  e. Manifestations in older adults
     1. Change in behavior
     2. Acute confusion
     3. Incontinence
     4. General deterioration in condition
3. Chronic pyelonephritis
  a. Involves chronic inflammation and scarring of tubules and interstitial tissues of kidney
  b. Common cause of chronic renal failure
  c. May develop from chronic hypertension, vascular conditions, severe vesicoureteral reflux, obstruction of urinary tract
  d. Behaviors
     1. Asymptomatic
     2. Mild behaviors: urinary frequency, dysuria, flank pain
4. Collaborative Care
  a. Eliminate causative agent
  b. Prevent relapse
  c. Correct contributing factors
5. Diagnostic Tests
  a. Urinalysis: assess pyuria, bacteria, blood cells in urine; Bacterial count > 100,000/ml indicative of infection
  b. Rapid tests for bacteria in urine
     1. Nitrite dipstick (turning pink = presence of bacteria)
     2. Leukocyte esterase test (identifies WBC in urine)
  c. Gram stain of urine: identify by shape and characteristic (gram positive or negative); obtain by clean catch urine or catheterization
  d. Urine culture and sensitivity: identify infecting organism and most effective antibiotic; culture requires 24–72 hours for results; obtain by clean catch urine or catheterization
  e. WBC with differential: leukocytosis and increased number of neutrophils
6. Diagnostic Tests for adults who have recurrent infections or persistent bacteriuria
  a. Intravenous pyelography (IVP) or excretory urography
     1. Evaluates structure and excretory function of kidneys, ureters, bladder
     2. Kidneys clear an intravenously injected contrast medium and outline kidneys, ureters, bladder, and vesicoureteral reflux
     3. Check for allergy to iodine, seafood, radiologic contrast medium; if client has allergy, hold testing and notify physician or radiologist
  b. Voiding cystourethrography: instill contrast medium into bladder and use x-ray to assess bladder and urethra when filled and during voiding
  c. Cystoscopy
     1. Direct visualization of urethra and bladder through cystoscope
     2. Used for diagnostic, tissue biopsy, interventions
     3. Client receives local or general anesthesia
  d. Manual pelvic or prostate examinations to assess structural changes of genitourinary tract, such as prostatic enlargement, cystocele, rectocele
7. Medications
  a. Short-course therapy: 3 day course of antibiotics for uncomplicated lower urinary tract infection (single dose associated with recurrent infection)
  b. 7–10 days course of treatment: for pyelonephritis, urinary tract abnormalities or stones, or history of previous infection with antibiotic-resistant infections; clients with severe illness may need hospitalization and intravenous antibiotics
  c. Antibiotics commonly used for short and longer course therapy include trimethoprim-sulfamethoxazole (TMP-SMZ), or quinolone antibiotic such as ciprofloxacin (Cipro)
  d. Intravenous antibiotics used include ciprofloxacin, gentamycin, ceftriaxone (Rocephin), ampicillin
  e. Possible outcomes of treatment for UTI, determined by follow-up urinalysis and culture
     1. Cure: no pathogens in urine
     2. Unresolved bacteriuria: pathogens remain

3. Persistent bacteriuria or relapse: persistent source of infection causes repeated infection after initial cure
4. Reinfection: development of new infection with different pathogen
    f. Prophylactic antibiotic therapy with TMP-SMZ, TMP alone or nitrofurantoin (Furadantin, Nitrofan) may be used with clients who experience frequent symptomatic UTI
    g. Catheter-associated UTI: removal of indwelling catheter followed by 10–14 day course of antibiotic therapy
8. Surgery
    a. Surgical removal of large calculus from renal pelvis or cystoscopic removal of bladder calculi which serve as irritant and source of bacterial colonization; may also use percutaneous ultrasonic pyelolithotomy or extracorporeal shock wave lithotripsy (ESWL)
    b. Ureteroplasty: surgical repair of ureter for stricture or structural abnormality; reimplantation if vesicoureteral reflux; clients usually return from surgery with catheter and ureteral stent in place for 3–5 days
9. Nursing Care: Health promotion to prevent UTI
    a. Fluid intake 2–2.5 L daily, more if hot weather or strenuous activity is involved
    b. Empty bladder every 3–4 hours
    c. Females
        1. Cleanse perineal area from front to back
        2. Void before and after sexual intercourse
        3. Maintain integrity of perineal tissues
            a. Avoid use of commercial feminine hygiene products or douches
            b. Wear cotton underwear
    d. Maintain acidity of urine (use of cranberry juice, take Vitamin C, avoid excess milk, milk products, and sodium bicarbonate)
10. Nursing Diagnoses
    a. Pain: Additional interventions include warmth, analgesic, urinary analgesics, antispasmodic medications
    b. Impaired Urinary Elimination

    c. Ineffective Health Maintenance: Clients must complete full course of antibiotic therapy
11. Home Care: Teaching prevention of infection and use alternatives to indwelling catheter whenever possible
II. Client with Urinary Calculi
    A. Background
        1. Urinary calculi are stones in urinary tract
            a. Nephrolithiasis: stones form in kidneys
            b. Urolithiasis: stones form in urinary tract outside kidneys
        2. Highest incidence in southern and Midwestern states
        3. Males more often affected than females (4:1)
        4. Most common in young and middle adults
    B. Risk factors
        1. Majority of stones are idiopathic (no demonstrable cause)
        2. Prior personal or family history of urinary calculi
        3. Dehydration: increased urine concentration
        4. Immobility
        5. Excess dietary intake of calcium, oxalate, protein
        6. Gout, hyperparathyroidism, urinary stasis, repeated UTI infection
    C. Pathophysiology
        1. Factors leading to lithiasis include supersaturation (high concentration of insoluble salt in urine), pH of urine
        2. Types of calculi
            a. Calcium stones (calcium oxalate, calcium phosphate)
                1. Associated with high concentrations of calcium in blood or urine
                2. Genetic link
            b. Uric acid stones
                1. Associated with high concentration of uric acid in urine
                2. Genetic link
                3. More common in males
                4. Associated with gout
            c. Sturvite stones
                1. Associated with UTI caused by bacteria *Proteus*
                2. Stones are very large
                3. Staghorn stones in renal pelvis and calyces
            d. Cystine stones: Associated with genetic defect

D. Manifestations: depends upon size and location of stones
  1. Calculi affecting kidney calices, pelvis
    a. Few symptoms unless obstructed flow
    b. Dull, aching flank pain
  2. Calculi affecting bladder
    a. Few symptoms
    b. Dull suprapubic pain with exercise or post voiding
    c. Possibly gross hematuria
  3. Calculi affecting ureter, causing ureteral spasm
    a. Renal colic: acute, severe flank pain of affected side, radiates to suprapubic region, groin, and external genitals
    b. Nausea, vomiting, pallor, cool, clammy skin
  4. Manifestations of UTI may occur with urinary calculi
E. Complications
  1. Obstruction: manifestations depend upon speed of obstruction development; can ultimately lead to renal failure
  2. Hydronephrosis: distention of renal pelvis and calyces; unrelieved pressure can damage kidney (collecting tubules, proximal tubules, glomeruli) leading to gradual loss of renal function
    a. Acute: colicky pain on affected side
    b. Chronic: few manifestations: dull ache in back or flank
    c. Other manifestations: hematuria, signs of UTI, GI symptoms
F. Collaborative Care
  1. Relief of acute symptoms
  2. Remove or destroy stone
  3. Prevent future stone formation
G. Diagnostic Tests
  1. Urinalysis: hematuria, possible WBCs and crystal fragments, urine pH helpful to diagnose stone type
  2. Chemical analysis of stone: All urine must be strained and saved; stones or sediment sent for analysis
  3. 24-urine collection for calcium, uric acid, oxalate to identify possible cause of lithiasis
  4. Serum calcium, phosphorus, uric acid: identify factors in calculi formation
  5. KUB x-ray (kidney, ureters, bladder): flat plate to identify presence and location of opacities
  6. Renal ultrasonography: sound waves to detect stones and detect hydronephrosis
  7. CT scan of kidney: identify calculi, obstruction, disorders
  8. IVP
  9. Cystoscopy: visualize and possibly remove calculi from urinary bladder and distal ureters
H. Medications
  1. Treatment of acute renal colic: analgesia and hydration
  2. Narcotic such as intravenous morphine sulfate, NSAID, large amounts of fluid by oral or intravenous routes
  3. Medications to inhibit further lithiasis according to analysis of stone:
    a. Thiazide diuretics: promotes reduction of urinary calcium excretion
    b. Potassium citrate: used to alkalinize urine for stones formed in acidic urine (uric acid, cystine, and some calcium stones)
I. Dietary Management: Prescribed to change character of urine and prevent further lithiasis
  1. Increased fluid intake to 2–2.5 liters daily, spaced throughout day
  2. Limited intake of calcium and Vitamin D sources if calcium stones
  3. Phosphorus and/or oxalate may be limited with calcium stones
  4. Low purine (rich meats) diet for clients with uric acid stones
  5. Control of pH to maintain pH that inhibits lithiasis
    a. Promote alkaline urine for clients with uric acid or cystine stones
    b. Promote acid urine for clients with calcium stones or urinary tract infections
J. Lithotripsy: Use of sound or shock waves to crush stones
  1. Extracorporeal shock-wave lithotripsy: acoustic shock waves aimed under fluoroscopic guidance to pulverize stone into fragments small enough to be eliminated in urine; sedation or TENS used to maintain comfort during procedure
  2. Percutaneous ultrasonic lithotripsy: nephroscope inserted into kidney pelvis through small flank incision; stone fragmented using small ultrasonic transducer and fragments removed through nephroscope
  3. Laser lithotripsy: stone is disintegrated by use of laser beams; nephroscope or ureteroscope used to guide laser probe

4. Stent may be inserted into affected ureter after procedure to maintain patency after lithotripsy procedures

K. Surgery
1. May be indicated as treatment depending on stone location, severe obstruction, infection, serious bleeding
2. Types:
    a. Ureterolithotomy: incision into affected ureter to remove calculus
    b. Pyelolithotomy: incision into and removal of stone from kidney pelvis
    c. Nephrolithotomy: surgery to remove staghorn calculus in calices and renal parenchyma
    d. Cystoscopy: crushing and removal of bladder stones through cystocope; stone fragments irrigated out of bladder with acid solution

L. Nursing Care
1. Focus on comfort during renal colic, diagnostic procedures, ensure adequate urine output, prevent future stone formation
2. Health promotion: adequate fluid intake for all clients, adequate weight-bearing activity to prevent bone resorption, hypercalcuria, prevention of UTI

M. Nursing Diagnoses
1. Acute Pain
    a. Adequate pain management
    b. Intensity of pain can cause vaso-vagal response; client may experience hypotension, syncope; client safety must be maintained
2. Impaired Urinary Elimination
    a. Teaching client and strain all urine; send recovered stones for analysis
    b. Complete obstruction causes hydronephrosis on involved side; other kidney continues forming urine; monitor BUN, Creatinine
    c. Maintain patency and integrity of all catheters; all catheters need to be labeled, secured, and sterility maintained
3. Knowledge Deficient: Client participation in treatment and prevention

N. Home Care
1. Education regarding management current treatment and prevention
2. Clients may be discharged with catheters, tubes, dressings; home care referral

III. Client with a Urinary Tract Tumor
A. Background

1. Malignancies in urinary tract: 90% bladder; 8% renal pelvis; 2% ureter, urethral; 5 year survival rate for bladder cancer is 94%
2. Bladder cancer: 4 times higher in males than females; 2 times higher in whites than blacks; occurs over age 60

B. Risk factors
1. Carcinogens in urine
    a. Cigarette smoking
    b. Occupational exposure to chemicals and dyes
2. Chronic inflammation or infection of bladder mucosa

C. Pathophysiology
1. Tumors arise from epithelial tissue which composes the lining
2. Tumors arise as flat or papillary lesions
3. Poorly differentiated flat tumor invades directly and has poorer prognosis
4. Metastasis commonly involves pelvic lymph nodes, lungs, bones, liver

D. Manifestations
1. Painless hematuria is presenting sign in 75% cases; may be gross or microscopic and may be intermittent
2. Inflammation may cause manifestations of UTI
3. May have few outward signs until obstructed urine flow or renal failure occurs

E. Collaborative Care
1. Removal or destruction of cancerous tissue
2. Prevent invasion or metastasis
3. Maintain renal and urinary function

F. Diagnostic Tests
1. Urinalysis: diagnosis of hematuria
2. Urine cytology: microscopic examination of cells for tumor or pre-tumor cells in urine
3. Ultrasound of bladder: detection of bladder tumor
4. IVP: evaluation of structure and function of kidneys, ureters, bladder
5. Cystoscopy, ureteroscopy: direct visualization, assessment, and biopsy of lesion(s)
6. CT scan or MRI: determine tumor invasion, metastasis

G. Medications
1. Immunologic or chemotherapeutic agent administered by intravesical instillation used as primary treatment of bladder cancer or to prevent recurrence following endoscopic removal of tumor

2. Agents include Bacillus Calmette-Guerin (BCGLive, TheraCys), doxorubicin, mitomycin C
3. Adverse reactions include bladder irritation, frequency, dysuria, contact dermatitis

H. Radiation Therapy
1. Adjunctive therapy used for treatment of urinary tumors
2. Used to reduce tumor size prior to surgery, palliative treatment

I. Surgery
1. Cystoscopic tumor resection by
   a. Excision
   b. Fulguration: destruction of tissue using high frequency electric current
   c. Laser photocoagulation: light energy to destroy tumor
2. Radical cystectomy: standard treatment to treat invasive cancers; removal of bladder and adjacent muscles and tissues
   a. Males: includes prostate and seminal vessels
   b. Females: hysterectomy, salpingo-oophorectomy
3. Client needs to have urinary diversion done to provide for urine collection and drainage through ileal conduit or continent urinary diversion (ureters are implanted in portion of ileum which is surgically made into a reservoir for urine and stoma brought to surface of abdomen)

J. Nursing Care
1. Treatment with recovery from initial treatment
2. Continual care for recurrence
3. Management for elimination
4. Coping with cancer diagnosis

K. Health Promotion
1. Encouragement of clients not to smoke
2. Smoking cessation programs
3. Periodic examination of urinalysis and possibly urine cytology

L. Nursing Diagnoses
1. Impaired Urinary Elimination
2. Risk for Impaired Skin Integrity (clients with urinary diversions)
   a. Urine is irritating to skin around stoma
   b. Care includes using appliance with adhesives and sealants
   c. Urine will have shreds of mucus in it from bowel
   d. Collection bag emptied frequently (every 2 hours) during day
   e. Connected to bedside drainage bag while asleep

3. Disturbed Body Image
   a. Abdominal stoma requiring drainage appliance or regular catheterization of stoma to drain urine
   b. Removal of reproductive organs has made client sterile
   c. Side effects from chemotherapy or radiation
4. Risk for Infection

M. Home Care
1. Involves continual surveillance for cancer recurrence
2. If client has had urinary diversion surgery requires teaching regarding stoma and skin care
3. Home care referral
4. Smoking cessation

IV. Client with Urinary Retention
A. Definition
1. Incomplete emptying of bladder leading to overdistention of bladder
2. Poor bladder contractility
3. Inability to urinate
4. May develop hydronephrosis

B. Pathophysiology
1. Mechanical obstruction of bladder outlet or functional problem leads to urinary retention including
   a. Benign prostatic hypertrophy (BPH)
   b. Acute inflammation associated with infection or trauma of bladder
   c. Status post abdominal or pelvic surgery disrupting detrusor muscle function
   d. Anticholinergic medications
   e. Failure to void regularly, resulting in bladder overfill and loss of detrusor muscle tone
2. Client may experience overflow voiding or incontinence 25–50 ml at frequent intervals

C. Collaborative Care: Treatment focuses on removing or repairing obstruction, e.g., prostrate gland resection

D. Treatment may include
1. Catheterization indwelling or intermittent
2. Cholinergic medications such as bethanechol chloride (Urecholine) promoting detrusor muscle contraction and bladder emptying
3. Elimination of medications with anti-cholinergic effects

E. Nursing Care
1. Focus on monitoring urine output of at risk clients including those receiving

medications which interfere with detrusor muscle function

2. With acute urinary retention, catheterization may be necessary; if bladder is overdistended, drain only 500 ml at 5–10 minute intervals to prevent vaso-vagal response and hematuria

F. Home Care: Specific teaching depends on prescribed treatment which may include
   1. Intermittent self-catheterization
   2. Care with over the counter medications which may have anticholinergic effects
   3. Double voiding; scheduled voiding
   4. Indwelling catheter

V. Client with Neurogenic Bladder
   A. Definition: Disruption of central or peripheral nervous system that interferes with normal mechanisms involved with bladder filling, perception of fullness, need to void, bladder emptying
   B. Spastic Bladder Dysfunction
      1. Normal physiology: simple reflex between bladder and spinal cord (S2–S4): stimulus of > 400 ml of urine in bladder causes reflex contraction of detrusor muscle and bladder emptying unless voluntary control suppresses it
      2. Pathophysiology includes disruption of CNS transmission above sacral spinal cord segment; bladder filling causes frequent spontaneous detrusor muscle contraction and involuntary bladder emptying
      3. Causes include: spinal cord injury, multiple sclerosis, stroke
   C. Flaccid Bladder Dysfunction
      1. Client cannot perceive bladder fullness; loss of detrusor muscle tone and bladder overdistends: occurs in clients with myelomeningocele and during spinal shock stage post spinal cord injury above sacral region
      2. Peripheral neuropathies lead to incomplete bladder emptying with large residual volumes after voiding; occurs in clients with diabetes mellitus, multiple sclerosis, prolonged overdistension of bladder
   D. Collaborative Care
      1. Maintenance of continence
      2. Voiding complications
      3. Client self-care
   E. Diagnostic Tests
      1. Urine culture: determine UTI
      2. Urinalysis (presence of albumin, RBC's), BUN, Creatinine to determine renal function

3. Post-void catheterization for residual urine: should be < 50 ml.
4. Cystometrography: testing to evaluate bladder filling and detrusor muscle done and function

F. Medications
   1. To improve detrusor muscle contraction with flaccid bladder, such as post-operatively or after childbirth, with bladder training:
      a. Cholinergic drug (e.g., Bethanechol)
      b. Anticholinesterase drugs (e.g., neostigmine (Prostigmin))
   2. To relax detrusor muscle and contract internal sphincter, increasing bladder capacity in clients with spastic bladder:
      a. Anticholinergic medications
         1. Oxybutynin (Ditropan)
         2. Tolterodine (Detrol)
         3. Propantheline (Pro-Banthine)
         4. Flavoxate (Urispas)
      b. Adverse effects include dry mouth, blurred vision, constipation

G. Dietary management
   1. Moderate to high fluid intake, timing to promote continence
   2. Acidify urine to prevent UTI with cranberry juice

H. Bladder Retraining
   1. Scheduled toileting with stimulated reflex voiding by using trigger points, e.g., stroke or pinch abdomen, inner thighs for clients with spastic bladder
   2. Crede method: applying pressure to suprapubic region, manual pressure on abdomen, Valsalva maneuver to promote bladder emptying with either type or neurogenic bladder (Do not use with spinal cord injury clients: at risk for autonomic dysreflexia)
   3. Intermittent catheterization

I. Surgery
   1. May be used with clients unresponsive to other therapies
   2. Includes rhizotomy (destruction of nerves supplying detrusor muscle) with spasticity
   3. Urinary diversion

J. Nursing Diagnoses
   1. Impaired Urinary Elimination
   2. Self-care Deficit
   3. Risk for Infection

K. Home care: Involves teaching client, family about methods to control voiding, promote bladder emptying, medications, manifestations of UTI, reducing complications

VI. Client with Urinary Incontinence
   A. Background
      1. Urinary incontinence is involuntary urination; leads to
         a. Physical problems including skin breakdown and infection
         b. Psychosocial aspects: embarrassment, isolation, depression
      2. Up to 30% older women in community have incontinence; 50% of long-term care and home-bound populations
   B. Pathophysiology
      1. Pressure within the urinary bladder exceeds urethral resistance
      2. Conditions leading to incontinence include
         a. Relaxation of pelvic musculature
         b. Disruption of cerebral and nervous system control
         c. Disturbances in bladder and its musculature
      3. Acquired, irreversible causes include chronic neurological conditions
      4. Acute, reversible causes include confusion, effects of medications, prostatic enlargement, vaginal and urethral atrophy, UTI, fecal impaction
      5. Categories include
         a. Stress incontinence
         b. Urge incontinence (overactive bladder)
         c. Overflow incontinence
         d. Functional incontinence
         e. Mixed incontinence (stress and urge)
      6. Incontinency associated with increased risk for falls, pressure ulcers, UTI, depression, caregiver stress, and cause for institutionalizing client
   C. Collaborative Care
      1. Focus is identification and correction of cause if possible; otherwise management of urinary output
      2. Evaluation includes history including duration, frequency, volume and circumstances associated with incontinence (e.g., prostatic enlargement, cystocele, rectocele); voiding diary
   D. Diagnostic Tests
      1. Urinalysis and urine culture: assess for UTI
      2. Postvoiding residual: < 50 ml is expected; > 100 ml indicates need for further testing
      3. Cystometrography: evaluation of neuromuscular function of bladder;

normally urge to void occurs at 150–450 ml; bladder feels full at 300–500 ml.
      4. Uroflowmetry: noninvasive test to evaluate voiding pattern
      5. IVP: evaluates structure and function of urinary tract
      6. Cystoscopy or ultrasound: identify structural disorders
   E. Medications
      1. Mild stress incontinence may be improved by using medications that contract smooth muscles of bladder neck such as phenylpropanolamine which is often used in over the counter decongestants and diet aids
      2. Incontinence with postmenopausal atrophic vaginitis responds to topical estrogen therapy
      3. Urge incontinence treated with medications that increase bladder capacity: oxybutynin (Ditropan), tolterodine (Detrol)
      4. Clients may have other medical conditions adversely affected by medications used to treat incontinence
   F. Surgery: Treatments for stress incontinence
      1. Suspension of bladder neck by laparoscopic, vaginal, or abdominal approach treats stress incontinence associated with cystocele
      2. Prostatectomy may be used to treat enlarged prostate gland and urethral obstruction
   G. Complementary Therapies: Biofeedback and relaxation techniques
   H. Nursing Care
      1. Health promotion includes education that incontinence is not normal with aging
      2. Educate females about pelvic floor exercises
      3. Educate males about treatment for prostatic enlargement
      4. Availability of therapies and health practitioners
   I. Nursing Diagnoses
      1. Urinary Incontinence, stress and/or urge
         a. Clients with difficulty emptying bladder should not stop flow while voiding
         b. Limit fluids that are irritating to bladder: caffeine, alcohol, citrus juices, artificial sweeteners
      2. Self-care Deficit: Toileting
         a. Assist client in independence
         b. Planned toileting schedule
      3. Social Isolation

J. Home Care
1. Assisting clients to deal effectively with incontinence lessens risk for institutionalization; address causes, availability of treatment, management interventions

2. Assess toileting environment for safety and assist to obtain mobility aids such as safety bar, raised toilet seat
3. Clients who have had bladder neck suspension surgery often are discharged with catheter in place; client and family teaching, home health referral

FOCUSED STUDY TIPS

- Care for an incontinent client in the clinical setting. Formulate nursing interventions that meet the psychosocial needs of this client. Share them with your instructor.
- Practice urinary catheterization in the skills lab. Critique a classmate's aseptic technique. Describe why aseptic technique is necessary to prevent urinary tract complications.
- Demonstrate urinary hygiene teaching. Describe the relationship between urinary hygiene and urinary health.
- Create instructions for the collection of a clean-catch urine specimen. Evaluate the instructions for ease of understanding and optimal specimen collection.

CASE STUDY

The physician orders an indwelling catheter for a client for whom you are caring. As you prepare for the procedure, the client asks what risks are involved in the procedure. What do you tell him? What are the risk factors for urinary catheterization of hospitalized clients? Describe your nursing interventions that will eliminate as many risk factors and/or complications as possible for this client.

CARE PLAN CRITICAL THINKING ACTIVITY

The client with urinary tract infection is at increased risk for future UTI. Identify measures to be included in a teaching plan to help clients prevent recurrent infection. Be sure to include dietary, hygiene, and lifestyle measures.

NCLEX TEST QUESTIONS

1. Phenazopyridine (Pyridium) is sometimes ordered for the client with a urinary tract infection. Which of the following should be explained to a male client?
   a. "This is an antibiotic that is commonly used."
   b. "This drug may discolor the urine and semen orange."
   c. "The drug will cure the urinary tract infection and takes the place of increasing fluids."
   d. "This drug is good, but very nephrotoxic."
2. An 80-year-old female is brought to the office by her daughter complaining of decreased appetite and confusion. The nurse knows that these complaints may be symptoms of
   a. dementia.
   b. cerebral vascular accident (CVA).
   c. urinary tract infection (UTI).
   d. constipation.
3. A client has had a cystectomy and ureteroileostomy (ileal conduit). The nurse

observes this client for complications in the postoperative period. Which of the following symptoms indicates an unexpected outcome and requires priority care?
   a. Edema of the stoma
   b. Mucus in the drainage appliance
   c. Redness of the stoma
   d. Feces in the drainage appliance
4. A 64-year-old client is admitted to the hospital with acute urinary retention. The primary treatment for this condition after conservative nursing measures have been exhausted is to
   a. catheterize the client.
   b. perform a transurethral prostate resection.
   c. introduce a cystostomy tube.
   d. decrease oral intake and perform an IVP.
5. The nurse is preparing a teaching plan for the client with a urinary stone. Fluid intake is an important preventive measure and should be between 2,500–3,000 mL/day. A client with

which of the following disorders would have to decrease fluid intake in spite of this recommendation?

a. arthritis.

b. systemic lupus.

c. congestive heart failure (CHF).

d. diabetes.

6. A client has a routine physical and the urinalysis returns with microscopic hematuria. Which other signs or symptoms would likely be present in a client with a urinary tract tumor?

a. Colicky pain

b. Burning on urination

c. Infection

d. Polyuria

7. A Foley catheter was removed after being in place for 2 days. The response considered to be normal at this time is

a. dribbling after the first several voidings.

b. urgency and frequency for several days.

c. frequent voidings in small amounts.

d. retention of urine for 10- to 12-hour periods.

8. A female client with recurrent cystitis has been instructed to follow an acid-ash diet. The client

demonstrates understanding of diet instruction if she states to avoid which of the following foods?

a. Fish

b. Corn

c. Eggs

d. Milk

9. A client seen in the emergency department complains of painful urination, frequency, and urgency. Which of the following conditions would the nurse suspect?

a. Renal calculi

b. Cystitis

c. Glomerulonephritis

d. Polycystic kidney disease

10. A client complains of inability to inhibit urine flow long enough to reach the toilet. The nurse documents the presence of which type of urinary incontinence?

a. Stress

b. Reflex

c. Urge

d. Functional

CHAPTER 27

NURSING CARE OF CLIENTS WITH KIDNEY DISORDERS

LEARNING OUTCOMES

After completing this chapter, you will be able to:

- Relate the pathophysiology of common kidney disorders to normal renal physiology (see Chapter 25).
- Relate manifestations of kidney disease to the pathophysiology of the disorder.
- Discuss diagnostic studies used to identify disorders of the kidneys.
- Discuss the nursing implications for medications used to treat clients with kidney disorders.
- Identify specific dietary modifications ordered for clients with kidney disorders.
- Compare and contrast dialysis procedures used to manage acute and chronic renal failure.
- Discuss nursing care of the client undergoing dialysis.
- Provide appropriate nursing care for the client who has had kidney surgery or a renal transplant.
- Use the nursing process to plan and provide individualized care to clients with renal disorders.

KEY TOPICS

- Pathophysiology of kidney disorders
- Medical management of kidney disorders
- Comparison of dialysis treatments for kidney failure
- Nursing care of clients with kidney disorders
- Nursing care of clients with kidney transplant surgery
- Nursing care of clients undergoing dialysis

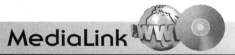

MediaLink

www.prenhall.com/lemone

Additional resources for this chapter can be found on the Student CD-ROM accompanying this textbook, and on the Companion Website at www.prenhall.com/lemone. Click on Chapter 27 to select the activities for this chapter.

CD-ROM
- Audio Glossary
- NCLEX Review

Animations
- Furosemide

Companion Website
- More NCLEX Review
- Case Study
  Acute Glomerulonephritis
- Care Plan Activity
  Acute Glomerulonephritis
- MediaLink Application
  Kidney Disorders

195

LECTURE OUTLINE

I. Age-Related Changes in Kidney Function
   A. Decline in glomerular filtration rate (GFR) to half or less related to
      1. Arteriosclerosis
      2. Decreased renal vascularity
      3. Decreased cardiac output
   B. Reduced clearance of drugs excreted through kidneys: prolonged half life of such medications as
      1. Cardiac drugs: digoxin, procainamide
      2. Antibiotics: aminoglycosides, tetracyclines, cephalosporins
      3. Histamine H_2 antagonists: cimetidine
      4. Antidiabetic agents: chlorpropamide
   C. Increased risk for fluid and electrolyte imbalance
      1. Decreased ability to concentrate urine and compensate for altered salt intake
      2. Decreased effectiveness of antidiuretic hormone (ADH) and reduced thirst response
      3. Decreased potassium excretion due to lower aldosterone levels
II. Client with a Congenital Kidney Malformation
   A. Affects form and function of kidney
      1. Agenesis: absence of kidney; renal function normal as long as other kidney is functioning
      2. Hypoplasia: underdevelopment of kidney; renal function normal as long as other kidney is functioning
      3. Horseshoe kidney: embryonic kidney fails to ascend normally and results in single horseshoe-shaped organ; increased risk for hydronephrosis and recurrent UTI, renal calculi
   B. Education is important to maintain and prevent renal complications from developing
III. Client with Polycystic Kidney Disease
   A. Definition
      1. Hereditary disease characterized by cyst formation and massive kidney enlargement
      2. Adult form of disorder is autosomal dominant polycystic kidney disease and accounts for 10% of persons in End Stage Renal Disease (ESRD)
   B. Pathophysiology
      1. Renal cysts are fluid-filled sacs affecting nephrons; cysts fill, enlarge, multiply thus compressing and obstructing kidney tissue; renal parenchyma atrophies, becomes fibrotic

2. Cysts occur elsewhere in body including liver, spleen
   C. Manifestations
      1. Disease is slowly progressive; symptoms develop in age 30–40's
      2. Common manifestations include
         a. Flank pain
         b. Microscopic or gross hematuria
         c. Proteinuria
         d. Polyuria and nocturia (impaired ability to concentrate urine)
         e. UTI and renal calculi are common
         f. Hypertension from disrupted renal vessels
         g. Kidneys become palpable, enlarged, knobby
         h. Symptoms of renal insufficiency and chronic renal failure by age of 50–60
   D. Collaborative Care: Determine extent of polycystic kidney disease
   E. Diagnostic Tests
      1. Renal ultrasonography: primary choice for diagnostic; assesses kidney size, identifies and locates renal masses: cysts, tumors, calculi
      2. Intravenous pyelography (IVP): evaluate structure and excretory function of kidneys, ureters, bladder
      3. CT scan of kidneys: detects and differentiates renal masses
   F. Management
      1. Mainly supportive: prevent further renal damage from UTI, nephrotoxic substances, obstruction, hypertension
      2. Fluid intake of 2000–2500 ml to prevent UTI, calculi
      3. Control of hypertension with ACE inhibitors and other antihypertensive agents
      4. Eventually require dialysis or transplantation (typically good candidates)
   G. Nursing Care and Nursing Diagnoses
      1. Risk for Ineffective Coping: address genetic counseling and screening for family members
      2. Excess Fluid Volume
      3. Anticipatory Grieving
      4. Knowledge Deficit: of measures to preserve kidney function
IV. Client with a Glomerular Disorder
   A. Definition
      1. Leading cause of chronic renal failure in U.S.

2. Primary disorders involve mainly kidney
   a. Immunologic
   b. Idiopathic
3. Secondary disorders relate to inherited or multisystem disease
   a. Diabetes mellitus
   b. Systemic lupus erythematosus (SLE)
   c. Goodpasture's syndrome
B. Pathophysiology
   1. Glomerular disease affects structure and function of glomerulus affecting filtration and increasing permeability in glomerulus
   2. Results in manifestations:
      a. Hematuria
      b. Proteinuria (most important indicator; increases progressively with glomerular damage)
      c. Edema (results from hypoalbuminemia)
   3. GFR falls resulting in azotemia (increased blood level of nitrogenous waste products) and hypertension
   4. Involvement may be diffuse (all glomeruli) or focal (some glomeruli)
   5. Oliguria (urine output < 400 ml in 24 ml)
C. Primary glomerular disorders:
   1. Acute glomerulonephritis
      a. Inflammation of glomerular capillary membrane
      b. Most common form is poststreptococcal glomerulonephritis
      c. Circulating antigen-antibody immune complexes formed in primary infection are trapped in glomerular membrane; complement system activated; glomeruli inflamed and increasingly permeable
      d. Manifestations
         1. Abrupt onset of hematuria, proteinuria, salt and water retention, azotemia 10–14 days post initial infection
         2. Urine is cocoa or coffee-colored
         3. Edema noted in face, particularly periorbital, dependent edema in hands and upper extremities
         4. Fatigue, anorexia, nausea, vomiting
         5. Older adults have less apparent symptoms: nausea, malaise, arthralgias, proteinuria, pulmonary infiltrates
      e. Adults: 60% recover fully; remainder have persistent symptoms and permanent kidney damage

2. Rapidly progressive glomerulonephritis (RPGN)
   a. Severe glomerular damage without specific identifiable cause
   b. Primary or secondary to SLE or Goodpasture's syndrome
   c. Diffuse glomerular damage with rapid progressive disease with irreversible renal failure over weeks to months
   d. May have flulike illness preceding onset resulting in oliguria, abdominal or flank pain, moderate hypertension, hematuria, proteinuria
3. Chronic glomerulonephritis
   a. Typically end stage of other glomerular disorders (RPGN, lupus nephritis, diabetic nephropathy)
   b. Symptoms develop insidiously, may be unrecognized until signs of renal failure develop
   c. Course of disease varies with time between diagnosis and development of end-stage renal failure
4. Nephrotic syndrome
   a. Group of clinical findings, not specific disorder
   b. Characterized by
      1. Massive proteinuria
      2. Hypoalbuminemia
      3. Hyperlipidemia
      4. Edema (often facial and periorbital)
   c. Several disorders affect glomerular capillary membrane
   d. Clients have increased risk for atherosclerosis
   e. Complication is thromboemboli leading to renal vein and deep vein thrombosis, pulmonary embolism
   f. Adults: < 50% recover; remainder develop persistent proteinuria and progress to ESRD
D. Common secondary forms of glomerular disease
   1. Diabetic nephropathy
      a. Leading cause of ESRD in U.S.
      b. 30% of clients with Diabetes Type 1; 20% of clients with Diabetes Type 2
      c. Initial evidence is microproteinuria typically seen 10–15 years after onset of diabetes; nephropathy develops within 15–20 years after initial diagnosis
      d. Characteristic lesion is glomerulosclerosis and thickening of glomerular basement membrane

e. Arteriosclerosis and hypertension contribute to disease
2. Lupus nephritis
    a. 40–85% of clients develop manifestations of nephritis
    b. Immune complexes trigger glomerular injury
    c. Manifestations range from microscopic hematuria to massive proteinuria; progression varies form slow and chronic to fulminant
    d. Improved management, dialysis and transplantation has improved prognosis
E. Collaborative Care
1. Identification of underlying disease process
2. Preservation of renal function
F. Diagnostic Tests
1. Throat or skin cultures: detect group A beta-hemolytic streptococci; used with identification of poststreptococcal glomerulonephritis
2. Antistreptolysin O (ASO) titer: detect streptococcal exoenzymes; used with identification of poststreptococcal glomerulonephritis
3. Erythrocyte sedimentation rate (ESR): indicator of inflammatory response as with poststreptococcal glomerulonephritis or lupus nephritis
4. KUB (kidney, ureters, bladder) abdominal x-ray: evaluate kidney size; enlarged with acute glomerulonephritis; small with chronic glomerulonephritis
5. Kidney scan: nuclear medicine procedure reveals delayed uptake with glomerular disease
6. Biopsy: microscopic examination of kidney tissue most reliable diagnostic procedure for glomerular disorders; determines type, prognosis, and appropriate treatment of glomerulonephritis
7. Serum BUN, Creatinine: evaluate kidney function; creatinine is good indicator of kidney function since entirely excreted by kidneys
8. Urine creatinine: levels decrease with impaired renal function
9. Creatinine clearance: very specific indicator of renal function and GFR
10. Serum electrolytes: evaluate values affected by impaired kidney function, especially serum potassium

11. Urinalysis: shows red blood cells, abnormal protein
12. 24 hour urine for protein: determine amount of protein in urine
G. Medications
1. Not curative but treatment for underlying disorders, decrease inflammation, symptom management
2. Antibiotics: treatment for poststreptococcal glomerulonephritis if any remaining bacteria (avoid nephrotoxic antibiotics)
3. Immunosuppressive therapy: aggressively treat acute inflammatory processes (RPGN), Goodpasture's syndrome, SLE
    a. Prednisone, glucocorticoid in large doses
    b. Cyclophosphamide (Cytoxan) or azathioprine (Imuran)
    c. ACE inhibitors to reduce protein loss associated with nephrotic syndrome, diabetic nephropathy
    d. Antihypertensive medications
H. Treatment
1. Bedrest: treatment of acute phase of poststreptococcal glomerulonephritis
2. Sodium restriction to 1–2 gm/day with nephrotic syndrome
3. Protein intake may be restricted and should be of high biologic value (complete proteins: have all essential amino acids)
4. Plasmapheresis: procedure to remove damaging antibodies
5. Dialysis procedures
I. Nursing Care: Health Promotion
1. Effective treatment of streptococcal infections with completion of full course of antibiotics
2. Effective management of chronic conditions such as diabetes mellitus and SLE and hypertension
3. Avoiding potentially nephrotoxic medications
J. Nursing Diagnoses
1. Fluid Volume Excess: monitor effects on cardiac workload, blood pressure, respiratory status
2. Fatigue: manifestation of anemia, hypoproteinemia, anorexia, nausea
3. Ineffective Protection: increased risk for infection
4. Ineffective Role Performance
K. Home Care
1. Teach clients that glomerular disorders are self-limiting or progressive

2. Course is lengthy
3. Self-management is essential
V. Client with a Vascular Kidney Disorder
  A. Hypertension
    1. Sustained elevation of systemic blood pressure results from or causes kidney disease
    2. Damages walls of arterioles and accelerates process of atherosclerosis including afferent and efferent arterioles and glomerular capillaries in kidney
    3. Untreated malignant hypertension can lead to rapid decline in renal function
  B. Renal Artery Occlusion
    1. Pathophysiology
      a. Primary process affecting renal vessels
      b. Result from emboli, clots, other foreign materials
    2. Risk factors acute renal artery thrombosis
      a. Severe abdominal trauma
      b. Vessel trauma from surgery or angiography
      c. Aortic or renal artery aneurysms
      d. Severe aortic or renal artery atherosclerosis
      e. Emboli from atrial fibrillation, post myocardial infarction, vegetative growth on heart valves from bacterial endocarditis, fatty plaque in aorta
    3. Manifestations
      a. Slow onset may be asymptomatic
      b. Acute occlusion: severe localized flank pain, nausea, vomiting, fever, hypertension, hematuria, oliguria
      c. In older client, new onset or worsening of hypertension
    4. Diagnostic tests
      a. WBC: leukocytosis
      b. Elevated renal enzymes: aspartate transaminase (AST), lactic dehydrogenase (LDH)
      c. Tests showing acute renal failure if bilateral arterial occlusion and infarction
    5. Treatment
      a. Surgery to restore blood flow to affected kidney with acute occlusion
      b. Management includes anticoagulant therapy, hypertension control, supportive treatment
  C. Renal Vein Occlusion
    1. In adults usually occurs with nephrotic syndrome
    2. Gradual or acute deterioration of renal function is only manifestation

    3. If thrombus breaks loose, results in pulmonary embolism
    4. Diagnosis: visualization of thrombus on renal venography
    5. Treatment: thrombolytic drugs to dissolve clot; anticoagulant therapy
  D. Renal Artery Stenosis
    1. Causes 2–5% of cases of hypertension affecting one or both kidneys; in males: atherosclerosis with gradual occlusion of renal artery; in females, fibromuscular dysplasia
    2. Manifestations
      a. Hypertension before age 30 or after 50 without prior history
      b. Epigastric bruit
    3. Diagnostic tests
      a. Renal ultrasound shows small and atrophied kidney
      b. Captopril test for renin activity shows higher levels of renin
      c. Renal angiography visualizes renal stenosis
    4. Treatment
      a. Dilation of stenotic vessel by percutaneous transluminal angioplasty
      b. Surgery: bypass graft of renal artery beyond stenosis
VI. Client with Kidney Trauma
  A. Pathophysiology
    1. Kidneys damaged by blunt force or penetrating injury
    2. Minor injuries: contusion, small hematoma, capsule or cortex laceration
    3. Major injuries:
      a. Kidney fragment or "shatter": significant blood loss, urine extravasation
      b. Tearing of renal artery or vein
      c. Renal artery, vein, or pelvis laceration
  B. Manifestations
    1. Hematuria, gross or microscopic
    2. Flank or abdominal pain
    3. Localized swelling, tenderness, ecchymoses in flank region
    4. Turner's sign: bluish discoloration of flank
    5. Acute blood loss: signs of shock: hypotension, tachycardia, tachypnea, cool and pale skin, altered level of consciousness
  C. Diagnostic Tests
    1. Falling hemoglobin and hematocrit levels
    2. Urinalysis: hematuria
    3. AST levels rise

4. Renal ultrasound: reveal renal bleeding and damage
5. CT scan
6. IVP
7. Renal arteriography
D. Treatment
  1. Minor kidney injuries
     a. Conservative treatment: bedrest and observation
     b. Minimal bleeding and self-limiting
  2. Major kidney injuries
     a. Immediate treatment to control hemorrhage, prevent and treat shock
     b. Surgery including surgical repair, partial or total nephrectomy
     c. Percutaneous arterial embolization during angiography
E. Nursing Care
  1. Accurate assessment
  2. Interventions
  3. Prevention of complications
VII. Client with a Renal Tumor
A. Definition/Pathophysiology
  1. Primary renal tumors are renal cell carcinomas
     a. Account for 2% adult cancers
     b. Often metastasized when diagnosed
     c. Metastasis tends to occur in lungs, bone, lymph nodes, liver, and brain
  2. Tumor may produce hormones resulting in hypercalcemia, hypertension, hyperglycemia
  3. Increased incidence in males, over age 55
B. Risk factors
  1. Smoking
  2. Obesity
  3. Renal calculi
  4. Genetic factors
C. Manifestations
  1. Often few manifestations
  2. Gross hematuria
  3. Flank pain
  4. Palpable abdominal mass
  5. Systemic: fever without infection, fatigue, weight loss
D. Diagnostic tests
  1. Renal ultrasonography: detect renal masses
  2. CT scan: determine tumor size, extension, regional lymph node or vascular involvement
  3. IVP and MRI: evaluate renal structure and function
  4. Renal angiography to evaluate extent of vascular involvement

5. Chest x-ray, bone scan, liver function tests to identify metastases
E. Treatment
  1. Radical nephrectomy is treatment of choice with regional lymph node resection
  2. No effective treatment for metastases, attempt biologic therapies or chemotherapy
F. Nursing Care: Focus on needs related to diagnosis and surgical intervention
G. Nursing Diagnoses (surgery and cancer diagnosis)
  1. Pain
  2. Ineffective Breathing Pattern
  3. Risk for Impaired Urinary Elimination
  4. Anticipatory Grieving
H. Home Care: Focus on protecting remaining kidney, monitor for recurrence
VIII. Clients with Renal Failure
A. Definition
  1. Condition in which kidneys are unable to remove accumulated metabolites from blood which leads to altered fluid, electrolyte and acid-base balance
  2. May be due to kidney (primary disorder) or resulting from another disease in another organ or systemic (secondary disorder)
  3. Classified as acute (abrupt onset and may be reversible) or chronic (develops slowly and insidiously with few symptoms until kidneys are severely damaged and unable to meet body's excretory needs)
  4. Common and costly disease with people with End Stage Renal Disease requiring dialysis or transplant to live
  5. 5-year survival rate for clients on dialysis is 31.3%
B. Acute Renal Failure (ARF)
  1. Definition
     a. Rapid decline in renal function with azotemia, fluid and electrolyte imbalances
     b. High mortality rate but is related to clients being seriously ill and aged
  2. Risk factors
     a. Major surgery or trauma
     b. Infection
     c. Hemorrhage
     d. Severe heart failure, liver disease
     e. Lower urinary tract obstruction
     f. Use of nephrotoxic contrast media and medications

3. Pathophysiology involved with cause categories
  a. Prerenal
    1. 55–60% cases of ARF
    2. Causes: Conditions that affect renal blood flow and perfusion
      a. Decrease vascular volume
      b. Decrease cardiac output
      c. Decrease vascular resistance
  b. Intrarenal
    1. 35–40% cases of ARF
    2. Cause: Acute damage to renal parenchyma and nephron
      a. Acute glomerulonephritis
      b. Vascular disorders including vasculitis, malignant hypertension, arterial or venous occlusion
      c. Acute Tubular Necrosis (ATN): Destruction of tubular epithelial cell with abrupt decline in renal function from
        1. Prolonged ischemia (> 2 hours) as with surgery, severe hypovolemia, sepsis, trauma, burns
        2. Nephrotoxins
          a. Aminoglycoside antibiotics
          b. Radiologic contrast media
          c. Other potential drugs: NSAIDs, heavy metals, ethylene glycol (antifreeze)
        3. Nephrotoxins have increased risk with clients with preexisting renal insufficiency or state of dehydration
        4. Rhabdomyolysis: excess myoglobin from skeletal muscle injury clogs renal tubules (muscle trauma, drug overdose, infection)
        5. Hemolysis: red blood cell destruction
  d. Postrenal
    1. < 5% cases of ARF
    2. Cause: Obstructive; prevents urine excretion
      a. Benign prostatic hypertrophy
      b. Renal or urinary tract calculi or tumors

4. Course and Manifestations of ARF in 3 phases
  a. Initiation phase
    1. Lasts hours to day
    2. Begins with initiating event until maintenance phase begins
    3. Good prognosis if treated at this phase
    4. Few manifestations; identified when maintenance phase begins
  b. Maintenance phase
    1. Characterized by significant fall in GFR and tubular necrosis
    2. Oliguric or non-oliguric but kidneys not eliminating wastes, water, electrolytes, acids: azotemia, fluid retention, electrolyte imbalances (hyperkalemia, hypocalcemia, hyperphosphatemia), acidosis (impaired hydrogen ion elimination)
    3. Anemia after several days due to suppressed erythropoetin secretion; impaired immune function
    4. Salt and water retention leading to hypertension and risk for heart failure and pulmonary edema
    5. Hyperkalemia: cardiac dysrhythmias and EKG changes, muscle weakness, nausea, diarrhea
    6. Confusion, disorientation, agitation or lethargy, hyperreflexia, possible seizures, coma
    7. Vomiting, decreased or absent bowel sounds
  c. Recovery phase
    1. Progressive tubule cell repair and regeneration; return of GFR to pre-ARF levels
    2. Diuresis occurs as kidney recover but BUN, creatinine, potassium and phosphate remain high
    3. Renal function improves rapidly first 5–25 days but improvement may continue for up to a year
5. Collaborative Care
  a. Prevention of ARF is goal for all clients, especially those at high risk
    1. Preserve kidney perfusion by adequate vascular volume, cardiac output and blood pressure
    2. Limiting use of nephrotoxic medications or using minimal effective dose, maintaining hydration, monitoring renal function tests

b. Treatment goals
   1. Identify and correct underlying cause
   2. Prevent additional renal damage
   3. Restore urine output and kidney function
   4. Compensate for impaired renal function: maintain fluid and electrolyte balance
6. Diagnostic tests to identify ARF
   a. Urinalysis
      1. Fixed specific gravity 1.010 (low)
      2. Proteinuria if glomerular damage
      3. Presence of red blood cells (glomerular dysfunction), white blood cells (inflammation), renal tubule epithelial cells (ATN)
      4. Cell casts (protein and cellular debris molded in shape of tubular lumen); brown color may indicate hemoglobinuria or myoglobinuria
   b. Serum BUN and creatinine
      1. Creatinine rises rapidly (24–48 hours) and peaks in 5–10 days; rise is slower if output maintained
      2. Halt in rise of BUN and creatinine signals onset of recovery
   c. Serum electrolytes
      1. Monitored to determine whether to initiate dialysis
      2. Moderate rise in potassium
      3. Hyponatremia related to water excess
   d. CBC showed moderate anemia and low hematocrit (Iron and folate may be low and add to anemia)
   e. Renal ultrasound: used to identify any obstruction, identify acute from chronic renal failure
   f. CT scan: identify obstruction and kidney size
   g. IVP, retrograde pyelography, or antegrade pyelography
      1. Assess renal structure and function
      2. Retrograde and antegrade testing less toxicity from contrast media
   h. Renal biopsy: determine cause, differentiate acute from chronic
7. Medications
   a. Intravenous fluids and blood volume expanders to restore renal perfusion
   b. Low dose dopamine (Intropin) intravenous infusion to increase renal blood flow and improve cardiac output

c. Diuretics: Furosemide (Lasix) or osmotic diuretic such as mannitol along with intravenous fluids; "washes out" nephrons, prevents oliguria reducing azotemia and electrolyte imbalance
d. Antihypertensive medications including ACE inhibitors to limit renal injury
e. Medications to prevent possible complications
   1. Prevention of gastrointestinal bleeding (at risk due to stress, impaired platelet function)
      a. Antacids
      b. H_2 receptor antagonists
      c. Proton-pump inhibitors
   2. Treatment of hyperkalemia: serum K > 6.5 mEq/L puts client at risk for cardiac arrest
      a. Calcium chlorides
      b. Bicarbonate
      c. Insulin and glucose
      d. Sodium polystyrene sulfonate (Kayexalete)
         1. Removes potassium from body primarily in large intestine
         2. If given orally, is combined with sorbitol
         3. May be given as retention enema with tap water enema to follow after 30–60 minutes
   3. Treatment of hyperphosphatemia
      a. Aluminum hydroxide (AlternaGEL, Amphojel, Nephrox)
      b. Binds with phosphates in GI tract and is eliminated from bowel
8. Fluid management
   a. Once vascular volume and renal perfusion restored, fluids are restricted
   b. Often intake is calculated by adding output from previous 24 hours and 500 ml for insensible losses
   c. Fluid balance monitored by daily weights and serum Na level
9. Dietary management
   a. Renal insufficiency and underlying disease creates increased rate of catabolism (breakdown of body proteins) and decreased rate of anabolism (tissue repair)
   b. Client needs adequate nutrition and calories to prevent catabolism but protein intake needs to be limited to minimize azotemia

    c. Protein limited to 0.6 g/kg body weight per day; protein should be of high biologic value (contains all essential amino acids)

    d. Carbohydrate intake is increased for adequate calories and protein-sparing effect

10. Dialysis

    a. Dialysis is the diffusion of solute molecules across semipermeable membrane from area of higher solute concentration to lower concentration

    b. Dialysis used to remove excess fluid, waste products from client with renal failure; can rapidly remove nephrotoxins from blood

11. Hemodialysis

    a. In this type of dialysis blood is taken from client via vascular access and pumped into a dialyzer; blood is separated from the dialysate (dialysis solution) by semipermeable membrane

    b. Processes of diffusion and ultrafiltration remove waste products, electrolytes, excess water

    c. Glucose, electrolytes, water can pass through but larger molecules (protein, red blood cells) are blocked

    d. Substances can be added to dialysate to diffuse into the blood of the client

    e. A client with ARF may undergo hemodialysis daily initially then 3–4 times/week according to client condition; 3–4 hours at a time

12. Complications associated with hemodialysis

    a. Hypotension, most common, related to changes in osmolality, rapid removal from vascular department, vasodilation

    b. Bleeding related to platelet function and use of heparin during dialysis

    c. Infection, local or systemic; Staphylococcus aureus septicemia associated with infected vascular access site; higher rates of hepatitis B and C, cytomegalovirus, HIV in hemodialysis clients

13. Continuous Renal Replacement Therapy (CRRT)

    a. Technique used: which allows more gradual fluid and solute removal than hemodialysis; used for clients with ARF unable to tolerate hemodialysis

    b. Done over period of 12 hours or more

14. Vascular access for hemodialysis

    a. Acute or temporary access is gained by inserting double lumen catheter into subclavian, jugular, or femerol vein

    b. Blood is drawn from proximal portion of catheter and returned to circulation through distal end of catheter

    c. Arteriovenous (AV) fistula created for longer term access for dialysis

        1. Surgical anastomosis of artery and vein in non-dominant arm, usually radial artery and cephalic vein

        2. Usually cannot use fistula for hemodialysis access for a month while it matures

        3. Nurse or client can assess functional fistula for complications:

            a. Thrombosis (clotted off): check for palpable thrill, audible bruit

            b. Infection: check for redness, drainage

        4. Venipunctures and blood pressures should not be done in arm with the AV fistula

        5. AV fistulas are commonly used for vascular access for dialysis clients with chronic renal failure

15. Peritoneal dialysis:

    a. Peritoneal membrane of client is used as dialyzing surface

    b. Warmed sterile dialysate instilled into peritoneal cavity through a catheter that has been inserted into peritoneal cavity

    c. Metabolic waste products and excessive electrolytes diffuse into dialysate while it remains in abdomen

    d. The water diffusion is controlled by glucose in the dialysate which acts as an osmotic agent

    e. Fluid is drained off by gravity into sterile bag at set intervals, thus removing waste products and excess fluid

16. Disadvantages of peritoneal dialysis

    a. Dialysis is more gradual and may be slow for ARF

    b. Risk of peritonitis

    c. Contraindicated for clients with abdominal surgery, peritonitis, significant lung disease

17. Health promotion: Prevention of ARF

    a. Maintenance of fluid volume and cardiac output

    b. Reduce risk of exposure to nephrotoxins

c. Report output < 30 ml per hour in clients at risk

d. Report dehydration, monitor renal function tests in clients receiving nephrotoxic medications

e. Observe clients for signs of transfusion reactions

18. Nursing Diagnoses for clients in ARF
   a. Fluid Volume Excess
   b. Imbalanced Nutrition: Less than body requirements
   c. Knowledge Deficit

19. Home care: Client who is recovering from ARF will need teaching for prescribed diet and fluid intake, avoidance of nephrotoxins, prevention of infection, continue under medical supervision

C. Client with Chronic Renal Failure (CRF)
   1. Definition
      a. Progressive renal tissue destruction and loss of function
      b. May progress over many years without being recognized until kidneys are unable to excrete metabolic wastes and regulate fluid and electrolytes: End-stage Renal Disease (ESRD)
      c. Incidence is increasing especially in older adults; higher in African Americans, Native Americans
      d. Conditions causing chronic renal failure diffuse bilateral disease of kidneys with progressive destruction and scarring; diabetes is leading cause of ESRD; then hypertension

   2. Pathophysiology and Manifestations of Stages
      a. Decreased renal reserve: Early Stage
         1. Unaffected nephrons compensate for lost nephrons
         2. GFR is about 50% of normal
         3. Client is asymptomatic
         4. BUN and serum creatinine are normal
      b. Renal insufficiency
         1. GRF falls to 20–50% of normal
         2. Azotemia and some manifestations
         3. Insult to kidneys could precipitate onset renal failure (infection, dehydration, exposure to nephrotoxins, urinary tract obstructions)
      c. Renal failure
         1. GRF < 20% of normal
         2. BUN and serum creatinine rise sharply
         3. Oliguria, manifestations of uremia

      d. End-stage renal disease (ESRD)
         1. GRF < 5% of normal
         2. Renal replacement therapy necessary to sustain life

   3. ESRD: Uremia ("urine in blood")
      a. Early manifestations
         1. Nausea, apathy, weakness, fatigue
         2. Progresses to frequent vomiting, increasing weakness, lethargy, confusion
      b. Fluid and electrolyte effects
         1. Urine less concentrated with proteinuria and hematuria
         2. Sodium and water retention
         3. Hyperkalemia (muscle weakness, paresthesia, EKG changes)
         4. Hyperphosphatemia, hypocalcemia, hypermagesemia
         5. Metabolic acidosis
      c. Cardiovascular effects
         1. Systemic hypertension
         2. Edema and heart failure; pulmonary edema
         3. Pericarditis: metabolic toxins irritate pericardial sac, less often now with dialysis
         4. Cardiac tamponade: fluid in pericardial sac
      d. Hematologic effects
         1. Anemia contributing to fatigue, weakness, depression, impaired cognition, impaired cardiac function
         2. Impaired platelet function
      e. Immune system effects
         1. WBC declines
         2. Humoral and cell-mediated immunity impaired
         3. Fever suppressed
      f. Gastrointestinal effects
         1. Anorexia, nausea, vomiting, hiccups
         2. GI ulcerations, increased risk for GI bleeding
         3. Uremic fetor: urinelike breath odor
      g. Neurologic effects
         1. Changes in mentation, poor concentration
         2. Fatigue, insomnia
         3. Psychotic symptoms, seizures, coma
         4. Peripheral neuropathy: "restless leg syndrome," sensations of crawling, prickling
         5. Muscle weakness, decreased deep tendon reflexes, gait disturbances

h. Musculoskeletal effects
　　1. Renal osteodystrophy (renal rickets) characterized by osteomalacia (bone softening) and osteoporosis
　　2. Bone tenderness and pain
i. Endocrine and metabolic effects
　　1. Elevated uric acid levels; risk for gout
　　2. Resistance to insulin, glucose intolerance
　　3. High triglyceride and < HDL levels resulting in accelerated atherosclerotic process
　　4. Menstrual irregularities; reduced testosterone levels
j. Dermatologic effects
　　1. Yellowish hue to skin
　　2. Dry skin with poor turgor
　　3. Pruritis due to metabolic wastes deposited in skin
　　4. Uremic frost crystallized deposits of urea on skin

4. Collaborative Care
　a. Eliminate factors which further decrease renal function
　b. Maintenance of nutritional status with minimal toxic waste products
　c. Identify and treat complications of CRF
　d. Preparation for dialysis or renal transplantation

5. Diagnostic tests: Identify CRF and monitor renal function by following levels of metabolic wastes and electrolytes
　a. Urinalysis: fixed specific gravity at 1.010; excess protein, blood cells, cellular casts
　b. Urine culture: identify infection
　c. BUN and serum creatinine: evaluate kidney function
　　1. BUN levels
　　　a. Mild azotemia: 20–50 mg/dL
　　　b. Severe renal impairment: > 100 mg/dL
　　　c. Uremic symptoms: > 200 mg/dL
　　2. Creatinine levels > 4 mg/dL indicates serious renal impairment
　d. Creatinine clearance: evaluates GFR and renal function
　　1. Decreased renal reserve: 32.5–130 mL/min
　　2. Renal insufficiency: 10–30 mL/min
　　3. ESRD: 5–10 mL/min
　e. Serum electrolytes: monitored throughout course of CRF

f. CBC: moderately severe anemia with hematocrit 20–30%, low hemoglobin; reduced RBCs and platelets
g. Renal ultrasonography: CRF: decreased kidney size
h. Kidney biopsy: diagnose underlying disease process; differentiate acute from chronic

6. Medications
　a. General effects of CRF on medication effects
　　1. Increased half-life and plasma levels of meds excreted by kidneys
　　2. Decreased drug absorption if phosphate-binding agents administered concurrently
　　3. Low plasma protein levels can lead to toxicity when protein-bound drugs are given
　　4. Avoid nephrotoxic meds or given with extreme caution
　b. Diuretics (furosemide, other loop diuretics)
　　1. Reduce edema
　　2. Reduce blood pressure
　　3. Lower potassium
　c. Antihypertensive medications: ACE inhibitors preferred
　d. Sodium bicarbonate or calcium carbonate correct mild acidosis
　e. Oral phosphorus binding agents (calcium carbonate, calcium acetate) to lower phosphate levels and normalize calcium levels
　f. Aluminum hydroxide for acute treatment of hyperphosphatemia
　g. Vitamin D supplements to improve calcium absorption
　h. Treat dangerously high potassium levels
　　1. Intravenous bicarbonate, insulin, glucose
　　2. Sodium polystyrene sulfonate (Kayexalate)
　i. Folic acid, iron supplements to combat anemia
　j. Multiple vitamin supplement

7. Dietary and fluid management
　a. Early in course of CRF: diet modifications to slow kidney failure, uremic symptoms, and complications
　b. Restrict proteins (40 gm/day) of high biologic value
　c. Increase carbohydrate intake (35 kcal/kg/day)

    d. Limit fluid to 1–2 L per day; limit sodium to 2 g/day

    e. Restrict potassium (60–70 mEq/day); no salt substitutes

    f. Restrict phosphorus foods (meat, eggs, dairy products)

8. Renal replacement therapies: considered when medications and dietary modifications are no longer effective

    a. Hemodialysis: establish vascular access (create AV fistula) months ahead

    b. Peritoneal dialysis: can be initiated when indicated; training client and/or family involved

    c. Transplantation: tissue typing and identification of living related potential donors including health assessment of donor

9. Dialysis

    a. Considerations

        1. Dialysis manages ESRD but does not cure it

        2. Hemodialysis or peritoneal dialysis is constant factor of life

        3. Depending on individual client situation and total health, client may prefer death to dialysis

    b. Hemodialysis for ESRD

        1. Treatment are 3 times per week for total of 9–12 hours

        2. Specific dialysis orders according to body size, residual renal function (based on that day's current lab test results), dietary intake, concurrent illnesses

        3. Complications during treatment are hypotension and muscle cramps; dialysis disequilibrium syndrome

        4. Long term complications are infection and vascular access problems

        5. Cardiovascular disease is leading cause of death for hemodialysis clients; higher death rate than clients on peritoneal dialysis or transplanted

    c. Peritoneal dialysis for ESRD

        1. Continuous ambulatory peritoneal dialysis (CAPD) most common

        2. 2 liters of dialysate instilled into peritoneal cavity and catheter sealed; empty and replace every 4–6 hours

        3. Continuous cyclic peritoneal dialysis (CCPD) uses delivery device during nighttime hours and continuous dwell during day

    4. Advantages over hemodialysis

        a. Eliminates vascular access and heparinization

        b. Avoids rapid fluctuation in extracellular fluid

        c. Diet intake is more liberal with fluids and nutrients

        d. Regular insulin can be added to dialysate to manage hyperglycemia for diabetics

        e. Client more able to self-manage

    5. Disadvantages of peritoneal dialysis

        a. Less effective metabolite elimination

        b. Risk for infection (peritonitis: dialysate returns cloudy; should be straw colored)

        c. Serum triglyceride levels increase

        d. Altered body image with peritoneal catheter

10. Kidney transplant

    a. Background

        1. Treatment of choice for ESRD

        2. Primarily limited by availability of kidneys

        3. Many persons on waiting list for kidney

        4. Improves survival and quality of life for ESRD client

    b. Organ donors

        1. Majority are from cadavers

        2. Transplants from living donors increasing

        3. Close match between blood and tissue type desired; HLA are compared; 6 in common is perfect match

        4. Living donors must be in good physical health; nephrectomy is major surgery and remaining kidney must be healthy

    c. Cadaver donors

        1. Cadaver kidney from persons who

            a. Meet criteria for brain death

            b. Age < 65 years old

            c. Free of systemic disease, malignancy, or infection including HIV, hepatitis B, C

        2. Kidney removed and preserved by hypothermia

            a. Transplant in 24–48 hours

            b. Use technique: continuous hypothermic pulsatile perfusion, and transplant up to 3 days

3. Donor kidney placed in lower abdominal cavity, renal artery, vein, and ureter are anastomosed
d. Immunosuppressive therapy
  1. Necessary to block immune response that would reject transplanted organ
  2. Medications include
    a. Glucocorticoids: prednisone and methylprednisolone used for maintenance and treatment of acute rejection episodes
    b. Azathioprine: inhibits cellular and humoral immunity; metabolized by liver
    c. Mycophenolate mofetil: more potent and minimal bone marrow suppression
    d. Cyclosporine: affects cellular immunity; is hepatotoxic and nephrotoxic
e. Rejection
  1. Can occur at any time
  2. Acute rejection
    a. Occurs within months of transplant
    b. Cellular immune response with T cells
    c. Few manifestations:
      1. Rise in serum creatinine
      2. Possibly oliguria
    d. Treatment
      1. Methylprednisolone
      2. OKT3 monoclonal antibody
  3. Chronic rejection
    a. Develops months to years post transplant
    b. Major cause of graft loss
    c. Involves both humoral and cellular immune response
    d. Manifestations (same as renal failure)

    1. Progressive azotemia
    2. Proteinuria
    3. Hypertension
f. Complications of kidney transplant
  1. Hypertension
  2. Glomerular lesions with manifestations of nephrosis
  3. Increased risk for myocardial infarction and stroke
g. Complications associated with long-term immunosuppression
  1. Infection: bacterial, viral, fungal in blood, lung, CNS
  2. Tumors: carcinoma in situ in cervix, lymphomas, skin cancers
  3. Steroid use leads to bone problems, peptic ulcer disease, cataract formation
11. Health Promotion
  a. Ensure all clients with impaired renal function are well hydrated, especially while receiving nephrotoxic drugs
  b. Encourage clients with ESRD to explore transplant options
12. Nursing Diagnoses
  a. Impaired Tissue Perfusion: Renal
  b. Imbalanced Nutrition: Less than body requirements
  c. Risk for Infection
  d. Disturbed Body Image
13. Home Care
  a. CRF and ESRD are long-term processes requiring client management
  b. Extensive teaching required
    1. Monitoring health status
    2. Compliance with fluid and dietary restriction and medications
    3. Care involved with hemodialysis, peritoneal dialysis, or living with transplant

FOCUSED STUDY TIPS

- Visit a kidney dialysis center. Speak with a client undergoing dialysis. Assess level of knowledge regarding the dialysis process. Observe symptoms of ESRD (end-stage renal disease) that he or she manifests. Share this information with classmates.
- Read labels on food items in the grocery store. Prepare a list of commonly bought items that are high in potassium. Describe the relationship between high dietary potassium and ESRD.
- Describe and discuss ESRD with a family member. Present medical treatment options. Elicit a treatment preference from the family member. Ask him or her to describe why the treatment chosen is preferred.

CASE STUDY

A client with ESRD who has been on hemodialysis for 10 years and is not a kidney transplant candidate states, "To-day is my last treatment. I am not going through this any more. I realize I will die, and I am ready to do so." How do you respond? What must you assess first?

Describe your words as well as your actions. If, indeed, the client refuses further treatment, what physiological changes can be anticipated as this client approaches death? For what must the nurse plan?

CARE PLAN CRITICAL THINKING ACTIVITY

Compare and contrast a nursing care plan for a client with ESRD utilizing hemodialysis as a kidney replacement therapy and a care plan for a client utilizing CAPD (continuous ambulatory peritoneal dialysis). How do they differ? What nursing diagnoses are common to both? What nursing interventions are common to both? When evaluating the effectiveness of both therapies, what does the nurse need to assess?

NCLEX TEST QUESTIONS

1. A client in renal failure has an abnormally high potassium level. Which of the following is a priority nursing intervention?
   a. obtain an electrocardiogram (ECG)
   b. evaluate level of consciousness
   c. measure urinary output
   d. draw arterial blood gases

2. Which of the following findings relative to calcium would the nurse expect to see in a client in renal failure?
   a. increased calcium levels and decreased phosphate levels
   b. increased calcium excretion and phosphate retention
   c. decreased calcium and potassium
   d. increased calcium and decreased creatinine levels

3. A 54-year-old female client who has recently begun hemodialysis states, "Now I can eat anything I want." How would the nurse respond to this client statement?
   a. "As long as you don't overdo, there are very few dietary restrictions that you will have to follow."
   b. "Caloric intake will have to be increased by 3,000 kcalories in order to meet nutritional goals."
   c. "You will still have to follow certain dietary restrictions because hemodialysis is a treatment modality and does not correct the underlying problem of kidney disease."
   d. "No fluids will be given on the day you receive hemodialysis therapy in order to prevent fluid overload."

4. A 39-year-old client has been admitted to the hospital with clinical manifestations indicating acute renal failure. A precipitating factor seems to be a viral infection of the upper respiratory tract. Considering the diagnosis while completing a physical assessment, the nurse would expect to observe:
   a. urine output of 400 mL/day, dyspnea, neck vein distention.
   b. anuria, bradycardia, tachypnea.
   c. urine specific gravity of 1.010, decreased creatinine levels, hypokalemia.
   d. hypomagnesemia, nausea, vomiting, weakness.

5. Which of the following statements made by a client who has received a renal transplant indicates that the desired outcome of the discharge teaching plan has been met?
   a. "I will double my prednisone dose if my urine output is less than 300 mL/day."
   b. "I will need to avoid crowds and prevent infection."
   c. "Now I can eat whatever I want as long as I watch how much salt I use."
   d. "Since I have not yet rejected the transplant, I never have to worry about rejection anymore."

6. A 45-year-old male client comes to the clinic for evaluation. He is receiving continuous ambulatory peritoneal dialysis. For the past three cycles, he has retained between 250 and 400 cc with each cycle. He has no urine output and has not moved his bowels in 3 days. The effluent is clear. The nurse should:

a. add glucose to the solution to help pull off excess fluid.

b. cap the catheter and notify the physician.

c. assess the client for possible constipation.

d. allow the solution to drain with the next cycle.

7. A client has an arteriovenous fistula as an access site for hemodialysis. Which assessment finding indicates that the fistula is patent?

a. Palpation of a pulse distal to the fistula

b. Normal capillary refill distal to the fistula

c. Auscultation of a bruit over the fistula

d. Absence of edema or redness over the fistula

8. Which nursing diagnosis should receive the highest priority in a client with acute renal failure?

a. Altered nutrition: less than body requirements related to anorexia

b. Risk for trauma related to decreased alertness

c. Activity intolerance related to fatigue and muscle cramps

d. Fluid volume excess related to oliguria

9. A 54-year-old female is admitted with acute tubular necrosis. As a result of the acute renal failure, she has developed hyperkalemia. She does not yet have a vascular access for dialysis. Which of the following therapies could be used to treat hyperkalemia prior to the use of dialysis?

a. Ammonium chloride resin

b. Kayexalate

c. Calcium chloride 500 mg

d. Sodium chloride 500 mL fluid bolus

10. A client undergoes a partial nephrectomy. In planning for the post-operative care of this client, the nurse institutes aggressive measures to prevent atelectasis and pneumonia because

a. the nephrectomy involves paralyzing the intercostal muscles.

b. the surgery involves an upper abdominal incision.

c. the client must be maintained in a flat position for 24 hours.

d. intraoperative surgical contamination of the pulmonary structures is unavoidable.

CHAPTER 28

ASSESSING CLIENTS WITH CARDIAC DISORDERS

LEARNING OUTCOMES

After completing this chapter, you will be able to:

- Review the anatomy and physiology of the heart.
- Trace the circulation of blood through the heart and coronary vessels.
- Identify the normal heart sounds and relate them to the corresponding events in the cardiac cycle.
- Name and locate the elements of the heart's conduction system.
- Define cardiac output and explain the influence of various factors in its regulation.
- Identify specific topics for consideration during a health history interview of the client with health problems involving cardiac function.
- Describe physical assessment techniques for cardiac function.
- Identify abnormal findings that may indicate cardiac malfunction.

KEY TOPICS

- Review of anatomy and physiology of the cardiac system
- Assessing cardiac functioning

LECTURE OUTLINE

I. Background of Anatomy and Physiology
    A. Heart
        1. Size of adult's fist, weight < 1 pound
        2. Located in mediastinum, between vertebral column and sternum
        3. 2/3 of heart mass is left of sternum; upper base is beneath second rib; pointed apex lies approximately with fifth intercostal space, mid-clavicular

B. Pericardium
    1. Covering of double layered fibroserous membrane, forming pericardial sac
    2. Layers of pericardium:
        a. Parietal pericardium: outermost layer
        b. Visceral pericardium (epicardium) adheres to heart surface

MediaLink

www.prenhall.com/lemone

Additional resources for this chapter can be found on the Student CD-ROM accompanying this textbook, and on the Companion Website at www.prenhall.com/lemone. Click on Chapter 28 to select the activities for this chapter.

CD-ROM
- Audio Glossary
- NCLEX Review

Animations
- Cardiac A&P
- Dysrhythmias

Companion Website
- More NCLEX Review
- Functional Health Pattern Assessment
- Case Study
   Chest Pain
- MediaLink Application
   Heart Sounds

3. Small space between layers is pericardial cavity which contains small amount of serous lubricating fluid that cushions heart as it beats

C. Layers of Heart Wall
   1. Epicardium: same as visceral pericardium
   2. Myocardium: specialized cardiac muscle cells provide bulk of contractile heart muscle
   3. Endocardium: sheath of endothelium that is lining inside heart's chambers and great vessels

D. Chambers and Valves
   1. Four hollow chambers: two upper atria, two lower ventricles; separated lengthwise by interventricular septum
      a. Right atrium: receives deoxygenated blood from veins of body
         1. Superior vena cava: blood from body above diaphragm
         2. Inferior vena cava: blood from body below diaphragm
         3. Coronary sinus: blood from heart
      b. Left atrium: receives freshly oxygenated blood from lungs via pulmonary veins
      c. Right ventricle: receives deoxygenated blood from right atrium and pumps it to lungs for oxygenation via pulmonary artery
      d. Left ventricle: receives freshly oxygenated blood from left atrium and pumps it to arterial circulation via aorta
   2. Valves separate each chamber of heart allowing unidirectional blood flow
      a. Atrioventricular (AV) valves: between atrium and ventricle; flaps of valves anchored to papillary muscles of ventricles by chordae tendineae
         1. Tricuspid: right side
         2. Mitral (biscuspid): left side
      b. Semilunar valves: connect ventricles to great vessels
         1. Pulmonary: right side; joins right ventricle and pulmonary artery
         2. Aortic: left side; joins left ventricle and aorta
      c. Heart sounds associated with closure of valves
         1. S_1 ("lub"): first heart sound; closure of AV valves
         2. S_2 ("dub"): second heart sound; closure of semilunar valves at onset of relaxation

E. Systemic Circulation
   1. Pulmonary circulation begins with right heart: deoxygenated blood from superior and inferior vena cavae is transported to lungs via pulmonary artery and branches
   2. In lungs, oxygen and carbon dioxide are exchanged in capillaries of lungs, and blood returns to left atrium through several pulmonary veins
   3. Blood pumped out of left ventricle through aorta and major branches to all body tissues

F. Coronary Circulation (Circulation for heart)
   1. Left and right coronary arteries originate at base of aorta and branch out to encircle myocardium
   2. During ventricular relaxation coronary arteries fill with oxygen-rich blood
   3. Blood perfuses heart muscle and cardiac veins drain blood into coronary sinus which empties into right atrium

G. Cardiac Cycle and Cardiac Output
   1. Cardiac cycle: one heartbeat involving contraction and relaxation of heart
   2. Systole: phase during which ventricles contract and eject blood into pulmonary and systemic circuits
   3. Diastole: phase during which ventricles relax and refill with blood; atria contract and myocardium is perfused
   4. Heart Rate (HR): number of cardiac cycles in a minute (normal 70–80)
   5. Stroke Volume (SV): volume of blood ejected with each contraction
   6. Ejection Fraction (EF): percentage of total blood in ventricle at the end of diastole ejected from heart with each beat; normal ejection fraction is 50%–70%
   7. Cardiac Output (CO): amount of blood pumped by ventricles into pulmonary and systemic circulations in 1 minute
      a. Formula ($HR \times SV = CO$)
      b. Average cardiac output is 4–8 liters per minute (L/min)
      c. Indicator of pump function of heart; if heart is ineffective pump, then cardiac output and tissue perfusion are decreased; body tissues become ischemic (deprived of oxygen)
      d. Cardiac output is influenced by
         1. Activity level
         2. Metabolic rate
         3. Physiologic and psychologic stress responses
         4. Age
         5. Body size

e. Cardiac reserve: ability of heart to respond to body's changing need for cardiac output

8. Cardiac output is determined by interaction of four factors
  a. Heart rate: affected by direct and indirect autonomic nervous system stimulation
    1. Sympathetic nervous system: increases heart rate
    2. Parasympathetic nervous system: decreases heart rate
    3. Reflex regulation occurs in response to systemic blood pressure through activation of baroreceptors or pressure receptors (located in carotid sinus, aortic arch, venae cavae, pulmonary veins)
    4. Very rapid heart rate decreases cardiac output and coronary artery perfusion due to decreased filling time
    5. Bradycardia decreases cardiac output if stroke volume stays the same
  b. Preload: amount of cardiac muscle fiber tension or stretch and the end of diastole (right before contraction of ventricles)
    1. Influenced by venous return and ventricular compliance
    2. Starling's Law of the heart: Greater the volume, the greater the stretch of cardiac muscle fibers, and greater the force with which fibers contract to accomplish emptying
    3. Physiologic limit to Starling's Law: overstretching of cardiac muscle fibers results in ineffective contraction
      a. Like continuous overstretching of rubber band
      b. Disorders which result in increased preload:
        1. Congestive heart failure
        2. Renal disease
        3. Vasoconstriction
      c. Disorders which result in decreased preload:
        1. Decreased circulating blood volume
        2. Hemorrhage
        3. Third-spacing
  c. Afterload: force the ventricles must overcome to eject their blood volume
    1. Pressure in arterial system ahead of ventricles
      a. Right ventricle: generates enough tension to open pulmonary valve, eject its volume into low-pressure pulmonary arteries: Pulmonary Vascular Resistance (PVR)
      b. Left ventricle: ejects load by overcoming pressure behind aortic valve: systemic vascular resistance (SVR); much greater than right ventricle
    2. Alterations in vascular tone affect afterload and ventricular work
      a. As PVR and SVR increase, work of ventricles increase and consumption of myocardial oxygen increases
      b. Very low afterload decreases forward flow of blood into systemic and coronary circulation
  d. Contractility: inherent capability of cardiac muscle fibers to shorten
    1. Poor contractility
      a. Reduces forward flow of blood from heart
      b. Increases ventricular pressure from accumulated blood volume
      c. Reduces cardiac output
    2. Increased contractility: overtaxes heart

9. Conduction system
  a. Cardiac muscle cells have inherent characteristic of self-excitation: can initiate and transmit impulses independent of stimulus
  b. Conduction system
    1. Sinoatrial (SA) node: located junction of superior vena cava and right atrium
      a. Acts as normal pacemaker of heart
      b. Inherent rate: 60–100 times/minute
    2. Impulse travels across atria via internodal pathways to Atrioventricular (AV) node: located floor of interatrial septum; fibers of AV node slightly delay transmission to ventricles
    3. Impulse travels through bundle of His at atrioventricular junction and down interventricular septum

through right and left bundle branches out to Purkinje fibers in ventricular muscle walls
  c. Path of electrical transmission produces series of changes in ion concentration across membrane of each cardiac muscle cell
    1. Electrical stimulus: increases permeability of cell membrane, creates action (electrical) potential
    2. Exchange of sodium, potassium, and calcium ions across cell membrane; intracellular electrical state: positive charge; depolarization (myocardial contraction)
    3. Ion exchange reverses; cell returns to resting state; electrical state: negative; repolarization (cardiac muscle relaxes)
  10. Cardiac Index
    a. Cardiac output adjusted for client's body size which is the Body Surface Area (BSA)
    b. More accurate indicator of ability of heart to effectively circulate blood
    c. BSA is stated in square meters (m^2); Cardiac index calculated by dividing cardiac output by BSA: $CI = CO \div BSA$
    d. Normal CI is 2.5–4.2 L/min/m^2
II. Assessing Cardiac Function
  A. Health assessment interview to collect subjective data
    1. Explore client's chief complaint
    2. Description of client's symptom regarding
      a. Location
      b. Quality or character
      c. Timing
      d. Setting or precipitating factors
      e. Severity
      f. Aggravating and relieving factors
      g. Associated symptoms
    3. Explore client history for
      a. Heart disorders
        1. Angina
        2. Myocardial infarction (Heart attack)
        3. Congestive Heart Failure (CHF)
        4. Hypertension (HTN)
        5. Valvular Disease
      b. Previous heart surgeries or related illnesses
        1. Rheumatic fever
        2. Scarlet fever

        3. Recurrent streptococcal throat infection
      c. Pertinent other chronic illnesses
        1. Diabetes Mellitus
        2. Bleeding disorders
        3. Endocrine disorders
      d. Client family history for specific heart conditions
        1. Coronary artery disease (CAD)
        2. HTN
        3. Stroke
        4. Hyperlipidemia
        5. Diabetes Mellitus
        6. Congenital heart disease
        7. Sudden death
    4. Past or present occurrence of cardiac symptoms
      a. Chest pain
      b. Shortness of breath
      c. Difficulty breathing, cough
      d. Palpitations
      e. Fatigue
      f. Light-headedness or fainting
      g. Heart murmur
      h. Blood clots
      i. Swelling
    5. Personal habits and nutritional history
      a. Body weight
      b. Eating patterns: usual intake of fats, salt, fluids
      c. Restrictions, food intolerances
      d. Use of alcohol and caffeine
    6. Use of tobacco products, type, duration, amount, efforts to quit
    7. Use of street drugs, type, efforts to quit
    8. Activity level and tolerance, recreation and relaxation habits
    9. Sleep patterns; interruptions due to dyspnea, cough, discomfort, urination, stress
    10. Pillows used to sleep
    11. Psychosocial factors
    12. Personality type
    13. Perception of health or illness, compliance with treatment
  B. Physical assessment to collect objective data
    1. Apical impulse assessment with abnormal findings
      a. Positioning lateral to midclavicular line or below fifth left intercostal space: enlarged or displaced heart
      b. Increased size, amplitude, duration of point of maximal impulse (PMI)
        1. Left ventricular volume overload (increased preload): HTN, aortic stenosis

2. Pressure overload (increased afterload): aortic or mitral regurgitation
  c. Increased amplitude alone: hyperkinetic states; anxiety, hyperthyroidism, anemia
  d. Decreased amplitude: dilated heart in cardiomyopathy
  e. Displacement alone: dextrocardia, diaphragmatic hernia, gastric distention, chronic lung disease
  f. Thrill (palpable vibration over precordium or artery): severe valve stenosis
  g. Marked increase in amplitude of PMI at right ventricular area: right ventricular volume overload in atrial septal defect
  h. Increase in amplitude and duration with right ventricular pressure overload (also lift, heave): pulmonary stenosis, pulmonary hypertension, chronic lung disease
  i. Palpable thrill: ventricular septal defect
2. Subxyphoid area
  a. Downward pulsation: right ventricular enlargement
  b. Accentuated pulsation at pulmonary area: hyperkinetic states
  c. Prominent pulsation: increased flow or dilation of pulmonary artery
  d. Thrill: aortic or pulmonary stenosis, pulmonary HTN, atrial septal defect
  e. Increased pulsation at aortic area: aortic aneurysm
  f. Palpable second heart sound (S_2): systemic HTN
3. Cardiac rate and rhythm with abnormal findings
  a. Heart rate > 100: tachycardia
  b. Heart rate < 60: bradycardia
  c. Pulse deficit (Radial pulse < than apical when checked simultaneously): weak ineffective contractions of left ventricle
  d. Irregular rhythm: frequent ectopic beats such as premature ventricular beats, atrial fibrillation
  e. Gradual increase and decrease in heart rate correlated with respirations: sinus arrhythmia
4. Heart sounds assessment with abnormal findings

  a. S_1
    1. Accentuation: tachycardia, states of high cardiac output such as fever, exercise, hyperthyroidism
    2. Diminishment: mitral regurgitation, CHF, CAD, pulmonary or systemic HTN, obesity, emphysema, pericardial effusion
    3. Splitting: right bundle branch block, premature ventricular contractions
  b. S_2
    1. Accentuation: HTN, exercise, excitement, conditions of pulmonary HTN (mitral stenosis, CHF, cor pulmonale)
    2. Diminishment: aortic stenosis, shock, pulmonary stenosis, increased anterioposterior chest diameter
    3. Splitting:
      a. Fixed: atrial septal defect, right ventricular failure
      b. Paradoxical: left bundle branch block
  c. Extra heart sounds in systole
    1. Clicks: aortic and pulmonic stenosis
    2. Midsystolic: mitral valve prolapse (MVP)
  d. Extra heart sounds in diastole:
    1. Opening snap: opening sound of a stenotic mitral valve
    2. S_3 (ventricular gallop): myocardial failure and ventricular volume overload (CHF, mitral or tricuspid regurgitation)
    3. S_4 (atrial gallop): increased resistance to ventricular filling after atrial contraction (HTN, CAD, aortic stenosis, cardiomyopathy)
    4. S_4 (right-sided): less common, occurs with pulmonary HTN and pulmonary stenosis
    5. Combined S_3 and S_4 (summation gallop): severe CHF
  e. Pericardial friction rub: inflammation of pericardial sac as with pericarditis, occurs during systole and diastole
5. Murmur assessment with abnormal findings
  a. Midsystolic murmurs: aortic and pulmonic stenosis; hypertrophic cardiomyopathy
  b. Pansystolic (holosystolic) murmurs: mitral and tricuspid regurgitation, ventricular septal defect

   c. Late systolic murmur: MVP

   d. Early diastolic murmur: aortic regurgitation

   e. Middiastolic and presystolic murmurs: mitral stenosis

   f. Continuous murmurs throughout systole and all or part of diastole: patent ductus arteriosus

FOCUSED STUDY TIPS

- Teach a group of children at a day care center or preschool how to use a stethoscope and listen to their hearts. Explain at their level of understanding what they are hearing.
- Assist with a 12-lead EKG (electrocardiogram). Observe each lead as it is printed. Visualize the path of the signal through the heart's conduction system.
- Describe to a classmate the difference between *preload* and *afterload*. Evaluate each other's understanding.

CASE STUDY

T. C. is admitted to the coronary care unit. He is extremely anxious and is questioning everything staff attempts to do for him. What information would be important to provide T. C. before attaching him to a cardiac monitor?

CARE PLAN CRITICAL THINKING ACTIVITY

A client has been prescribed a drug that reduces preload. He asks you what the drug will do for him. Describe your answer.

NCLEX TEST QUESTIONS

1. The client presents to the clinic for a routine check-up. The nurse notes that the blood pressure (BP) is 180/96. The client denies any history of hypertension. The client is a 50-year-old male with a strong family history of CAD. The nurse would include which of the following in the teaching about modifiable risk factors?

   a. age

   b. gender

   c. family history

   d. hypertension

2. The client presents to the emergency department complaining of "palpitations." The client's heart rate is 180 bpm and blood pressure is 108/50. The nurse would expect his pulse to be

   a. full and bounding.

   b. weak and thready.

   c. weak and bounding.

   d. full and thready.

3. Which of the following clients is at high risk for developing coronary artery disease (CAD) that may not be responsive to diet and exercise alone? A client who

   a. has diabetes.

   b. has a strong family history of cardiovascular disease.

   c. is overweight and 55 years old.

   d. has a history of hyperlipidemia.

4. A client with congestive heart failure (CHF) has been advised to follow a low-sodium diet. Which statement by the client indicates to the nurse that diet teaching has been effective?

   a. "If I stop adding table salt, I shouldn't have any problems."

   b. "I need to avoid eating processed foods and canned meats and vegetables."

   c. "I can still use a small amount of table salt in cooking."

   d. "I only have to worry about salty-tasting foods like potato chips."

5. A simple, noninvasive method to assess adequacy of tissue perfusion is:

   a. echocardiography.

   b. capillary refill.

   c. serum electrolyte monitoring.

   d. arterial blood gas monitoring.

6. When evaluating the initial rate and rhythm of a client's apical pulse, the nurse should count for:
   a. 15 seconds.
   b. 30 seconds.
   c. 60 seconds.
   d. 120 seconds.

7. Assessing for hypokalemia, the nurse will observe for ECG changes of:
   a. peaked T waves.
   b. depressed P waves.
   c. PVCs (premature ventricular contractions).
   d. narrowed QT interval.

8. The client arrives in the emergency department with a heart rate of 130 bpm. The client appears anxious and is tachypneic. What part of the central nervous system is most likely responsible for this increased heart rate?
   a. parasympathetic nervous system (PSNS)
   b. sympathetic nervous system (SNS)
   c. acetylcholine-cholinesterase feedback
   d. vagus nerve

9. After the client has recovered from coronary bypass surgery, her physician has advised a low-cholesterol diet. The nurse will know that the client understands this diet when she includes foods such as:
   a. meats, especially organ meats, and dairy products.
   b. eggs, cheese, fruits, and vegetables.
   c. vegetables, fruits, lean meats, and vegetable oils.
   d. raw or cooked vegetables, fruits, and red meat.

10. The client who has peripheral edema during the day states he wakes up in bed at night with difficulty breathing. He is most likely experiencing:
    a. angina pectoris.
    b. orthopnea caused by recumbent position.
    c. a sinus infection.
    d. sleep apnea.

CHAPTER 29

NURSING CARE OF CLIENTS WITH CORONARY HEART DISEASE

LEARNING OUTCOMES

After completing this chapter, you will be able to:

- Use knowledge of the normal anatomy and physiology of the heart in caring for clients with coronary heart disease.
- Discuss the coronary circulation and electrical properties of the heart.
- Compare and contrast the pathophysiology and manifestations of coronary heart disease and common cardiac dysrhythmias.
- Identify diagnostic tests and procedures used for clients with coronary heart disease and/or dysrhythmias.
- Discuss nursing implications for drugs used to prevent and treat coronary heart disease and dysrhythmias.
- Describe nursing care for the client undergoing diagnostic testing, an interventional procedure, or surgery for coronary heart disease or a dysrhythmia.
- Use the nursing process to plan and implement individualized nursing care and teaching for clients with coronary heart disease or dysrhythmias.

KEY TOPICS

- Disorders of myocardial perfusion
- Cardiac rhythm disorders
- Nursing care of clients with coronary heart disease

LECTURE OUTLINE

I. Cardiovascular disease (CVD)
   A. Definition
      1. Generic term for disorders of heart and blood vessels

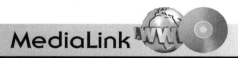

MediaLink

2. Leading cause of death and disability in U.S.; includes > 60 million persons

3. Incidence of new CVD cases per year is decreasing; mortality rate has had slow but steady decline since 1963
B. Disorders of Myocardial Perfusion
   1. Coronary heart disease (CHD) or Coronary artery disease (CAD)
   2. Angina Pectoris
   3. Acute Myocardial Infarction (AMI)
   4. Cardiac Dysrhythmia
   5. Sudden Cardiac Death (SCD)
II. Client with Coronary Heart Disease (CHD) or Coronary Artery Disease (CAD)
   A. Definition
      1. Heart disease caused by impaired blood flow to myocardium
      2. Cause is accumulation of atherosclerotic plaque in coronary arteries (blood supply of heart)
      3. May be asymptomatic or cause angina pectoris, myocardial infarction (heart attack), dysrhythmias, heart failure, sudden death
      4. Leading cause of death for all U.S. ethnic groups except Asian females
         a. Highest incidence in white males > 45
         b. Post menopause women's risk equal to risk of men
   B. Risk factors (research obtained from Framingham Heart Study)
      1. Non-modifiable
         a. Age: > 50% are 65 or older; 80% of deaths
         b. Gender: male
         c. Race: African Americans have higher rates of HPT
         d. Genetic factors: occurs in families
      2. Modifiable: Life-style factors and pathologic conditions predispose client to development of CHD
         a. Pathologic conditions
            1. Hypertension (HPT)
               a. Blood pressure reading > 140 systolic mmHg/90 diastolic mmHg
               b. Affects > third of persons over age of 50 in U.S.
            2. Diabetes mellitus
               a. Associated with higher blood lipid levels, incidence of HPT, obesity
               b. Contributes to process of atherosclerosis
            3. Hyperlipidemia
               a. Abnormal high level of blood lipids and lipoproteins
               b. Elevated LDL (low density lipoproteins) and triglycerides on VLDL (very-low-density-lipoprotein) contribute to risk for CHD
               c. HDL (high density lipoproteins) above 35 mg/dL reduce risk of CHD
            4. Elevated homocystine levels
               a. Research links elevation with CHD
               b. Negatively correlated with serum folate and dietary intake of folate
            5. Metabolic syndrome: research is showing individual with abdominal obesity, hyperlipidemia, HPT, insulin resistance, increased tendency for clotting and inflammation risk for premature CHD
            6. Female risk factors: (Research from Women's Health Initiative)
               a. Premature menopause
               b. Oral contraceptive use
               c. Hormone replacement therapy (HRT)
         b. Life-style factors
            1. Cigarette smoking: independent risk factor
               a. Carbon monoxide damages vascular endothelium promoting cholesterol deposition
               b. Nicotine stimulates catecholamine release: increasing blood pressure, heart rate, myocardial oxygen use
               c. Nicotine is vaso-constrictor
               d. Nicotine reduces HDL levels; increases platelet aggregation
            2. Obesity (body weight > 30% ideal body weight)
               a. Higher rates associated with HPT, diabetes, hyperlipidemia
               b. Central obesity (intra-abdominal fat) increased risk for CHD indicated by waist circumference
                  1. Waist to hip ratio > 0.8 female
                  2. Waist to hip ratio > 0.9 male
                  3. Physical inactivity: regular activity less prone to CHD than sedentary
                  4. Diet: protective effect from diets high in fruits, vegetables, whole grains, unsaturated fatty acids

C. Coronary blood flow regulated by
   1. Aortic pressure
   2. Heart rate
   3. Metabolic activity of heart
   4. Blood vessel tone (constriction)
   5. Collateral circulation: alternative routes for blood through connections between smaller arteries
D. Pathophysiology of atherosclerosis
   1. Progressive disease characterized by atheroma (plaque formation)
   2. Affecting intimal and medial layers of large and medium sized arteries
   3. Initiated by unknown precipitating factors that cause lipoproteins and fibrous tissue to accumulate in arterial wall
   4. Begins with injury or inflammation of endothelial cells lining artery promoting platelet adhesion and aggregation, wbc's go to area
   5. At injury site, lipoproteins collect in intimal lining contact with platelets, cholesterol, blood components to stimulate smooth muscle cells and connective tissue to proliferate within vessel wall
   6. Fibrous plaque develops and blood lipids accumulate
   7. Developing plaque gradually occludes vessel lumen and impairs ability of vessel to dilate; occurs at bifurcations, curves, narrowed areas
   8. Plaque expands to create stenosis or total occlusion of artery
   9. Development of atheromas which become calcified and can ulcerate or rupture, stimulating thrombosis; can be occluded by thrombus or can embolize to distal vessel
   10. Manifestations of process do not appear until 75% of lumen occluded
E. Myocardial Ischemia
   1. Myocardial cells are ischemic when oxygen supply inadequate for metabolic demands and is dependent upon
      a. Coronary perfusion
      b. Myocardial workload
      c. Oxygen content of blood (contributing factor)
   2. Process: myocardial cells have limited supplies of adenosine triphosphate (ATP) for energy storage; if stores are depleted contractility is affected
   3. Cellular metabolism switches from efficient aerobic process to anaerobic metabolism and lactic acid is produced

   4. If blood flow restored within 20 minutes: aerobic metabolism and contractility are restored and cellular repair begins
   5. Continued ischemia results in cellular necrosis and death
F. Coronary Heart Disease: 2 categories
   1. Chronic ischemic heart disease: stable and vasospastic angina, silent myocardial ischemia
   2. Acute coronary syndromes: range from unstable angina to myocardial infarction
G. Collaborative Care: Care focused on aggressive risk factor management to
   1. Slow down atherosclerotic process
   2. Maintain myocardial perfusion
H. Diagnostic Tests
   1. Assessment of risk factors
      a. Total serum cholesterol: elevated in hyperlipidemia
      b. Lipid profile: includes triglyceride, HDL, LDL level and ratio of HDL to total cholesterol
         1. Dietary cholesterol intake should be consistent for 3 weeks prior to testing
         2. Client fast 10–12 hours prior to sample
         3. Affected by alcohol and medications
         4. HDL: Total Cholesterol Ratio: at least 1:5; 1:3 is ideal
   2. Tests to identify subclinical (asymptomatic) CHD when multiple risk factors are present:
      a. Ankle-brachial blood pressure index (ABI)
      b. Exercise ECG
         1. ECG assesses the response to increased cardiac workload induced by exercise
         2. Positive for CHD if
            a. ST depression on ECG > 3 mm
            b. Client develops chest pain
            c. Test stopped due to excessive fatigue, dysrhythmias or symptoms before maximal heart rate attained
      c. Electron beam computed tomography (EBCT) Creates 3-dimensional image of heart and coronary arteries to reveal plaque and any abnormalities
      d. Myocardial perfusion imaging: evaluate myocardial blood flow and perfusion at rest and during stress testing

I. Risk Factor Management: Conservative management of CHD
  1. Smoking
     a. Quitting reduces risk by 50% regardless of time spent smoking
     b. Improvement of HDL levels
     c. Lower LDL levels
     d. Reduces blood viscosity
  2. Diet
     a. Reduce saturated fat and cholesterol intake
     b. Strategies to lower LDL
        1. Avoid saturated fats (whole-milk products, red meats, coconut oil); solidified vegetable fats which contain trans fatty acids
        2. Include nonfat dairy products, fish, poultry as protein sources; use monosaturated fats (olive, canola, peanut oil); include cold water fish
        3. Increase intake of soluble fiber (oats, psyllium, pectin-rich fruit, beans) and insoluble fiber (whole grains, vegetables, fruit)
        4. Folic acid, Vitamin B_6 and B_{12} reduce serum homocystine levels
        5. In older adults moderate alcohol use may decrease risk of CHD (males 2 drinks; females 1 drink)
        6. Overweight or obese person encouraged to lose weight through reduced calorie intake and increased exercise
  3. Exercise
     a. Done regularly lowers VLDL, LDL, triglycerides; raises HDL
     b. Reduces blood pressure and insulin resistance
     c. 30 minutes 5–6 times/week
  4. Hypertension: control > 140/90 mm HG by reduction of sodium intake, increasing calcium intake, stress management, medications
  5. Diabetes
     a. Causes acceleration of atherosclerotic process
     b. Control will decrease risk of CHD
     c. Involves weight loss if needed, reduced fat intake and regular exercise
  6. Medications
     a. Cholesterol-lowering drugs: goal to lower LDL < 130 mg/dL
        1. Statins
           a. First line drugs
           b. Can cause myopathy or increase liver enzymes
        2. Bile acid sequestrants
        3. Nicotinic acid
        4. Fibrates
     b. Meds other than statins are used in combination to effectively lower cholesterol levels
     c. Low-dose aspirin
        1. For persons at high-risk for MI
        2. Dosage: 30–325 mg
     d. ACE inhibitors prescribed for clients at high risk including diabetics
  7. Complementary Therapies
 J. Health Promotion: Education
  1. Avoid smoking and all tobacco use
  2. Benefits of regular exercise
  3. Diet for healthy weight and optimal cholesterol
  4. Regular screenings for HPT, diabetes, hyperlipidemia
 K. Nursing Diagnoses
  1. Imbalanced Nutrition: More than body requirements: Assist client with setting reasonable goals for weight loss
  2. Ineffective Health Maintenance: Interventions to lower or remove risk factors
 L. Home Care: Participation in cardiac rehabilitation program: lower risk for CHD
III. Client with Angina Pectoris (Angina)
 A. Definition
  1. Chest pain resulting from reduced coronary blood flow causing a temporary imbalance between myocardial blood supply and demand
  2. Due to CHD, atherosclerosis or vessel constriction that impairs blood supply to myocardium
  3. Precipitating factors
     a. Hypermetabolic conditions
        1. Exercise
        2. Thyrotoxicosis, hyperthyroidism
        3. Stimulant abuse (cocaine)
        4. Emotional stress
     b. Factors affecting blood and oxygen supplies
        1. Anemia
        2. Heart failure
        3. Pulmonary disease
 B. Pathophysiology
  1. Temporary and reversible myocardial ischemia caused by partial obstruction of coronary artery, coronary artery spasm or thrombus

2. Cells in region supplied by artery are deprived of essential oxygen and nutrients for metabolic processes compromising cellular processes
3. Cells switch to anaerobic metabolism causing lactic acid to build up in cells
4. Cell membranes release histamine, kinins, specific enzymes stimulating nerve fibers in cardiac muscle that send pain impulses to CNS
5. Pain radiates to upper body because heart shares same dermatome as this region
6. Return of adequate circulation provides nutrients and clears away waste products
7. > 30 minutes of ischemia irreversible damages myocardial cells or necrosis

C. Types of Angina
1. Stable angina
   a. Most common and predictable angina; occurs with predictable amount of activity or stress
   b. Common manifestation of CHD
   c. Occurs when work of heart is increased by physical exertion, exposure to cold, stress
   d. Relieved by rest and nitrates
2. Prinzmetal's (variant) angina
   a. Atypical angina occurs unpredictably: not related to activity and often at night
   b. Caused by spasm of coronary artery with or without atherosclerotic lesion
   c. Exact cause unknown
      1. May result from hyperactive sympathetic nervous system responses
      2. May result from altered calcium flow in smooth muscle
      3. May result from reduced prostaglandins causing vasoconstriction
3. Unstable angina
   a. Occurs with increasing frequency, severity, duration
   b. Pain is unpredictable and occurs with rest, low activity, stress
   c. At risk for myocardial infarction
4. Silent myocardial ischemia
   a. Asymptomatic ischemia, thought to be very common with CHD
   b. May occur with activity or mental stress

D. Manifestations
1. Chest pain
   a. Typically precipitated by identifiable event such as physical activity, strong emotion, stress, eating a heavy meal, exposure to cold
   b. Classic sequence: activity, pain, rest, relief
   c. Description of pain: tight, squeezing, heavy pressure, constricting sensation beginning beneath sternum and may radiate to jaw, neck, or arm
   d. Pain may just be in jaw, epigastric region, or back
   e. Pain usually lasts M < 15 minutes; relieved by rest
2. Other manifestations: dyspnea, pallor, tachycardia, great anxiety or fear

E. Collaborative Care
1. Pain relief
2. Restoration of coronary blood flow

F. Diagnostic Tests
1. Diagnosis based on
   a. Past medical history and family history
   b. Comprehensive description of pain
   c. Physical assessment findings
   d. Laboratory tests confirm presence of risk factors
   e. Diagnostic tests: information about overall cardiac function
2. Electrocardiography
   a. Resting ECG: may be normal, show nonspecific changes in ST segment and T wave; signs of previous myocardial infarction
   b. ECG changes consistent with anginal episodes: ST segment is depressed or downsloping; T wave flattened or inverted
   c. Ischemic changes reverse when ischemia is relieved
3. Stress electrocardiography
   a. Exercise Stress Tests
   b. Uses ECG to monitor cardiac response to increased workload during progressive exercise
4. Radionuclide testing
   a. Noninvasive, injection of small amount of radioisotope
   b. Evaluates myocardial perfusion and left ventricular function
   c. May be combined with pharmacologic stress testing for clients physically unable to exercise or to detect subclinical myocardial ischemia
5. Echocardiography
   a. Uses ultrasound to evaluate cardiac structure and function

b. Evaluation of myocardial wall for ischemia or infarction
c. Transesophageal echocardiography (TEE)
  1. Probe is on tip of endoscope inserted into esophagus
  2. Gives posterior view (left atrium, aorta)
6. Coronary angiography
  a. Evaluation of coronary arteries; guided by fluoroscopy, catheter introduced into femoral or brachial artery and threaded into coronary arteries and dye injected; main coronary branches are visualized
  b. Abnormalities may include
    1. Obstruction or stenosis
    2. Significant lesions are > 50%
    3. Lesions causing symptoms are > 70%
  c. Mapping of coronary artery provides guide for tracking disease progression and elective treatment such as angioplasty or cardiac surgery
  d. Nursing care of client having coronary angiography
    1. Before procedure
      a. Assessment of allergy to contrast media, iodine, seafood; renal function tests
      b. Baseline assessment including peripheral pulses
      c. Teaching regarding procedure, sense of warmth and metallic taste with injection of dye, lying flat post procedure
    2. Post procedure
      a. Maintenance of bedrest with head elevated 30 degrees; monitoring vital signs, catheterization site for bleeding, hematoma, peripheral pulses, neurovascular status per protocol; report significant deviations
      b. Minimal flexion or hyperextension of affected extremity
      c. Maintenance of adequate fluid intake (IV and/or oral)
      d. Discharge teaching
G. Medications: to reduce oxygen demand and increase oxygen supply to myocardium
  1. Nitrates
    a. Includes nitroglycerine (sublingual or buccal spray for acute angina relief)

and longer-acting nitrate preparations (prevention of angina)
  b. Description
    1. Sublingual
    2. Drug of choice to treat acute angina
    3. Acts within 1–2 minutes
    4. Decreases myocardial work and oxygen demand through arterial and venous dilation
    5. Improves oxygenation by dilating collateral blood vessels
  c. Longer acting preparations are available as oral tablets, ointment, transdermal patches to prevent angina
  d. Tolerance: decreasing effect from same dose of medication
    1. Can develop with long-term nitrate use
    2. Limit tolerance by allowing nitrate-free period at least 8–10 hours per day
  e. Side effects: headache, nausea, dizziness, hypotension
2. Beta-blockers (e.g., propranolol)
  a. First-line drugs to treat stable angina
  b. Description
    1. Blocks cardiac-stimulating effects of norepinephrine and epinephrine
    2. Prevents anginal attacks by reducing heart rate, myocardial contractility, and blood pressure
    3. Reduces myocardial oxygen demand
  c. Contraindicated for clients with asthma or severe COPD (severe bronchospasm)
  d. Not used for clients with significant bradycardia or AV conduction blocks (further slows heart rate)
  e. Worsens Prinzmetal's angina
3. Calcium channel blockers (e.g., diltiazem)
  a. Description
    1. Reduces myocardial oxygen demand
    2. Increases myocardial blood and oxygen supply
    3. Acts by lowering blood pressure and heart rate
    4. Reduces myocardial contractility
  b. Potent coronary vasodilators
  c. Long term prophylaxis of angina
  d. Used cautiously in clients with dysrhythmias, heart failure, hypotension

4. Aspirin: Low dose prescribed to reduce risk of platelet aggregation and thrombus formation

H. Revascularization Procedures

1. Percutaneous Coronary Revascularization (PCR)
   a. Invasive procedures used to restore blood flow to ischemic myocardium
   b. Used to treat moderately severe chronic stable angina unrelieved by medication, coronary ischemia; unstable angina; acute myocardial infarction
   c. Catheter introduced into narrowed coronary artery and procedure performed to restore circulation
   d. Percutaneous Transluminal Balloon Angioplasty (PTCA)
      1. Balloon positioned across area of narrowing and inflated to decrease vessel obstruction to less than 50% of arterial lumen
      2. Usually used in combination with stent placement (metallic scaffolds to maintain an open arterial lumen, in 70–80% PCR procedures)
      3. Antiplatelet medications (aspirin and ticlopidine) to reduce thrombus formation
   e. Atherectomy procedure
      1. Removes plaque from identified lesion by shaving plaque off vessel wall
      2. Laser athrectomy uses laser energy to remove plaque
   f. Complications post PCR procedures
      1. Hematoma at catheter insertion site
      2. Pseudoaneurysm
      3. Embolism
      4. Dysrhythmias
      5. Bleeding, vessel perforation
      6. Reocclusion of treated vessel
   g. Nursing care of client having PCR procedures
      1. Before procedure: Education
         a. Procedure including sedation and medications
         b. Sensations with contrast dye injection
         c. Chest pain balloon inflation
      2. Post procedure
         a. Head to toe assessment and maintain femoral sheath or pressure post removal at site, bedrest with head of bed elevated 30 degrees or less; maintenance of infusions usually heparin, nitroglycerine
         b. Monitoring of vital signs and cardiac rhythm continuously; insertion site for bleeding, hematoma, circulation and neurovascular status of leg
         c. Monitor and treat chest pain (could occur with ischemia or infarction)
         d. Monitor intake/output, lab values (electrolytes, renal function tests, CBC, cardiac enzymes, PTT)
         e. Monitor and treat vasovagal reaction during removal of femoral sheath

2. Coronary Artery Bypass Grafting (CABG)
   a. Surgery involves using section of vein or artery to create connection between aorta and coronary artery beyond obstruction, i.e., revascularization
   b. Blood perfuses ischemic sections of heart
   c. Internal mammary artery in chest and saphenous vein from legs are vessels commonly used for cardiac bypass grafts
   d. Recommended treatment for clients with multiple vessel disease, impaired ventricular function, diabetes, clients with significant obstruction of left main coronary artery
   e. Surgery involves medial sternotomy; heart often stopped during surgery and circulation is maintained by cardiopulmonary bypass pump which oxygenates blood and perfuses organs while heart is stopped
   f. Hypothermia during surgery reduces metabolic rate and need for oxygen
   g. Grafting done by anastomosis of graft to aorta and coronary artery distal to occlusion; internal mammary artery (IMA) has only distal end excised and anastomosed to coronary artery
   h. Temporary pacemaker wires inserted and sutured in place brought to outside; chest tubes placed in pleural space and mediastinum
   i. Rewarming heart stimulates heart to resume beating
   j. Nursing Diagnoses

1. Decreased cardiac output
   a. Continuous assessment with hemodynamic and rhythm monitoring
   b. Monitoring intake (intravenous at first) output (urinary, chest tubes)
   c. Cardiac pacing, if necessary
2. Hypothermia
3. Acute pain
4. Ineffective Airway Clearance/Impaired Gas Exchange: client initially intubated and on ventilator
5. Risk for Infection
6. Disturbed Thought Processes

3. Minimally Invasive Coronary Artery Surgery
   a. Alternative to CABG done in some centers
   b. Only small surgical incision and several chest wall ports to perform surgery
4. Transmyocardial Laser Revascularization
   a. Laser used to drilled tiny holes in myocardial muscle to provide collateral blood flow to ischemic muscle
   b. Procedure for clients with too diffuse disease for CABG

I. Nursing Diagnoses for clients with angina
   1. Ineffective Tissue Perfusion: Cardiac
   2. Risk for Ineffective Therapeutic Regimen Management
J. Home Care: Education
   1. Understand angina and management
   2. Lower risk factors for CHD
   3. Medications
   4. Participation in rehabilitation

IV. Client with Acute Myocardial Infarction (AMI)
   A. Definition
      1. Necrosis of myocardial cells is life-threatening event
      2. Loss of functional myocardium affects heart ability to maintain effective cardiac output
      3. Heart disease is leading cause of death in U.S.; AMI and other ischemic heart diseases cause majority of deaths
      4. Majority of deaths from MI occur during initial period post symptoms: 60% within first hour; 40% prior to hospitalization
      5. Need to educate public to seek immediate medical assistance with symptoms; train public in cardiopulmonary resuscitation (CPR) techniques
      6. Risks for MI are the same as for CHD

   B. Pathophysiology
      1. Develops from atherosclerotic plaques in coronary arteries
         a. Stable lesions: gradual occlusion of vessel lumen; cause angina
         b. Unstable (complicated) lesions: lead to acute coronary syndromes or acute ischemic heart diseases (unstable angina, myocardial infarction, sudden cardiac death)
      2. Occurs when blood flow to portion of cardiac muscle is blocked from prolonged tissue ischemia and irreversible cell damage
      3. Sequence of events
         a. Ulceration or rupture of complicated atherosclerotic lesion
         b. Substances released which lead to platelet aggregation, thrombin generation, local vasomotor tone
         c. Formation of clot which occludes vessel and blocks blood to myocardium distal to obstruction
         d. Prolonged ischemia (> 20–45 minutes): irreversible hypoxemic damage
         e. Cellular metabolism shifts from aerobic to anaerobic metabolism producing hydrogen ions and lactic acid
      4. Dysrhythmias and decreased myocardial contractility cause decreased stroke volume, cardiac output, blood pressure and tissue perfusion
      5. Depth of infarction
         a. Subendocardial or non-Q-wave infarction
            1. Damage is limited to subendocardial tissue
            2. Occurs within 20 minutes of injury
            3. Common complication is recurrent ischemia
         b. Transmural infarction
            1. All layers of myocardium to epicardium affected within 1 to 6 hours
            2. Common complication is heart failure
      6. Surrounding tissue: areas of injured and ischemic tissues
         a. Ischemic tissues: potentially viable and minimal damaged if perfusion restored
         b. Injured tissues: undergo metabolic changes

1. Stunned: impaired contractility for hours to days following reperfusion
2. Hibernating: myocytes protected until perfusion restored
3. Myocardial remodeling: cellular hypertrophy with loss of contractility in areas distant from infarction
   c. Collateral circulation development: smaller arteries in coronary system dilate to maintain blood flow to cardiac muscle; degree of collateral circulation limits size of MI
7. Areas of heart
   a. Particular coronary artery occluded determines area of damage
   b. The specific infarct site predicts possible complications and dictates appropriate therapy
   c. Specific artery and affected area of heart
      1. Left anterior descending (LAD) artery: anterior wall of left ventricle and part of interventricular septum
      2. Left circumflex artery (LCA): lateral MI
      3. Right coronary artery (RCA) and posterior descending artery (PDA): right ventricular, inferior, and posterior infarct
      4. Left main coronary artery: entire left ventricle and a grave prognosis
8. Cocaine intoxication can cause acute MI secondary to sympathetic nervous system stimulation resulting in over-stimulation of the heart, dysrhythmias and vasoconstriction
C. Manifestations
   1. Pain: classic manifestation
      a. Chest pain differs from angina in duration and continuous nature
         1. Lasts > 15–20 minutes
         2. Unrelieved by rest or nitroglycerine
      b. Onset sudden and usually not associated with activity
      c. Described as crushing and severe; as a pressure, heavy or squeezing sensation; tightness or burning in the chest
      d. Location: center of chest (substernal) and may radiate to shoulders, neck, jaw, arms
      e. Women and older adults have atypical chest pain with complaints of indigestion, heartburn, nausea, vomiting

   f. No chest discomfort in 25% of clients with acute MI
   2. Additional symptoms relate to sympathetic nervous system stimulation
      a. Cool, clammy, mottled skin
      b. Tachypnea
      c. Sense of impending doom and death
   3. Depending on location and amount of infarct
      a. Hypertension or hypotension
      b. Signs of heart failure
      c. Nausea and vomiting, bradycardia
      d. Hiccoughs
      e. Sudden death (large blood vessel involvement)
   4. Complications
      a. Dysrhythmias
         1. Disturbances or irregularities of heart rhythm; most frequent
         2. Infarcted tissue generates and conducts electrical impulses
         3. Common dysrhythmias
            a. Premature ventricular contractions (PVC's)
               1. Occurs in 90% of clients with acute MI
               2. May lead to dangerous dysrhythmias
            b. Ventricular tachycardia or fibrillation: fibrillation risk greatest first hour post MI and frequent cause of sudden death with acute MI
            c. Atrioventricular (AV) blocks
            d. Bradydysrhythmias
      b. Pump failure
         1. Greatest risk when large portions of left ventricle infarcted
         2. More severe with anterior MI: manifestations of left sided heart failure
         3. Inferior or right ventricular MI: manifestations of right-sided heart failure
         4. Hemodynamic monitoring indicated
      c. Cardiogenic shock
         1. Impaired tissue perfusion due to pump failure (functioning myocardial muscle mass < by more than 40%)
         2. Heart as pump cannot meet needs of body (low cardiac output); impaired perfusion of coronary arteries and myocardium

3. Mortality is > 70% (reduced if prompt revasculization procedures)
4. Hemodynamic monitoring indicated
d. Infarct extension
1. 10% clients reinfarct or extend area of original MI in first 10–14 days
2. Extension or expansion of MI manifestations: continuing chest pain, hemodynamic compromise, worsening heart failure
e. Structural defects
1. Scar tissue replacing area of infarct is thinner
2. Can lead to complications:
a. Ventricular aneurysm: outpouching of ventricular wall (client at risk for intramural clots)
b. Rupture of interventricular septum or papillary muscle
c. Myocardial rupture (risk between days 7–14 post MI)
f. Pericarditis
1. Inflammation of pericardial tissue around heart from tissue necrosis; complication of acute MI within 2–3 days
2. Manifestations: chest pain (aching, or sharp, aggravated by movement or deep breathing); pericardial friction rub
3. Dressler's syndrome: hypersensitivity response to necrotic tissue resulting in fever, chest pain, dyspnea days to weeks post acute MI; may resolve or recur over months
D. Collaborative Care
1. Treatment goals
a. Relieve chest pain
b. Reduce extent of myocardial damage
c. Maintain cardiovascular stability
d. Decrease cardiac workload
e. Prevent complications
2. Rapid assessment and early diagnosis key
a. "Time is muscle"
b. Initiation of definitive treatment within 1 hour of entry into health care system
c. Major problem: delay in seeking medical care post onset of symptoms (44% wait > 4 hours to seek treatment)
d. Reasons for delay
1. Denial
2. Advanced age

3. Lack of perception of seriousness of symptoms
4. Availability of emergency response system
5. In-hospital delay
E. Diagnostic Tests
1. Serum cardiac markers: Proteins released from necrotic heart muscle; ordered on admission and for 3 succeeding days
a. Creatine phosphokinase (CK)
1. Enzyme found in cardiac and skeletal muscle
2. Appears 4–6 hours post acute MI; peaks 12–24 hours; declines over next 48–72 hours
3. Level correlates with size of infarction: greater amount of infarcted tissue, higher the serum CK level
b. CK-MB: subset of CK specific to cardiac muscle
1. Isoenzyme of CK most sensitive indicator of MI
2. CK-MB elevation > 5% positive indicator of MI
c. Cardiac-specific troponin T (cT_nT) and cardiac-specific troponin I (cT_nI)
1. Proteins released during myocardial infarction; sensitive indicators for myocardial damage
2. Released and levels rise with necrosis of cardiac muscle
3. Sensitive enough to detect very small infarction and remain in blood 10–14 days post MI
2. Other laboratory tests
a. CBC, Erythrocyte Sedimentation Rate: WBC and ESR elevated because of inflammation
b. Arterial Blood Gases (ABG's): assessment of blood oxygen levels and acid-base balance secondary to physical effects of MI
3. Electrocardiography: ECG reflects changes in conduction due to myocardial ischemia and necrosis
a. Changes seen with acute MI
1. T wave inversion
2. Elevation of S-T segment
3. Formation of Q wave (transmural infarction)
b. Location of MI reflected in which leads of 12-lead ECG show the changes

4. Echocardiography
   a. Can be done at bedside
   b. Evaluates cardiac wall motion and left ventricular function
5. Radionuclide imaging
   a. Evaluation of myocardial perfusion
   b. Identification of specific areas of myocardial ischemia and damage; does not differentiate between acute MI and old scar tissue
   c. Isotope: Thallium-201: ischemic areas "cold spots"
   d. Isotope: Technetium-99m: (technetium-99m) pyrophosphate ischemic areas "hot spots"
6. Hemodynamic monitoring: initiated when acute MI leads to changes in cardiac output and hemodynamic status
F. Medications: used to reduce oxygen demand and increase oxygen supply
1. Thrombolytic Therapy
   a. Drugs break up blood clots and restore blood flow to obstructed artery
   b. Early (within first 6 hours of MI)
      1. Limits infarct size
      2. Reduces heart damage
      3. Improves outcome
   c. Complications involved from activating fibrinolytic system, including serious bleeding
   d. Contraindications
      1. Known bleeding disorders
      2. History cerebrovascular disease
      3. Uncontrolled HPT
      4. Pregnancy
      5. Recent trauma or surgery
   e. Thrombolytic agents
      1. Streptokinase: risk of hypersensitivity reaction
      2. Anisolylated plasminogen streptokinase activator complex (APSAC)
      3. Tissue plasminogen activator (t-PA): more effective with reestablishing perfusion when pain has lasted more than 3 hours
      4. Reteplase: more effective with reestablishing perfusion when pain has lasted more than 3 hours
2. Analgesia
   a. Pain relief important to decrease myocardial workload (sympathetic nervous system stimulation increases heart rate and blood pressure)
   b. Morphine sulfate: drug of choice for pain and sedation
      1. Initial intravenous dose of 4–8 mg followed by 2–4 mg every 5 minutes until pain relieved
      2. Frequent pain assessment and observation for over-sedation or respiratory depression
   c. Sublingual nitroglycerine (3 0.4 mg doses at 5 minute intervals)
      1. Decreases myocardial oxygen demand
      2. Dilates collateral circulation improving oxygen supply
3. Antidysrhythmics
   a. Common complication of acute MI, especially first 12–24 hours
   b. Dysrhythmias
      1. Ventricular
      2. Symptomatic bradycardia (treated with IV atropine 0.5–1 mg)
      3. Supraventricular tachydysrhythmias (treated with IV verapamil, short-acting beta blockers)
4. Other medications
   a. Beta blockers reduce heart rate, cardiac work and myocardial oxygen demand thus
      1. Reduce pain
      2. Limit infarct size
      3. Decrease serious ventricular dysrhythmias
      4. Oral therapy continued to reduce risk of re-infarction and death from cardiovascular causes
   b. Angiotensin-converting enzyme (ACE) inhibitors reduce ventricular remodeling post MI thus
      1. Reduce risk for development of heart failure
      2. Reduce risk of re-infarction
   c. Intravenous nitroglycerine for first 24–48 hours
      1. Reduces myocardial work by reducing afterload by vasodilation which also increases coronary blood flow
      2. Observe for excessive reflex tachycardia or excessive hypotension
   d. Aspirin
      1. Platelet inhibitor
      2. 160–325 mg given by emergency personnel at onset of symptoms
      3. Daily thereafter

e. Anticoagulants and antiplatelet medications to maintain coronary artery patency post thrombolysis or revascularization procedure
　　1. Abciximab (ReoPro) suppresses platelet aggregation
　　2. Heparin, standard or low-molecular-weight
f. Dopamine
　　1. Low dose ($<$ 5 mcg/kg/min) improving renal perfusion
　　2. Higher doses to treat hypotension and low cardiac output
g. Antilipemic agents
h. Stool softeners

G. Medical Management
1. Continuous observation for suspected or confirmed MI in intensive coronary care unit
　a. Continuous rhythm monitoring
　b. Bed rest for first 12 hours with gradual increase in activity as condition allows
　c. Continuous oxygen at 2–5 L for optimum oxygenation
　d. Liquid diet advanced to low fat, cholesterol diet with small frequent feedings, quiet calm environment
2. Revascularization procedures
　a. Percutaneous coronary revascularization (PCR) with angioplasty and stent placement (may follow thrombolytic therapy)
　b. CABG surgery may be performed in some cases
3. Other invasive procedures as indicated: with large MI's and pump failure, devices to take over function of heart while myocardium heals
　a. Intra-aortic balloon pump (IABP) or intra-aortic balloon counterpulsation
　　1. Catheter with 30–40 ml balloon introduced into aorta via femoral artery
　　2. Balloon inflates during diastole to increase perfusion of coronary and renal arteries; deflates during systole: decreases afterload and cardiac work
　　3. Inflation-deflation sequence triggered by ECG pattern
　　4. Most acute cases, balloon activates with each heart beat (1:1 ratio); as condition improves ratio is weaned (e.g., 1:2; 1:4; 1:8)
　　5. Removed when no longer needed

b. Ventricular assist devices (VADs)
　1. Becoming more common with advanced technology
　2. Used temporary or complete assist with cardiogenic shock
　3. Complications include risk for infection, pneumonia
　4. Mechanical failure is life-threatening event
4. Cardiac rehabilitation
　a. Long-term program of medical evaluation, risk factor modification, education and counseling to limit effects of cardiac illness and improve quality of life
　b. Phases
　　1. Inpatient phase
　　　a. Client assessment
　　　b. Activity from bedrest to independent ADLs and ambulation inside
　　2. Immediate outpatient rehabilitation phase
　　　a. Begins within 3 weeks of cardiac event
　　　b. Increase activity and capacity
　　　c. Improve psychosocial state
　　　d. Education and support for risk factor reduction
　　3. Final Phase: Continuation phase
　　　a. Transition to independent exercise
　　　b. Exercise maintenance

H. Nursing Care
1. Risk factor management
2. Use of prescribed medications
3. Cardiac rehabilitation to reduce risk of complications or future infarcts

I. Nursing Diagnoses
1. Acute pain
2. Ineffective Tissue Perfusion: obtain 12-lead ECG to assess significant chest pain
3. Ineffective Coping: peruse of denial may interfere with learning and compliance with treatment
4. Fear

J. Home Care
1. Cardiac rehabilitation
2. Education program
3. Community resources including CPR training

V. Client with a Cardiac Dysrhythmia
A. Background
1. Dysrhythmias can occur as natural consequence of emotion, body demand

for oxygen, or sympathetic nervous
system stimulation, athletic training,
aging
2. Physiology
a. Cardiac muscle is unique in that it can
generate electrical impulse and
contraction independent of nervous
system
b. Cardiac conduction system: network
of specialized cells and conduction
pathways that initiate and spread
electrical impulses causing heart to
beat
c. Electrical stimulation of heart muscle
always precedes mechanical
contraction
d. Pacemaker cells of heart
1. Sinoatrial (SA) or sinus node:
intrinsic rate 60–100 bpm
2. Atrioventricular (AV) node:
intrinsic rate 40–60 bpm
3. Purkinje fibers (of ventricle
conduction system): intrinsic rate
15–40 bpm
e. Electrophysiologic properties: unique
properties of cardiac cells allow
effective heart function
1. Automaticity: ability of pacemaker
cells to spontaneously initiate
electrical stimulation (SA node)
2. Excitability: ability of myocardial
cells to respond to stimuli generated
by pacemaker cells
3. Conductivity: ability to transmit
impulse from cell to cell
4. Contractility: ability of myocardial
fibers to shorten in response to
stimulus; "All or nothing" manner:
stimulation of one muscle fiber
causes entire muscle mass to
contract to fullest extent as one unit
f. Action potential
1. Electrical activity produces
waveforms on ECG strips because
of ion movement across cell
membranes stimulating muscle
contraction
2. Stages
a. Resting State: polarized state
1. Positive and negative ions
align on either side of cell
membrane
2. Relatively negative charge
within cell and positive
extracellularly

3. Negative resting membrane
potential maintained at −90
millivolts (mV)
b. Depolarization
1. Resting cell stimulated by
charge
2. Na ions enter cell rapidly
through fast sodium channels
3. Calcium enter cells via slow
calcium-sodium channels
4. Membrane less permeable to
K ions
5. Membrane potential changes
to slightly positive at +20 −
+30 mV
c. Threshold potential
1. As cell becomes more
positive a point is reached
and action potential is
generated
2. Causes chemical reaction of
Ca within cell
3. Actin and myosin filaments
slide together producing
cardiac muscle contraction
4. Once myocardium
completely depolarized,
repolarization begins
d. Repolarization
1. Cell returns to resting,
polarized state
2. Fast sodium channels close
abruptly
3. Cell regains negative charge
(rapid repolarization)
4. Muscle contraction prolongs
as slow calcium-sodium
channels remain open
(plateau phase)
5. Once closed sodium-
potassium pump restores ion
concentration and cell
membrane is polarized again
3. Refractory period
a. Myocardial cells are resistive to
stimulation; dysrhythmias
triggered during relative
refractory and supernormal
periods
b. Three periods
1. Absolute refractory period:
no depolarization can occur
2. Relative refractory period:
greater than normal stimulus
required for depolarization

3. Supernormal period: mild stimulus will cause depolarization
3. Electrocardiography
   a. Graphic recording of electrical activity of heart detected by electrodes on surface of body
   b. Electrodes applied to body surface and detect magnitude and direction of electrical current produced by heart
   c. Standard 12-lead ECG simultaneous recording of 6 limb leads and 6 precordial leads
      1. Limb leads: bipolar leads (I, II, III); unipolar leads: aV_R, aV_L, aV_F
      2. Precordial leads (chest leads): V_1, V_2, V_3, V_4, V_5, V_6
      3. Waveforms reflect direction of electrical flow
         a. Positive (upward) waveform is toward the positive electrode
         b. Negative (downward) waveform is away from positive electrode
         c. Biphasic (both positive and negative) waveform shows perpendicular to positive pole
         d. Isoelectric line (straight line) absence of electrical activity
      4. ECG waveforms recorded on paper with marking representative of time
         a. Each small box = 0.04 seconds (sec)
         b. One large box (5 small boxes) = 0.20 sec.
         c. 5 large boxes measure 1 second
         d. Vertically, each small box = 0.1 millivolt (mV)
      5. Cardiac cycle depicted as series of waveforms
         a. P wave: atrial depolarization and contraction
         b. PR interval
            1. Time for sinus impulse to travel from SA node to AV node and into bundle branches (beginning of P wave to beginning of QRS complex)
            2. Normal 0.12–0.20 seconds
         c. QRS complex
            1. Ventricular depolarization and contraction
            2. Transmission of impulse through ventricular conduction system
            3. Normal 0.06–0.10 seconds
      d. ST segment
         1. Beginning of ventricular repolarization
         2. End of QRS complex to beginning of T wave
         3. Should be isoelectric
      e. T wave
         1. Ventricular repolarization
         2. Smooth and round < 10 mm tall
         3. Same direction as QRS complex
         4. Abnormalities indicate myocardial injury or ischemia, electrolyte imbalances
      f. QT interval
         1. Total time of ventricular depolarization and repolarization
         2. Beginning of QRS complex to end of T wave
         3. Normal: 0.32–0.44 seconds
         4. Prolonged QT: prolonged relative refractory period and greater risk for dysrhythmias
         5. Shortened QT: due to medications or electrolyte imbalance
      g. U wave
         1. Not normally seen but thought to signify repolarization of terminal Purkinje fibers
         2. Same direction as T wave
         3. Seen commonly with hypokalemia
B. Pathophysiology
   1. 2 major mechanisms for dysrhythmia development
      a. Altered impulse formation
         1. Tachydysrhythmias (rapid heart rates)
         2. Bradydysrhythmia (slow heart rates)
         3. Ectopic rhythms (impulses originate outside normal conduction pathways)
      b. Altered conductivity
         1. Block in normal conduction pathway
         2. Varying degrees of heart block at AV node
         3. Bundle branch blocks
   2. Re-entry phenomenon

a. Cause of tachydysrhythmias
b. Impulse delayed in one area of heart but conducted normally through the rest and part of heart repolarized and able to conduct impulse again
c. Dysrhythmia propagates itself

C. Classifications: according to site of impulse formation

1. Supraventricular rhythms (above ventricles)
   a. Normal sinus rhythm
      1. Normal conduction
      2. Rhythm originates in SA node
      3. Rate 60–100 bpm
   b. Sinus arrhythmia
      1. Sinus rhythm which has rate variations according to respirations
      2. Rate increases with inspiration; rate decreases with expiration
      3. Common in very young and very old
   c. Sinus tachycardia
      1. Normal conduction
      2. Rate is greater than 100 bpm
      3. Causes
         a. Sympathetic nervous system stimulation
         b. Blockage of vagal activity
         c. Body response to condition or event that requires increase in oxygen and/or nutrition
      4. Manifestations
         a. Palpitations
         b. Shortness of breath
         c. Dizziness
   d. Sinus bradycardia
      1. Normal conduction
      2. Rate is slower than 60 bpm
      3. Causes
         a. Increased vagal (parasympathetic) activity
         b. Injury or ischemia to sinus node
         c. Normal (athletic heart syndrome, asleep)
         d. Inferior wall damage with acute MI
         e. Increased intracranial pressure
         f. Hypothermia
      4. Manifestations
         a. Asymptomatic (none)
         b. Symptomatic: decreased level of consciousness, syncope, hypotension
   e. Sick Sinus Syndrome—SSS (sinus node dysfunction)

1. Causes
   a. Dysfunction of sinus node often with aging
   b. Use of medications which slow heart (e.g., digitalis, beta blockers)
2. Rhythm changes
   a. Sinus bradycardia or arrhythmias
   b. Sinus pauses or arrest
   c. Atrial tachydysrhythmias such as atrial fibrillation, flutter, or tachycardia
   d. Bradycardia-tachycardia syndrome: paroxysmal tachyrhythms followed by sinus pauses and/or bradycardias
3. Manifestations
   a. Intermittent fatigue
   b. Dizziness
   c. Light-headedness
   d. Syncope

2. Supraventricular dysrhythmias
   a. Premature Atrial Contractions (PAC's)
      1. Ectopic atrial beat occurring earlier than next expected sinus beat
      2. Usually asymptomatic and benign
      3. Non-compensatory pause
   b. Paroxysmal Supraventricular Tachycardia (PSVT)
      1. Sudden onset and termination
      2. Often initiated by a reentry loop in or around AV node
      3. Precipitated by
         a. Sympathetic nervous system stimulation and stressors
            1. Fever
            2. Sepsis
            3. Hyperthyroidism
         b. Heart diseases
            1. CHD, myocardial infarction
            2. Rheumatic heart disease
            3. Myocarditis or acute pericarditis
            4. Wolff-Parkinson-White syndrome
      4. Manifestations
         a. Palpitations, "racing heart"
         b. Anxiety
         c. Dizziness
         d. Dyspnea, anginal pain
         e. Extreme fatigue, diaphoresis
         f. Polyuria
   c. Atrial Flutter

1. Rapid, regular atrial rhythm resulting from intra-atrial reentry mechanism
2. Causes
   a. Sympathetic nervous system stimulation
      1. Anxiety
      2. Caffeine and alcohol intake
   b. Thyrotoxicosis
   c. CHD
   d. Pulmonary embolism
   e. Wolff-Parkinson-White syndrome
   f. Rheumatic heart disease and/or valvular disease
3. Manifestations
   a. Palpitations or fluttering sensations in chest or throat
   b. If rapid ventricular response: hypotension, cool, clammy skin, decreased level of consciousness
4. ECG characteristics
   a. Sawtooth flutter waves at 300 bpm
   b. Constant conduction ratio gives regular ventricular rhythm
d. Atrial Fibrillation
   1. Disorganized atrial activity without discrete atrial contractions
   2. Extremely rapid atrial impulses result in irregular ventricular response
   3. Associated with heart failure, rheumatic heart disease, CHD, HPT, hyperthyroidism
   4. Manifestations (relate to ventricular response)
      a. Rapid response rates
         1. Hypotension
         2. Shortness of breath
         3. Fatigue
         4. Angina
      b. May develop syncope, heart failure
      c. Increased risk for thromboemboli; high incidence of stroke
   5. Irregular irregular rhythm without P waves
3. Junctional dysrhythmias
   a. Rhythms that originate in AV nodal tissue
   b. Junctional escape rhythm; due to drug toxicity, hyperkalemia, increased vagal tone, cardiac causes

c. Premature junctional contractions (PJCs) or Junctional Tachycardia: junctional rhythm with rate > 60 and usually < 140 bpm due to increased automaticity of AV nodal tissue; associated with
   1. Digitalis toxicity
   2. Hypoxia, ischemia
   3. Electrolyte imbalances
4. Ventricular dysrhythmias (originate in ventricles)
   a. Any disruption of ventricular rhythm can seriously impact cardiac output and tissue perfusion
   b. ECG Characteristics of ventricular rhythms
      1. Wide and bizarre QRS complex (> 0.12 sec)
      2. Increased amplitude of QRS complex
      3. No relationship to P wave; abnormal ST segment, T wave deflected opposite to QRS complex
   c. Premature Ventricular Contractions (PVCs)
      1. ECG Characteristics
         a. Occur before next expected beat
         b. Often followed by full compensatory pause
      2. ECG Descriptors
         a. Couplet or pair: 2 PVC's in a row
         b. Triplet or salvo: 3 PVC's in a row
         c. Bigeminy: PVC every other beat
         d. Trigeminy: PVC every third beat
         e. Unifocal PVC's: arise from one site
         f. Multifocal PVC's: from different ectopic sites
      3. Significance
         a. None in persons without heart disease
         b. Frequent, recurrent, multifocal PVC's associated with increased risk for lethal dysrhythmias
      4. Triggers
         a. Anxiety or stress
         b. Tobacco, alcohol, caffeine use
         c. Hypoxia, acidosis, electrolyte imbalance
         d. Sympathomimetic drugs
         e. Coronary heart disease, heart failure

f. Mechanical stimulation of heart (insertion of cardiac catheter)
g. Reperfusion after thrombolytic therapy
h. Post MI
5. Indicators of myocardial irritability and increased risk for lethal dysrhythmias
    a. PVC's occurring within 4 hours of MI
    b. Frequent (> 6 per minute)
    c. Couplets or triplets
    d. Multifocal PVC's
    e. R on T phenomenon (PVC's falling on T wave)
d. Ventricular Tachycardia (VT, V Tach)
    1. Rapid ventricular rhythm of 3 or more PVC's
    2. Rate > 100 with regular rhythm
    3. Result of re-entry phenomenon
    4. Manifestations if sustained VT
        a. Severe hypotension
        b. Weak or nonpalpable pulse
        c. Loss of consciousness
        d. Allowed to continue, deteriorates into ventricular fibrillation
e. Ventricular Fibrillation (VF, V fib)
    1. Extremely rapid, chaotic rhythm in which ventricles quiver and do not contract
    2. Cardiac arrest and death will result within 4 minutes if rhythm not terminated
    3. Triggers
        a. Severe myocardial ischemia or infarction
        b. Precipitated by PVC or V Tach
        c. Other causes
            1. Digitalis toxicity
            2. Reperfusion therapy
            3. Antidysrhythmic drugs
            4. Hypo and hyperkalemia
            5. Hypothermia
            6. Metabolic acidosis
            7. Mechanical stimulation
            8. Electric shock
    4. Manifestations
        a. Absence of palpable or audible pulse
        b. Loss of consciousness
        c. Without treatment, breathing stops
5. Atrioventricular (AV) Conduction Blocks
    a. Delayed or block transmission of sinus impulse through AV node

b. Causes
    1. Tissue injury or disease
    2. Increased vagal tone
    3. Drug effects
c. Types of AV blocks
    1. First-degree AV block
        a. Slowed conduction
        b. PR interval is > 0.20 sec
        c. Benign, no ill effects
    2. Second-degree AV block
        a. Characterized by failure to conduct one or more impulses from atria to ventricles
        b. Type 1 AV block (Mobitz type I, Wenckebach phenomenon)
            1. Usually transient
            2. Associated with acute MI or drug intoxication
            3. Rarely progresses
        c. Type 2 AV block (Mobitz type II)
            1. Intermittent failure of AV node to conduct impulse
            2. Frequently associated with acute anterior MI and high mortality rate
            3. Pacemaker may be required
    3. Third-degree AV block (complete heart block)
        a. Atrial impulses blocked at AV node and fail to reach ventricles
        b. Atria and ventricles have separate rates and rhythms
        c. Rhythm from junctional fibers (rate 40–60 bpm) or ventricular (< 30 bpm)
        d. Causes
            1. Inferior or anteroseptal MI
            2. Congenital, active, or degenerative cardiac disease
            3. Drug effects
            4. Electrolyte imbalances
    4. AV Dissociation
        a. Severe sinus bradycardia and lower pacemakers have competing rhythms
        b. Causes
            1. Acute MI
            2. Cardiac surgery
            3. Drug effects
    5. Ventricular Conduction Blocks
        a. Conduction through right or left bundle branches of ventricle is impaired
        b. Prolonged QRS complex

D. Collaborative Care
1. Focus
   a. Recognition and identification of dysrhythmia
   b. Evaluating the effects, especially lethality
   c. Treatment of underlying causes
2. ECG rhythm analysis process
   a. Rate determination
   b. Regularity determination
   c. P wave assessment
   d. Assessment of P to QRS relationship
   e. Determination of intervals
      1. PR interval
      2. QRS complex duration
      3. QT interval
   f. Identification of abnormalities
E. Diagnostic Tests
1. 12 lead Electrocardiogram
   a. Identification of rhythm
   b. Information about underlying disease processes
   c. Monitor effects of treatment
2. Cardiac monitoring
   a. Continuous cardiac monitoring: observed during hospitalization including telemetry while client is ambulatory
   b. Ambulatory or Holter monitoring
      1. Identification of intermittent dysrhythmias
      2. Monitor effects of treatments
      3. Client records symptoms and events in a journal
3. Electrophysiology Studies
   a. Diagnostic procedures used to identify dysrhythmias and cause
   b. Evaluation of treatment effectiveness
   c. Invasive procedure in which electrode catheters introduced into heart
   d. Timing and sequence of electrical activity noted during normal and abnormal rhythms
   e. May involve treatment of dysrhythmia by overdrive pacing or perform ablative therapy to destroy ectopic site
   f. Nursing care is similar to that for coronary angiogram
   g. Possible complications
      1. Ventricular fibrillation
      2. Cardiac perforation
      3. Venous thrombosis
F. Medications
1. Goal of therapy: suppression of dysrhythmia and rhythm stabilization and effective cardiac output

2. All have prodysrhythmic effects: may worsen existing dysrhythmias or precipitate new ones
3. Classifications according to effects of cardiac action potential
   a. Class I: fast sodium channel blockers; subclasses are A, B, C
   b. Class II: beta-blockers
      1. Decrease SA note automaticity
      2. AV conduction velocity
      3. Myocardial contractility
   c. Class III: block potassium channels
      1. Delay repolarization
      2. Prolong relative refractory period
   d. Class IV: calcium channel blockers
   e. Not classified
      1. Adenosine, Digoxin: reduce SA node automaticity, slow AV conduction
      2. Drugs affecting autonomic nervous system
         a. Epinephrine
         b. Atropine
         c. Magnesium for v tach
G. Countershock
1. Interrupts cardiac rhythms that compromise cardiac output and client's well being
2. Delivery of direct current depolarizes all cells simultaneously
3. Types of countershock
   a. Synchronized cardioversion
      1. Direct electrical current synchronized with client's heart rhythm
      2. Avoids shock during vulnerable period of repolarization
      3. Elective procedure to treat supraventricular tachycardia, atrial fibrillation or flutter, hemodynamically stable v. tachy
      4. Clients in atrial fibrillation should be anticoagulated for several weeks before cardioversion to decrease risk for thromboembolism post cardioversion
   b. Defibrillation
      1. Emergency delivery of direct current without regard to cardiac cycle
      2. Performed immediately rhythm is recognized
      3. Performed externally or internally (surgery, open chest); also automatic external defibrillators

H. Pacemaker Therapy
   1. Pulse generator provide electrical stimulus to heart when heart fails to generate or conduct own at a rate for adequate cardiac output
   2. Conditions that can be treated with pacemaker
      a. Third-degree AV block
      b. Bradydysrhythmias
      c. Tachydysrhythmias
   3. Types
      a. Temporary
         1. External pulse generator attached to lead threaded into right ventricle
         2. Pacer wires implanted during surgery or as external conductive pads for emergency pacing
      b. Permanent
         1. Pulse generator is placed surgically in a subcutaneous pocket (often subclavian space) and leads are placed either
            a. Directly onto heart (epicardial with a thoracotomy)
            b. Transvenously into heart (endocardial)
         2. Local anesthesia used with transvenous insertion
      c. Single-chamber pacing (atria or ventricles are stimulated) or dual-chamber pacing (both are stimulated)
      d. Most commonly used pacemakers are
         1. Pacemakers which sense activity in and pace ventricles only
         2. Pacemakers which sense activity in and pace both atria and ventricles: atrioventricular sequential pacing stimulates in sequence that imitates normal sequence of atrial contraction followed by ventricular contraction
      e. ECG characteristics
         1. Pacing detected by presence of pacing artifact which is a sharp spike occurring before P wave in atrial pacing or before QRS complex in ventricular pacing
         2. Capture is noted by contraction of chamber following the spike (seen as P wave in atrial pacing or QRS complex in ventricular pacing)
      f. Nursing care
         1. Monitoring pacemaker function
         2. Maintaining safety
         3. Preventing infection and complications

I. Implantable Cardioverter-defibrillator (ICD)
   1. Pulse generator is implanted surgically into client with lead electrodes for rhythm detection and current delivery
   2. ICD senses life-threatening rhythm changes and delivers automatically electric shock to convert dysrhythmia
   3. ICD
      a. Provides pacing on demand
      b. Stores ECG records of rhythms
      c. May be reprogrammed at bedside when necessary
      d. Needs surgically replaced every 5 years
   4. Use of ICD indicated for clients with
      a. Sudden death survivors
      b. Recurrent ventricular tachycardia
      c. Significant risk factors for sudden death

J. Cardiac Mapping and Catheter Ablation
   1. Involves location and destruction of ectopic foci in heart which cause life-threatening dysrhythmias
   2. Diagnosed in electrophysiology lab and performed in cardiac catheterization laboratory
   3. Cardiac mapping: identification of sites where impulse initiated in atria or ventricles with use of internal or external catheters
   4. Ablation: destruction of ectopic focus using radiofrequency energy with catheters; anticoagulant therapy may be started afterward to decrease risk of clot forming at ablation site

K. Other measures to stop dysrhythmias
   1. Vagal maneuvers in which client "bears down": a forced exhalation against a closed glottis to slow heart rate
   2. Carotid sinus massage with continuous monitoring done by physician only

L. Nursing Care
   1. Decrease risk for CHD which is major risk for dysrhythmias
   2. Reduce sympathetic nervous system stimulants like caffeine

M. Nursing Diagnoses
   1. Decreased Cardiac Output
      a. Always assess the client before treating the dysrhythmia
      b. Monitor vital signs, ECG, and oxygen saturation frequently during antidysrhythmic drug infusions
      c. Nurses caring for clients with dysrhythmias need to be competent in CPR and ACLS

2. Ineffective Tissue Perfusion
3. Anxiety
N. Home care
   1. Education about implanted devices such as pacemakers and ICDs
   2. Self monitoring of pulse and rhythm
   3. Medication regimens
   4. CPR training for families
VI. Client with Sudden Cardiac Death (SCD)
A. Definition
   1. Unexpected death occurring within 1 hour of onset of cardiovascular symptoms
   2. Cardiac arrest: sudden collapse, loss of consciousness, cessation of effective circulation
   3. Half of all cardiac arrest victims die before reaching hospital
   4. Ventricular fibrillation is most common dysrhythmia associated with sudden cardiac death; other rhythms include severe bradydysrhythmias, asystole, pulseless electrical activity
B. Pathophysiology
   1. Findings in 75% of SCD victims: CHD with significant atherosclerosis and narrowing of 2 or more major coronary arteries
   2. Acute change in cardiovascular status precedes cardiac arrest by up to 1 hour
      a. Onset is abrupt: tachycardia with increased PVC's
      b. Then ventricular tachycardia deteriorating into ventricular fibrillation

3. Other factors include abnormalities of myocardial structure or function
C. Collaborative Care
   1. Goal: restore cardiac output and tissue perfusion
   2. Basic and advanced cardiac life support measures instituted within 2–4 minutes
      a. Use of automated external defibrillator (AED)
      b. CPR performed according to AHA protocol
      c. ACLS including endotracheal intubation, intravenous drugs following protocols, additional interventions: repeated defibrillation, cardiac pacing
      d. Postresuscitation care
         1. Clients who experience SCD associated with ventricular fibrillation and acute MI
         2. Risk for recurrent SCD is high for survivors; extensive diagnostic testing and interventions (angioplasty, CABG, ablation or ICD)
D. Nursing Diagnoses
   1. Ineffective Tissue Perfusion: Cerebral
   2. Impaired Spontaneous Ventilation related to cardiac arrest
   3. Spiritual Distress
   4. Disturbed Thought Processes related to compromised cerebral circulation

FOCUSED STUDY TIPS

- Evaluate your personal risk factors for coronary heart disease. Compare your risk factors with a classmate's. Identify differences in risk factors. Identify which factors are modifiable and which are nonmodifiable. Create a plan to modify those risk factors that are modifiable.
- Visit the coronary care unit of a hospital. Ask for sample rhythm strips from clients experiencing cardiac rhythm disturbances. Study them for understanding of cardiac dysfunction. Share the strips with classmates.
- Compare and contrast advanced directives and do-not-resuscitate orders with family members. Encourage verbalization of preferences. Document preferences and encourage discussion of these topics with the family physician.

CASE STUDY

T. T. is scheduled for placement of a permanent pacemaker. Preoperatively, he expresses concern regarding lifestyle changes after the procedure. What impact will pacer therapy have on his lifestyle? What must he and family members know and understand before his discharge from the hospital?

CARE PLAN CRITICAL THINKING ACTIVITY

Develop a care plan for a client who has just undergone successful synchronized cardioversion for the treatment of atrial fibrillation. For what is the client most at risk? What nursing assessments and interventions are necessary to prevent, as well as detect, this major complication? What teaching is necessary before the client is discharged from the hospital?

NCLEX TEST QUESTIONS

1. Which one of the following statements reflects that a client with coronary artery disease (CAD) has been compliant with dietary teaching to decrease fat intake?

   a. "I have been limiting my fiber intake to 10 g/day and drinking more fluids."

   b. "I eat tuna once a week."

   c. "I use butter and partially hydrogenated cooking oils."

   d. "I eat chicken nuggets several times a week."

2. A client with chest pain is given nitroglycerin (NTG) 1/150 sublingual for complaint of angina pectoris. Prior to the NTG, his blood pressure was 110/78. After 5 minutes, he says the chest pain is better but not gone. The nurse's most immediate action is to:

   a. give another NTG.

   b. check the pulse rate.

   c. give morphine sulfate instead of NTG.

   d. check the blood pressure (BP).

3. Which breakfast option indicates to the nurse that the client with coronary artery disease requires further diet instruction?

   a. orange juice, shredded wheat, skim milk, toast with jelly

   b. grapefruit juice, oatmeal, 1% milk, bagel with jelly

   c. canned peaches, egg omelet, whole milk, fruited yogurt

   d. applesauce, bagel with margarine, egg-white omelet, skim milk

4. A male client is being discharged from the hospital following a short hospitalization for angina. He will be sent home on the drug propranolol hydrochloride (Inderal). Which of the following statements would indicate to the nurse that he understands the actions of the drug?

   a. "I will need to have laboratory tests done every month."

   b. "I will monitor my blood pressure before each dose of the drug."

   c. "I will need to take additional potassium supplements."

   d. "I will not discontinue the drug suddenly."

5. When evaluating the client who is taking sublingual nitroglycerin for coronary artery disease, which of the following client statements indicates an understanding of this medication?

   a. "I can expect to get a headache after I take this medication."

   b. "I should obtain relief from the chest pain in 15 to 20 minutes."

   c. "I need to take this medication several times a day for prevention."

   d. "I should keep a 1-year supply of this medication in the house for emergencies."

6. A 22-year-old female is admitted for treatment of supraventricular tachycardia. Which of the following medications may be ordered to try to treat this dysrhythmia?

   a. lidocaine

   b. bretylium

   c. epinephrine

   d. adenosine

7. The nurse would recognize that a client in atrial fibrillation has a decreased cardiac output when the client demonstrates:

   a. a difference between apical and radial pulse rates.

   b. increased blood pressure from his baseline.

   c. a difference between the right side and left side blood pressure.

   d. a decrease in respiratory rate from baseline.

8. The nurse is caring for a client who is in the immediate post procedure period following a cardiac catheterization. The client insists on getting up to go to the bathroom to urinate immediately when he is brought back to his room. Which of the following would be the nurse's best response?

   a. "You can't walk yet. You may be too weak after the procedure and may fall."

b. "If you bend your leg, you will risk bleeding from the insertion site. It is an artery, and it could lead to complications."

c. "If you get out of bed, you may have an arrhythmia from the catheterization. Your heart has to rest after this procedure."

d. "The doctor has ordered that you stay on bedrest for the next 6 hours. It is important that you follow these orders."

9. A client awakens with severe substernal chest pressure and dyspnea. He takes two nitroglycerin tablets without relief. In 5 minutes, he takes two more without relief. He calls his physician, who instructs him to go directly to the hospital. Understanding the rationale for the physician's instructions, the nurse knows that sudden death (outside the hospital) in association with coronary artery disease is most often due to:

a. acute myocardial infarction.

b. pump failure accompanied by pulmonary congestion.

c. arrhythmias.

d. papillary muscle dysfunction.

10. A goal for a client with chronic atrial fibrillation is to prevent clot formation and possible stroke. The nurse would anticipate which of the following medication orders to achieve this goal?

a. coumadin

b. vitamin K

c. heparin

d. erythropoietin

CHAPTER 30

NURSING CARE OF CLIENTS WITH CARDIAC DISORDERS

LEARNING OUTCOMES

After completing this chapter, you will be able to:

- Apply knowledge of normal cardiac anatomy and physiology and assessment techniques in caring for clients with cardiac disorders.
- Compare and contrast the pathophysiology and manifestations of common cardiac disorders, including heart failure, structural disorders, and inflammatory disorders.
- Identify common diagnostic tests used for cardiac disorders and their nursing implications.
- Discuss indications for and management of clients with hemodynamic monitoring.
- Discuss nursing implications for medications commonly prescribed for clients with cardiac disorders.
- Describe nursing care for the client undergoing cardiac surgery or cardiac transplant.
- Use the nursing process to provide individualized care for clients with cardiac disorders.
- Provide appropriate teaching and home care for clients with cardiac disorders and their families.

KEY TOPICS

- Assessment techniques of clients with cardiac disorders
- Pathophysiology of cardiac disorders
- Medical management of cardiac disorders
- Nursing care of clients with cardiac disorders
- Nursing care of clients undergoing cardiac surgery or cardiac transplantation

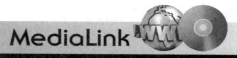

MediaLink

www.prenhall.com/lemone

Additional resources for this chapter can be found on the Student CD-ROM accompanying this textbook, and on the Companion Website at www.prenhall.com/lemone. Click on Chapter 30 to select the activities for this chapter.

CD-ROM
- Audio Glossary
- NCLEX Review

Animations
- Cardiac A&P
- Digoxin
- Dopamine

Companion Website
- More NCLEX Review
- Case Study
    Rheumatic Fever
- Care Plan Activity
    Acute Pulmonary Edema
- MediaLink Application
    Heart Failure

LECTURE OUTLINE

I. Care of client with heart failure
   A. Definition
      1. Inability of heart to pump sufficient blood to meet metabolic demands of body resulting in decreased tissue perfusion
      2. May be acute or chronic
      3. Common terminology used is Congestive Heart Failure (CHF)
      4. Leading causes are HPT and CHD
      5. Affects 5 million persons in U.S.; 6–10% of persons older than 65
   B. Etiology
      1. Impaired myocardial contraction
         a. CAD and myocardial infarction resulting in left ventricular damage
         b. Inflammatory conditions: cardiomyopathy, myocarditis
      2. Long-standing excessive workload
         a. Valvular disorders or congenital heart defects
         b. HPT
      3. Acute excess demands
         a. Volume overload
         b. Hyperthyroidism
         c. Massive pulmonary embolism
   C. Pathophysiology
      1. With heart failure, body responses by compensation
         a. Frank-Starling mechanism: Increased ventricular filling and myocardial stretch eventually results in ineffective contraction
         b. Activation of sympathetic nervous system and renin-angiotensin system
            1. Release of norepinephrine increases heart rate and contractility; arterial and venous vasoconstriction
            2. Decreased renal perfusion (blood is redistributed to maintain adequate circulation to brain and heart) activates renin release from kidneys
            3. Renin-angiotensin system results in salt and water retention; somewhat offset by atrial natriuretic factor (ANF)
         c. Myocardial hypertrophy
            1. Ventricular remodeling: chambers dilate to adapt to excess fluid volume
            2. Ventricular hypertrophy occurs as muscle cells enlarge
      2. Initially compensation improves cardiac output but long-term results in

deterioration of cardiac function and decompensation
      3. With heart function deterioration, decrease in tissue and heart perfusion leads to further weakening of heart, and cycle perpetuates
      4. The normal heart can adjust output to meet increased demands up to 5 times basic level; clients with heart failure have minimal to no cardiac reserve which results in activity intolerance
   D. Classifications of heart failure
      1. Systolic versus Diastolic Failure
         a. Systolic failure: ventricle fails to contract adequately to eject sufficient blood
            1. Due to loss of myocardial cells as with ischemia, infarction, cardiomyopathy, inflammation
            2. Results in decreased cardiac output: fatigue, decreased exercise tolerance
         b. Diastolic failure: heart cannot completely relax resulting in less than normal filling
            1. Due to decreased ventricular compliance
            2. Manifestations from increased pressure and congestion behind ventricle
               a. Left ventricle: shortness of breath, tachypnea, audible crackles
               b. Right ventricle: neck vein distension, liver enlargement, anorexia, nausea
               c. Often components of systolic and diastolic failure are present
      2. Left-sided versus right-sided failure
         a. Depending on cause, one ventricle may be primarily affected
            1. Left sided: results from CAD, HPT
            2. Right sided: results from restricted blood flow to lungs, as with acute or chronic pulmonary disease
            3. In chronic heart failure, both sides are involved
            4. Left sided failure can lead to right sided failure
         b. Manifestations of left-sided heart failure result from
            1. Decreased cardiac output: dizziness and syncope

2. Pulmonary congestion: dyspnea, shortness of breath, cough, orthopnea (difficulty breathing lying flat)
3. Assessment: cyanosis, breath sounds include crackles and wheezes, S_3
   c. Manifestations of right-sided heart failure result from
   1. Right sided heart distension: distended neck veins, peripheral tissue edema seen in dependent tissues: feet and legs or sacrum if client bedridden
   2. GI congestion: nausea and anorexia,
   3. Liver engorgement: RUQ pain
3. High-output versus low-output failure
   a. Occurs in situations requiring increased cardiac output, but heart is unable to meet increased oxygen demands
   b. Occurs with hypermetabolic states
   1. Hyperthyroidism
   2. Infection
   3. Anemia
   4. Pregnancy
4. Acute versus chronic failure
   a. Acute failure: Abrupt onset with sudden decrease cardiac function and decreased cardiac output, e.g., massive MI
   b. Chronic failure: Progressive deterioration of heart due to underlying condition, e.g., CHD
E. Manifestations (additional to those already listed with classifications)
   1. Related to increased salt and water retention
      a. Nocturia: voids more than once during night as fluid reabsorbed from dependent tissues when client is supine
      b. Paroxymal nocturnal dyspnea (PND): client awakens with acute shortness of breath that occurs when fluid is reabsorbed into circulation while client is supine
      c. Dyspnea at rest (little or no cardiac reserve)
      d. Audible S_3 and S_4
   2. Related to compensatory mechanisms
      a. Hepatomegaly and splenomegaly
      1. Ascites
      2. Impaired liver function: nausea, vomiting, anorexia

   b. Myocardial distention
      1. Dysrhythmias
      2. Pleural effusion
      3. Acute pulmonary edema
F. Collaborative Care
   1. Slow progression of heart failure
   2. Reduce cardiac workload
   3. Improve cardiac function
   4. Control fluid retention
G. Diagnostic Tests
   1. Diagnosis based on client history, physical examination and diagnostic findings
   2. Atrial natriuretic factor (ANF), atrial natriuretic hormone (ANH), B-type natriuretic peptide (BNP): hormones released by heart muscle in response to changes in blood volume; blood levels elevated with heart failure
   3. Serum electrolytes and osmolarity: monitoring of electrolytes to evaluate treatment; osmolarity may be decreased with fluid retention
   4. Urinalysis, BUN, Creatinine: renal function evaluation
   5. Liver function tests: effects of heart failure on liver function
   6. Arterial blood gases: evaluation of effectiveness of gas exchange
   7. Chest x-ray: show pulmonary vascular congestion, cardiomegaly
   8. Electrocardiography: changes associated with ventricular enlargement and dysrhythmias, ischemia, infarction
   9. Echocardiography with Doppler flow studies: evaluation of left ventricular function; blood flow across valves and great vessels
   10. Radionuclide imaging: evaluation of ventricular function and size
H. Hemodynamic monitoring
   1. Involves assessment of cardiovascular function in critically ill or unstable clients and response to interventions by studying forces involved in blood circulation
   2. Heart parameters
      a. Heart rate
      b. Arterial blood pressure
      c. Central venous pressure
      d. Pulmonary pressures
      e. Cardiac output
   3. Direct parameters are heart rate, arterial and venous pressures
   4. Indirect or derived measurements include cardiac index, mean arterial blood pressure (MAP), stroke volume

5. Consists of system which measures pressure within a vessel by use of a transducer which translates pressures into an electrical signal that is relayed to monitor
6. Complications associated with hemodynamic monitoring
   a. Infection
   b. Thrombosis from rupture of balloon or persistent wedging of Swan Ganz catheter
7. Types of monitoring
   a. Intra-arterial pressure monitoring
      1. Indwelling arterial line (art line, a line)
      2. Allows direct and continuous monitoring of systolic, diastolic and mean arterial blood pressure, easy access for arterial blood sampling
      3. Arterial blood pressure reflects cardiac output and resistance to flow by arterial walls (Systemic Vascular Resistance or SVR)
      4. Systolic blood pressure (normal 120 mm Hg): pressure generated during ventricular systole
      5. Diastolic blood pressure (normal 90 mm Hg): pressure within arteries to maintain blood flow through capillary beds
      6. Mean arterial blood pressure (desirable: 70–90 mm Hg)
         a. Formula: MAP = CO × SVR
         b. MAP ≤ 50: severely jeopardized perfusion to vital organs
         c. MAP > 105: indicates HPT or vasoconstriction
   b. Central venous pressure monitoring
      1. Measure of blood volume and venous return and reflects right heart filling pressures
      2. Used to monitor fluid volume status
      3. Catheter is inserted into the internal jugular or subclavian vein and distal end is positioned in the superior vena cava just above right atrium
      4. Measured in cm of water with manometer (normal: 2–8 cm) or mm Hg if connected to transducer (normal: 2–6 mm Hg)
      5. Decreased CVP: hypovolemia, shock
      6. Increased CVP: fluid overload, vasoconstriction, cardiac tamponade

   c. Pulmonary artery pressure monitoring
      1. Pulmonary artery (PA) catheter (Swan Ganz catheter) is flow-directed, balloon tipped catheter used to evaluate left ventricular and overall cardiac function
         a. Catheter inserted into central vein and threaded into right atrium
         b. Balloon inflated and drawn into right ventricle and into pulmonary artery
         c. Carried forward until wedges in a small branch of pulmonary vasculature
         d. Balloon deflated and multiple lumens of catheter allow for pressure readings in right atrium, pulmonary artery (PA), left ventricle
      2. Normal PA pressure: 25/10
         a. Mean is 15 mm Hg
         b. Elevated with left-sided heart failure
      3. Inflation of balloon blocks pressure from behind
         a. Allows measurement of pressure generated by left ventricle
         b. Pulmonary Artery Wedge Pressure (PAWP), which assesses left ventricular function
      4. Normal PAWP: 8–12 mm Hg
         a. Increased PAWP: left ventricular failure and pericardial tamponade
         b. Decreased PAWP: hypovolemia
      5. Cardiac output measurement
         a. Measured with PA catheter using thermodilution
         b. Cardiac index (calculation of cardiac output per square meter of body surface area) is calculated
         c. Normal cardiac index is 2.8–4.2 L/min/m^2

I. Medications used for clients with heart failure
   1. Action of Angiotensin-converting enzyme (ACE) inhibitors
      a. Block renin-angiotensin system activity, decrease cardiac work and increase cardiac output
      b. Reduce manifestations and progression of heart failure

2. Action of beta-blockers
   a. Prevents deleterious effects of sympathetic nervous system stimulation
   b. Used in low doses since reduce the force of myocardial contraction
3. Action of diuretics
   a. Relieve symptoms related to fluid retention
   b. May cause serious electrolyte imbalance and rapid fluid loss
   c. Types
      1. Loop diuretics: used with severe heart failure i.e., furosemide (Lasix), bumetanide (Bumex), torsemide (Demadex), Ethacrynic acid (Edecrin)
      2. Thiazide diuretics: used to treat less severe heart failure
4. Action of vasodilators
   a. Arterial dilation: reduces PVR and afterload
   b. Venous dilation: reduces venous return and preload
   c. Pulmonary vascular relaxation: allows reabsorption of fluid from interstitial tissues and alveoli
   d. Types
      1. Nitrates (intravenous sodium nitroprusside in treatment of acute heart failure)
      2. Hydralazine
      3. Prazosin (alpha-adrenergic blocker)
5. Action of inotropic medications
   a. Increases the strength of myocardial contraction by increasing intracellular calcium concentration
   b. Digitalis glycosides
      1. Decreases SA node automaticity and slows conduction through AV node, increasing ventricular filling time
      2. Has narrow therapeutic range, excreted through kidneys
      3. Digitalis toxicity
         a. Early manifestations: anorexia, nausea and vomiting, headache, altered vision, confusion
         b. Dysrhythmias: sinus arrest, supraventricular and ventricular tachycardia, high AV blocks
         c. Risk increased by hypokalemia, hypomagnesia, hypercalcemia, increased age

6. Action of anti-dysrhythmic medications
   a. PVC's with heart failure frequently left untreated
   b. Amiodarone is drug of choice for nonsustained ventricular tachycardia
J. Diet and Activity
   1. Sodium-restricted diet moderate at 1.5–2 gm of sodium
   2. Moderate, progressive activity program to improve myocardial function, but bed rest may be necessary during acute episodes
K. Heart Transplantation
   1. Currently only effective treatment for end-stage heart failure
   2. Survival rates: 80% at one year; 70% at five years
   3. Chief causes of mortality with transplants: infection and rejection
   4. Client treated with immunosuppressive drugs even with good match
   5. Donor heart is denervated and will not respond to position changes, stress, exercise, and some drugs
L. Other Surgical Procedures
   1. Cardiomyoplasty
   2. Ventricular reduction surgery
M. Complementary Therapies: Hawthorn and Coenzyme Q 10
N. End of Life Care
   1. Chronic heart failure usually a terminal disease
   2. Discussion regarding advance directives to prevent prolonged life support without reasonable expectation of functional recovery
   3. Hospice services including management of severe dyspnea with narcotic analgesics and intravenous diuretics and/or continuous infusion of inotropic agents
O. Nursing Care/Health Promotion
   1. Decreasing risk factors for CHD
   2. Screening and effective management of HPT and diabetes
P. Nursing Diagnoses
   1. Decreased Cardiac Output
   2. Fluid Volume Excess: monitoring daily weight: 1 liter of fluid = 1 kg or 2.2 lb of weight
   3. Activity Intolerance: providing nursing care and teaching client and family to function with frequent rest periods
   4. Knowledge Deficit regarding low sodium diet and medications

Q. Home Care: Education
   1. Regarding self monitoring for cardiac decompensation
   2. Regarding daily weights (notify physician if 2 pound gain in daily weight)
   3. Maintaining medications, diet, progressive exercise with rest periods, cardiac rehabilitation, continued medical care

II. Client with Pulmonary Edema
   A. Definition
      1. Abnormal accumulation of fluid in the interstitial tissue and alveoli of the lung
      2. Medical emergency with onset either gradual or acute
      3. Causes
         a. Cardiac
            1. Acute myocardial infarction
            2. Acute heart failure
            3. Valvular disease
         b. Non-cardiac causes
            1. Acute respiratory distress syndrome (ARDS)
            2. Trauma
            3. Sepsis
            4. Drug overdose or neurologic sequellae
   B. Pathophysiology
      1. Severe impairment of left ventricular contractility
      2. Ejection fraction falls with rise in end-diastolic volume and pressure
      3. Pulmonary pressure rises; fluid leaks from pulmonary capillaries into interstitial tissues, decreasing lung compliance and interfering with gas exchange
      4. Fluid enters alveoli disrupting ventilation and gas exchange
   C. Manifestations
      1. Dyspnea, shortness of breath, orthopnea
      2. Skin is cyanotic, cool, clammy, and diaphoretic
      3. Productive cough: pink, frothy sputum
      4. Audible crackles with lung sounds
      5. Mental changes: often restless and highly anxious, may be confused or lethargic
   D. Collaborative Care
      1. Restoration of effective gas exchange
      2. Reduction of fluid and pressure in pulmonary vascular system
      3. Intervention: Upright, sitting position with legs dependent
   E. Diagnostic Tests
      1. Arterial blood gases
      2. Continuous monitoring of oxygen saturation

      3. Chest x-ray
      4. Hemodynamic monitoring (PAWP often > 25 mm Hg)
   F. Medication and Treatment
      1. Medication: intravenous morphine to allay anxiety, improve breathing, to vasodilate, which reduces venous return and left atrial pressure
      2. Oxygen administration to achieve 100% oxygen concentration
      3. Continuous positive airway pressure (CPAP) with mask
      4. Intubation and mechanical ventilation
      5. Other medications
         a. Loop diuretics for rapid diuresis
         b. Vasodilators such as intravenous nitroprusside to reduce afterload and improve cardiac output
         c. Dopamine or dobutamine infusion or digoxin to improve myocardial contractility
         d. Intravenous aminophylline cautiously to reduce bronchospasm and decrease wheezing
   G. Nursing Care
      1. Improve oxygenation
      2. Reduce fluid volume
      3. Support emotionally
      4. Involves early recognition and initiation of treatment; emergent care is ABC (Airway, Breathing, Circulation)
   H. Nursing Diagnoses
      1. Impaired Gas Exchange: work of breathing is increased which leads to fatigue and decreased effort
      2. Decreased Cardiac Output
         a. When cardiogenic in nature, cause is acute decrease in myocardial contractility or increased workload for left ventricle
         b. Accurate intake and output with indwelling catheter
      3. Fear
   I. Home Care: Teaching related to cause, usually CHD or acute MI

III. Client with Rheumatic Fever and Rheumatic Heart Disease
   A. Definition
      1. Rheumatic fever is systemic inflammatory disease caused by immune response to pharyngeal infection by group A beta-hemolytic streptococci
      2. Rheumatic fever is self-limiting disorder usually occurring between 5–15 years of age

3. 10% persons with rheumatic fever develop rheumatic heart disease
4. Rheumatic heart disease damages heart valves and is major cause of mitral and aortic valve disorders
B. Pathophysiology
1. Rheumatic fever thought to result from abnormal immune response to M proteins or group A beta-hemolytic streptococcal bacteria
2. Immune response results in inflammation in connective tissues on heart, joints, and skin
   a. Carditis: in all layers of heart tissue in 50% persons with rheumatic fever
   b. Aschoff bodies are localized areas of tissue necrosis surrounded by immune cells develop in cardiac tissue
   c. Endocardial inflammation results in fibrous scarring of valve leaflets causing deformity
3. Rheumatic heart disease (RHD)
   a. Slowly progressive valvular deformity following acute or repeated episodes of rheumatic fever
   b. Usually affects valves on left side of heart especially mitral valve
      1. Stenosis of valve: narrowed fused valve obstructs forward blood flow
      2. Regurgitation occurs with incompetent valve (fails to close properly) and allows blood to flow back through it
C. Manifestations of rheumatic fever (2–3 weeks post strep infection)
1. Initially fever, migratory joint pain (knees, hips, ankles, elbows)
2. Erythema marginatum: temporary skin rash characterized by red circumscribed lesions with blanched centers on trunk and proximal extremities
3. Manifestations of carditis: chest pain, tachycardia, pericardial friction rub or manifestations of heart failure; may develop S_3, S_4 or murmur, cardiomegaly, pericardial effusion
D. Collaborative Care
1. Eradicating the streptococcal infection
2. Managing manifestations of disease
3. Limiting activities, generally
E. Diagnostic Tests
1. History and physical examination
2. CBC and erythrocyte sedimentation rate (ESR): WBC and ESR are elevated signifying the inflammatory process

3. C-reactive protein (CRP): positive for active inflammatory process
4. Antistreptolysin titer (ASO) titer: test for streptococcal antibodies; rises within 2 months of onset and is positive with rheumatic fever
5. Throat culture: positive for group A beta-hemolytic streptococcus in 25–40% of clients with acute rheumatic fever
F. Medications
1. Penicillin antibiotic of choice to treat infection; course of 10 days
2. If client allergic to penicillin, erythromycin or clindamycin prescribed
3. Prophylactic antibiotic therapy continued for 5–10 years to prevent recurrences (Penicillin G, 1.2 million units I.M. every 3–4 weeks prophylaxis of choice; oral antibiotics may be used)
4. Joint pain and fever treated with aspirin or other NSAID; corticosteroids may be used for severe pain with inflammation or carditis
G. Nursing Care/Health Promotion
1. Prompt identification and treatment of streptococcal throat infections
2. Understanding that full course of antibiotics should be completed
H. Nursing Diagnoses
1. Acute Pain
2. Activity Intolerance
   a. Activities are limited during acute phase of carditis to reduce workload of heart
   b. Gradual activity progression encouraged as condition improves
I. Home Care
1. Most clients recuperate at home and need teaching for acute care and prevention of recurrences
2. Client must complete full course of antibiotic therapy and continue antibiotic prophylaxis
3. Preventive dental care and good oral hygiene
4. Recognition of streptococcal sore throat and early manifestations of heart failure and seek medical attention
5. Follow prescribed activity and diet (usually high carbohydrate, high protein with possible sodium restriction)
IV. Client with Infective Endocarditis
A. Definition
1. Inflammation of endocardium, endothelial lining of heart

2. Usually affects valves with colonization by pathogen
B. Risk factors
 1. Previous heart damage such as deformed valves, valve prostheses, areas of heart damaged by congenital or ischemic disease (left-sided valves, especially mitral)
 2. Intravenous illicit drug use (right-sided valves usually affected)
 3. Invasive catheters (central venous lines, indwelling urinary catheters)
 4. Dental procedures, poor dental health
 5. Recent heart surgery
C. Classifications
 1. Acute infective endocarditis
  a. Abrupt onset, rapidly progressive severe disease
  b. *Staphylococcus aureus* most common infective organism
 2. Subacute infective endocarditis
  a. Gradual onset with systemic manifestation
  b. Occurs with preexisting heart disease
  c. Organisms include *Streptococcus viridans,* enterococci, yeasts, fungi
 3. Prosthetic valve endocarditis (PVE)
  a. Occurs in clients with mechanical or tissue valve replacement during early postoperative period (within 2 months after surgery)
  b. More frequently associated with aortic valve prostheses
  c. Early onset is usually due to contamination during surgery or preoperative bacteremia and has high mortality rate
  d. Late onset is similar to subacute endocarditis
D. Pathophysiology
 1. Pathogens enter bloodstream through dental work, invasive procedures and vegetation forms on damaged endothelium
 2. Organisms colonize the vegetations and become covered with platelets and fibrin
 3. Friable vegetations break off and embolize and travel through blood stream to other organ systems
 4. Emboli lodge in small vessels causing hemorrhages, infarcts, abscesses
 5. Vegetation scars and deforms valves and cause turbulent blood flow through the heart

E. Manifestations
 1. Temperature above 101.5° F. (39.4° C) with flulike symptoms (cough, shortness of breath, joint pain)
 2. Acute staphylococcal endocarditis may present with sudden onset of chills and high fever
 3. Heart murmurs occur (new or worsening)
 4. Embolic complications
  a. Splenomegaly with chronic disease
  b. Peripheral manifestations
   1. Petechiae
   2. Splinter hemorrhages (hemorrhagic streaks under finger or toenails)
   3. Osler's nodes: small, reddened painful raised growths on finger and toe pads
   4. Janeway lesions: small nontender purplish red macular lesions on palms of hands or soles of feet
   5. Roth's spots, small whitish spots seen on retina
 5. Complications include heart failure, organ infarction
F. Collaborative Care
 1. Eradication of the infected organism with antibiotics
 2. Minimizing valve damage and complications
G. Diagnostic Tests
 1. Blood cultures: considered positive if infecting organism is identified from 2 or more separate blood cultures (different sites, different times)
 2. Echocardiography: visualization of vegetations and evaluation of valve function
 3. Serologic immune testing: test for circulating antigens to infective organisms
H. Medications
 1. Antibiotic prophylaxis for pre-existing valve damage or heart disease prior to high risk procedures
 2. Infective endocarditis involves extended course of multiple intravenous antibiotics (2–8 weeks); repeat blood cultures
 3. Prosthetic valve endocarditis includes extended treatment (6–8 weeks) with combination of antibiotics
I. Surgery
 1. Surgery may be part of treatment
  a. To replace damaged valve
  b. To remove large vegetation
  c. To remove valve that is source of infection not responding to antibiotics and replace

2. Surgery usually indicated for clients with valvular regurgitation causing heart failure that does not respond to antibiotic therapy; also fungal endocarditis

J. Nursing Care/Health Promotion
1. Prevention, including education, against intravenous drug use
2. Preventive measures for clients with risk
3. Aseptic technique for all invasive procedures
4. Monitoring of central venous line sites for infection

K. Nursing Diagnoses
1. Risk for Imbalanced Body Temperature
2. Risk for Ineffective Tissue Perfusion
3. Ineffective Health Maintenance

L. Home Care: Teaching includes
1. Use of medications
2. Notifying health practitioners of need for prophylaxis with all invasive procedures
3. Dental care and hygiene
4. Maintaining follow-up with physician

V. Client with Myocarditis
A. Definition
1. Inflammation of heart muscle from infectious process, immunologic response to radiation, toxins, medications
2. In U.S. most myocarditis is viral due to coxsakie virus B
3. More common in clients with altered immunity
4. Viral myocarditis usually self-limiting, but can become chronic and lead to dilated cardiomyopathy

B. Pathophysiology
1. Myocardial cells damaged by inflammation and invading pathogens
2. Extent of damage determines outcome

C. Manifestations
1. Dependent on degree of myocardial damage
2. Range is from asymptomatic to heart failure
3. Non-specific: fever, fatigue, general malaise, dyspnea, palpitations, arthralgias (may be preceded by nonspecific febrile illness or upper respiratory infection)
4. Heart sounds: muffled S_1, S_3, murmur, pericardial friction rub
5. Manifestations of heart failure, chest pain

D. Collaborative Care: resolution of inflammatory process to prevent further damage

E. Diagnostic Tests
1. Electrocardiography: may show ST segment and T wave changes, dysrhythmias, possible heart block

2. Cardiac markers (Creatinine kinase, troponin T and I) may be elevated
3. Endomyocardial biopsy for definitive diagnosis

F. Treatment
1. Medications to eradicate infecting organism, including interferon-alpha for virus
2. Immunosuppressive therapy may be instituted with corticosteroids
3. Other medications may include: ACE inhibitors for heart failure; anti-dysrhythmic agents, if indicated; anticoagulants, to prevent emboli
4. Bedrest and restricted activity during the acute inflammatory process

G. Nursing Care: decreasing myocardial work and maintaining cardiac output

H. Nursing Diagnoses
1. Activity Intolerance
2. Decreased Cardiac Output
3. Fatigue
4. Anxiety
5. Fluid Volume Excess

I. Home Care: Teaching includes
1. Activity restriction
2. Recognition of early manifestations of heart failure
3. Medications, diet modifications
4. Continue follow-up with medical care

VI. Client with Pericarditis
A. Definition
1. Inflammation of pericardium
2. Types include acute, which is usually viral in nature
3. Can result from end-stage renal disease and uremia, post-MI, post-open heart surgery

B. Pathophysiology
1. Damage occurs to pericardial tissue leading to inflammation
2. Increased capillary permeability and plasma proteins seep into pericardial space forming exudate
3. Scar tissue or adhesions may form between pericardial layers
4. Chronic inflammation may cause pericardium to become rigid

C. Manifestations (acute)
1. Chest pain: aggravated by respiratory movement, changes in body position; sitting upright and leaning forward may reduce the pain
2. Pericardial friction rub: leathery grating sound produced by inflamed layers

rubbing together; heard most clearly at left lower sternal border with client sitting and leaning forward during expiration
3. Fever (low grade) with dyspnea and tachycardia
D. Complications
1. Pericardial effusion
a. Abnormal collection of fluid in pericardial space that threatens normal cardiac function
b. Fluid may be pus, blood, serum, lymph or combination
c. Rate at which effusion develops effects manifestations
1. Slow build up causes no immediate effects
2. Rapid buildup can compress heart interfering with myocardial function (tamponade)
d. May have distant or muffled heart sounds, cough, mild dyspnea
2. Cardiac tamponade
a. Medical emergency; rapid collection of fluid interferes with ventricular filling and pumping, reducing cardiac output
b. Manifestations
1. Paradoxical pulse (pulsus paradoxus): pulse has markedly decrease in amplitude during inspiration
2. Paradoxical pulse indicated by drop in systolic blood pressure of more than 10 mm HG during inspiration
3. Muffled heart sounds
4. Dyspnea and tachypnea
5. Narrowed pulse pressure
6. Distended neck veins
3. Chronic Constrictive Pericarditis
a. Scar tissue forms between pericardial layers and restricts heart movement and filling
b. May follow viral infection, radiation therapy, heart surgery
c. Manifestations
1. Dyspnea
2. Fatigue, weakness
3. Ascites
4. Neck vein distension during inspiration (Kussmaul's sign)
E. Collaborative Care
1. Identify cause
2. Reduce inflammation
3. Relieve symptoms
4. Prevent complications

F. Diagnostic Tests: to differentiate from myocardial infarction
1. CBC and ESR: Elevated WBC and ESR reflect acute inflammation
2. Cardiac enzymes: elevation is lower than as with MI
3. Electrocardiography: diffuse ST segment elevation in all leads which resolves more quickly than as with MI; Q waves and T wave changes associated with MI do not occur
4. Echocardiography: assesses heart motion, pericardial effusion and any restricted movement
5. Hemodynamic monitoring: assesses pressures and cardiac output
6. Chest x-ray: cardiac enlargement if pericardial effusion is present
7. CT scan or MRI to identify effusion or constrictive pericarditis
G. Medications
1. Aspirin or acetaminophen to reduce fever
2. NSAIDS for comfort
3. Corticosteroids for severe or recurrent pericarditis
H. Pericardiocentesis
1. Removal of fluid from pericardial sac for diagnostic or therapeutic purposes
2. Involves needle insertion into pericardial sac and withdrawal of fluid
3. Emergency procedure for cardiac tamponade
I. Surgery
1. Pericardial Window: excision of rectangular piece of pericardium to allow fluid to drain into pleural space with recurrent pericarditis or effusion
2. Partial or total pericardectomy with constrictive pericarditis
J. Nursing Care/Health Promotion: early identification and treatment
K. Nursing Diagnoses
1. Acute Pain
2. Ineffective Breathing Pattern
3. Risk for Decreased Cardiac Output
4. Activity Intolerance
L. Home Care: Education
1. Regarding anti-inflammatory medications
2. Activity restriction
3. Manifestations of recurrent pericarditis and seeking treatment
VII. Client with Valvular Heart Disease
A. Definition
1. Conditions which involve interference with blood flow to and from heart involving valves of heart

2. Include acquired valvular disorders resulting from acute conditions (infective endocarditis) and chronic conditions (rheumatic heart disease)
3. Causes of valvular heart disease
   a. Rheumatic heart disease: most common cause
   b. Damage from acute MI, which involves papillary muscles that affect valve leaf function
   c. Congenital heart disease: often manifests in adulthood
   d. Effects of aging: changes in heart structure and function
B. Pathophysiology
   1. Stenosis
      a. Valve leaflets fuse together and are unable to open or close completely
      b. Valve becomes scarred from endocarditis, infarction and calcium deposits form leading to stenosis
      c. Results in
         1. Impedance of forward flow of blood
         2. Decreased cardiac output from impaired ventricular filling, or ejection and stroke volume
   2. Regurgitation (also called insufficient or incompetent valves)
      a. Valves do not close completely allowing backflow of blood into area it just left
      b. Valve becomes incompetent due to deformity or erosion of valve cusps, as from endocarditis, myocardial infarction or cardiac dilation (enlargement), in which annulus supporting ring of valve is stretched and no longer allows complete closure
   3. Changes resulting from valvular disorders
      a. Blood volume and pressure are reduced in front of involved valve
      b. Blood volume and pressure are increased behind involved valve
      c. Higher pressures and compensatory changes to maintain cardiac output lead to remodeling and hypertrophy of heart muscle
      d. Eventually leads to pulmonary complications or heart failure
      e. Increased muscle mass and size can increase myocardial oxygen consumption that may lead to ischemia and chest pain

f. Murmur: results from interference with smooth blood flow through heart
g. Increased risk for infective endocarditis due to damage from jet stream effect as blood forced through defective valve into next chamber
C. Specific valvular disorders
   1. Mitral stenosis
      a. Narrowed mitral valve obstructing blood flow from left atrium to left ventricle during diastole
      b. Usually caused by rheumatic heart disease or bacterial endocarditis
      c. Chronic and progressive
      d. Untreated results in
         1. Left atrial hypertrophy with pressure reflected back and causing pulmonary hypertension
         2. Leading to right ventricular dilation and hypertrophy and heart failure
      e. Manifestations: asymptomatic or severely impaired
         1. Dyspnea on exertion (DOE): earliest manifestation
         2. Cough, hemoptysis, frequent pulmonary infections, paroxysmal nocturnal dyspnea, orthopnea, weakness, fatigue, palpitations
         3. Progresses to right heart failure: jugular vein distension, hepatomegaly, ascites, peripheral edema
         4. On auscultation of heart sounds: loud S_1, split S_2, mitral opening snap; diastolic murmur is low-pitched, rumbling, crescendo-decrescendo heard with bell in apical region
         5. Atrial dysrhythmias especially atrial fibrillation which may cause mural thrombi and then emboli to brain, coronary arteries, kidneys, spleen, extremities
         6. Women may be asymptomatic until pregnancy when heart is unable to adequately compensate for circulatory changes
   2. Mitral regurgitation (insufficiency)
      a. Mitral valve does not close fully and allows blood to flow back into left atrium during systole
      b. Causes include
         1. Rheumatic heart disease (common)
         2. Degenerative calcification of mitral annulus (older women)

3. Left ventricular hypertrophy and/or MI dilating the mitral annulus or supporting structures
4. Congenital defects
   c. Mitral incompetency leads to increased left atrial volume and then dilation of left atrium
   d. Manifestations
      1. Range from asymptomatic to left sided heart failure
      2. Fatigue, weakness, exertional dyspnea, orthopnea
      3. Behaviors of left-sided heart failure (pulmonary congestion, edema) and lead to right sided heart failure
      4. Murmur is loud, high-pitched, rumbling, holosystolic heard most clearly at apex, with palpable thrill; musical quality
3. Mitral valve prolapse
   a. Type of mitral insufficiency occurring when one or both mitral valve cusps billow into atrium during ventricular systole
   b. Most common in women aged 14–30
   c. Cause is often unclear; can result from rheumatic heart disease, ischemic heart disease, inherited connective tissue disorders such as Marfans
   d. Usually benign, but if thickened, mitral leaflets can cause morbidity and sudden death
   e. Manifestations
      1. Usually asymptomatic
      2. Midsystolic ejection click or murmur may be auscultated
      3. May develop high-pitched late systolic murmur with development of regurgitation of blood through valve
      4. Most common symptom: atypical chest pain: left sided or substernal pain related to fatigue, not exertion
      5. Tachydysrhythmias causing palpitations, lightheadedness, and syncope with sense of anxiety
   f. Complications
      1. Increases risk for bacterial endocarditis
      2. With regurgitation, development of heart failure
      3. Development of thrombi with embolization leading to transient ischemic attacks (TIAs)

4. Aortic stenosis
   a. Blood flow is obstructed from left ventricle into aorta during systole
   b. Causes include
      1. Idiopathic
      2. Congenital defect
      3. Rheumatic damage (often also has mitral valve disease)
      4. Degenerative disease (associated with aging)
   c. Valve annulus decreases in size, increasing work of left ventricle with left ventricle hypertrophy resulting in
      1. Myocardial ischemia (increased oxygen consumption, decreased coronary blood flow)
      2. Pulmonary vascular congestion and edema
   d. Manifestations
      1. May be asymptomatic for years
      2. Classic manifestations include
         a. Dyspnea on exertion
         b. Angina
         c. Syncope
      3. Narrow pulse pressure
      4. Harsh systolic crescendo-decrescendo murmur heard best in second intercostal space right of sternum with palpable thrill; may radiate to carotid arteries
   e. Untreated
      1. Pulmonary hypertension and right ventricular failure develop
      2. Increased risk for sudden cardiac death
5. Aortic Regurgitation (Aortic insufficiency)
   a. Allows blood to flow back into left ventricle from aorta during diastole
   b. Mostly results from rheumatic heart disease
   c. Other causes
      1. Congenital disorder
      2. Infective endocarditis
      3. Blunt chest trauma
      4. Aortic aneurysm
      5. Syphilis
      6. Marfan syndrome
      7. Chronic hypertension
   d. Leads to increased diastolic left ventricular pressure
   e. Manifestations
      1. May be asymptomatic for years
      2. Complaints of persistent palpitations; throbbing pulse visible in arteries of neck

3. May have characteristic head bob (Musset's sign) that shakes the whole body
4. Dizziness, exercise intolerance, angina, fatigue, paroxysmal nocturnal dyspnea
5. Murmur heard during diastole; "blowing" high-pitched; may have palpable thrill and ventricular heave
6. Wide pulse pressure, "water-hammer" pulse

6. Tricuspid valve disorders
   a. Tricuspid stenosis
      1. Blood flow is obstructed from right atrium to right ventricle
      2. Usually results from rheumatic heart disease and occurs with mitral stenosis
      3. Manifestations
         a. Increased jugular venous distention, ascites, hepatomegaly, peripheral edema
         b. Fatigue, weakness
         c. Murmur heard during diastole, low-pitched and rumbling heard in 4th intercostals space at left sternal border or xiphoid process
   b. Tricuspid regurgitation
      1. Blood flows back into right atrium during systole
      2. Results from right ventricular dilation as with left ventricular failure, pulmonary hypertension
      3. Manifestations
         a. As with right sided failure
         b. Atrial fibrillation
         c. Systolic murmur is high-pitched, blowing and heard over tricuspid or xiphoid area

7. Pulmonic valve disorders
   a. Pulmonic stenosis
      1. Obstruction of blood flow from right ventricle into pulmonary system
      2. Cause is usually congenital, but also can result from rheumatic heart disease or cancer
      3. Manifestations
         a. Asymptomatic, unless severe
         b. Dyspnea on exertion, fatigue progressing to right sided heart failure
         c. Murmur is harsh, crescendo-decrescendo heard in pulmonic area, second left intercostals space

   b. Pulmonic regurgitation
      1. Blood flows back into right ventricle during diastole decreasing blood flow into pulmonary circulation
      2. Results from pulmonary hypertension and also infective endocarditis, pulmonary artery aneurysm, syphilis
      3. Manifestations
         a. As with right side heart failure
         b. Murmur is diastolic, high-pitched, decrescendo and blowing best heard along left sternal border

D. Collaborative Care
   1. After diagnosis (usually murmur heard on physical exam)
      a. Close observation for progression of disease
      b. Prophylactic therapy (antibiotics before invasive procedures such as dental cleaning) to prevent infection
   2. Management of heart failure with diet and medications or surgical treatment

E. Diagnostic Tests
   1. Echocardiography: identifies valve leaflets abnormalities, myocardial function, chamber size
   2. Chest x-ray
      a. Identifies cardiac and blood vessel hypertrophy
      b. Identifies calcifications of valve leaflets and annular openings
   3. Electrocardiography
      a. Identifies atrial and ventricular hypertrophy
      b. Identifies associated conduction defects or dysrhythmias
   4. Cardiac catheterization
      a. Assessment of cardiac contractility
      b. Measure pressure gradients across heart valves, heart chambers, and within pulmonary system

F. Medications
   1. Heart failure resulting from valvular disease
      a. Diuretics
      b. ACE inhibitors
      c. Digitalis: increases force of myocardial contraction; controls ventricular response with atrial fibrillation
   2. Potential for clot and embolus formation from atrial fibrillation: Anticoagulants

3. Risk for infective bacteriocarditis: Antibiotic prophylaxis prior to dental work, invasive procedures, surgery

G. Percutaneous balloon valvuloplasty
1. Invasive procedure done in cardiac catheterization laboratory with balloon catheter under fluoroscopy
2. Procedure used to divide fused leaflets of valve and enlarge orifice of valve
3. Treatment of choice for symptomatic mitral stenosis
4. Used to treat aortic stenosis in children and young adults; "bridge to surgery" for older adults who are poor surgical risks
5. Post-procedural care similar to angioplasty

H. Surgery
1. Repair or replacement of diseased valve
2. Should be done before cardiopulmonary function is severely compromised
3. Repair done, if risk too great with valve replacement
4. Procedures
  a. Valvuloplasty: Reconstruction or repair of heart valve
    1. Open commissurotomy
    2. Annuloplasty
  b. Valve replacement
    1. Outcome determined by
      a. Heart function at time of surgery
      b. Intraoperative and postoperative care
      c. Characteristics and durability of replacement valve
    2. Increases risk of endocarditis, but incidence overall low
    3. Types of prosthetic heart valves
      a. Mechanical valves
        1. Advantage: Long term durability
        2. Disadvantage: Lifetime anticoagulation to prevent clot formation on valve
      b. Biological tissue valves
        1. Advantages: More normal blood flow and low risk of thrombus formation
        2. Disadvantages: Less durable than mechanical: 50% need replacement in 15 years
        3. Types
          a. Heterografts (pig, calf pericardium)
          b. Homografts (from human cadaver or during transplant)

4. Nursing care of client undergoing valve surgery is similar to care for clients having open-heart surgery (emphasis on adequate anticoagulation, prevention of endocarditis)

I. Health Promotion
1. Prevention of rheumatic heart disease through early and adequate treatment of strep throat (complete course of antibiotics)
2. Prophylactic antibiotic therapy before invasive procedures for clients with pre-existing heart disease

J. Nursing Diagnoses
1. Decreased Cardiac Output
2. Activity Intolerance: Monitor vital signs before and after activities
3. Risk for Infection
4. Ineffective Protection

K. Home Care
1. Client must be vigilant in self care and continuing medical follow-up
2. Education includes
  a. Adequate rest to prevent fatigue
  b. Diet management, medications
  c. Notify health practitioners about need for antibiotic prophylaxis before invasive procedures or dental work
  d. Report manifestations of heart failure, transient ischemic attacks, bleeding immediately to health care providers

VIII. Client with Cardiomyopathy
A. Definition
1. Disorders affecting heart muscle and systolic and diastolic functions
2. Origin
  a. Primary: idiopathic—cause unknown
  b. Secondary: result of other processes including
    1. Ischemia
    2. Infectious disease
    3. Exposure to toxins
    4. Connective tissue disorders
    5. Metabolic disorders
    6. Nutritional deficiencies
3. Mortality higher in older adults, men, and African Americans

B. Categories according to pathophysiology and presentation
1. Dilated cardiomyopathy
  a. Incidence
    1. Most common type (87% cases)
    2. Cause is often unknown but seems related to alcohol and cocaine

abuse, chemotherapeutic drugs, pregnancy, HPT; some cases are genetic
  b. Pathophysiology
     1. Heart chambers dilate and ventricular contraction is impaired
     2. Decreased cardiac output
     3. Extensive interstitial fibrosis (scarring)
  c. Manifestations (develop gradually)
     1. Same as associated with left- and right-sided heart failure
     2. S_3, S_4, AV regurgitation murmur
     3. Dysrhythmias are common: supraventricular tachycardias, atrial fibrillation, complex ventricular tachycardias
  d. Complications
     1. Sudden death (dysrhythmias)
     2. Mural thrombi (secondary to dysrhythmias)
  e. Outcome: Progressive worsening with 50% mortality within 5 years of diagnosis
2. Hypertropic cardiomyopathy
  a. Pathophysiology
     1. Decreased compliance of left ventricle and hypertrophy of ventricular muscle mass
     2. Impaired ventricular filling and low cardiac output
     3. Half of clients have family history
  b. Hypertrophic subaortic stenosis (IHSS): interventricular septal mass enlarges obstructing blood flow from ventricle through aorta
  c. Manifestations
     1. Asymptomatic for many years
     2. With increase in oxygen demand as with physical activity; sudden cardiac death in children, young adults (and some young athletes)
     3. Usual manifestations: dyspnea, angina, syncope
     4. Fatigue, dizziness, palpitations
     5. Harsh crescendo-decrescendo systolic murmur, S_4
3. Restrictive cardiomyopathy
  a. Ventricular walls become rigid and impair filling during diastole
  b. Causes include myocardial fibrosis and infiltrative processes
  c. Decrease in ventricular size occurs with decreased cardiac output
  d. Manifestations

     1. Those associated with heart failure and decreased tissue perfusion
     2. Exertional dyspnea, exercise intolerance
     3. Audible S_3 and S_4
C. Collaborative care
   1. Treatment of underlying cause, if known
   2. Management of heart failure and treatment of dysrhythmias
   3. Avoidance of strenuous activity, which may precipitate sudden cardiac death
D. Diagnostic Tests
   1. History and physical assessment
   2. Tests to rule out other known causes of heart failure
   3. Echocardiography
      a. Assessment of heart chamber size and thickness
      b. Ventricular wall motion
      c. Systolic and diastolic function
   4. Electrocardiography and ambulatory rhythm monitoring
      a. Detection of cardiac enlargement
      b. Detection of dysrhythmia
   5. Chest x-ray: Detection of cardiomegaly, pulmonary congestion or edema
   6. Hemodynamic studies: Assessment of cardiac output and pressures within heart
   7. Radionuclear scans to assess ventricular volume and mass, perfusion
   8. Cardiac catheterization and coronary angiography
   9. Myocardial biopsy to analyze cells regarding infiltration, fibrosis, inflammation
E. Medications
   1. Treatment for dilated and restrictive cardiomyopathy
      a. ACE inhibitors
      b. Vasodilators
      c. Digitalis
      d. Beta-blockers: used cautiously with dilated cardiomyopathy
      e. Anticoagulants: decrease risk of thrombus formation and embolization
      f. Antidysrhythmic medications cautiously since may precipitate other further dysrhythmias
   2. Treatment for hypertrophic cardiomyopathy
      a. Beta-blockers
         1. Reduce angina and syncopal episodes
         2. Decrease myocardial contractility and obstruction of outflow tract

3. Decrease heart rate and increase ventricular compliance
   b. Amiodarone: often used to treat ventricular dysrhythmias
F. Surgery
   1. Heart transplantation: only definitive treatment for dilated cardiomyopathy; not option for restrictive cardiomyopathy
   2. Excess muscle may be surgically resected in clients with obstructive hypertrophic cardiomyopathy
   3. Insertion of implantable cardioverter-defibrillator (ICD) to treat lethal dysrhythmias
G. Nursing care
   1. Education about disease process and management including
      a. Activity restriction for conservation of energy
      b. Coping skills and adaptation to changes in life-style

2. Support and education regarding cardiac transplantation
3. Abstinence from alcohol
4. Education about treatment and medication of heart failure
H. Nursing Diagnoses
   1. Decreased Cardiac Output
   2. Fatigue
   3. Ineffective Breathing Pattern
   4. Fear (related to risk of sudden death)
   5. Ineffective Role Performance
   6. Anticipatory Grieving
I. Home Care
   1. Clients have chronic disease and are managed in home and community settings with need for education about medications and heart failure management and continuing medical follow-up
   2. Clients and family needs may include support through cardiac transplantation, CPR training, hospice care

FOCUSED STUDY TIPS

- Care for a client in the clinical setting with the diagnosis of "heart failure." Read the client's medical record, especially the H & P (history and physical), medication record, laboratory results, and diagnostic procedure results. Determine if you are able to describe the client's diagnosis of "heart failure" more specifically after reading this information.
- Interview a client with a cardiac disorder. Describe differences in lifestyle before and after diagnosis.
- Observe hemodynamic monitoring in the clinical setting. Observe nursing management of these clients.

CASE STUDY

As part of case management protocol, you are asked to describe an "art line" or "A line" (arterial line) to a group of preoperative cardiac clients. Describe the purpose of the line and how it may be utilized. Describe advantages as well as disadvantages.

CARE PLAN CRITICAL THINKING ACTIVITY

Anticoagulant therapy is commonly prescribed for clients following valve replacement surgery. Develop a discharge teaching plan for a client receiving chronic anticoagulant therapy. Include descriptions of INR (International Normalized Ratio) and PT (prothrombin time) and reasons for close monitoring and adjustment of medications.

NCLEX TEST QUESTIONS

1. A 56-year-old client with a history of heart failure and hypertension is hospitalized following abdominal surgery. Vital signs have been stable and $D_5$1/2NS is infusing at 80 mL/hour. The client awakens in the middle of the night complaining of trouble breathing.

Which assessment by the nurse should take priority at this time?
   a. review intake and output record
   b. assess extremities for edema
   c. count apical heart rate
   d. auscultate lung fields

2. Which of the following findings most likely reflects edema related to inadequate heart pumping action?

   a. swollen feet and sacral area of an elderly client upon awakening in the morning

   b. swelling of legs and feet in a 45-year-old client after a 10-hour airplane flight

   c. ankle swelling in a 40-year-old waitress that resolves after sleeping all night

   d. swelling in the arm of a client who has had axillary lymph nodes removed

3. A 58-year-old client has been treated for fluid volume excess and mild pulmonary edema for 24 hours. Which of the following findings is most indicative of improvement in response to therapy?

   a. slightly decreased hematocrit (HCT) and blood urea nitrogen (BUN)

   b. no weight loss or gain in 24 hours

   c. jugular veins flat sitting at 45- and 90-degree angles

   d. pulse oximetry 92% on room air

4. Which of the following potassium levels would be of greatest concern in a client who is taking furosemide (Lasix)?

   a. 5.4 mEq/L

   b. 6.2 mEq/L

   c. 4.3 mEq/L

   d. 3.2 mEq/L

5. The client admitted with right-sided congestive heart failure is treated with diuretics, and his edema cleared quickly on the second day. On day 3, he has a relatively normal head-to-toe assessment at 8:00 A.M. Around 10:00 A.M., the client reports he is having trouble breathing, upon assessment, the nurse notes his respirations are 42 and labored. The nurse also notes that he has marked rales and rhonchi, an S_3 heart sound, and frothy pink sputum. The nurse suspects

   a. return of right-sided heart failure.

   b. development of mild left-sided heart failure.

   c. tamponade.

   d. pulmonary edema.

6. A client on the telemetry unit with a diagnosis of congestive heart failure and atrial fibrillation has an order for digoxin (Lanoxin). The client's pulse is 112 and irregular. The nurse should:

   a. give the dose as ordered.

   b. hold the dose and call the physician.

   c. call the physician immediately.

   d. give the dose and monitor vital signs every 15 minutes.

7. The signs of pacemaker malfunction that the nurse would include in discharge teaching for a client with a new pacemaker are:

   a. increased urine output, headache.

   b. regular, slow pulse.

   c. weakness, fatigue.

   d. disorientation, confusion.

8. The best position to facilitate breathing in a client with a diagnosis of pericarditis, would be to place her:

   a. in the prone position.

   b. onto her left side.

   c. in a low Fowler's position.

   d. in an upright position.

9. A client's demand pacemaker is programmed for a ventricular rate of 72. When the nurse takes the client's apical pulse, it is 84 and regular. The nursing action is to:

   a. report this finding immediately.

   b. obtain an electrocardiogram.

   c. place the client on bedrest.

   d. do nothing more at this time.

10. The nurse is caring for a client with a diagnosis of aortic stenosis. The client reports episodes of angina and states passing out recently at home. The client has scheduled surgery in 2 weeks. Which of the following would be the nurse's most appropriate instruction regarding activity at this time?

    a. "It is best to avoid strenuous exercise, stairs, or lifting."

    b. "Take short walks three times daily to prepare for postoperative rehabilitation."

    c. "There are no activity restrictions unless the angina reoccurs."

    d. "Gradually increase your activity while waiting for surgery."

CHAPTER 31

ASSESSING CLIENTS WITH PERIPHERAL VASCULAR AND LYMPHATIC DISORDERS

LEARNING OUTCOMES

After completing this chapter, you will be able to:

- Review the structures and functions of the arterial and venous networks of the peripheral vascular system and the lymphatic system.
- Describe the physiologic dynamics of blood flow, peripheral resistance, and blood pressure.
- Describe the major factors influencing arterial blood pressure.
- Identify interview questions pertinent to the assessment of the peripheral vascular and lymphatic systems.
- Describe physical assessment techniques for peripheral vascular and lymphatic function.
- Identify manifestations of impairment in the function of the peripheral vascular and lymphatic systems.

KEY TOPICS

- Review of anatomy and physiology of the peripheral vascular and lymphatic systems
- Assessing peripheral vascular and lymphatic functioning

LECTURE OUTLINE

I. Background of Anatomy and Physiology
  A. Peripheral vascular system
    1. Arterial network
      a. Aorta (blood contains oxygen and nutrients)
      b. Major arteries
      c. Smaller arteries
      d. Arterioles

MediaLink

www.prenhall.com/lemone

Additional resources for this chapter can be found on the Student CD-ROM accompanying this textbook, and on the Companion Website at www.prenhall.com/lemone. Click on Chapter 31 to select the activities for this chapter.

CD-ROM
- Audio Glossary
- NCLEX Review

Animations
- Lymphatic System
- The Immune Response

Companion Website
- More NCLEX Review
- Functional Health Pattern Assessment
- Case Study
    Arterial Blood Pressure

    e. Capillary beds: oxygen and nutrients are exchanged for metabolic waste products
    2. Venous network
      a. Capillary beds: oxygen and nutrients are exchanged for metabolic waste products
      b. Venules

      c. Small veins
      d. Large veins
      e. Superior and inferior vena cavae
        (return blood to right atrium)
  B. Structure of blood vessels: Most, except smallest vessels, have 3 layers
    1. Tunica intima
      a. Innermost layer composed of endothelium (squamous epithelium)
      b. Provides slick surface to facilitate blood flow
    2. Tunica media
      a. Middle layer composed of smooth muscle
      b. Thicker in arteries making arteries more elastic than veins
      c. Allows arteries to alternately expand and recoil as heart contracts and relaxes with each beat (felt as pulse)
      d. Arterioles are less elastic than arteries but contain more smooth muscle
        1. Allows for constriction and dilation
        2. Arterioles exert major control over arterial blood pressure
    3. Tunica adventitia
      a. Outermost layer composed of connective tissue which protects and anchors vessel
      b. Thicker in veins than arteries
  C. Veins
    1. Much lower blood pressure than in arteries
    2. Have thinner walls, larger lumen and greater capacity
    3. Have valves which help blood flow against gravity back to heart
      a. Muscular pump: "milking" action of skeletal muscle contraction
      b. Respiratory pump: changes in abdominal and thoracic pressures occur with breathing
  D. Capillaries
    1. Connects arterioles and venules
    2. Consists of only one thin layer of tunica intima
    3. Permeable to gases and molecules exchanged between blood and tissue cells
    4. Found in interwoven networks
    5. Filter and shunt blood from terminal arterioles to postcapillary venules
  E. Factors affecting Arterial Circulation
    1. Blood flow
      a. Volume of blood transported in vessel, organ or throughout entire circulation in a given period of time

      b. Expressed in liters or milliliters per minute or cubic centimeters per second
    2. Peripheral vascular resistance (PVR)
      a. Opposing forces or impedance to blood flow as arterial channels are more distant from heart
      b. Determined by 3 factors
        1. Blood viscosity: thickness of blood; greater viscosity the greater resistance to moving and flowing
        2. Length of vessel: longer the vessel, the greater the resistance to blood flow
        3. Diameter of vessel: smaller the diameter of vessel, the greater the friction against the walls of the vessel and greater impedance to blood flow
    3. Blood pressure
      a. Force exerted against the walls of arteries by blood as it is pumped from heart (mean arterial pressure—MAP)
        1. Highest pressure: peak of ventricular contraction or systole (systolic blood pressure)
        2. Lowest pressure: exerted during ventricular relaxation (diastolic blood pressure)
      b. Mean arterial pressure (MAP): calculated by formula
MAP = CO (cardiac output) × PVR
      c. Estimated clinical calculation of MAP: diastolic blood pressure plus 1/3 of pulse pressure (difference between systolic and diastolic blood pressures)
      d. Other factors regulating blood pressure
        1. Sympathetic and parasympathetic nervous systems
          a. Sympathetic stimulation: vasoconstriction of arterioles, increasing blood pressure
          b. Parasympathetic stimulation: vasodilation of arterioles, lowering blood pressure
          c. Baroreceptors and chemoreceptors in aortic arch, carotid sinus and other large vessels: sensitive to pressure and chemical changes causing reflex sympathetic stimulation
            1. Vasoconstriction
            2. Increased heart rate and blood pressure
        2. Action of kidneys to excrete or conserve sodium and water

a. Kidneys initiate renin-angiotensin mechanism in response to decrease in blood pressure
   1. Release of aldosterone from adrenal cortex
   2. Sodium ion reabsorption and water retention
b. Kidneys reabsorb water in response to pituitary release of antidiuretic hormone
c. Increase in blood volume and therefore increase in cardiac output and blood pressure
3. Temperature
   a. Cold causes vasoconstriction
   b. Warmth causes vasodilation
4. Chemicals, hormones, drugs
   a. Vasoconstriction
      1. Epinephrine
      2. Endothelin (chemical released by blood vessel inner lining)
      3. Nicotine
   b. Vasodilation
      1. Prostaglandins
      2. Alcohol and histamine
5. Dietary Factors: including salt, saturated fats, cholesterol
6. Other factors: race, gender, age, weight, time of day, position, exercise and emotional state

F. Lymphatic System
1. Composed of lymphatic vessels and lymphoid organs
   a. Lymphatics form network around arterial and venous channels and interweave at capillary beds
   b. Lymph (tissue fluid) leaks from cardiovascular system and accumulates at end of capillary bed
   c. Fluid returned to heart through lymphatic veins and venules that drain into right lymphatic duct and left thoracic duct which empty into subclavian veins
   d. Low pressure system that depends on rhythmic contraction of smooth muscle and muscular and respiratory pumps
2. Organs of lymphatic system
   a. Lymph nodes
      1. Special cells of immune system that remove foreign material, infectious organism, tumor cells from lymph

      2. Distributed along lymphatic vessels forming clusters in regions of neck, axilla, groin
   b. Spleen
      1. Filters blood by breaking down old red blood cells; stores or releases to liver by-products such as iron
      2. Synthesizes lymphocytes
      3. Stores platelets for blood clotting
      4. Serves as reservoir for blood
   c. Thymus: active in childhood and produces hormones facilitating the immune action of lymphocytes
   d. Tonsils: protect upper respiratory tract
   e. Peyer's patches of small intestine: protect digestive tract

II. Assessing Peripheral Vascular and Lymphatic Function
A. Assessment of Peripheral Vascular System
1. Health assessment interview to collect subjective data
   a. Client's chief complaint
   b. Description of client's symptom regarding
      1. Onset
      2. Characteristics and course
      3. Severity
      4. Precipitating and relieving factors
      5. Associated symptoms (noting timing and circumstances)
   c. Client's medical and family history for cardiovascular disorders or chronic illness, such as diabetes
   d. Past surgery of heart or blood vessels, tests results that evaluate function, such as cardiac catheterization, angiography of lower extremities, medications affecting circulation or blood pressure
   e. Review of symptoms
      1. Pain, burning, numbness, tingling in limbs or digits
      2. Leg fatigue or cramps
      3. Changes in skin color or temperature
      4. Texture of hair
      5. Ulcerations or skin irritations
      6. Varicose veins, phlebitis, or swelling
   f. Review of nutritional history: intake of protein, vitamins, minerals, salt, fat, fluid
   g. Consumption of caffeine, alcohol, history of smoking (packs/years) and other types of tobacco

h. Client's activity level for exercise habits and tolerance

i. Socioeconomic factors and occupational factors

j. Psychosocial factors including stress level and emotional state

2. Physical assessment of peripheral vascular system

a. Blood pressure and pulse pressure assessment with abnormal findings

1. Auscultate blood pressure in each arm with client seated

a. Hypertension (HTN): readings over 140/90 under age 40

b. Hypotension: readings under 90/60

c. Ausculatory gap (temporary disappearance of sound between systolic and diastolic BP); may be normal, or associated with HTN or drop diastolic BP due to aortic stenosis

d. Korotkoff's sounds may be heard down to zero with cardiac valve replacements, hyperkinetic states, thyrotoxicosis, severe anemia, after vigorous exercise

e. Sounds of aortic regurgitation may obscure diastolic BP

f. Difference > 10 mm Hg between arms suggests arterial compression on side of lower BP reading, aortic dissection, coarctation of aorta

g. Orthostatic hypotension: decrease in systolic BP 10–15 mm Hg from sitting to standing due to antihypertensive medications, volume depletion, peripheral neurovascular disease, prolonged bed rest, aging

2. Pulse pressure: difference between systolic and diastolic BP's; normally one-third the systolic measurement

a. Widened with elevated systolic BP: occurs with exercise, arteriosclerosis, severe anemia, thyrotoxicosis, increased intracranial pressure

b. Narrowed with decreased systolic BP: occurs with shock, cardiac failure, pulmonary embolus

b. Skin assessment with abnormal findings

1. Pallor: reflects constriction of peripheral blood flow (as with shock, syncope) or decreased circulating oxyhemoglobin (as with anemia)

2. Central cyanosis of lips, earlobes, oral mucosa, tongue as with chronic cardiopulmonary disease

c. Artery and vein assessment with abnormal findings

1. Redness, swelling, nodularity over temporal arteries and variations in temporal artery pulses may occur with temporal arteritis

2. Carotid artery abnormalities

a. Unilateral pulsating bulge: tortuous or kinked carotid artery

b. Alterations in pulse rate or rhythm: cardiac dysrhythmias

c. Absent pulse: arterial occlusion

d. Weak, hypokinetic pulse: decreased stroke volume as with congestive heart failure, aortic stenosis, hypovolemia; increased peripheral resistance as with cold temperatures, arterial narrowing as with atherosclerosis

e. Hyperkinetic (bounding) pulse: increased stroke volume or decreased peripheral resistance as with high cardiac output, aortic regurgitation, anemia, hyperthyroidism, bradycardia; reduced compliance as with atherosclerosis

f. Bigeminal pulse (decreased amplitude every other beat): premature contractions (usually ventricular)

g. Pulsus alternans: regular pulse with alternating strong and weak beats as with left ventricular failure and severe HTN

h. Water-hammer pulse (collapsing pulse): greater than normal amplitude with sharp rise and fall as with aortic insufficiency

i. Pulsus bisferiens ("double beat"): combined aortic stenosis and regurgitation, pericardial effusion, constrictive pericarditis

j. Pulsus paradoxus (pulse in which amplitude is diminished or absent during inspiration and exaggerated during expiration): cardiac tamponade, constrictive pericarditis, severe chronic lung disease

k. Palpable thrill: suggests arterial narrowing as with atherosclerosis

l. Murmuring or blowing sound (bruit) heart over blood vessel suggests atherosclerosis

3. Jugular vein assessment with abnormal findings

a. Increase in jugular venous pressure > 3 cm and above sternal angle reflects right atrial pressure: right ventricular failure, constrictive pericarditis, tricuspid stenosis, superior venae caval obstruction

b. Decrease in venous pressure: reduced left ventricular output or blood volume

c. Unilateral neck vein distention: local compression or anatomic anomaly

d. Rise in column of neck vein distention over 1 cm with liver compression: right heart failure

4. Upper extremity assessment with abnormal findings

a. Unilateral swelling with venous prominence: venous obstruction

b. Extreme localized pallor of fingers: Raynaud's disease

c. Cyanosis of nailbeds: chronic cardiopulmonary disease

d. Cold temperature of hands and fingers: vasoconstriction

e. Delayed capillary refill: reflects circulatory compromise as with hypovolemia, anemia

f. Distended hand veins at elevations over 9 cm above heart level: increase in systemic venous pressure

g. Altered pulse rate or rhythm: cardiac dysrhythmias

h. Pulse deficit: dysrhythmias and CHF

i. Diminished or absent radial pulses: acute arterial occlusion or thromboangitis obliterans (Buerger's disease)

j. Weak, thready pulse: tachycardia (decreased cardiac output)

k. Bounding pulse: hyperkinetic states and atherosclerosis

l. Unequal pulses between extremities: arterial narrowing or obstruction on one side

m. Pulse rate increases with inspiration and decreases with expiration: as with sinus dysrhythmia

n. Persistent pallor with Allen's test: suggests ulnar artery occlusion

5. Lower extremity assessment with abnormal findings

a. Signs of arterial insufficiency

1. Diminished or absent pulses

2. Pallor, dependent rubor (dusky redness)

3. Cool to cold temperature

4. Atrophic changes: loss of hair growth, shiny and smooth skin, thickened nails, sensory loss, slowed capillary refill, muscle atrophy

5. Ulcers with symmetric margins, deep base, necrotic tissue with absence of bleeding over pressure points, on toes, heels, lateral malleolar or tibial area, side or sole of foot, metatarsal heads

6. Pregangrenous color changes: deep cyanosis and purple-black discoloration

7. Gangrene: black, dry, hard skin

b. Signs of venous insufficiency

1. Swelling

2. Thickened skin

3. Cyanosis

4. Stasis dermatitis: brown pigmentation, erythema, scaling

5. Superficial ankle ulcers often located at medial malleolus with uneven margins, ruddy granulation tissue, bleeding

6. Presence of varicose veins: dilated, tortuous, thickened veins more prominent in dependent position

c. Increased and widened femoral and popliteal pulsations suggest aneurysm

d. Absence of posterior tibial pulse with signs of arterial insufficiency often due to acute occlusion due to thrombus or embolus

e. Diminished or absent pedal pulses often due to popliteal occlusion associated with diabetes mellitus

f. Postural color changes suggest arterial insufficiency

g. Presence of femoral bruit: suggest arterial narrowing as with arteriosclerosis

h. Thrombophlebitis or deep vein thrombosis (DVT): redness, warmth, swelling, tenderness, cords along a superficial vein

i. Presence of edema occurs with
   1. Cardiovascular system disease (CHF), renal, hepatic, or lymphatic problems, infection
   2. DVT (lower leg or ankle edema)
   3. Iliofemoral thrombosis (entire leg edema)

6. Abdominal assessment with abnormal findings
   a. Pulsating mass in upper abdomen suggests aortic aneurysm especially in older adult
   b. Bruits
      1. Abdominal: partial arterial occlusion
      2. Over aorta: aneurysm
      3. Over epigastrium and radiating laterally suggests renal artery stenosis
      4. Lower abdominal quadrants suggests partial occlusion of iliac arteries

B. Assessment of Lymphatic System
   1. Health assessment interview to collect subjective data
      a. Review of specific lymphatic findings: lymph node enlargement, infection or impaired immunity (fever, fatigue, weight loss)
      b. Description of client's health problem regarding
         1. Onset
         2. Characteristics
         3. Severity
         4. Precipitating and relieving factors

5. Associated symptoms (noting timing and circumstances)

c. Explore client's history for
   1. Chronic illnesses: Cardiovascular or renal disease, cancer, tuberculosis, HIV infection
   2. Predisposing factors: Surgery, trauma, infection, blood transfusions, intravenous drug use
   3. Environmental exposure: Radiation, toxic chemicals, travel-related infectious diseases

d. Family history: Cancer, anemia, blood dyscrasias

e. Past or present bleeding: From nose, gums, mouth; vomiting, from rectum, areas of bruising

f. Associated symptoms: Pallor, dizziness, fatigue, difficulty breathing

g. Lymph node changes: Enlargement, pain or tenderness, itching, warmth

h. Swelling of extremities

i. Recurrent irritations or infections

j. Socioeconomic status, life-style, intravenous drug use, sexual practices

2. Physical assessment of lymphatic system: Assessment usually integrated into assessment of other body systems
   a. Skin over regional lymph nodes, noting any edema, erythema, red streaks, skin lesions
      1. Lymphangitis (inflammation of lymph vessel): red streak with hardness following course of lymphatic collecting duct
      2. Lymphedema (swelling due to lymphatic obstruction) as with congenital lymphatic anomaly, trauma to area as with surgery (arm lymphedema after radical mastectomy) or metastasis
   b. Lymph node assessment
      1. Lymphadenopathy: enlargement over 1 cm with or without tenderness indicates inflammation, infection, or malignancy of nodes or region drained by nodes
      2. Lymphadenitis (inflammation): enlargement with tenderness; bacterial infection may cause warm and localized swelling
      3. Malignant or metastatic nodes: hard as with lymphoma, rubbery as with Hodgkin's disease, fixed to adjacent structures; usually non-tender

4. Specific areas of lymph node enlargement
   a. Preauricular and cervical nodes: ear infections, scalp and face lesions
   b. Anterior cervical nodes: streptococcal pharyngitis or mononucleosis
   c. Occipital nodes: can occur with brain tumors
   d. Supraclavicular nodes, especially on left: suggestive of metastatic disease
   e. Axillary nodes: associated with breast cancer
   f. Inguinal nodes: lesions of genitals
5. Persistent generalized lymphadenopathy: associated AIDS and AIDS-related complex (ARC)
   c. Spleen assessment with abnormal findings: Splenic enlargement may be associated with cancer, blood dyscrasias, viral infection such as mononucleosis

FOCUSED STUDY TIPS

- Trace throughout the venous system of the body a drop of normal saline injected into an antecubital vein. Identify major veins the drop travels through. Reflect on this routing when learning to administer IV (intravenous) medications.
- Practice assessing the lymphatic system with classmates in the skills lab. Identify lymph nodes. Compare and contrast assessment findings. Practice documenting assessment findings.
- Trace a drop of blood through the arterial system of the body. Name every major artery through which the blood travels. Identify organs each artery supplies.

CASE STUDY

Arterial insufficiency of the upper extremities is suspected in R. J., a client for whom you have been assigned care. An Allen test is indicated. How do you explain the test to R. J.? Describe how you will administer the test. Indicate normal and abnormal findings that might result from this test.

CARE PLAN CRITICAL THINKING ACTIVITY

When assessing a client with suspected lymphatic disorder, describe how you would carry out a physical assessment of the client. What areas of the body would you inspect and palpate? What added equipment might be useful and why?

NCLEX TEST QUESTIONS

1. In the process of a physical examination of an adult client with a possible diagnosis of hypertension, the nurse should gather data through the use of which method?
   a. blood pressure from one arm only
   b. orthostatic blood pressure with 2 minutes between each reading
   c. blood pressure from both arms taken 5 minutes apart
   d. cuff and doppler blood pressure in both arms
2. The nurse should discuss which of the following as nonmodifiable risk factors influencing hypertension?
   a. ethnicity and stress
   b. obesity and substance abuse
   c. nutrition and occupation
   d. family history and gender
3. An elderly gentleman enters the emergency department with complaints of back pain and feeling fatigued. Upon examination, his blood pressure is 200/110, pulse is 120, and hematocrit and hemoglobin are both low. The nurse palpates the abdomen which is soft, nontender, and auscultates an abdominal pulse. The most likely diagnosis is:
   a. secondary hypertension.
   b. aneurysm.

c. congestive heart failure (CHF).

d. Buerger's disease.

4. Assessment of a client to detect the presence of a deep vein thrombosis is done by pulling up on the toes while gently holding down on the knee. The client complains of extreme pain in the calf. This should be documented as a

a. positive tourniquet test.

b. positive Homan's sign.

c. negative Homan's sign.

d. negative tourniquet test.

5. The nursing management of Raynaud's disease has as its highest priority to:

a. provide rest during the periods of intermittent claudication.

b. provide opioid analgesics for pain.

c. keep the client's hands and feet warm and injury-free.

d. teach the client stress management.

6. To assess the peripheral pulses of a client's lower extremities, which of the following areas would the nurse palpate?

a. the dorsalis pedis, posterior tibial, and brachial

b. the radial, femoral, and popliteal

c. the ulnar, brachial, and radial

d. the popliteal, dorsalis pedis, and posterior tibial

7. A male client complaining of pain when he tries to walk in order to exercise three times a week is seen in the clinic. Upon examination, his feet are noted to be dusky and purplish while dangling from the stretcher. The pedal pulse is palpable but diminished, and he states his feet "tingle on occasion." The nurse has him lie supine on the stretcher with the foot of the stretcher elevated for about 30 minutes, after which his feet show pallor. The client is probably suffering from:

a. varicose veins.

b. thrombophlebitis.

c. Raynaud's disease.

d. peripheral vascular disease (PVD).

8. When assessing a client, the nurse determines capillary refill time to be 7 seconds. The nurse determines the client may be experiencing:

a. normal signs of aging.

b. impending stroke.

c. decreased cardiac output.

d. hypokalemia.

9. When assessing a client with peripheral arterial disease, the nurse anticipates signs and symptoms of ischemia, which include:

a. warm, pink extremities.

b. increased pulse pressure.

c. intermittent claudication.

d. bounding pulse.

10. Which of the following is the nurse likely to assess in a client with varicose veins of the lower extremity?

a. dry, necrotic ulcers on the feet

b. veins that become more prominent when the leg is in a dependent position

c. decreased or diminished peripheral pulses

d. extensive pallor when the leg is elevated

CHAPTER 32

NURSING CARE OF CLIENTS WITH HEMATOLOGIC DISORDERS

LEARNING OUTCOMES

After completing this chapter, you will be able to:

- Relate the physiology and assessment of the hematologic system and related systems (see Chapter 31) to commonly occurring hematologic disorders.
- Describe the pathophysiology of common hematologic disorders.
- Identify diagnostic tests commonly used for hematologic disorders.
- Discuss nursing implications for medications prescribed for hematologic disorders.
- Discuss nursing implications for bone marrow transplantation, chemotherapy, and radiation for hematologic disorders.
- Compare and contrast bleeding disorders.
- Describe the major types of leukemia and the most common treatment modalities and nursing interventions.
- Differentiate Hodgkin's disease from non-Hodgkin's lymphomas.
- Use the nursing process to provide individualized care to clients with hematologic disorders.

KEY TOPICS

- Pathophysiology of hematological disorders
- Medical management of hematological disorders
- Nursing care of clients experiencing hematological disorders

LECTURE OUTLINE

I. Hematopoietic (blood-forming) system
    A. Composition
        1. Bone marrow (myeloid) tissues where blood cells are formed

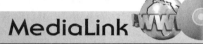

MediaLink

www.prenhall.com/lemone

Additional resources for this chapter can be found on the Student CD-ROM accompanying this textbook, and on the Companion Website at www.prenhall.com/lemone. Click on Chapter 32 to select the activities for this chapter.

CD-ROM
- Audio Glossary
- NCLEX Review

Animations
- Sickle Cell Anemia

Companion Website
- More NCLEX Review
- Case Study
    Immune Thrombocytopenic Purpura
- Care Plan Activity
    Acute Myelocytic Leukemia
- Media Link Applications
    Stem Cell Transplant
    Sickle Cell Anemia

        2. Lymphoid tissue of lymph nodes where white blood cells mature and circulate
    B. Stem cells (hemocytoblasts)
        1. Cells in bone marrow from which all blood cells originate

2. Differentiate into parent cells which give rise to RBCs, WBC's, platelets

II. Red blood cell disorders

A. Physiology Background

1. Erythrocyte (red blood cell or RBC): biconcave disk that increases surface area and allows cell to pass through small capillaries

2. Contains hemoglobin which is oxygen-carrying protein which allows transport of oxygen as oxyhemoglobin to cells

3. Erythropoiesis (RBC production) begins in red bone marrow of vertebrae, sternum, ribs, pelvis and is completed in the blood or spleen

4. Erythroblasts begin forming hemoglobin while still in bone marrow; differentiate into normoblasts that have no nucleus and assume biconcave shape

5. Cells enter circulation as reticulocytes which fully mature in 48 hours

6. Sequence from stem cells to RBC takes 3–5 days

7. Stimulus for RBC production is tissue hypoxia

   a. Hormone, erythropoietin, is released by kidneys in response to hypoxia

   b. Erythropoietin stimulates bone marrow to produce RBCs

8. Increased percentage of reticulocytes over mature cells occurs during periods of increased RBC production

9. Life span of RBC is 120 days; old or damaged RBCs are lysed by phagocytes in spleen, liver, bone marrow, lymph nodes; process is called hemolysis

10. Most of iron from heme units is converted to bilirubin

    a. Orange-yellow pigment removed from blood by liver and excreted in bile

    b. Jaundice occurs with increased hemolysis or impaired liver function

B. Client with Anemia

1. Definition

   a. Abnormally low number of circulating RBCs, hemoglobin concentration or both

   b. Usual cause of decrease
      1. Blood loss
      2. Inadequate production
      3. Increased RBC destruction

   c. Insufficient or defective hemoglobin contributes to anemia

   d. Depending on severity, anemia affects all major organ systems

2. Pathophysiology

   a. Altered hemoglobin synthesis such as iron deficiency

   b. Altered DNA synthesis such as Vitamin B_{12} or folic acid deficiency

   c. Bone marrow failure such as aplastic anemia (stem cell dysfunction)

   d. Increased RBC loss or destruction
      1. Acute or chronic blood loss
      2. Increased hemolysis such as sickle cell anemia, infection

3. Manifestations

   a. Pallor of skin, mucous membranes, conjunctiva, nail beds

   b. Increased heart and respiratory rates as body compensates

   c. Angina, fatigue, dyspnea on exertion, night cramps

   d. Increased erythropoietin activity may cause bone pain

   e. Cerebral hypoxia: headache, dizziness, dim vision

   f. Heart failure with severe anemia

   g. Signs of circulatory shock with rapid blood loss

   h. Systolic heart murmur with chronic blood loss due to decreased viscosity of blood

4. Categories of Anemia

   a. Blood loss anemia
      1. Acute blood loss
         a. Circulating blood volume decreases and fluid shifts from interstitial space into vascular bed
         b. Circulating RBCs are of normal size and shape; hemoglobin and hematocrit are reduced
      2. Chronic blood loss
         a. Depletion of iron stores as RBC production attempts to maintain supply
         b. RBCs are microcytic (small) and hypochromic (pale)

   b. Nutritional anemias
      1. Affect RBC formation or hemoglobin synthesis
      2. Causes include inadequate diet, malabsorption, increased nutrition need
      3. Common types
         a. Iron deficiency anemia
         b. Vitamin B_{12} anemia
         c. Folic acid deficiency anemia
      4. Megaloblastic anemias (enlarged nucleated RBCs) occur with

Vitamin B$_{12}$ anemia and folic acid deficiency anemia
  c. Iron deficiency anemia
    1. Most common type of anemia
    2. With inadequate supply of iron; body cannot synthesize hemoglobin
    3. Fewer number of RBCs which are microcytic, hypochromic and malformed (poikilocytosis)
    4. Due to inadequate dietary iron intake, malabsorption, increased iron needs as with pregnancy and lactation
    5. Due to chronic bleeding
      a. Menstrual blood loss
      b. Chronic occult (hidden) blood loss in older adults: slowly bleeding ulcers, GI inflammation, hemorrhoids, cancer
    6. Additional manifestations
      a. Brittle, spoon-shaped nails
      b. Cheilosis (cracks at corners of mouth)
      c. Smooth sore tongue
      d. Pica (craving for unusual substances such as clay, starch)
  d. Vitamin B$_{12}$ deficiency anemia
    1. Vitamin B$_{12}$ necessary for DNA synthesis
    2. Food sources of Vitamin B$_{12}$ occur in foods derived from animals
    3. RBCs
      a. Macrocytic (large) misshapened (oval) with thin membranes
      b. Fragile, have shortened life span
      c. Do not carry adequate oxygen
    4. Pernicious anemia
      a. Failure to absorb dietary Vitamin B$_{12}$ due to lack of intrinsic factor which is secreted by gastric mucosa
      b. Intrinsic factor binds with Vitamin B$_{12}$ and is absorbed in ileum
      c. Occurs in clients who have stomach or ileal resections, loss of pancreatic secretions, chronic gastritis
      d. Strict vegetarians
    5. Manifestations: gradual onset
      a. Pallor, slight jaundice
      b. Sore beefy red tongue and diarrhea
      c. Impaired neurologic functioning

      1. Paresthesias (numbness and tingling) in extremities
      2. Proprioception (position sense)
      3. Difficulty with balance
      4. Treatment of CNS manifestations within 6 months or may become permanent
    6. Treatment
      a. Increase intake of meats, eggs, dairy products; supplements for vegetarians
      b. Parenteral Vitamin B$_{12}$ replacement for malabsorption disorders or lack of intrinsic factor
  e. Folic acid deficiency anemia
    1. Folic acid is required for DNA synthesis and normal maturation of RBCs
    2. Characterized by fragile megaloblastic cells
    3. Causes
      a. Inadequate intake
        1. Chronically malnourished
          a. Older adults
          b. Alcoholics
          c. Drug addicted persons
        2. Increased need
          a. Pregnant women at greatest risk; Deficiency associated with neural tube defects in fetus
          b. Persons experiencing rapid growth
      b. Malabsorption disorders
        1. Celiac sprue
        2. Persons taking methotrexate and other chemotherapy
    4. Manifestations (develop gradually)
      a. Pallor, progressive weakness and fatigue, shortness of breath, palpitations
      b. Glossitis, cheilosis, diarrhea
      c. No neurological symptoms, but may co-exist with Vitamin B$_{12}$ deficiency
    5. Treatment
      a. Diet high in green leafy vegetables, fruits, cereals, meats
      b. Supplementation with folic acid
  f. Hemolytic anemias
    1. Characterized by premature lysis of RBCs within circulation or by

phagocytosis within reticuloendothelial system
2. Increased hematopoietic activity of bone marrow causing increased number of circulating reticulocytes
3. Characterized by normocytic and normochromic RBCs
4. Causes
   a. Intrinsic (within RBC)
   b. Extrinsic (outside RBC): including drugs, bacteria infections and toxins, trauma
g. Sickle cell anemia
1. Hereditary, chronic hemolytic anemia
2. Characterized by episodes of sickling in which RBC become abnormally crescent shaped
3. Autosomal recessive genetic defect causing abnormal form of hemoglobin (HbS) within RBC
4. Most common among persons of African descent
   a. 7–13% of American blacks carry defective gene (sickle cell trait) in which 40% of hemoglobin is HbS
   b. Asymptomatic unless stressed by severe hypoxemia
   c. < 1% of American blacks are homozygous and have sickle cell disease and nearly all hemoglobin is HbS
5. Pathophysiology
   a. HbS becomes deoxygenated under hypoxemia and RBC deform into crescent or sickle shape
   b. Sickled cells clump together and obstruct capillary blood flow leading to ischemia and possible infarction of surrounding tissue
   c. Under normal oxygen tension, sickled RBCs regain normal shape and unsickle
   d. Repeated episodes weakens RBC and they are hemolyzed; RBCs have shortened life span
6. Manifestations
   a. Occur with episodic sickling episodes known as sickle cell crises, triggered by
      1. Hypoxia
      2. Low environmental or body temperature

3. Excessive exercise
4. Anesthesia
5. Dehydration
6. Infection
7. Acidosis
   b. General manifestations: pallor, fatigue, jaundice, irritability
   c. With vaso-occlusive crises (4–6 days): Painful swelling hands and feet, large joints, priapism (persistent, painful erection), abdominal pain, stroke
   d. Aplastic anemia: due to shortened life span or RBC and compromised erythropoiesis
   e. Sequestration crises: pooling of large amounts of blood in liver and spleen occurring more in children
7. Treatment
   a. Largely supportive: rest, oxygen, pain management, adequate hydration
   b. Treat precipitating factors
   c. Folic acid supplementation
   d. Blood transfusions
   e. Genetic counseling
h. Thalassemia
1. Inherited disorder of hemoglobin synthesis in which alpha or beta chains of hemoglobin are missing or defective
2. Fragile hypochromic microcytic RBCs called target cells because of "bull's eye" appearance
3. Types of thalassemia
   a. Beta-defect thalassemia (Cooley's anemia) affects persons of Mediterranean descent (southern Italy and Greece)
   b. Alpha-defect thalassemia affects persons of Asian ancestry
   c. Both alpha and beta defect occur in African and African Americans
   d. Beta-thalassemia minor: one defective beta gene; mild symptoms
   e. Beta-thalassemia major: two defective beta genes; more severe symptoms
4. Manifestations
   a. Minor: asymptomatic; may develop mild anemia and

splenomegaly, bronze skin coloring, bone marrow hyperplasia
   b. Major: severe anemia, heart failure, liver and spleen enlargement; may have fractures of long bones, ribs, vertebrae
   c. May accumulate iron from repeated transfusions and develop failure of organs such as liver
i. Acquired hemolytic anemia
   1. Causes include
      a. Mechanical trauma to RBC such as with prosthetic heart valves
      b. Autoimmune disorders
      c. Bacterial or protozoan infection
      d. Immune system-mediated responses (transfusion reactions)
      e. Drugs, toxins, chemical agents, venoms
   2. Manifestations
      a. Dependent on extent of hemolysis and ability of body to replace RBCs
      b. Anemia is mild to moderate
      c. May develop splenomegaly, jaundice, pathologic fractures
j. Glucose-6-Phosphate Dehydrogenase (G6PD) Anemia
   1. Hereditary defect in RBC metabolism
      a. Relatively common in people of African and Mediterranean descent
      b. Males more common than females
   2. Direct oxidation of hemoglobin damages RBC; occurs when person exposed to stressors such as medications: aspirin, sulfonamides, Vitamin K derivatives
   3. Body responds in 7–12 days and manifestations occur several days post stressor exposure: pallor, jaundice, hemoglobinuria, elevated reticulocyte count
k. Aplastic anemia
   1. Bone marrow failure
      a. Resulting in pancytopenia (low levels of RBC, WBC, platelets)
      b. Marrow replaced with fat
   2. Causes are idiopathic
      a. Viral infections
      b. Stem cell damage from radiation

   c. Exposure to chemicals
   d. Certain antibiotics (chloramphenicol)
   e. Chemotherapeutic drugs
3. Manifestations: vary with onset and severity of pancytopenia
   a. Pallor, fatigue, headache, exertional dyspnea, tachycardia, heart failure
   b. Bleeding due to low platelet levels
   c. Fever, increased infection risk due to low WBC
4. Treatment
   a. Removal of causative agent
   b. Blood transfusions
   c. Bone marrow transplant
5. Collaborative Care
   a. Ensure adequate tissue oxygenation
   b. Treatment determined by underlying cause
6. Diagnostic Tests
   a. CBC: blood cell count, hemoglobin, hematocrit, RBC indices
   b. Iron levels and total iron-binding capacity (TIBC): deficits occur with iron deficiency anemia
   c. Serum ferritin
      1. Low with depletion of total iron reserves
      2. Ferritin is iron-storage protein produced by liver, spleen, bone marrow
   d. Sickle cell test: screening test to evaluate hemolytic anemia, detect HbS
   e. Hemoglobin electrophoresis: separation of normal from abnormal forms of hemoglobin
   f. Schilling Test
      1. Measures vitamin B_{12} absorption before and after intrinsic factor administration
      2. Includes 24-hour urine collection
      3. Used to differentiate between pernicious anemia and intestinal malabsorption
   g. Bone marrow examination: diagnosis of aplastic anemia
   h. Quantitative assay of G6PD: diagnosis of G6PD deficiency

7. Medications: Specific medications are indicated based on cause of anemia
   a. Iron supplements, oral or parenteral
   b. Vitamin B_{12} parenterally
   c. Folic acid for pregnant women, clients with sickle cell disease, folic acid deficiency
   d. Hydroxyurea: promotes fetal hemoglobin production and reduces crises for clients with sickle cell disease
   e. Immunosuppressive therapy for clients with aplastic anemia
8. Diet Therapy: Diet modifications for nutritional deficiency anemias
9. Blood Transfusions: Treatment of anemias from major blood loss and severe anemias
10. Complementary Therapies: Use of specific plant enzymes
11. Nursing Care: Health promotion
    a. Prevention by teaching all clients good dietary habits
    b. Concurrent intake of Vitamin C with iron enhances iron absorption
12. Nursing Diagnoses
    a. Activity Intolerance
       1. Measures for conservation of energy
       2. Discontinue activities with onset of angina, breathlessness, smoking cessation
    b. Impaired Oral Mucous Membrane
    c. Risk for Decreased Cardiac Output
    d. Self Care Deficit
13. Home Care
    a. Usually are treated in community
    b. Education regarding diet, medications, energy conservation
    c. Continue with medical care
C. Client with Polycythemia (Erythrocytosis)
   1. Definition: Excess of RBC with hematocrit > 55%
   2. Types
      a. Primary (polycythemia vera—PV): uncommon affecting males of European Jewish ancestry aged 40–70
         1. Myeloproliferative disorder: RBC produced in absence of erythropoietin
         2. Manifestations
            a. Initially asymptomatic
            b. Hypertension is common
            c. Plethora, ruddy coloration of face, hands, feet, mucous membranes; painful pruritis of fingers and toes
            d. Hypermetabolism: weight loss, night sweats
         3. Complications: Thrombosis, hemorrhage
      b. Secondary
         1. Response to elevated erythropoietin levels occurring as compensation to hypoxia (living in high altitude, smoking, chronic lung disease)
         2. Similar to primary polycythemia
      c. Relative: RBC count is normal but fluid loss increases their concentration
   3. Treatment
      a. Treat underlying cause; smoking cessation
      b. Periodic phlebotomy, removing 300–500 ml of blood
      c. Primary polycythemia may be treated with medications
         1. Hydroxyurea: to suppress bone marrow function
         2. Antihistamines for pruritis
         3. Aspirin to decrease risk of thrombosis
   4. Nursing Care
      a. Preventative measures include education not to smoke
      b. Clients with chronic condition need education
         1. Maintenance of adequate hydration
         2. Prevention of blood stasis
         3. Recognition of manifestations of thrombosis and bleeding
         4. Continue with medical care
III. Platelet and Coagulation Disorders
   A. Physiology background
      1. Platelets (thrombocytes)
         a. Produced in bone marrow as portions of large megakaryocytes
         b. Produce ATP and release mediators required for clotting
         c. Live in circulation after being released from spleen for 10 days
         d. Thrombocytosis: excessive number
         e. Thrombocytopenia: deficit of platelets

2. Hemostasis mechanism
   a. Stage 1: Vessel spasm lasting for about a minute
   b. Stage 2: Formation of platelet plug
      1. Platelets are attracted to damaged vessel
      2. Fibrinogen converts to fibrin
   c. Stage 3: Development of insoluble fibrin clot
      1. Coagulation occurs with many interactive reactions
      2. Two clotting pathways
   d. Stage 4: Clot retraction
      1. Clot stabilizes
      2. Trapped platelets in clot contract pulling broken portions of blood vessel together, tissue repair
   e. Stage 5: Clot dissolution
      1. Fibinolysis, clot dissolution
      2. Restores blood flow, tissue repair
B. Client with Thrombocytopenia
   1. Definition
      a. Platelet count < 100,000 per ml of blood: abnormal bleeding
      b. If platelet count < 20,000 per ml of blood: spontaneous bleeding and hemorrhage from minor trauma
      c. < 10,000 serious or fatal bleeding can occur
      d. Usually bleeding occurs in small vessels resulting in
         1. Petechiae: very small red or purple spots on skin
         2. Purpura: purple bruising
      e. Areas prone to bleeding include mucous membranes, of nose, mouth, GI tract, vagina
   2. Mechanisms leading to thrombocytopenia
      a. Decreased production
      b. Increased sequestration in spleen
      c. Accelerated destruction
   3. Primary thrombocytopenia
      a. Immune thrombocytopenic purpura (ITP) or idiopathic thrombocytopenic purpura
         1. Autoimmune disorder with accelerated platelet destruction
            a. Chronic form affects adults aged 20–40 mostly females
            b. Acute form lasts 1–2 months
         2. Pathophysiology
            a. Platelets stimulate antibody production (IgG)

   b. Function normally but destroyed by spleen after 1–3 days of circulation
      3. Manifestations
         a. Petechiae and purpura on chest, arms, neck, oral mucous membranes
         b. Epistaxis, excessive menstrual bleeding, bleeding gums, hematuria
   b. Thrombotic thrombocytopenic purpura (TTP)
      1. Rare disorder in which thrombi occlude arterioles and capillaries of microcirculation and client develops hemolytic anemia
      2. Manifestations include purpura, petechiae and neurologic symptoms
      3. Can be fatal without treatment
   c. Diagnostic Tests for primary thrombocytopenias
      1. CBC
      2. Platelet Count: decreased
      3. Antinuclear antibodies (ANA): assess antibodies
      4. Serologic studies for hepatitis viruses, cytomegalovirus, Epstein-Barr virus, toxoplasma, HIV
      5. Bone marrow examination
   d. Medications: Immunosuppressive medications including glucocorticoids, azathioprine, cyclophosphamide, cyclosporine
   e. Treatments
      1. Platelet transfusions for acute bleeding (Expected increase is 10,000/ml per unit transfused)
      2. Plasmapheresis for acute TTP
   f. Surgery
      1. Splenectomy treatment of choice for ITP, which relapsed after glucocorticoids were stopped
      2. Often curative
   g. Nursing Diagnoses
      1. Ineffective Protection
         a. Monitoring platelet counts and early recognition of bleeding
         b. Minimize invasive procedures including rectal temperatures, use small bore needles and apply pressure to any puncture sites
      2. Impaired Oral Mucous Membranes
   h. Home Care: Client and family education regarding disease

management and continued medical care

C. Client with Disseminated Intravascular Coagulation (DIC)
  1. Definition
    a. Disruption of hemostasis characterized by widespread intravascular clotting and bleeding
    b. May be acute and life threatening or mild
    c. Clinical syndrome that develops as complication to
      1. Sepsis (most common)
      2. Trauma
      3. Obstetrical complications
      4. Fat emboli
  2. Pathophysiology
    a. Endothelial damage occurs leading to extensive thrombin entering systemic circulation and unrestricted clot formation
    b. Widespread clotting consumes clotting factors and activates fibrinolytic process with hemorrhage resulting
  3. Manifestations
    a. Include both clotting and bleeding
    b. Bleeding ranging from oozing from puncture sites to frank hemorrhage from every body orifice
  4. Collaborative Care
    a. Treat underlying disorder
    b. Prevent further bleeding or massive thrombosis
  5. Diagnostic Tests
    a. CBC and platelet count: platelet count is decreased; may note fragmented RBC (schistocytes) due to cell trapping and damage
    b. Coagulation studies
      1. Prolonged PT, PTT, thrombin time
      2. Low fibrinogen level (depleted clotting factors) as level falls risk of bleeding increases
    c. Fibrin degradation products (FDP) or fibrin split products (FSP): increased due to fibrinolysis that occurs with DIC
  6. Treatment
    a. Fresh frozen plasma and platelet concentrates administration to restore clotting factors and platelets
    b. Heparin (controversial): interfere with clotting cascade and block further clotting factor consumption with uncontrolled thrombosis

  7. Nursing Care
    a. Awareness of early manifestations
    b. Facilitating timely intervention
  8. Nursing Diagnoses (clients are often critically ill)
    a. Ineffective Tissue Perfusion
    b. Impaired Gas Exchange
    c. Pain (recognition of arterial occlusion to extremity)
    d. Fear
  9. Home Care
    a. Clients who recover may have impaired tissue integrity of distal extremities
    b. Some clients with chronic DIC may require home heparin therapy
    c. Clients need to continue with medical care
D. Client with Hemophilia
  1. Definition
    a. Group of hereditary clotting factor disorders causing persistent and sometimes severe bleeding
    b. May be diagnosed in adult
    c. Majority of types include deficiencies of clotting factors VIII, IX, XI
    d. Types
      1. Hemophilia A (Classic hemophilia)
        a. Deficiency or dysfunction in clotting factor VIII
        b. Transmitted as X-linked recessive disorder from mothers to sons
        c. Severity varies from mild to severe
      2. Hemophilia B (Christmas disease)
        a. Factor IX deficiency
        b. Transmitted as X-linked recessive disorder from mothers to sons
      3. Von Willebrand disease
        a. Deficit or defective von Willebrand factor, a protein mediating platelet adhesion
        b. Transmission is autosomal dominant and affects men and women equally
        c. Often diagnosed when prolonged bleeding follows surgery or dental extraction
      4. Hemophilia C
        a. Deficiency in factor XI
        b. Mild disorder
        c. Autosomal recessive pattern affecting Ashkenazi Jews

2. Pathophysiology
   a. Clients are able to form a platelet plug at the site of bleeding
   b. Unable to form a stable fibrin clot
   c. Results in prolonged or excessive bleeding
3. Manifestations
   a. Hemarthrosis: spontaneous bleeding into joints
   b. Easy bruising and cutaneous hematoma with minor injury
   c. Prolonged bleeding from minor cuts or injuries
   d. Bleeding from gums, GI tract, hematuria, epistaxis
   e. Pain or paralysis from pressure of hematomas on nerves
   f. Intracranial hemorrhage
4. Collaborative Care
   a. Prevention and treatment of bleeding
   b. Prevent acquisition of blood borne diseases such as hepatitis or HIV infection
5. Diagnostic Tests
   a. Serum platelet levels (usually normal)
   b. Coagulation studies (APTT, PT, bleeding time) as screening tests
   c. Factor assays: measurement of blood factors
   d. Amniocentesis or chorionic villus sampling: option for parents who have family history of hemophilia
6. Medications
   a. Clotting factors may be self-administered
      1. Taken on regular or intermittent schedules
      2. Prior to surgery or dental procedures
   b. Fresh frozen plasma: replaces all clotting factors except platelets; given without definitive diagnosis
   c. Factor VIII as heat-treated concentrate or recombinant (decrease risk of blood borne diseases): for clients with Hemophilia A
   d. Desmopressin acetate (DDAVP, Stimate) prior to minor surgeries for mild hemophilia A or von Willebrand disease
   e. Factor IX
   f. All clients with hemophilia should avoid aspirin
7. Health Promotion: Clients need education about genetic counseling

8. Nursing Diagnoses
   a. Ineffective Protection: Prevention of injury and protect skin from damage
   b. Risk for Ineffective Health Maintenance: Education for self care, medication administration and continued medical care
9. Home Care: Education of manifestations and treatments
   a. Application of cold, immobilization for 24–48 hours if hemarthrosis occurs
   b. Avoidance of injury
   c. Wearing MedicAlert bracelet
   d. Preparation and administration of intravenous medications
IV. White Blood Cell and Lymphoid Tissue Disorders
   A. Physiology Review
      1. Leukocytes (WBC) are part of body's defense against microorganisms
      2. Normal WBC 5000–10000 per cubic ml
         a. Leukocytosis: increased WBC
         b. Leukopenia: decreased WBC
      3. WBC's produced from stem cells in bone marrow
      4. Types of WBC's
         a. Granulocytes (contain large granules in cytoplasm)
            1. Stimulated by GM-CSF and G-CSF
            2. Mature in bone marrow before being released into blood
            3. Types:
               a. Neutrophils (60–70% total)
               b. Eosinophils (1–3%)
               c. Basophils ($<$ 1%)
         b. Non-granulocytes
            1. Enter blood before final maturation
            2. Types
               a. Monocytes (3–8%)
               b. Lymphocytes (20–30%)
      5. Lymphoid tissues and organs
         a. Central (primary) lymphoid organs: where lymphocytes are created and differentiated
            1. Bone marrow
            2. Thymus
         b. Peripheral (secondary) lymphoid organs: active role in immune function
            1. Lymph nodes and associated lymphoid tissues
            2. Spleen
   B. Client with Neutropenia
      1. Decrease in circulating neutrophils which affects immune function and increases

risk of infection (bacterial, fungal, protozoan)

2. Cause can be congenital or acquired, developing secondarily to prolonged infection, hematologic disorders, starvation, or autoimmune disorders
3. Can result from chemotherapy or other drugs which suppress bone marrow
4. Treated with hematopoietic growth factors such as GM-CSF

C. Client with Infectious Mononucleosis
1. Characterized by invasion of B-cells in oropharyngeal lymphoid tissues by Epstein-Barr virus (EBV)
2. Usually benign and self limiting affecting adults 15–30
3. Spread through saliva: "kissing disease"
4. Incubation is 4–8 weeks
5. Insidious onset
    a. Headache, malaise, fatigue
    b. Fever, sore throat
    c. Cervical lymphadenopathy for 1–3 weeks;
    d. 50% of persons develop splenomegaly
6. Diagnostic Tests
    a. Increase in monocytes and lymphocytes, some atypical
    b. Increased WBC, low platelet count
7. Recovery in 2–3 weeks; debility and lethargy for up to 3 months
8. Treatment includes bedrest and analgesia

D. Client with Leukemia
1. Definition
    a. Group of chronic malignant disorder of white blood cells and their precursors
    b. Characterized by
        1. Replacement of bone marrow by malignant immature WBC's
        2. Abnormal circulating WBC's
        3. Infiltration of abnormal WBC's into liver, spleen, and lymph nodes
    c. Occurs more frequently in adults than children; half of cases are acute, half chronic
2. Risk Factors
    a. Down syndrome and other genetic disorders
    b. Exposure to ionizing radiation, certain chemicals, e.g., benzene
    c. Treatment for other cancers
    d. Some caused by a retrovirus, human T-cell leukemia/lymphoma virus-1
3. Classifications
    a. According to acuity

1. Acute leukemias
    a. Acute onset
    b. Rapid disease progression
    c. Immature or undifferentiated blast cells
2. Chronic leukemias
    a. Gradual onset
    b. Prolonged course
    c. Abnormal mature-appearing cells
b. According to predominant cell type involved
    1. Lymphocytic (lymphoblastic)
        a. Involve immature lymphocytes and their precursors in bone marrow
        b. Infiltrate spleen, lymph nodes, CNS
    2. Myelocytic (myeloblastic)
        a. Involve myeloid stem cells in bone marrow
        b. Interfere with maturation of all types of blood cells (granulocytes, RBC's, thrombocytes)
4. Common leukemias in adult clients
    a. Acute myeloblastic leukemia (AML)
    b. Chronic lymphocytic leukemia (CLL)
5. Prognosis
    a. Without treatment leukemia is fatal from infiltrates in bone marrow and vital organs (hemorrhage, infection)
    b. With treatment prognosis varies; 5-year survival rate is 46%
6. Pathophysiology
    a. Malignant transformation of single stem cell; proliferate but do not differentiate normally
    b. Proliferate in bone marrow edging out normal blood cells
    c. Leukemic WBC are ineffective in inflammatory and immune functions
    d. Decrease in RBC and platelets leads to anemia, splenomegaly, bleeding problems
    e. Leukemic circulate and infiltrate other body tissues
    f. Can lead to death from hemorrhage, infection
7. Manifestations
    a. Anemia
        1. Pallor
        2. Fatigue, malaise, lethargy
        3. Tachycardia
        4. Dyspnea on exertion (exertional dyspnea)

b. Infection
   1. Fever, night sweats
   2. Oral ulcerations
   3. Frequent infections (respiratory, skin, urinary)
c. Bleeding (thrombocytopenia)
   1. Bruising, petechiae
   2. Bleeding gums, other organ/tissue bleeding
d. From leukemic cell infiltrates of organs, body systems
   1. Pain in liver, spleen, lymph nodes, bones
   2. Meningeal: signs of increased intracranial pressure
   3. Decreased renal function
   4. Increased metabolism: weight loss, dyspnea on exertion, tachycardia
   5. Increased levels of uric acid (occurs with WBC destruction) causing renal insufficiency

8. Specific types of leukemias
   a. Acute myeloblastic leukemia (AML)
      1. Uncontrolled proliferation of myeloblasts
      2. Hyperplasia of bone marrow and spleen
      3. Treatment induces remission in 70%
      4. 25% achieve long-term remission or cure
   b. Chronic myelogenous leukemia (CML)
      1. Uncontrolled proliferation of all bone marrow elements
      2. Most cases associated with chromosome abnormality, Philadelphia chromosome
         a. Accounts for 20% adult leukemias
         b. More males than females
         c. Associated with radiation or chemical exposure
      3. Prognosis
         a. Asymptomatic in early stages
         b. Becomes more aggressive in 3–4 years
         c. Evolves to acute leukemia with 2–4 month survival
   c. Acute lymphoblastic leukemia (ALL)
      1. Most common in children and young adults
      2. Abnormal proliferation of lymphoblasts with acute onset

   3. Combination chemotherapy induces complete remission in 80–90% of adults
   d. Chronic lymphocytic leukemia (CLL)
      1. Proliferation of small abnormal mature lymphocytes usually B-lymphocytes
      2. Occurs in older adults (median age 65)
      3. Abnormal cells present with elevated or reduced WBC counts
      4. Slow onset and years elapse before treatment required

9. Collaborative Care: Focus is achieving remission or cure and relief of symptoms
10. Diagnostic Tests
   a. CBC with differential: evaluate cell counts, hemoglobin and hematocrit, number, distribution and morphology of WBC's
   b. Platelets: identify thrombocytopenia, risk of bleeding
   c. Bone marrow examination: type of cells within marrow, type of erythropoiesis, maturity of erythropoietic and leukopoietic cells
11. Chemotherapy
   a. Includes single agent or combination chemotherapy to eradicate leukemic cells and produce remission
   b. Combination therapy reduces drug resistance and toxicity; interrupts cell growth at various stages of cell cycle
   c. Phases
      1. Induction phase
         a. High doses of drugs to eradicate leukemic cells from bone marrow and suppress bone marrow
         b. Followed by colony stimulating factors (CSFs) to rescue bone marrow (usually factors that support neutrophil maturation GM-CSF and G-CSF)
      2. Post-remission chemotherapy
         a. Continues to eradicate additional leukemic cells, prevent relapse, prolong survival
         b. Includes single agent, combination therapy, bone marrow transplant
12. Radiation Therapy
   a. Damages cellular DNA which blocks cell's ability to divide and multiply

b. Radiosensitive cells (bone marrow and cancer cells) respond to radiation

c. Normal cells recover from damage better than cancer cells

13. Bone Marrow Transplant (BMT)

  a. Treatment of choice for some leukemias

  b. Used in conjunction with or post chemotherapy or radiation

  c. Categories of BMT

    1. Allogeneic BMT

      a. Bone marrow cells from donor (sibling or unrelated donor with closely matched tissue antigens)

      b. Prior to BMT, high dose chemotherapy and/or total body irradiation to destroy leukemic cells in bone marrow of client

      c. Donor marrow infused through central venous line

      d. Client is critically ill prior and during re-establishment of bone marrow

      e. Potential risk for

        1. Infection

        2. Bleeding

        3. Graft-versus-host disease (GVHD)

    2. Autologous BMT

      a. Bone marrow rescue: Client's own bone marrow used to restore bone marrow function after chemotherapy or radiation

      b. During client's period of remission, 1 L of bone aspirated from iliac crests, frozen and stored for use after relapse

      c. After relapse client is given lethal doses of chemotherapy and radiation to prepare space for new cells in bone marrow

      d. Client's saved bone marrow is thawed, and given intravenously through central line

      e. Client is critically ill during bone marrow destruction and immunosuppression

      f. Potential complications include malnutrition, bleeding, and infection

14. Stem Cell Transplant (SCT)

  a. Allogeneic SCT is alternative to BMT: replacement of recipient's blood cell lines with cells from donor stem cells

  b. Donors are closely matched to recipient, treated with hematopoietic growth factors prior to harvesting of peripheral blood; WBC are separated from plasma and administered to client via central line

  c. Stem cells can also be obtained from umbilical cord blood which can be stored and used in some cases

  d. Client preparation and risks are similar to those for BMT

15. Biologic Therapy

  a. Cytokines such as interferons and interleukins are biologic agents used to treat leukemias by modifying body's response to cancers

  b. Interleukin side effects include flulike symptoms, persistent fatigue and lethargy, weight loss, muscle and joint pain

16. Complementary Therapies: None have been shown to be beneficial

17. Nursing Care: Health promotion includes decreasing risk factors for leukemia (smoking, exposure to chemical and ionizing radiation)

18. Nursing Diagnoses

  a. Risk for Infection

    1. Impaired immune response so may have masked signs of infection until fully septic

    2. Need to monitor neutrophil counts

  b. Imbalanced Nutrition: Less than body requirements

    1. Increased needs

    2. Nausea and vomiting with chemotherapy

    3. Painful mucous membranes

  c. Impaired Oral Mucous Membrane

    1. Need inspection of oral lesions

    2. Need anti fungal agents, oral care with non-alcohol agents, topical anesthetics, bland foods

  d. Ineffective Protection

    1. Early identification of bleeding

    2. Avoidance of invasive procedures

    3. Care with venipunctures (small gauge needles, pressure to injection sites)

  e. Anticipatory Grieving: reaction to life threatening illness and losses related to illness

19. Home Care: Continued medical care and education regarding

a. Promotion of self care
b. Information about leukemia and treatment options
c. Prevention of infection and injury
d. Promotion of nutrition

E. Client with Multiple Myeloma
1. Definition
   a. Malignancy in which plasma cells (B-cell lymphocytes that produce antibodies) multiply uncontrollably and infiltrate bone marrow, lymph nodes, spleen and tissues
   b. Affects males more than females, blacks at twice the rate of whites, rarely occurs before age of 40
   c. Usually develops into chronic progressive disease with remissions and relapses with pancytopenia and widespread organ infiltration in the final stage
2. Pathophysiology
   a. Malignant plasma cells produce abnormally large amounts of a particular immunoglobin called the M protein
   b. M protein interferes with normal antibody production, impairs immune response and damages kidney tubules
   c. Myeloma cells proliferate and replace bone marrow and infiltrate bone causing bone destruction
   d. Leads to pathologic fractures of vertebrae, ribs, skull, pelvis, femur, clavicle, scapula
3. Manifestations (slow onset)
   a. Bone pain is common presenting symptom
   b. Hypercalcemia (from bone destruction) with neurologic dysfunction: lethargy, confusion, weakness
   c. Recurrent infections (suppressed immunity)
   d. Bence Jones proteins found in urine and may lead to renal failure
4. Diagnostic Tests
   a. X-rays and other radiologic studies reveal multiple punched-out lesions of bones
   b. Bone marrow examination: abnormal number of immature plasma cells
   c. CBC: moderate to severe anemia
   d. Urinalysis: Bence-Jones protein in urine
   e. Biopsy of myeloma lesion considered diagnostic

5. Treatment
   a. Systemic chemotherapy to stop progression
   b. Supportive care to prevent complications
      1. Management of hypercalcemia
      2. Plasmapheresis to remove M proteins
6. Nursing Diagnoses
   a. Chronic Pain
   b. Impaired Physical Mobility
   c. Risk for Injury: often use of back braces to protect vertebral fractures

F. Client with Malignant Lymphoma
1. Definition
   a. Malignancies of lymphoid tissue characterized by proliferation of lymphocytes, histocytes and precursors and derivatives
   b. Types categorized into 2 categories
      1. Hodgkin's disease
      2. Non-Hodgkin's disease
   c. Sixth leading cause of cancer deaths in U.S.
2. Risk Factors
   a. Immunosuppression due to drug therapy following organ transplant or HIV disease
   b. Viruses including HTLV-1 and Epstein-Barr
   c. Occupational herbicide or chemical exposure
3. Hodgkin's Disease
   a. Lymphatic cancer occurring in persons aged 15–35 and over 50; males more often than females
   b. Develops from single lymph node or chain of nodes and spreads to adjoining nodes
   c. Malignant cells are Reed-Sternberg cells which can invade almost any tissue in body (spleen, liver, lungs, digestive tract, CNS)
   d. Impaired immune response
   e. Manifestations
      1. Commonly painless enlarged lymph node in cervical or subclavicular region
      2. Persistent fever, night sweats, fatigue, weight loss
      3. Late manifestations include malaise, pruritus, anemia
      4. Involvement of spleen, lungs, GI tract
   f. One of most curable cancers

4. Non-Hodgkin's Disease
   a. Diverse group of lymphoid tissue malignancies that do not contain Reed Sternberg cells
   b. Arise in peripheral lymph nodes and spread early to tissues throughout body
   c. Affects older adults, males more than females
   d. Associated with genetic and environmental factors
   e. Begins as single transformed cell (T or B-lymphocyte, histocyte); different types develop in different regions
   f. Spreads early to lymphoid tissues and organs including nasopharynx, GI tract, bone, CNS
   g. Prognosis ranges from excellent to poor, dependent on cell type and grade of differentiation; low grade and better differentiated tumors are more curable
   h. Manifestations
      1. Early painless lymphadenopathy, local or wide-spread
      2. Less often than with Hodgkins: fever, night sweats, fatigue, weight loss
      3. GI involvement: abdominal pain, nausea, vomiting
      4. CNS involvement: neurological signs, headache
5. Collaborative Care
   a. Treatment includes chemotherapy and radiation
   b. Investigative treatments include monoclonal antibodies, bone marrow and stem cell transplants
6. Diagnostic Tests
   a. CBC
      1. Hodgkins disease: anemia, leukocytosis with high neutrophil and eosinophil counts, elevated sedimentation rate
      2. Non-Hodgkins lymphoma: CBC normal until late in disease, then pancytopenia
   b. Chest x-ray: identify enlarged mediastinal lymph nodes and pulmonary involvement
   c. Chest or abdominal CT scan: abnormal or enlarged nodes
   d. Bipedal lymphangiography: radiographic dye injected into lymphatic channels of lower legs to identify extent of lymph node involvement
   e. Biopsy of largest most central lymph node to establish diagnosis
7. Staging
   a. Determines extent of disease and appropriate treatment
   b. Delineation of extent of lymph node involvement above and below diaphragm and extra-nodal disease, presence of systemic symptoms
8. Treatment
   a. Combination chemotherapy used to treat Hodgkins and non-Hodgkins lymphoma depending on stage of disease and client's age and general condition
   b. Radiation therapy
      1. Primary treatment for early stage Hodgkin's disease; (later stage Hodgkin's disease and non-Hodgkin's lymphoma with chemotherapy)
      2. Involved areas are radiated and unaffected areas are shielded to minimize radiation burns and normal cell damage
   c. Long term effects of chemotherapy and radiation therapy
      1. Permanent sterility
      2. Bone marrow depression leading to anemia, bleeding and immunosuppression
      3. Secondary cancers and cardiac injury
      4. Increased risk of acute leukemia
      5. Thoracic radiation: CHD and hypothyroidism
9. Nursing Diagnoses
   a. Ineffective Protection
   b. Fatigue
   c. Nausea
   d. Disturbed Body Image, including dealing with alopecia
   e. Sexual Dysfunction
   f. Risk for Impaired Skin Integrity, including radiation burns
10. Home Care
   a. Education regarding disease, treatment, symptoms to report to physician
   b. Referrals to home health care agencies and local chapter of American Cancer Society

FOCUSED STUDY TIPS

- Visit the laboratory in your clinical setting. Ask to see centrifuged blood. Identify blood layers and components. Ask to observe red blood cells and white blood cells under the microscope. Visualize their differences.
- Visit a local blood bank with classmates. Observe how blood donations are obtained and what happens to blood once it is donated. Identify the many services blood banks provide for the medical community.
- Identify the nurse's role in blood banking. Become a blood donor. Share your experience with others and encourage others to become donors.

CASE STUDY

W. B. is receiving chemotherapy for non-Hodgkin's lymphoma. His most recent laboratory studies show that he has profound leukopenia. Based on these results, what assessments or observations can be made?

CARE PLAN CRITICAL THINKING ACTIVITY

K. A. is suspected of having a hematological disorder and is scheduled for many diagnostic tests. A priority nursing diagnosis of many hematological disorders is "Risk for infection." What universal precautions are observed, and what nursing interventions are utilized when assisting the physician with tests that involve blood or bone marrow?

NCLEX TEST QUESTIONS

1. A client is being treated with cryoprecipitate for factor VIII deficiency, hemophilia A. Which of the following laboratory test result changes should the nurse expect to see?
   a. increased platelets
   b. increased prothrombin time (PT)
   c. decreased partial thromboplastin time (PTT)
   d. decreased fibrinogen

2. A client diagnosed with anemia and is being treated with iron replacement therapy is not responding to clinical treatment and reports tingling and paresthesias of the extremities. Which of the following might account for this poor response to therapy?
   a. client compliance with iron replacement therapy
   b. underlying medical condition of diabetes that is complicating course of treatment
   c. client may also have a vitamin B_{12} deficiency that may account for presentation of neuropathy symptoms
   d. client may be taking vitamin C supplements that may account for presentation of neuropathy symptoms

3. A client has an order for an iron preparation to be administered by the parenteral route. The nurse plans to give the medication by:
   a. intermittent infusion.
   b. deep gluteal intramuscular (IM) injection, using the Z-track method.

   c. intramuscular in the deltoid to promote medication dissipation through muscle contraction.
   d. subcutaneous injection with weekly site rotation.

4. A client with a history of sickle cell anemia begins to complain of pain. The nurse suspects that the client is going into sickle cell crisis because of the pain, which signals:
   a. vasoocclusion by sickled cells.
   b. viscosity of the blood.
   c. spasms caused by thickened blood.
   d. cells in the marrow causing bone pain.

5. The nursing care plan for a client newly diagnosed with idiopathic thrombocytopenia purpura (ITP) takes into account which of the following therapies for this disorder?
   a. alkylating chemotherapy
   b. platelet transfusions
   c. corticosteroid therapy
   d. bone marrow transplant

6. A client presents with acute myelogenous leukemia (AML). Her white blood cell (WBC) count is 1,000/mm³, hemoglobin is 8.0 g/dL, hematocrit is 20 percent, and platelet count is 80,000/mm³. Which of the following interventions is appropriate?
   a. prevent contact with visitors or personnel with colds

b. administer pain medicine with aspirin or aspirin-containing products

c. keep the client pain-free with intramuscular pain medications

d. monitor the client's respirations every 4 hours

7. For clients with severe thrombocytopenia, bleeding precautions would include allowing them to:

a. shave with a regular razor.

b. brush their teeth with a soft sponge or toothbrush.

c. have their temperature taken rectally.

d. eat a low-fiber diet.

8. Clients prescribed to take ferrous sulfate for iron-deficiency anemia should be instructed by the nurse to:

a. take the medication with meals.

b. take the medication before meals.

c. take the medication after meals.

d. take the medication between meals.

9. What type of treatment is needed for a client who has been diagnosed with pernicious anemia?

a. lifetime niacin supplementation

b. lifetime vitamin B_{12} injections

c. one injection of ferrous sulfate to correct this nutritional anemia

d. surgical correction of the intestines to repair the loss of intrinsic factor

10. A nurse caring for a client who has experienced a bone marrow biopsy and aspiration should assess for which of the following as the most serious complication?

a. hemorrhage

b. pain

c. shock

d. splintering of bone marrow fragments

CHAPTER 33

NURSING CARE OF CLIENTS WITH PERIPHERAL VASCULAR AND LYMPHATIC DISORDERS

LEARNING OUTCOMES

After completing this chapter, you will be able to:

- Relate the anatomy, physiology, and assessment of the peripheral vascular and lymphatic systems discussed in Chapter 31 to common disorders of these systems.
- Describe the pathophysiology of common peripheral vascular and lymphatic disorders.
- Identify tests used to diagnose and assess peripheral vascular and lymphatic disorders.
- Explain the nursing implications for medications used to treat clients with peripheral vascular and lymphatic disorders.
- Describe preoperative and postoperative nursing care of clients having vascular surgery.
- Provide client and family teaching to promote, maintain, and restore health in clients with common peripheral vascular and lymphatic disorders.
- Use the nursing process to plan and provide individualized care for clients with peripheral vascular and lymphatic disorders.

KEY TOPICS

- Pathophysiology of common peripheral vascular and lymphatic disorders
- Medical management of peripheral vascular and lymphatic disorders
- Preoperative and postoperative care of clients having vascular surgery
- Nursing care of clients with peripheral vascular and lymphatic disorders

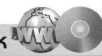

MediaLink

www.prenhall.com/lemone

Additional resources for this chapter can be found on the Student CD-ROM accompanying this textbook, and on the Companion Website at www.prenhall.com/lemone. Click on Chapter 33 to select the activities for this chapter.

CD-ROM
- Audio Glossary
- NCLEX Review

Animations
- Lisinopril
- Warfarin

Companion Website
- More NCLEX Review
- Case Study
    Abdominal Aortic Aneurysm
- Care Plan Activity
    Lymphedema
- MediaLink Application
    Peripheral Vascular Disease

LECTURE OUTLINE

I. Disorders of Blood Pressure Regulation
  A. Blood pressure: tension or pressure exerted by blood against arterial walls
  B. Hypertension (HPT): excess pressure in arterial portion of systemic circulation
II. Client with Primary Hypertension (essential hypertension)
  A. Definition
    1. Systolic BP of 140 mm Hg or >, or diastolic BP 90 mm Hg or higher, based on average of 3 or more readings on separate occasions, or initial reading of 210 mm Hg or > systolic, and 120 mm Hg or > diastolic
    2. Affects 50 million persons in U.S. with more than 90% of cases without identifiable cause; majority are persons middle aged and older
    3. "Silent killer": most persons are asymptomatic
    4. Prevalence of HPT higher in blacks, equally distributed between sexes; in whites and Hispanics, more males than females
  B. Risk factors of primary HPT
    1. Family history: genetic link in 30–40%
    2. Age: incidence increases with age
    3. Race: more common and severe with blacks
    4. Mineral intake
      a. High sodium intake (fluid retention)
      b. Low potassium, calcium, magnesium intake
    5. Obesity: central obesity (fat deposits in abdomen)
    6. Insulin resistance (hyperinsulinemia)
    7. Excessive alcohol consumption: intake of 3 or > drinks per day
    8. Smoking: correlates with serum norepinephrine levels
    9. Stress: physical and emotional
  C. Pathophysiology
    1. Primary HPT thought to develop from physiological interactions resulting in increased blood volume and peripheral resistance
      a. Sympathetic nervous system overactivity
      b. Renin-angiotensin-aldosterone system overactivity
      c. Chemical mediators of vasomotor tone and blood volume including atrial natriuretic peptide factor
      d. Interaction between insulin resistance and endothelial function
    2. Sustained HPT affects other body systems:
      a. Accelerates rate of atherosclerosis, increasing risk of CHD and stroke
      b. Workload of left ventricle increases leading to left ventricle hypertrophy and increasing the risk of CHD, dysrhythmias and heart failure
      c. Leads to nephrosclerosis and renal insufficiency
  D. Manifestations
    1. Early: typically no symptoms
    2. Later may develop vague symptoms: headache near back of head and neck occurs when awakened and subsides during day
    3. May develop symptoms if other organs affected: nocturia, confusion, nausea, vomiting, visual disturbances
    4. Eye exam reveals narrowed arterioles, hemorrhages, papilledema
  E. Collaborative Care
    1. Reduction of BP < 140 mm Hg systolic, < 90 mm Hg diastolic
    2. Prevention of complications including stroke, heart failure, and renal failure
    3. No cure available but control is possible
  F. Diagnostic Tests
    1. No tests for essential HPT
    2. But test for possible causes of secondary HPT
    3. Tests for assessment of target organ damage and cardiovascular risk factors
  G. Lifestyle Modifications
    1. Weight loss if overweight or obese
    2. Diet
      a. Mild to moderate restriction of sodium
      b. DASH diet (rich in fruits and vegetables, low fat)
    3. Limited alcohol intake and smoking cessation
    4. Increase physical activity: aerobic exercise 30–45 minutes most days
    5. Stress reduction through regular moderate exercise, relaxation techniques
  H. Medications and Treatment
    1. Classifications of medications used to treat HPT
      a. Diuretics
      b. Beta-adrenergic blockers
      c. Centrally acting sympatholytics

d. Vasodilators
e. ACE inhibitors
f. Calcium channel blockers
2. Treatment
   a. Initiated with single antihypertensive drug at low dose
   b. Dose increased slowly until BP control achieved
   c. Other drugs may be substituted
   d. Second or more classes of drugs may be added until control achieved
3. General pharmacologic guidelines followed in pharmacologic control of HPT
   a. Thiazide diuretics widely used to control HPT; single therapy used in 50% of clients in studies; effective in black, older, or obese clients
   b. Beta-blockers preferred for clients with concurrent CHD and angina, contraindicated for clients with asthma or depression
   c. ACE inhibitors used for diabetic clients, those with heart failure of history of MI
   d. Diuretics and calcium channel blockers are more effective to treat HPT in black clients
   e. If average BP > 200/120 requires immediate treatment and possible hospitalization
   f. Step-down therapy: after a year of effective BP control, effort to reduce dosage and number of drugs with careful BP monitoring
I. Nursing Care: Health promotion focus is on modifying risk factors including diet, exercise, and not smoking
J. Nursing Diagnoses
   1. Ineffective Health Maintenance: motivation of clients to continue treatment and lifestyle modification
   2. Risk for Noncompliance
      a. Mutual goal setting
      b. Client involvement addressing adverse drug effects
      c. BP monitoring by client
   3. Imbalanced Nutrition: More than body requirements
   4. Fluid Volume Excess
K. Home Care: Client needs to take active role in disease management
   1. Regular BP monitoring
   2. Taking prescribed medications
   3. Diet, stop smoking, stress management

III. Client with secondary hypertension
A. Definition
   1. Elevated blood pressure resulting from identifiable underlying condition; accounts for 5–10% cases
   2. Conditions associated with secondary hypertension
      a. Kidney disease: any condition affecting renal blood flow or function may disrupt renin-angiotensin-aldosterone system
      b. Coarctation of aorta
         1. Narrowing of aorta just distal to subclavian arteries results in reduced renal and peripheral blood flow
         2. Associated with marked difference in pressure in upper and lower extremities, weak pulses and capillary refill in lower extremities
      c. Endocrine disorders including Cushing's syndrome, primary aldosteronism, pheochromocytoma
      d. Neurologic disorders: increased intracranial pressure
      e. Drug use: estrogen; oral contraceptives; stimulants: cocaine, methamphetamines
      f. Pregnancy: affects 10% of women pregnant
B. Diagnostic Tests
   1. Renal function studies, urinalysis
   2. Blood chemistries: detection of endocrine and cardiovascular disease
   3. Intravenous pyelography, renal ultrasound or arteriography, CT or MRI
IV. Client with Hypertensive Crisis
A. Malignant HPT: diastolic pressure > 120
B. Emergency situation: requires rapid diagnosis and aggressive treatment to prevent encephalopathy, cardiac, and renal failure
C. Cerebral edema often develops with behaviors
   1. Headache, confusion
   2. Blurred vision, papilledema
   3. Restlessness
   4. Motor and sensory deficits
D. Treatment goal: reduction of BP no more than 25% within minutes to 2 hours, and toward 160/100 within 2–6 hours
E. Treatment
   1. Parenteral administration of rapidly acting antihypertensive, such as sodium nitroprusside (Nipride)
   2. Continuous frequent monitoring of BP

F. Renal function studies are monitored after BP is controlled to determine if renal damage and/or acute renal failure

G. Clients, usually between ages of 30–50 will need continued medical care and monitoring of BP

V. Client with an Aneurysm

A. Definition

1. Aneurysm is abnormal dilation of blood vessel at site of weakness or tear in vessel wall under high pressure, often aorta and peripheral arteries

2. Arterial aneurysms more common in males over age of 50

3. HPT is major contributing factor

4. Most asymptomatic

B. Pathophysiology

1. True aneurysms

a. Caused by gradual weakening of arterial wall due to effects of atherosclerosis and HPT

b. Affect all 3 layers of vessel wall

c. Types

1. Fusiform: spindle-shaped and tapered at both ends

2. Circumferential: involving entire diameter of vessel

2. False aneurysms (traumatic aneurysms)

a. Caused by traumatic break in vessel wall rather than weakening

b. Types:

1. Saccular: shaped like small out-pouchings (sacs)

2. Berry: small sac caused by congenital weakness in tunica media

3. Dissecting

a. Develop where break or tear in tunica intima and media allow blood to dissect layers of vessel wall

b. Blood contained by adventitia forming longitudinal or saccular aneurysm

C. Types of aneurysms

1. Thoracic aortic aneurysm

a. Account for 10% of aortic aneurysms resulting from HPT, arteriosclerosis, trauma, tertiary syphilis, Marfan syndrome

b. Manifestations:

1. Usually asymptomatic

2. Symptoms vary by location, size, growth rate and pressure on adjacent structures

a. Substernal, neck, or back pain

b. Dyspnea, stridor, cough, difficult swallowing, hoarseness, edema of face and neck, distended neck veins

2. Abdominal aortic aneurysm (AAA)

a. Aneurysm occurs in abdominal aorta, > 90% develop below renal arteries where aorta branches form iliac arteries

b. Associated with arteriosclerosis, HPT, increasing age (> 70), smoking

c. Manifestations

1. Most asymptomatic; pulsating mass in mid and upper abdomen and bruit over mass found on exam

2. Pain is constant or intermittent, in mid abdominal region or lower back; severity increases with size and closeness to impending rupture

3. Emboli in lower extremities, if aneurysm contains thrombi which break off

4. Rupture results in hemorrhage and hypovolemic shock; survival rate of 10–20% of clients experiencing rupture of AAA

3. Popliteal and femoral aneurysms

a. Result from arteriosclerosis, occur in males and usually bilateral; may rupture

b. Popliteal aneurysms: asymptomatic or result in intermittent claudication (cramping or pain in leg brought on by exercise and relieved by rest), rest pain, numbness, pulsating mass behind knee

c. Femoral aneurysms: pulsating mass in femoral area

4. Aortic dissections

a. Life threatening emergency and can occur anywhere along aorta including ascending and descending aorta

b. Predisposing factors: HPT, older males, Marfan syndrome, aortitis, coarctation of aorta

c. Manifestations:

1. Sudden, excruciating pain often with ripping, tearing sensation

2. Chest or back pain

3. Syncope, dyspnea, weakness

4. If dissection occludes blood flow: rapidly falling or undetectable BP, no peripheral pulses

D. Diagnostic Tests: Establish diagnosis and determine size and location of aneurysm

1. Chest x-ray: visualize thoracic aneurysm

2. Abdominal ultrasonography: diagnose abdominal aneurysm

3. Transesophageal echocardiography (TEE): visualize thoracic or dissecting aneurysm
4. Contrast-enhanced CT or MRI: precise measurement of aneurysm
5. Angiography: visualize precise size and location of aneurysm

E. Medications
1. During asymptomatic and low risk for rupture, clients with aortic aneurysms are treated long term with beta-blockers and other antihypertensive drugs to control heart rate and blood pressure
2. Clients with dissection
   a. Treated with medication to control heart rate and blood pressure, to prevent rupture, and to stabilize client before aneurysm is repaired surgically
   b. Medications include intravenous beta-blockers and sodium nitroprusside (Nipride) and client has constant monitoring with hemodynamic monitoring
3. Post surgical correction, client is usually treated with anticoagulant therapy initially heparin, and long term with oral anticoagulants or low-dose aspirin

F. Surgery
1. Indications
   a. Symptomatic or rapidly expanding aneurysms
      1. Thoracic: > 6 cm diameter
      2. Abdominal: > 5 cm diameter
   b. Depends on client's operative risk factors; area and degree of dissections
2. Types of procedures
   a. Open surgical procedure
      1. Aneurysm is excised and replaced with synthetic fabric graft
      2. Thoracic repair more complex than abdominal and may utilize cardiopulmonary bypass
   b. Endovascular stent grafts
      1. Stent, metal sheath covered with polyester fabric is placed percutaneously under fluoroscopy
      2. Option for higher surgical risk clients
      3. Involves close monitoring of location of graft afterward on continuous basis

G. Nursing Diagnoses
1. Risk for Ineffective Tissue Perfusion
   a. Monitoring manifestations of dissection or rupture in preoperative client

   b. Monitoring for manifestations of arterial thrombosis
2. Risk for Injury: continuous monitoring of adequacy of arterial perfusion, renal perfusion
3. Anxiety

H. Home Care
1. Education regarding manifestations of increasing size, dissection, or rupture for clients who have not had repair of aneurysm and need to seek immediate medical attention; control of hypertension, smoking cessation
2. Education for clients who have had surgical repair include postoperative recovery, anticoagulation, meeting nutritional needs

VI. Disorders of Peripheral Arteries
A. Client with acute arterial occlusion
1. Pathophysiology
   a. Thrombus is blood clot that adheres to vessel in area where lumen is partially obstructed or wall damaged by atherosclerosis
   b. Conditions which prompt coagulation include infection, inflammation or pooling of blood
   c. Obstruction of circulation leads to ischemia of tissues supplied by artery; if gradual, collateral circulation often develops to compensate
   d. Embolism is sudden obstruction of blood vessel by debris
      1. Thrombus which breaks loose and moves is thromboembolus
      2. Other emboli include plaque, bacterial masses, cancer cells, bone marrow fat, foreign objects
   e. Arterial emboli may originate from left side of heart when client has myocardial infarction, valvular heart disease, left sided failure, atrial fibrillation, cardiac infection
      1. Emboli trapped in cerebral circulation result in neurological deficits
      2. Emboli in peripheral circulation lodge in areas where vessel lumen is narrowed or bifurcates
2. Manifestations
   a. Tissue ischemia: extremity if painful, pale, cool or cold
   b. Distal pulses are absent
   c. Paresthesia (numbness and tingling)
   d. Cyanosis, mottling
   e. Paralysis, muscle spasms

3. Collaborative Care: acute occlusions require emergency treatment to preserve limb and prevent tissue necrosis and subsequent gangrene
4. Diagnostic Tests
   a. Diagnosis often apparent based on manifestations
   b. Arteriography used to confirm diagnosis and locate specific site of occlusion
5. Medications
   a. Heparin intravenously to prevent further clot propagation
   b. Thrombolytic therapy with streptokinase, urokinase, t-PA
6. Surgery
   a. Embolectomy within 4–6 hours is treatment of choice to prevent tissue necrosis and gangrene
   b. Embolus in mesenteric circulation requires emergency laparotomy
7. Nursing Diagnoses
   a. Ineffective Tissue Perfusion: Peripheral: includes frequent circulation assessment often using Doppler stethoscope
   b. Anxiety
   c. Altered Protection: client at risk for further clot formation and bleeding from anticoagulant therapy
8. Home Care: Education
   a. Regarding wound care, anticoagulant therapy
   b. Reporting immediately if manifestations of occlusion or bleeding occur
   c. Lifestyle modification to slow atherosclerosis, HPT

B. Client with peripheral atherosclerosis
   1. Peripheral vascular disease (PVD)
      a. Arteriosclerotic and atherosclerotic changes occur in and impair circulation to lower extremities
      b. Usually affects persons in 60s and 70s, males more than females
      c. Risk factors similar to those for atherosclerosis and CHD
   2. Pathophysiology
      a. Lesions involve intimal and medial layers of arteries and develop in large and medium sized arteries
         1. Abdominal aorta and iliac arteries (30% of clients)
         2. Femoral and popliteal arteries (80–90% of clients)
         3. More distal arteries (40–50% of clients)
      b. Plaque tends to form at arterial bifurcations; client develops collateral circulation but is insufficient to meet increased metabolic demands during exercise
   3. Manifestations: develop when occlusion is 60% or >
      a. Pain, especially intermittent claudication: cramping or aching pain in calves, thighs, or buttocks that occurs with activity and is relieved by rest
      b. Rest pain: occurs during inactivity; burning sensation that increases with elevation and decreases with dependence, numb and cold feeling; diminished sensation and may have muscle atrophy
      c. Peripheral pulses are decreased or absent; bruit may be heard at site of occlusion (aorta, femoral artery); legs are pale when elevated; dark red when dependent (dependent rubor)
      d. Skin often thick, shiny, hairless, toenails thickened, ulcerations may be present
   4. Complications
      a. Gangrene
      b. Extremity amputation
      c. Possible infection, sepsis
   5. Collaborative Care
      a. Slowing arteriosclerotic process
      b. Maintaining tissue perfusion
   6. Diagnostic Tests
      a. Segmental pressure measurements: measurement and comparison of blood pressures in upper and lower extremities; normally similar; lower in legs than arms with PVD
      b. Stress testing: using treadmill, provides functional assessment, pressure at ankle declines further with exercise
      c. Doppler ultrasound: use of sound waves to evaluate blood flow in vessel; locate site of obstruction
      d. Duplex Doppler ultrasound: combines Doppler ultrasounds with ultrasound imaging identifying arterial or venous abnormalities
      e. Transcutaneous oximetry: determines oxygenation of tissues
      f. Angiography or magnetic resonance angiography: prior to revascularization procedures locates and quantifies

extent of arterial obstruction; Contrast media used with angiography; none with magnetic resonance angiography
7. Medications: drug treatment less effective than with CHD
   a. Inhibit platelet aggregation
      1. Aspirin
      2. Clopidogril (Plavix)
   b. Platelet inhibitor with vasodilator properties: Cilostazol (Pletal)
   c. Improve microcirculation: Pentoxifylliune (Trental)
8. Treatments
   a. Smoking cessation essential for client to preserve circulation
   b. Foot care to prevent ulceration, infection
   c. Progressive exercise to improve circulation
   d. Slow atherosclerosis: control of diabetes and HPT, lower cholesterol, weight loss if obese
9. Revascularization
   a. Procedures indicated if
      1. Symptoms are progressive, severe, disabling
      2. Rest pain, pre-gangrenous or gangrenous lesions
   b. Non-surgical procedures
      1. Percutaneous transluminal angioplasty (PTA)
      2. Stent placement
      3. Atherectomy
   c. Surgical procedures: Endarterectomy
      1. Remove plaque and bypass grafts
      2. Improved results, longer term than PTA
      3. Operative risks
10. Complementary Therapies
    a. Herb
    b. Yoga
    c. Vegetarian diet
    d. Antioxidants
11. Nursing Care/Health Promotion: to prevent and slow progression of atherosclerosis
    a. Not smoking
    b. Healthy diet
    c. Regular exercise
    d. Screenings for diabetes, HPT, and hyperlipidemia
12. Nursing Diagnoses
    a. Ineffective Tissue Perfusion: Peripheral
    b. Pain: avoidance of cold and stress to limit pain
    c. Impaired Skin Integrity

1. Teach daily inspection
2. Proper fitting shoes
3. Avoidance of pressure
   d. Activity Intolerance: encourage regular exercise with gradual increase in duration and intensity
13. Home Care: Education
    a. Regarding smoking cessation, avoiding second-hand smoke, and medications
    b. Regarding signs of thrombosis and needing to seek immediate medical care
    c. Continuing under medical supervision
C. Client with thromboangitis obliterans (Buerger's disease)
   1. Definition
      a. Occlusive vascular disease of small and medium sized arteries which become inflamed and spastic leading to clot formation; effects either upper or lower extremities
      b. Primarily affects men under 40 who smoke; higher incidence in Asians and persons of eastern European heritage; possible genetic link
      c. Course is intermittent with dramatic exacerbations and marked remissions; with progression of disease collateral vessels are involved
      d. With more intense and prolonged episodes, increased risk for tissue ulceration and gangrene
   2. Pathophysiology
      a. Inflammatory process in walls of arteries in feet and possibly hands
      b. Thrombus formation with vasospasms occurs and impairs blood flow
      c. Eventually results in scarred and fibrotic blood vessels
   3. Manifestations
      a. Pain in affected extremities, including claudication and rest pain
      b. Diminished sensation, thin and shiny skin, thickened nails
      c. Involved digits or extremities are pale, cyanotic or ruddy, cold
      d. Distal pulses are weak or absent
      e. Painful ulcers and gangrene occur; may necessitate amputation of necrotic tissues
   4. Diagnosis usually made by history and physical examination
   5. Collaborative Care
      a. Smoking cessation is imperative to slow progression

b. Medications such as calcium channel blockers or pentoxifylline (Trental) may provide some symptom relief
c. Surgical approaches
1. Sympathectomy: interrupting sympathetic nervous system input reduces vasoconstriction and spasms
2. Arterial bypass if larger arteries affected
3. Amputation of portions of digits or limbs
6. Nursing Care and Home Care: emphasis is on smoking cessation, foot care, continue medical care
D. Client with Raynaud's disease
1. Definition
a. Characterized by episodes of intense vasospasm in small arteries and arterioles of fingers and sometimes toes
1. Raynaud's disease: no identifiable cause
2. Raynaud's phenomenon: secondary to other disease such as collagen vascular disease like scleroderma; exposure to cold
b. Primarily affects young women ages 20–40, genetic predisposition
2. Pathophysiology
a. Spasms of small arteries in digits blocking arterial blood flow to fingers and toes
b. Initially just the tips
3. Manifestations
a. Intermittent occurrence
b. "Blue-white-red disease": digits turn blue due to vasospasm, white with less circulation; very red as spasm resolves
c. Accompanying numbness, stiffness, decreased sensation, aching pain
d. Episodes become more frequent and prolonged; fingertips thicken and nails become brittle
4. Diagnosis is by history and physical examination
5. Medications
a. Vasodilators to provide symptomatic relief
b. Low dose of sustained release calcium channel blockers, such as nifedipine (Procardia)
c. Alpha-adrenergic blocker prazosin (Minipres)
d. Transdermal nitroglycerine
6. Conservative measures are mainstay of treatment

a. Maintain warmth of hands with gloves, avoiding cold
b. Smoking cessation if client smokes
c. Stress reduction
7. Home Care: emphasis of client education on treatment measures
VII. Disorders of Venous Circulation
A. Client with venous thrombosis (thrombophlebitis)
1. Definition
a. Thrombus forms on wall of vein accompanied by inflammation of vein wall and some degree of obstructed blood flow
b. Deep venous thrombosis (DVT): thrombosis in deep veins of legs
c. Deep veins in calf and pelvis are most common sites involving popliteal and femoral veins
d. Risk Factors
1. Complication of surgery, immobilization
2. Certain cancers
3. Trauma
4. Pregnancy, use of oral contraceptives, hormone replacement therapy
2. Pathophysiology
a. Virchow's triad associated with thrombophlebitis
1. Stasis of blood
2. Vessel damage
3. Increased blood coagulability
b. Pieces of thrombus may break off and travel as embolus
c. Thrombus scars vein wall and permanently damages valve in vein
3. Manifestations
a. Asymptomatic
b. Calf pain as tightness or dull ache, especially with walking
c. Tenderness, swelling, warmth, erythema along course of involved vein
d. Positive homan's sign (pain in calf when foot is dorsiflexed) is unreliable indicator
e. Pulmonary embolus
4. Complications
a. Chronic venous insufficiency
b. Pulmonary embolism: clot breaks loose, moves through larger veins to right side of heart and becomes lodged in pulmonary circulation

5. Collaborative Care
   a. Establish diagnosis for proper treatment
   b. Prevent extension of clot and complications
   c. Address underlying cause
6. Diagnostic Tests
   a. Duplex venous ultrasonography: visualize vein and measure velocity of blood flow in veins
   b. Plethysmography: measures changes in blood flow of vein
   c. MRI: used when thrombosis of vena cavae or pelvic veins suspected
   d. Ascending contrast venography: involves injection of contrast medium to assess location and extent of venous thrombosis; more definitive in establishment of diagnosis
7. Prophylaxis (used with hospitalized clients at risk)
   a. Low-molecular weight heparin for clients undergoing general or orthopedic surgery, acute medical illness, or on prolonged bedrest
   b. Elevating foot of bed with knees slightly flexed to promote venous return, use of intermittent pneumatic compression devices, support stockings
   c. Early ambulation and leg exercises
   d. Oral anticoagulation for clients with fractures, orthopedic surgery
8. Anticoagulants as treatment
   a. Prevent clot extension and reduce risk of subsequent pulmonary embolism
   b. Unfractionated heparin as intravenous bolus and then continuous heparin infusion calculated according to PTT, usually about twice the control
   c. Oral anticoagulation with warfarin therapy (coumadin) initiated concurrently with heparin therapy
      1. Regulated according to Protime with INR at 2.0 to 3.0
      2. Heparin is stopped and client discharged on warfarin therapy for at least 3 months to prevent recurrent thrombosis
   d. Low-molecular weight heparin may be administered twice a day subcutaneously; no laboratory monitoring is necessary
9. Treatments
   a. Warm moist compresses to promote comfort and relieve inflammation with bedrest with legs elevated 15–20 degrees
   b. Elastic antiembolism stockings while walking
   c. Avoid long periods of standing or sitting
   d. Sit with legs elevated
   e. Avoid crossing legs, wearing restrictive clothing or stockings that bind
10. Surgery
    a. Filter insertion into vena cava may be done for clients with recurrent thrombosis and/or anticoagulant therapy is contraindicated
    b. Filter is inserted under fluoroscopy with local anesthesia (Greenfield filter commonly used)
    c. Extensive thrombosis of saphenous vein may necessitate ligation and division where it joins femoral vein
11. Nursing Care: education regarding prophylaxis of venous thrombosis
12. Nursing Diagnoses
    a. Pain
    b. Ineffective Tissue Perfusion: Peripheral
    c. Ineffective Protection: education for those on oral anticoagulants
    d. Impaired Physical Mobility
    e. Risk for Ineffective Tissue Perfusion: Cardiopulmonary
13. Home Care: Education
    a. Regarding activity, anticoagulant and laboratory studies
    b. Continuing medical supervision
B. Client with chronic venous insufficiency
   1. Definition
      a. Disorder of inadequate venous return over a prolonged period
      b. Causes include DVT, varicose veins, leg trauma
   2. Pathophysiology
      a. Post DVT, large veins remain occluded and pressure increases distending vein and damaging the valves within the veins
      b. Without competent venous valves, muscle pumping action during activity cannot effectively propel blood back to heart
      c. Blood collects in veins and results in venous stasis
      d. Increased pressure impairs arterial circulation
      e. Skin atrophies, breakdown of RBCs cause brown skin pigmentation and venous ulcers can develop

f. Congested venous circulation increases risk for infection
3. Manifestations
   a. Lower leg edema, itching
   b. Discomfort especially with prolonged standing
   c. Recurrent stasis ulcers develop above ankle on medial or anterior aspect of leg; heal poorly and scar tissue breaks down
   d. Tissue around ulcer is shiny, atrophic, cyanotic, pigmented
4. Collaborative Care
   a. Relief of symptoms
   b. Promotion of adequate circulation
   c. Promotion of healing
5. Diagnosis is based on history and physical examination
6. Conservative management
   a. Graduated compression hose
   b. Elevation of legs above level of heart during sleep
   c. Local treatment of stasis dermatitis, ulcers
7. Surgical treatment includes ligation of incompetent veins and excision of ulcer with skin graft
8. Nursing Care: education regarding promotion of venous return and proper foot care
C. Client with varicose veins
1. Definition
   a. Varicose veins are irregular tortuous veins with incompetent valves affecting lower extremities especially long saphenous vein
   b. Risk Factors
      1. Venous stasis related to pregnancy
      2. Persons in occupations that involve prolonged standing
   c. Contributing Factors
      1. Obesity
      2. Venous thrombosis
      3. Sustained pressure on abdominal veins
      4. Gravity
2. Pathophysiology
   a. Prolonged standing, gravity, lack of leg exercise, and incompetent valves weaken muscle pumping mechanism and reduce venous return
   b. Vessel wall is further stretched and valves become increasingly incompetent
3. Manifestations
   a. Severe aching leg pain, leg fatigue and heaviness

b. Obvious dilated tortuous veins; if long-standing skin is thin, discolored with brown pigmentation
4. Complications
   a. Venous insufficiency
   b. Stasis ulcers
5. Diagnostic Tests
   a. Often diagnosed by physical examination and history
   b. Doppler ultrasonography or duplex ultrasound
      1. Identify location of incompetent valves
      2. Useful before surgery to identify valves that allow reflux of blood
   c. Trendelenburg test: application of tourniquet around distal thigh to determine which veins, deep or superficial are incompetent
6. Treatments
   a. Properly fitted graduated compression stockings
   b. Regular daily walking routine
   c. Avoid prolonged sitting and standing
   d. Elevation of legs several times per day
7. Compression sclerotherapy
   a. Sclerosing solution injected into varicose vein and compression bandage applied for period of time which obliterates vein
   b. Used alone or in conjunction with varicose vein surgery
8. Surgery
   a. Usually involves ligation and stripping of greater and lesser saphenous veins with pressure bandaging afterward
   b. Legs are elevated postoperatively and standing and sitting are prohibited during recovery period
   c. Usually reserved for symptomatic or clients with stasis ulcers
9. Nursing Care/Health Promotion
   a. Educating on the benefits of regular exercise
   b. Avoiding prolonged standing or sitting
   c. Maintaining normal weight
10. Nursing Diagnoses
    a. Chronic Pain
    b. Ineffective Tissue Perfusion: Peripheral
    c. Risk for Impaired Skin Integrity
    d. Risk for Peripheral Neurovascular Dysfunction
11. Home Care: Education
    a. Effective self-care
    b. Information regarding elastic stockings

VIII. Disorder of lymphatic system
  A. Client with lymphadenopathy
    1. Clients who have palpable lymph nodes in one area are usually having a reaction to minor trauma or localized infection; generalized lymphadenopathy is associated with malignancy or disease
    2. Lymphangitis
      a. Inflammation of lymph vessels draining an infected area of body
      b. Characterized by red streak along inflamed vessels with heat, pain and swelling
      c. Local lymph nodes are swollen and tender
    3. Treatment
      a. Identification and specific treatment of underlying condition
      b. Elevation of body part and heat application
  B. Client with lymphedema
    1. Definition
      a. Condition resulting from inflammation, obstruction, removal of lymphatic vessels resulting in extremity edema due to lymph accumulation
      b. Types
        1. Primary: rare, may be associated with genetic disorder
        2. Secondary: acquired condition; in U.S. occurs with recurrent lymphangitis, obstruction of lymph vessels by tumors, surgical or radiation treatment of breast cancer
    2. Pathophysiology
      a. Obstruction of lymph drainage prevents return to circulation
      b. Protein molecules have osmotic pull which adds to edema which extends into soft tissues
    3. Manifestations
      a. Edema begins distally, progressing up limb to involve entire extremity
      b. Initially edema is soft and pitting; with chronic condition, subcutaneous

tissues become thick, fibrotic with woody texture: brawny edema
      c. Usually painless, but limb is heavy
    4. Collaborative Care
      a. Relieving edema
      b. Preventing or treating infection
      c. May be difficult to treat and leads to disability
    5. Diagnostic Test
      a. Lymphangiography: injection of contrast media to illustrate lymphatic vessels on x-ray
      b. Lymphoscintigraphy: injection of radioactively tagged substance into distal subcutaneous tissue and mapping flow through lymphatic system
    6. Treatments
      a. Meticulous skin and foot care
      b. Elastic compression stockings or sleeves, intermittent graduated pneumatic compression devices
      c. Antibiotic therapy to prevent and treat infection
      d. Diuretic therapy
      e. Surgery to re-establish channels for lymph drainage in cases not responding to conservative treatments
    7. Nursing Care/Health Promotion
      a. Teaching clients post mastectomy not to allow compression such as having BP taken or venipuncture in arm on affected side
      b. Educating clients on recognition of infection and edema and seeking medical attention
    8. Nursing Diagnoses
      a. Impaired Tissue Integrity
      b. Fluid Volume Excess
      c. Disturbed Body Image
    9. Home Care: Education
      a. Management of lymphedema and prevention of infection
      b. Continuation under medical supervision

FOCUSED STUDY TIPS

- Help with discharge teaching of a client with peripheral vascular disease. Identify client concerns. Observe and document the nurse's response to these concerns. Share this information with classmates.
- List nursing interventions specific to the prevention of peripheral vascular disease.
- Develop a holistic nursing care plan for the client with peripheral vascular disease that addresses pain control, improved circulation, promotion of healing, and prevention of tissue damage.

CASE STUDY

A. G. is 2 days postop right radical mastectomy. She has lymphedema of the right arm. She is scheduled to be discharged and expresses concern regarding her right arm's appearance, as well as how to care for it. What advice can you share with her?

CARE PLAN CRITICAL THINKING ACTIVITY

What sequence of nursing interventions might be utilized when a client is diagnosed with hypertension?

NCLEX TEST QUESTIONS

1. A client is being discharged on sodium warfarin (Coumadin) for treatment of a deep vein thrombosis. What dietary information should be provided to the client in order to maintain effective anticoagulant therapy?
   a. Maintain intake of green, leafy vegetables.
   b. Increase milk intake.
   c. Maintain consistent intake of foods that are high in vitamin K.
   d. Limit intake of vitamin K-rich foods in the diet.

2. The client has been following dietary and lifestyle modifications for management of hypertension. Which of the following blood pressure (BP) readings indicate to the nurse that the treatment has been successful?
   a. 132/84
   b. 150/90
   c. 168/88
   d. 140/96

3. A client has begun therapy with captopril (Capoten) for hypertension. Which of the following foods should the nurse caution the client to avoid?
   a. Oranges and bananas
   b. Cheese and yogurt
   c. Milk and milk products
   d. Bagels and oatmeal

4. What information would the nurse need prior to administering sodium warfarin (Coumadin) to a 38-year-old male client diagnosed with deep vein thrombosis (DVT) of the right leg?
   a. aPPT results from the day before are within normal range
   b. bleeding time
   c. daily weight
   d. PT/INR results seen and noted by the physician

5. When discussing the management of hypertension with the nurse, the client asks "What is the first thing I should do to lower my pressure?" The nurse would recommend that she:
   a. begin to diet to lose weight and restrict her sodium intake.
   b. take her medications when she feels she has fluid retention.
   c. restrict her sodium and potassium intake to decrease any swelling in her legs.
   d. change jobs to decrease the stress level in her life.

6. A compensatory mechanism of the body in a client with essential hypertension is the development of hypertrophy to increase the workload of the left ventricle. Over a long period, however, this increases the risk of which of the following?
   a. pulmonary embolus
   b. cardiac tamponade
   c. myocardial infarction
   d. congestive heart failure (CHF)

7. A client complains of pain and cramping after short periods of walking that stop when he rests. The nurse concludes he is describing which of the following symptoms of peripheral arterial disease?
   a. arterial-venous shunting
   b. phlebitis
   c. intermittent claudication
   d. Raynaud's phenomenon

8. A client with thrombophlebitis has orders for continuous heparin infusion. The nurse plans to have the antidote available, which is:
   a. vitamin K.
   b. protamine sulfate.
   c. Aqua-mephyton.
   d. calcium gluconate.

9. The client with Marfan syndrome plans on having children and asks the nurse what the risk is of his child having Marfan. The nurse's response is based on the fact that:
   a. Marfan is a multifactorial congenital syndrome with no singular known cause.
   b. Marfan is an autosomal dominant disorder with a 2:4 chance of having the disorder if the partner doesn't have the disorder.
   c. Marfan is an autosomal recessive disorder with a 1:4 chance of having the disorder if the partner is a carrier.
   d. Marfan is an autosomal dominant disorder with a 1:4 chance of carrier status.

10. A client has a strong family history of hypertension. He denies that he will get hypertension because he watches what he eats, gets plenty of exercise, and keeps his weight within normal range. When implementing the plan of care, you would include:
    a. praise and reassurance that these actions will prevent him from becoming hypertensive.
    b. emphasis that no matter what he does, he will eventually develop hypertension because of his family history.
    c. recognition of efforts towards a healthy lifestyle and emphasize that early detection is essential to prevent complications.
    d. recommendation that he be on antihypertensives prophylactically because of his family history.

CHAPTER 34

ASSESSING CLIENTS WITH RESPIRATORY DISORDERS

LEARNING OUTCOMES

After completing this chapter, you will be able to:

- Review the anatomy and physiology of the respiratory system.
- Explain the mechanics of ventilation.
- Describe factors affecting respiration.
- Identify specific topics for consideration during a health history interview of the client with health problems involving the respiratory system.
- Describe physical assessment techniques for respiratory function.
- Identify abnormal findings that may indicate impairment in the function of the respiratory system.

KEY TOPICS

- Review of anatomy and physiology of the respiratory system
- Assessment of respiratory function

LECTURE OUTLINE

I. Background of Anatomy and Physiology
   A. Events involved with respiration (provision of oxygen to cells, elimination of carbon dioxide)
      1. Pulmonary ventilation: air in and out of lungs
      2. External respiration: exchange of oxygen and carbon dioxide between alveoli and blood
      3. Gas transportation: oxygen and carbon dioxide transported to and from lungs and cells of body via blood
      4. Internal respiration: exchange of oxygen and carbon dioxide made between blood and cells
   B. Upper respiratory system
      1. Passageway for air moving into lungs and carbon dioxide moving to external environment

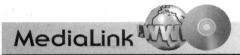

MediaLink

www.prenhall.com/lemone

Additional resources for this chapter can be found on the Student CD-ROM accompanying this textbook, and on the Companion Website at www.prenhall.com/lemone. Click on Chapter 34 to select the activities for this chapter.

CD-ROM
- Audio Glossary
- NCLEX Review

Animations
- Respiratory System
- Carbon Dioxide Transport
- Gas Exchange
- Oxygen Transport

Companion Website
- More NCLEX Review
- Functional Health Pattern Assessment
- Case Study
   Respiratory Assessment

293

2. Organs
   a. Nose: filters, warms, humidifies air; contains the turbinates where air passes and mucous traps debris
   b. Sinuses:
      1. Paranasal sinuses surround nasal cavity
      2. Frontal, sphenoid, ethmoid, and maxillary produce mucous which traps debris, assist in speech
   c. Pharynx
      1. Nasopharynx: passageway for air
         a. Contains ciliated epithelium
         b. Tonsils and adenoids located in mucosa in posterior wall; trap and destroy infectious agents
         c. Eustachian tubes open into nasopharynx
      2. Oropharynx: passageway for air and food
      3. Laryngeopharynx: passageway for air and food
   d. Larynx:
      1. Provides airway, routes air and food properly
      2. During swallowing moves upward and epiglottis covers opening to larynx; cough reflex further expels foreign substances from airway
   e. Trachea
      1. Begins at inferior larynx and descends anteriorly to esophagus to enter mediastinum, dividing into primary right and left bronchi of lung
      2. Composed of C-shaped cartilage rings; contains seromucous glands producing thick mucus which is moved toward throat by cilia
C. Lower respiratory system organs
   1. Lungs
      a. Lie on either side of the mediastinum (area containing heart, great blood vessels, bronchi, trachea, esophagus)
      b. Hilus: mediastinal surface of each lungs is where blood vessels of pulmonary and circulatory systems enter and exit; where primary bronchus enters
      c. Apex of each lung lies just below clavicle; base rests on diaphragm
      d. Two lungs differ in size and shape
         1. Left lung is smaller, has 2 lobes, 8 segments
         2. Right lung has 3 lobes, 10 segments

   e. Vascular system
      1. Pulmonary arteries and veins; pulmonary capillary network which surround the alveoli
      2. Bronchial arteries supply lung tissue and drained by bronchial and pulmonary veins
2. Pleura
   a. Double layered membrane covering lungs and inside thoracic cavities
      1. Parietal pleura: lines thoracic wall and mediastinum
      2. Visceral pleura: covers external lung surfaces
   b. Produce pleural fluid: lubricating serous fluid, which allows lungs to move easily over thoracic wall during breathing
   c. Layers cling together and hold lungs to thoracic wall
   d. Pleural structure creates slightly negative pressure in pleural space (normally just a potential space)
3. Bronchi and alveoli
   a. Bronchial or respiratory tree: right and left bronchi subdivide into secondary (lobar) bronchi and then branch into tertiary (segmental) bronchi ending in terminal bronchioles
   b. From terminal bronchioles air moves into air sacs which branch into alveolar ducts to alveolar sacs to the tiny alveoli
   c. During inspiration, air enters lungs moving through passageways to alveoli where external respiration occurs; during expiration carbon dioxide is expelled
   d. Alveoli cluster around alveolar sacs, which open into common chamber: atrium; alveoli provide enormous surface area for gas exchange
   e. External surface of alveoli covered with pulmonary capillaries which together form respiratory membrane where gas exchange occurs by simple diffusion
   f. Alveolar walls have cells, which secrete surfactant in fluid which maintains moist surface and reduces surface tension of alveolar fluid to prevent collapse of lungs
4. Rib cage and intercostal muscles
   a. Provide protection for lungs
   b. 12 pairs of ribs: first 7 articulate with body of sternum, ribs 8–10 articulate

with cartilage above ribs; ribs 11 and 12 are unattached

    c. Spaces between ribs are called intercostals spaces and named for rib above it

    d. Intercostal muscles between ribs and diaphragm called inspiratory muscles

D. Mechanics of ventilation

  1. Pulmonary ventilation depends on volume changes within thoracic cavity

    a. Change in air volume in thoracic cavity changes air pressure within cavity

    b. Resulting in gases flowing in or out of lungs to equalize pressure

  2. Pressures present in thoracic cavity

    a. Intrapulmonary pressure: within alveoli, rises and falls with inspiration and expiration

    b. Intrapleural pressure: rises and falls with acts of ventilation but always remains less (negative) to intrapulmonary pressure

    c. Pressures are necessary for lungs to expand and contract and not collapse

  3. Phases of pulmonary ventilation

    a. Inspiration: air flows into lungs (normally 1–1.5 seconds)

      1. Diaphragm contracts and contracts

      2. Intercostal muscles contact and expand diameter of thoracic cavity, decreasing intrapleural pressure

      3. Lungs stretch and intrapulmonary pressure decreases to slightly below atmospheric pressure

      4. Air rushes into lungs to equalize intrapulmonary and atmospheric pressures

    b. Expiration: air flows out of lungs (normally 2–3 seconds)

      1. Primarily passive process occurring as result of lung elasticity

      2. Inspiratory muscles relax, diaphragm rises, ribs descend, lungs recoil

      3. Increase in thoracic and intrapulmonary pressures compresses alveoli

      4. Intrapulmonary pressure is greater than atmospheric pressure and gases flow out of lungs

E. Factors affecting respiration (rate normally 12–20 per minute)

  1. Respiratory centers in medulla oblongata and pons of brain, chemoreceptors located medulla in carotid and aortic bodies control rate and depth of respirations in response to concentrations of oxygen, carbon dioxide, hydrogen ions in arterial blood

  2. Respiratory passageway resistance: as resistance increases, gas flow decreases, e.g., bronchial constriction

  3. Lung compliance: distensiblity of lungs dependent upon lung elasticity and flexibility of rib cage, e.g., pain limits breathing

  4. Lung elasticity: ability of lung to distend during inspiration and recoil during expiration, e.g., decrease of elasticity with emphysema

  5. Surfactant, a lipoprotein reduces surface tension in alveoli aiding lung recoil during expiration; insufficient surfactant increases work to reinflate lungs for inspiration

F. Respiratory volume and capacity (normal values)

  1. Tidal volume (TV): amount of air moved in and out of lungs with normal quiet respiration (500 mL)

  2. Inspiratory reserve volume (IRV): amount of air that can be forcibly inhaled over the tidal volume (2100–3100 mL)

  3. Expiratory reserve volume (ERV): air that can be forced out over tidal volume (1000 mL)

  4. Residual volume: volume of air remaining in lungs after forced expiration (1100 mL)

  5. Vital capacity: TV + IRV + ERB (4500 mL)

  6. Dead space volume: amount of air remaining in passageways (150 mL)

G. Oxygen transport and unloading

  1. Most oxygen carried in blood as oxyhemoglobin; each molecule of hemoglobin can carry 4 oxygen molecules

  2. Oxygen binding

    a. Rapid and reversible

    b. Affected by

      1. Temperature

      2. Blood pH

      3. Partial pressure of oxygen (PO_2) and of carbon dioxide (PCO_2)

      4. Serum concentration of 2,3-DPG

  3. Normally 97.4% of hemoglobin saturated with oxygen; hemoglobin fully saturated at PO_2 of 70 mmHg

    a. Temperature: affinity of oxygen and hemoglobin decreases as temperature of body increases above normal, oxygen unloading is enhanced; with chilling, oxygen unloading is inhibited

b. pH: oxygen-hemoglobin bond weakened by increased hydrogen ion concentration; more acidic, oxygen unloading is enhanced (also occurs with increase in P_{CO_2})

c. Organic chemical 2,3-DPG formed in RBCs enhances release of oxygen from hemoglobin during times of increased metabolism

H. Carbon dioxide transport
1. 200 mL of carbon dioxide produced and then excreted every minute by lungs
2. Transported in 3 forms in blood
   a. Dissolved in plasma
   b. Bound to hemoglobin
   c. As bicarbonate ions in plasma (majority in this form)
3. In systemic circulation, increase in carbon dioxide causes more oxygen to dissociate from hemoglobin allowing more carbon dioxide to combine with hemoglobin and more bicarbonate ions to be generated
4. In pulmonary circulation, the reverse situation: uptake of oxygen facilitates release of carbon dioxide

II. Assessment of Respiratory Function
A. Health assessment interview to collect subjective data
1. During interview observe client for
   a. Difficulty in breathing: pausing to breathe in mid sentence
   b. Hoarseness, change in voice quality, and cough
2. During interview obtain information whether client has
   a. Presence of pain in nose, throat, or chest
   b. Presence of cough
      1. Type and when it occurs
      2. Productive and type of sputum,
      3. What brings relief
   c. Dyspnea: association with activity, time of day
   d. Presence of chest pain
   e. Problems with swallowing, smelling, taste
   f. Nosebleed, nasal or sinus stuffiness or pain
   g. Current medication use, aerosols or inhalants, oxygen use
   h. Past medical history of
      1. Allergies
      2. Respiratory conditions: asthma, bronchitis, emphysema, pneumonia, tuberculosis, congestive heart failure

3. History of surgery, trauma to respiratory structures
4. Chronic illness
5. Use of medications to relieve nasal congestion, cough, dyspnea, chest pain
6. Family history of allergies, tuberculosis, emphysema, cancer

i. Lifestyle, environment, occupation
1. Smoking
2. Exposure to environmental chemicals: smog, dust, coal dust, animals, vapors, asbestos, fumes, pollen
3. Risk factors: sedentary lifestyle, obesity
4. Use of alcohol, injected or inhaled substances such as cocaine, marijuana

B. Physical assessment
1. Nasal assessment and abnormal findings
   a. Asymmetry of nose (previous surgery or trauma)
   b. Skin reddened around nostrils: red and swollen with allergies
   c. Nasal cavity
      1. Deviation of septum
      2. Perforation of septum: as with chronic cocaine use
      3. Red mucosa: infection
      4. Purulent drainage: nasal or sinus infection
      5. Watery nasal drainage, pale turbinate, polyps: allergies
   d. Changes in ability to smell: damage to olfactory nerve, chronic inflammation, zinc deficiency
2. Thoracic assessment with abnormal findings
   a. Respirations
      1. Tachypnea (rapid respiratory rate): atelectasis, pneumonia, asthma, pleural effusion, pneumothorax, congestive heart failure
      2. Bradypnea (low respiratory rate): circulatory and lung disorders, response to pain, medications
      3. Bradypnea and/or tachypnea: damage to brain stem from stroke, head injury
      4. Apnea (cessation of breathing lasting few seconds to minutes): post stroke or head trauma, side effect of medication, airway obstruction

b. Equal anteroposterior and transverse chest diameter (barrel chest): emphysema

c. Intercostal space retraction: asthma

d. Intercostal space bulging: pneumothorax

e. Decreased chest expansion on one side: atelectasis, pneumonia, pneumothorax, pleural effusion on affected side

f. Bilateral decreased chest expansion: emphysema

g. Tracheal shift to unaffected side: pleural effusion, pneumothorax

h. Tactile fremitus (palpable vibratory sensation when client says "99")
   1. Decreased: atelectasis, emphysema, asthma pleural effusion, pneumothorax
   2. Increased: pneumonia if bronchus is patent

i. Upon percussion of shoulder apices, intercostals spaces
   1. Dullness: atelectasis, lobar pneumonia, pleural effusion
   2. Hyperresonance: chronic asthma, pneumothorax

3. Breath assessment with abnormal findings
   a. Bronchial and/or bronchovesicular breath sounds over intercostals spaces: heard over lungs areas filled with fluid or solid tissue
   b. Decreased breath sounds: atelectasis, emphysema, asthma, pleural effusion, pneumothorax
   c. Increased breath sounds: lobar pneumonia
   d. Absent breath sounds: collapsed lung, pleural effusion, primary bronchus obstruction
   e. Crackles: pneumonia, bronchitis, congestive heart failure
   f. Wheezes: bronchitis, emphysema, asthma
   g. Friction rub: pleural inflammation
   h. Auscultate voice sounds: bronchophony (clients says "99"); whispered pectoriloquy (client whispers "1, 2, 3"); egophony: (client says "ee")
      1. Voice sounds decreased or absent: atelectasis, asthma, pleural effusion, pneumothorax
      2. Voice sounds increased and clearer: lobar pneumonia

FOCUSED STUDY TIPS

- Practice thoracic assessment in the skills laboratory. Utilize auscultation, palpation, and percussion techniques. Compare and contrast assessment findings. Practice documentation of assessment findings.

- Visit the respiratory therapy department in your clinical setting. Become familiar with commonly used respiratory equipment. Observe the functioning of this equipment.

- "Shadow" a respiratory therapist in your clinical setting. Observe assessment techniques utilized. Identify techniques that will be useful in your nursing practice.

CASE STUDY

When doing a health assessment interview, the client states he has noticed a disturbance in his sense of smell. What physical assessments does the nurse make? What can this symptom indicate?

CARE PLAN CRITICAL THINKING ACTIVITY

Describe how the nurse assesses a client's complaint of cough during a health assessment interview. How would the assessment findings be included in the nursing care plan? Name a potential nursing diagnosis utilized with cough.

NCLEX TEST QUESTIONS

1. The nurse is completing an admission assessment on a 67-year-old male client who has a long-standing history of asthma. Upon percussion of the lungs, the nurse expects to hear:

   a. dullness.
   b. resonance.
   c. tympany.
   d. hyperresonance.

2. A 57-year-old male is admitted with respiratory difficulty. He tells the nurse that he has trouble sleeping at night because of shortness of breath. Which question should the nurse ask next?

a. "How many pillows do you use at night?"

b. "Do you have a humidifier?"

c. "Have you traveled out of the country recently?"

d. "Do you sleep with the window open?"

3. When auscultating lung sounds in a client diagnosed with pneumonia, the nurse detects crackles. In order to better evaluate the sounds, the nurse should next ask the client to:

a. turn onto his left side.

b. hold his breath.

c. breathe through his nose.

d. cough.

4. An 81-year-old male client has begun Cheyne-Stokes respirations. The nurse understands that this respiratory pattern involves

a. periods of hyperpnea alternating with periods of apnea.

b. periods of tachypnea alternating with periods of apnea.

c. respirations characteristically increased in both rate and depth.

d. deep, regular, sighing respirations.

5. Which of the following requires immediate medical attention and emergency intervention? The client who

a. complains of sharp pain upon taking a deep breath and excessive coughing.

b. exhibits yellow, productive sputum, low-grade fever, and crackles.

c. has a shift of the trachea to the left, with no breath sounds on the right.

d. has asthma and complains of inability to "catch her breath" after exercise.

6. The diagnoses of asthma, COPD (chronic obstructive pulmonary disease), cystic fibrosis, and bronchiectasis all cause problems with obstruction to airflow out of the lungs. The nurse expects which of the following assessment findings to be present with these diagnoses?

a. wheezing

b. angina

c. orthopnea

d. anxiety

7. A client was involved in a motor vehicle accident (MVA) in which the seat belt was not worn. The client is exhibiting crepitus and decreased breath sounds on the left, complains of shortness of breath, and has a respiratory rate of 34/min. Which of the following assessment findings should concern the nurse the most?

a. temperature of 102°F and a productive cough

b. arterial blood gases (ABGs) with a PaO_2 of 92 and $PaCO_2$ of 40 mmHg

c. trachea deviating to the right

d. barrel-chested appearance

8. Physical assessment by the nurse is one of the keys to evaluation of therapy. During auscultation of the client's lungs, what should the nurse be aware of if a reduction in the degree of wheezing were to occur?

a. The client's condition may be worsening or improving.

b. Reduction in wheezing always indicates improvement.

c. Right-ventricular failure is developing.

d. Pulmonary hypertension is being alleviated.

9. A 50-year-old client with chronic obstructive pulmonary disease (COPD) who has smoked two packs of cigarettes a day is being cared for in the intensive care unit for an acute exacerbation of the disease. Which of the following should alert the nurse to the possibility of pulmonary hypertension?

a. pulmonary artery pressure of 30 mmHg

b. rust-colored sputum

c. thick, viscous mucus

d. absent breath sounds

10. When obtaining an infant's respiratory rate, the nurse should count his respirations for 1 full minute because

a. young infants are abdominal breathers.

b. infants do not expand their lungs fully with each respiration.

c. activity will increase the respiratory rate.

d. the rhythm of respiratory rate is irregular in infants.

CHAPTER 35

NURSING CARE OF CLIENTS WITH UPPER RESPIRATORY DISORDERS

LEARNING OUTCOMES

After completing this chapter, you will be able to:

- Relate anatomy, physiology, and assessment of the upper respiratory tract to commonly occurring disorders.
- Describe the pathophysiology of common upper respiratory tract disorders, relating their manifestations to the pathophysiologic process.
- Discuss nursing implications for diagnostic tests, medications, and other collaborative care measures to treat upper respiratory disorders.
- Provide care for clients having surgery involving the upper respiratory system.
- Identify nursing care needs for the client with a tracheostomy.
- Use the nursing process to assess needs, plan and implement individualized care, and evaluate responses for clients with upper respiratory disorders.

KEY TOPICS

- Pathophysiology of common upper respiratory tract disorders
- Medical management of upper respiratory tract disorders
- Surgeries involving the upper respiratory tract
- Nursing care of clients with upper respiratory disorders

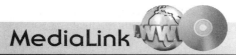

MediaLink

www.prenhall.com/lemone

Additional resources for this chapter can be found on the Student CD-ROM accompanying this textbook, and on the Companion Website at www.prenhall.com/lemone. Click on Chapter 35 to select the activities for this chapter.

CD-ROM
- Audio Glossary
- NCLEX Review

Companion Website
- More NCLEX Review
- Case Study
    Sleep Apnea
- Care Plan Activity
    Epistaxis
- MediaLink Applications
    Laryngectomy

LECTURE OUTLINE

I. Client with Viral Upper Respiratory Infection (URI)
  A. URI and common cold
    1. Most common respiratory tract infections

    2. Highly contagious
    3. Prevalent in school and work environments
    4. Most adults experience 2–4 colds per year

299

B. Pathophysiology
1. More than 200 strains of viruses cause URI; spread by aerosolized droplet nuclei during sneezing, coughing or direct contact.
2. Infected clients are highly contagious and shed virus few days before manifestations appear
C. Manifestations
1. Nasal mucous membranes red and boggy; nasal congestion
2. Coryza, rhinnorrhea: profuse nasal discharge
3. Sore throat
4. Systemic: low-grade fever, headache, malaise, muscle ache
5. Manifestations last from few days to 2 weeks, usually mild, self-limiting
D. Complications: More serious bacterial infections: sinusitis, otitis media
E. Usually self care unless complications require medical care
F. Symptomatic treatment
1. Rest
2. Maintain fluid intake
3. Avoid chilling
4. Covering mouth and nose
5. Avoid crowds
G. Medications
1. Mild decongestants
2. Over the counter antihistamines
3. Warm gargles
H. Complementary Therapies: Echinacea and garlic
I. Health Promotion
1. Frequent hand washing
2. Avoid exposure to crowds
II. Client with Influenza
A. Definition
1. Highly contagious viral respiratory disease characterized by coryza, fever, cough, headache and malaise
2. Occurs in epidemics; localized outbreaks occur every 1–3 years
3. Tends to be mild and self-limiting in healthy adults
4. Older persons and people with chronic heart or pulmonary disease have high incidence of complications
B. Pathophysiology
1. Influenza virus is transmitted by airborne droplet and direct contact
2. Influenza A virus is the cause of most infections and severe outbreaks
3. Incubation period is 18–72 hours

4. Causes respiratory epithelium necrosis which increases risk for secondary bacterial infection
C. Manifestations: one of 3 syndromes
1. Uncomplicated nasopharyngeal inflammation
2. Viral URI followed by bacterial infection
3. Viral pneumonia
D. Complications
1. Sinusitis, otitis media, tracheobronchitis
2. Increased incidence for pneumonia, especially older adults
3. Viral pneumonia develops within 48 hours and can cause hypoxemia and death within few days; also bacterial
4. Reye's syndrome: rare complication
E. Collaborative Care: Prevention by immunizing at-risk populations
1. Persons > 65
2. Residents of nursing homes
3. Adults and children with chronic cardiopulmonary disorders
4. Diabetics
5. Health care workers
F. Diagnostic Tests: to rule out complications
1. Clinical findings
2. History
3. Chest x-ray
4. WBC
G. Medications
1. Yearly immunizations
a. Only 30% of at-risk clients vaccinated yearly
b. 5% of persons immunized have reaction: low-grade fever, malaise, myalgia
c. Cannot be given to persons allergic to eggs
2. Amantadine (Symmetrel) or rimanadine (Flumadine) prophylaxis in unvaccinated persons exposed to virus (give within 48 hours)
3. Symptomatic relief: aspirin, acetaminophen, NSAIDs, antitussives
H. Nursing Diagnoses
1. Ineffective Breathing Pattern
2. Ineffective Airway Clearance
3. Disturbed Sleep Pattern
I. Home Care: Education includes
1. Rest
2. Liberal fluid intake
3. Symptomatic relief with over the counter drugs
4. Appropriate hygiene including frequent hand washing

5. Seek medical attention if manifestations of potential complications

III. Client with Sinusitis
   A. Definition
      1. Inflammation of mucous membranes of one or more sinuses, sequella of URI, influenza
      2. Frequent causative agents: streptococci, *S. pneumoniae, Haemophilus influenzae,* staphylococci
      3. Risk higher in persons immunosuppressed, including those with AIDS
   B. Pathophysiology
      1. Develops when nasal mucous membranes swell or sinus openings are blocked or drainage impaired
      2. In adults usually involves frontal and maxillary sinuses
      3. May be acute or chronic
   C. Manifestations
      1. Pain and tenderness across infected sinuses
      2. Headache, fever, malaise
      3. Intensity and location of headache changes as sinuses drain
      4. Nasal congestion, purulent nasal discharge, bad breath
   D. Complications
      1. Infections: periorbital abscess or cellulits
      2. Cavernous sinus thrombosis
      3. Meningitis
      4. Brain abscess
      5. Sepsis
      6. Hearing loss from Eustachean tube edema
   E. Collaborative Care
      1. Drainage of obstructed sinuses
      2. Controlling infection
      3. Pain relief
      4. Prevent complications
   F. Diagnostic Tests
      1. Sinus x-rays: normally translucent since air-filled
      2. CT scan and MRI
   G. Medications
      1. Antibiotic therapy directed at usual organisms; 2-week course
      2. Oral or topical decongestants
      3. Systemic mucolytic agents, aerobic exercise to promote mucous flow
   H. Surgery
      1. Endoscopic sinus surgery: remove obstruction, restore drainage; frequent nasal cleaning and irrigation
      2. Antral irrigation under local anesthesia
      3. Caldwell-Luc procedure: surgical incision to remove diseased mucous membrane create opening between nasal cavity and maxillary sinus; nasal packing postoperatively
   I. Home Care: education includes completion of antibiotic therapy, decongestants, liberal fluid intake

IV. Client with Pharyngitis or Tonsillitis
   A. Description
      1. Acute inflammation due to virus or bacteria
      2. Commonly group A beta-hemolytic streptococcus
   B. Pathophysiology
      1. Contagious, spread by droplet infection
      2. Incubation hours to few days
      3. Symptoms resolve within 3–10 days
      4. Viral and bacterial may not indistinguishable
   C. Manifestations
      1. Pain and fever
      2. Streptococcal pharyngitis
         a. Marked by abrupt onset with fever 101°F or higher; dysphagia, malaise, arthralgias and myalgias
         b. Anterior lymph nodes are enlarged and tender
         c. Exudate seen on pharynx and tonsils
      3. Viral pharyngitis
         a. More gradual onset, low-grade fever, sore throat, headache
         b. Infectious mononucleosis: presents with acute pharyngitis
   D. Complications
      1. Peritonsilar abscess (quinsy)
      2. 1–3% complications of strep pharyngitis and tonsillitis
         a. Acute glomerulonephritis (7–10 days post infection)
         b. Rheumatic fever (3–5 weeks post acute infection)
   E. Collaborative Care: Because of serious complications, efforts made to establish accurate diagnosis
   F. Diagnostic Tests
      1. Throat swab using LA or ELISA testing
         a. Test is positive: treat for strep throat
         b. Test is negative: swab is cultured to ensure no strep is present
      2. CBC: done on severely ill persons
   G. Treatment
      1. Antibiotics if group A streptococci is present: penicillin or another antibiotic if client allergic to PCN (penicillen) (complete course)

2. Antipyretics and mild analgesics
3. Incision and drainage under local anesthetic in case of peritonsilar abscess
4. Tonsillectomy: indicated for recurrent or chronic infections not responding to antibiotics, significant hypertrophy of tonsils
   a. Adenoid tissue usually also removed
   b. Bleeding most significant complication
   c. Post-tonsillectomy care
      1. Ensure patient airway, semi-Fowlers position
      2. Ice collar for pain and swelling
      3. Notify surgeon immediately for significant bleeding
H. Home Care for pharyngitis: Education includes
   1. Completion of antibiotic therapy
   2. Symptomatic treatment: aware of symptoms of strep infection and seek treatment

V. Client with Laryngeal Infection
A. Epiglottitis:
   1. Uncommon, presents as medical emergency usually caused by *H. influenzae*
   2. Rapidly progressive cellulitis which threatens airway
   3. Manifestations
      a. 1–2 day history of sore throat, painful swallowing
      b. Dyspnea
      c. Drooling, or stridor
   4. Diagnosis by flexible fiberoptic laryngoscopic exam
   5. May require nasotracheal intubation to maintain patent airway
   6. Treated with antibiotics, possibly corticosteroids
B. Laryngitis
   1. Mucous membrane lining of larynx is inflamed and vocal cords edematous: hoarseness, aphonia
   2. Treatment includes elimination of chemical irritants, voice rest
C. Diptheria
   1. Contagious disease caused by *Cornebacterium diptheriae* spread by droplet infection; most persons are immunized against this disease
   2. Tonsils and pharynx common sites of infections; thick grey pseudomembrane develops and interferes with eating, drinking, breathing; may need tracheostomy

3. Diagnosis confirmed by throat culture
4. Strict isolation required and treatment with diphtheria antitoxin and antibiotics
D. Pertussis (Whooping Cough)
   1. Highly contagious acute URI caused by *Bordetella pertusis;* persons usually immunized against disease in U.S.
   2. Toxins produced by bacteria lead to impaired clearance of respiratory secretions; milder course in adults
   3. Manifestations
      URI 7–10 days after exposure
      After 1–2 weeks, cough develops in paroxysms ending with audible whoop
      Vomiting often occurs after coughing
   4. Diagnosis by culture of nasopharyngeal secretions
   5. Erythromycin antibiotic of choice
VI. Client with Epistaxis
A. Nosebleed; precipitated by
   1. Trauma (blunt, picking the nose)
   2. Drying of nasal mucous membranes
   3. Infection
   4. Substance abuse (cocaine)
   5. Arteriosclerosis or HPT
   6. Bleeding disorder: acute leukemia, thrombocytopenia,
   7. Treatment with anticoagulant or antiplatelet drug
B. Pathophysiology
   1. Ninety percent nosebleeds arise in anterior nasal septum
   2. Posterior epistaxis develops secondarily to systemic disorders; usually more severely and more frequently in older adult
C. Collaborative Care
   1. Identify and control source of bleeding
   2. Anterior bleeding managed by simple first-aid measures
      a. Apply pressure (pinch nose at septum) for 5–10 minutes
      b. Apply ice packs to nose and forehead
      c. Sitting position and spit out blood; avoid swallowing
D. Medications
   1. Topical vasoconstrictors (cocaine 0.5%; phenylephrine or adrenaline) to control anterior bleeding; apply topically
   2. Chemical cauterization with use of Gelfoam, silver nitrate
   3. Topical anesthetic used prior to nasal packing
E. Nasal packing: petroleum gauze
   1. Anterior packs left in 24–72 hours
   2. Posterior nosebleeds more difficult to control

    a. Left in place 2–3 days
    b. Risk of respiratory and cardiovascular complications
    c. Foley catheter or inflatable nasal balloon alternative to packing
  F. Surgery
    1. Bleeding vessel cauterized by endoscopic approach
    2. Preferable to posterior packing
  G. Nursing Diagnoses
    1. Anxiety
    2. Risk for Aspiration
  H. Home Care: Education regarding prevention: limit activity, stress; humidification, first aid
VII. Nasal Trauma or Surgery
  A. Nose most common broken bone of face
    1. Bilateral fracture most common; displacement of both nasal bones to one side
    2. Often accompanied by soft tissue trauma including black eyes, swelling, bony crepitus
  B. Complications
    1. Septal hematoma and abscess formation, nasal obstruction
    2. Septal deviation; may lead to sinus obstruction or infection
    3. Accompanying facial trauma may include disruption of dura with CSF leakage or rhinorrhea (watery nasal drainage is positive for glucose if CSF)
  C. Collaborative Care: maintain airway and prevent deformity
  D. Diagnostic Tests
    1. Head and facial x-rays
    2. Intranasal cavity exam; rule out septal hematoma
    3. CT scan with CSF leak
  E. Treatments
    1. Early reduction with nasal splint
    2. Surgery may be indicated: Rhinoplasty: surgical reconstruction of nose with septoplasty or submucous resection (SMR)
  F. Nursing Care: Health promotion includes education of public about wearing helmets, face protectors, seatbelts
  G. Nursing Diagnoses
    1. Ineffective Airway Clearance
    2. Risk for Infection
  H. Home Care: Education of client includes ice application, rest, elevation of head
VIII. Client with Laryngeal Obstruction or Trauma
  A. Definition
    1. Larynx is narrowest portion of upper airway
    2. Obstruction is life-threatening emergency
    3. May occur with neck or head trauma

  B. Pathophysiology
    1. Full or partial obstruction may be due to
      a. Aspiration of food or foreign objects
      b. Laryngospasm
      c. Edema due to inflammation, injury, anaphylaxis
    2. Most common cause of obstruction is lodged ingested meat (café coronary); risk factors include
      a. Ingestion of large bolus of food with insufficient chewing
      b. Consuming alcohol
      c. Wearing dentures
  C. Manifestations of laryngeal obstruction
    1. Coughing, choking, gagging,
    2. Difficult breathing, using accessory muscles
    3. Stridor
  D. Laryngeal trauma
    1. May occur in motor vehicle accidents or assaults (strangulation attempt)
    2. Larynx can be traumatized during intubation, tracheotomy, soft tissue trauma
    3. Thyroid or cricoid cartilage can be fractured: obstructing airway
    4. Manifestations
      a. Subcutaneous emphysema or crepitus
      b. Voice change
      c. Dysphagia
      d. Painful swallowing
      e. Inspiratory stridor
      f. Hemoptysis and cough
  E. Collaborative Care: Treatments according to source of obstruction
    1. Removal of obstruction with Heimlich maneuver, laryngoscopic exam
    2. Endotracheal intubation; cricothyrotomy or tracheostomy
    3. Administration of epinephrine in case of anaphylaxis
    4. CT scan used to identify fracture but may need emergency treatment first
    5. Soft tissue management is initially conservative: humidification, intravenous fluids, antibiotics, corticosteroids
  F. Nursing Care
    1. Identify and closely monitor clients at high risk for laryngeal obstruction:
      a. Neck trauma
      b. Clients receiving medications high risk for anaphylaxis
    2. Observe for manifestations of obstruction
      a. Dyspnea and nasal flaring
      b. Tachypnea

c. Anxiety

d. Wheezing and stridor

3. Health promotion includes education regarding

    a. Recognition and early intervention

    b. Prevention

        1. Eating small bites

        2. Avoiding alcohol excess

        3. CPR and Heimlich maneuver

IX. **Client with Obstructive Sleep Apnea**

  A. Definition

    1. Intermittent absence of airflow through mouth and nose during sleep

    2. Affects middle age adults and is potentially life-threatening

    3. Leading cause of excessive daytime sleepiness

    4. Types

      a. Obstructive sleep apnea

        1. Respiratory drive intact but airflow ceases due to occlusion of oropharyngeal airway

        2. Risk Factors

          a. Increasing age

          b. Obesity

          c. Large neck circumference

          d. Use of alcohol and CNS depressants

      b. Central sleep apnea: neurological disorder involving transient impairment of neurology drive to respiratory muscles

    5. Pathophysiology

      a. During sleep, skeletal muscle tone decreases except diaphragm

      b. Most significant decrease occurs during REM (rapid eye movement) sleep and loss of pharyngeal tone and tongue tone and gravity result in airway obstruction

      c. Airway obstruction causes drop in oxygen saturation, PO_2, pH; rise in pCO_2

      d. Progressive asphyxia results causing brief arousal from sleep, thus restoring airway patency and airflow

      e. Occurs hundred of times each night

      f. Secondary physiologic effects

        1. Daytime sleepiness and impaired intellect

        2. Memory loss and personality changes

        3. Persons with CHD develop ischemia and angina

          a. Significant bradycardia, tachydysrhythmias

          b. Impaired ventricular function and heart failure

          c. Hypertension

    6. Manifestations

      a. Loud snoring during sleep

      b. Excessive daytime sleepiness

      c. Headache, irritability and restless sleep

    7. Collaborative Care: Goal is to restore airflow and prevent adverse effect

    8. Diagnostic Tests: Polysomnography (overnight sleep study):

      a. Electroencephalogram, measurements of ocular activity and muscle tone

      b. Recordings of ventilatory activity and airflow

      c. Continuous oxygen saturation readings

      d. Heart rate

      e. Transcutaneous arterial CO_2

    9. Treatment

      a. Mild to moderate sleep apnea treated with weight reduction (sustained), alcohol abstinence, improving nasal patency, avoid supine sleeping, use of oral appliances

      b. Nasal continuous positive airway pressure (CPAP): treatment of choice; consists of air compressor with tight-fitting nasal mask

      c. BiPaP ventilator delivers higher pressures during inhalation and lower pressures during expiration (provides less resistance to exhaling)

      d. Surgical treatments

        1. Tonsilectomy and adenoidectomy

        2. Uvulopolotopharyngoplasty (UPPP)

        3. Tracheostomy

  10. Nursing Diagnoses

    a. Disturbed Sleep Pattern

    b. Fatigue

    c. Ineffective Breathing Pattern

    d. Impaired Gas Exchange

    e. Risk for Injury

    f. Risk for Sexual Dysfunction (impotence)

  11. Home Care: Education regarding weight loss, use of CPAP, supplemental humidity

X. **Client with Nasal Polyps**

  A. Definition

    1. Benign grapelike growths of mucous membrane lining in nose interfering with air movement or obstructing sinus openings leading to sinusitis

    2. Affecting persons with chronic allergic rhinitis or asthma

B. Manifestations
1. Asymptomatic in some cases
2. Nasal obstruction, rhinorrhea, loss of smell
3. Nasal voice tone
4. Asthmatics may have associated aspirin allergy

C. Collaborative Care
1. Surgery (polypectomy) done under local anesthesia
2. Nasal packing to control bleeding
3. May use laser surgery

D. Nursing Care: Home care measures to reduce risk of bleeding
1. Use of cold or ice compresses
2. Avoid blowing for 24–48 hours after nasal packing removed
3. Avoid all straining, coughing, strenuous exercise

XI. Client with Laryngeal Tumor
A. Benign tumors
1. Occurs in clients with risks:
   a. Chronically shout, project or vocalize
   b. Vocal abuse
   c. Cigarette smoking
   d. Chronic irritation from industrial pollutants
2. Manifestations: hoarseness, breathy voice quality

B. Malignant tumors
1. Description
   a. Uncommon
   b. Curable if detected early
   c. Males affected more than females
   d. Age 50–70
   e. With advanced disease, often fatal
2. Risk Factors
   a. Smoking
   b. Alcohol consumption
   c. Poor nutrition
   d. Human papillovirus infection
   e. Exposure to asbestos and occupational pollutants
3. Pathophysiology
   a. Squamous cell carcinoma: most common
      1. Occurs over time with irritation
      2. Leukoplakia precancerous lesion develops into erythroplakia
      3. Cancer in situ: superficial layer involvement
      4. 30% of these lesions develop into carcinoma
   b. Manifestations vary with site of lesion
      1. Glottic: change in voice, hoarseness

2. Supraglottic: painful swallowing, sore throat, lump in throat
3. Subglottic: airway obstruction

4. Diagnostic Tests
a. Direct or indirect laryngoscopy visualize larynx
b. Biopsy: usually done under general anesthesia
c. CT scan, MRI, chest x-ray: evaluate size of mass, involvement of lymph nodes, determine metastasis

5. Treatment
a. Benign lesions are surgically excised and examined to rule out malignancy
b. Laryngeal cancer is staged: tumor size and location (T); lymph node involvement (N); presence or absence of metastases (M)
   1. Radiation therapy: treatment of choice early cancer
      a. Affects timber of voice
      b. Used in combination with chemotherapy in more advanced cases, palliative treatment
   2. Chemotherapy
      a. Used as primary treatment for some cancers
      b. Used to distant metastases and for palliation
   3. Surgery
      a. Partial laryngectomy: one half or more of larynx removed; voice generally preserved but changed
         1. Client receives several weeks of enteral or parenteral nutrition
         2. Client taught swallowing techniques to avoid aspiration
      b. Total laryngectomy: for cancers that extend beyond vocal cords
         1. Larnyx, epiglottis, thyroid cartilage, several tracheal rings and hyoid bone removed; no risk of aspiration
         2. Normal speech is lost
         3. Permanent tracheostomy
      c. Radical or modified neck dissection: if cervical lymph node involvement

6. Speech Rehabilitation
a. Tracheoesophageal puncture (TEP): small fistula created between posterior tracheal wall and anterior esophagus with one way shunt valve; by occluding tracheostomy stoma air

forced into esophagus and hypopharynx to create sound
   b. Esophageal speech: used swallowed air to create sound and form words; belchlike sound
   c. Use of speech generators; electrolarynx creates vibration and client forms words using normal muscles of speech
7. Health Promotion: Education regarding risks for laryngeal cancer: smoking and alcohol use
8. Nursing Diagnoses
   a. Risk for Impaired Airway Clearance: Have functioning suction available
   b. Impaired Verbal Communication
      1. Prior to surgery introduce nonverbal means to communicate: pencil and paper, magic slate, alphabet board
      2. Consultation with speech therapist

   c. Impaired Swallowing
      1. Maintain nutrition and fluid balance until normal eating is resumed
      2. Soft foods easier to handle than liquids
   d. Impaired Nutrition: Less than requirements
   e. Anticipatory Grieving: dealing with cancer diagnosis and possibly loss of speech, body image
9. Home Care: Client learning needs are determined by extent of treatment; may include
   a. Tracheostomy care
   b. Handling respiratory secretions
   c. Adapting to water near stoma
   d. Communication
   e. Nutrition
   f. Smoking cessation
   g. Referral to community Laryngectomy Club

FOCUSED STUDY TIPS

- Set up a nebulized medication administration utilizing normal saline for practice in the skills lab. Administer the nebulized treatment to a classmate. Describe and practice necessary assessments before and after treatment administration.
- Observe a nurse caring for a client with severe respiratory distress. Identify interventions made to minimize fear and anxiety. Evaluate their effectiveness.
- Work with a discharge planner in obtaining home respiratory equipment for therapy. Identify resources utilized and necessary referral information. Determine how these services are paid for. Identify baseline assessment information necessary for procurement of services.

CASE STUDY

B. T. is a client suffering from recurrent sinus infections. She has a history of unsuccessful endoscopic sinus surgery. She is scheduled for a Caldwell-Luc procedure. When doing her preoperative teaching, she indicates a knowledge deficit regarding postoperative expectations and care. What can you tell her to expect after surgery?

CARE PLAN CRITICAL THINKING ACTIVITY

Describe nursing care of a client with nasal packing. What can the nurse do to prevent aspiration? What can the nurse do to alleviate the fear experienced by these clients?

NCLEX TEST QUESTIONS

1. Clients with severe sleep apnea should be educated to plan frequent rest periods and activities around how well they feel in order to maximize energy because they may complain of which of the following during the day?
   a. Cardiac arrhythmias
   b. Fatigue
   c. Jaw pain
   d. Productive cough
2. The priority postoperative nursing action following nasal packing for epistaxis is
   a. providing frequent oral care.

b. ensuring adequate intake of oral fluids.

c. monitoring respiratory function and oxygen saturation.

d. administering analgesics as prescribed.

3. A 60-year-old male presents to the clinic complaining of hoarseness and a cough. His spouse states his voice has changed in the last few months. The nurse interprets that the client's symptoms are consistent with which of the following disorders?

   a. gastroesophageal reflux disease (GERD)

   b. coronary artery disease (CAD)

   c. laryngeal cancer

   d. chronic sinusitis

4. A client with chronic obstructive pulmonary disease (COPD), sleep apnea, and cardiac problems has been placed on continuous positive airway pressure (CPAP) at night at home to assist with the sleep apnea. He complains of having a nosebleed after about a week of the home oxygen therapy. What is the nurse's best explanation for this?

   a. The oxygen therapy is probably not the cause; other reasons should be investigated.

   b. The cardiac problems are more likely the cause of the nosebleed.

   c. The oxygen causes a vasodilating effect, which could enhance a nosebleed.

   d. The oxygen is drying to the nasal passage and could be irritating the membranes.

5. The clinic nurse should provide which of the following as the initial treatment for epistaxis?

   a. applying pressure on the anterior portion of the nose

   b. application of warm compresses to the nose

   c. insertion of nasal packing

   d. cauterization of the bleeding vessel

6. Over-the-counter (OTC) pseudoephedrine tablets and nasal sprays are used by a client to control symptoms of seasonal rhinitis. In teaching the client about the use of OTC allergy medications, the nurse advises the client that

   a. seasonal allergies should be treated only with prescription drugs.

   b. overmedication with decongestant nasal sprays may increase her nasal congestion and swelling.

   c. pseudoephedrine may cause drowsiness, and she should not drive or use machinery while taking it.

   d. she should take the pseudoephedrine continuously to prevent allergy symptoms from developing.

7. The priority intervention to ensure the best airway for a client having difficulty breathing is to position the client in the

   a. side-lying position.

   b. prone position.

   c. Fowler's position.

   d. supine position.

8. The census on the unit is 90 percent, and there are no private rooms available. An elderly client with influenza is admitted. Which of the following rooms would it be appropriate to assign this client?

   a. A double room with another client with the same diagnosis.

   b. A four-bed room with three clients who have had orthopedic surgery.

   c. A double room with an elderly client with a diagnosis of chicken pox.

   d. A double room with a client admitted for impetigo.

9. In addition to assessing for hemorrhage, the most important objective in client care following a tonsillectomy is prevention of

   a. coughing.

   b. swallowing blood.

   c. aspiration of mucus.

   d. airway constriction.

10. Which of the following viruses is most likely to be acquired through casual contact with an infected individual?

    a. influenza virus

    b. herpes virus

    c. cytomegalovirus (CMV)

    d. deficiency virus (HIV)

CHAPTER 36

NURSING CARE OF CLIENTS WITH LOWER RESPIRATORY DISORDERS

LEARNING OUTCOMES

After completing this chapter, you will be able to:

- Relate anatomy, physiology, and assessment of the lower respiratory tract and its function to common disorders affecting the lower respiratory system.
- Describe the pathophysiology and manifestations of common lower respiratory disorders.
- Identify tests used to diagnose disorders of the lower respiratory system.
- Discuss nursing implications for medications and treatments prescribed for lower respiratory disorders.
- Provide appropriate care for the client having thoracic surgery.
- Effectively teach clients with lower respiratory disorders and their families.
- Use the nursing process to assess, plan and implement individualized care, and evaluate responses for a client with a lower respiratory disorder.

KEY TOPICS

- Infections and inflammatory disorders of the lower respiratory tract
- Obstruction disorders of the airway
- Pulmonary vascular disorders
- Lung cancer
- Disorders of the pleura
- Trauma to the chest or lung
- Respiratory failure

© 2004 by Pearson Education, Inc.

LECTURE OUTLINE

I. Background
   A. Normal function of lower respiratory system depend on several organ systems
      1. Central nervous system: stimulates and controls breathing
      2. Chemoreceptors in brain, aortic arch, carotid bodies: monitor pH and oxygen content of blood
      3. Heart and circulatory system: provide blood supply and gas exchange
      4. Musculoskeletal system: provide intact thoracic cavity capable of expanding and contracting
      5. Lungs and bronchial tree: allow air movement and gas exchange
   B. Impaired function affects ventilation and respiration resulting in hypoxic tissues
   C. Lower respiratory tract normally sterile: protective forces include mucous, cilia, cough reflex, macrophages that reside in alveoli
II. Infectious or Inflammatory Conditions
   A. Client with acute bronchitis
      1. Inflammation of bronchi
         a. Acute
            1. Risks: impaired immunity, cigarette smoking
            2. Following viral URI
            3. Nonproductive cough that becomes productive occurring in paroxysms, aggravated by dry, cold, dusty air
            4. Chest pain, moderate fever, general malaise
         b. Chronic: component of chronic obstructive pulmonary disease (COPD)
      2. Collaborative Care
         a. Diagnosis based on history, clinical presentation
         b. Chest x-ray to rule out pneumonia
         c. Treatment
            1. Symptomatic: rest, increased fluid intake, aspirin or acetaminophen
            2. Broad-spectrum antibiotics (half of cases bacterial)
            3. Expectorant cough med during day; cough suppressant at night
   B. Client with pneumonia
      1. Inflammation of lung parenchyma (respiratory bronchioles and alveoli)
      2. Sixth leading cause of death in U.S.
      3. Incidence and mortality highest among older adults, persons with debilitating diseases

   4. Types
      a. Infectious: bacteria, viruses, fungi, protozoa, other microbes
      b. Noninfectious: aspiration of gastric contents, inhalation of toxic or irritating gases
      c. Community-acquired: *Streptococcus pneumoniae* most common
      d. Nosocomial (hospital-acquired): *Staphylococcus aureus, Klebsiella pneumoniae, Pseudomonas aeruginaosa, Escherichia coli*
      e. Opportunistic: *Pneumonocystis carinii* in immunocompromised persons
   5. Acute bacterial pneumonia
      a. Spread by droplet infection
      b. Bacteria cause inflammatory response: alveolar edema and formation of exudates, which fills alveoli and bronchioles; consolidation (solidification) of lung tissue
         1. Lobar: consolidation of large portion of entire lung lobe
         2. Bronchopneumonia: patchy consolidation involving several lobules
      c. Manifestations
         1. Acute onset with shaking chills, fever, productive cough or rust-colored or purulent sputum
         2. Pleuritic pain: sharp chest pain with cough and breaths
         3. Limited breath sounds, fine crackles, possible pleural rub
         4. Dyspnea and cyanosis if air exchange is impaired
         5. Bronchopneumonia has more insidious onset
         6. Older and debilitated clients may be atypical: little respiratory distress; more likely: fever, tachypnea, altered mentation or agitation
      d. Staph and gram-negative bacterial pneumonias cause extensive parenchymal damage: necrosis, lung abscess, empyema: accumulation of purulent exudates in pleural cavity
      e. Legionnaire's disease: bronchopneumonia caused by *Legionella pneumophila* found in warm standing water
         1. Clients at risk include smokers, older adults, persons with chronic

diseases, persons with impaired immunity
2. Manifestations
   a. Gradual onset: 2–10 days post exposure
   b. Chills, fever, cough, myalgias, arthralgias
   c. Lung consolidation
3. Mortality rate >30% without treatment
6. Primary atypical pneumonia
   a. Caused by mycoplasma pneumoniae primarily affected by college students, military recruits; "walking pneumonia"
   b. Highly contagious; resembles manifestations of viral pneumonia: fever, headache, myalgias, arthralgias; dry hacking cough; primarily systemic manifestations
7. Viral pneumonia
   a. Typically mild disease affecting older adults and those with chronic conditions
   b. Occurs with community epidemics
   c. Flulike manifestations
   d. Dry cough
8. *Pneumocystis carinii* pneumonia
   a. Occurs in 75–80% of persons with AIDS; immunocompromised persons
   b. Patchy involvement throughout lungs; severely impaired gas exchange
   c. Abrupt onset fever, shortness of breath, dry nonproductive cough
9. Aspiration pneumonia
   a. Aspiration of gastric contents into lungs resulting in chemical and bacterial pneumonia
   b. Risk factors: emergency surgery, depressed cough and gag reflexes, impaired swallowing
   c. Silent regurgitation of gastric contents may occur with decreased level of consciousness
   d. Low pH of gastric contents: severe inflammatory response in respiratory tract: pulmonary edema and respiratory failure
10. Collaborative Care: prevention is key component, especially with vulnerable populations
11. Diagnostic Tests
    a. Sputum gram stain, sputum culture and sensitivity

   b. CBC with WBC differential: leukocytosis, shift to left with bacterial pneumonias
   c. Arterial blood gases: evaluation of gas exchange
   d. Pulse oximetry: continuously monitor gas exchange
   e. Chest x-ray: extent and pattern of lung involvement; may show fluid infiltrates, consolidated lung tissue, atelectasis
   f. Fiberoptic bronchoscopy: obtain sputum specimen, remove secretions from bronchial tree
12. Immunization
    a. Pneumococcal vaccine: antigens from 23 types of pneumococcus, imparts life long immunity
    b. Influenza vaccine: recommended for high-risk populations
13. Medications
    a. Antibiotics: initially according to gram stain, pattern of lung involvement, then according to culture and sensitivity results
    b. Bronchodilators: improve ventilation, reduce hypoxia
       1. Sympathomimetics, i.e., albuterol, metaproterenol
       2. Methylxanthines, i.e., theophylline, aminophylline
    c. Expectorants: Acetylcysteine (Mucomyst) as inhalation; guaifenesin
14. Respiratory Treatments
    a. Incentive spirometry, suctioning
    b. Oxygen: according to client needs: range from cannula to intubation and mechanical ventilation
    c. Chest physiotherapy:
       1. Percussion: rhythmic clapping on chest wall to reduce lung consolidation, prevent atelectasis
       2. Vibration: application of pressure with repeated tensing of hand over involved areas to facilitate movement of secretions into larger airways
       3. Postural drainage: positioning client to facilitate drainage of secretions from lung segment
15. Complementary Therapies: Herbs: Echinacea, goldenseal, ma huang
16. Nursing Care/Health Promotion
    a. Vaccination against pneumonia
    b. Preventive measures in high risk groups

1. Increase mobility
2. Good hydration, nutrition
3. Prompt detection and treatment of pneumonia
17. Nursing Diagnoses
    a. Ineffective Airway Clearance
    b. Ineffective Breathing Pattern
    c. Activity Intolerance
18. Home Care
    a. Usually treated in community unless respiratory status compromised
    b. Preventative measures
    c. Recognition of manifestations
    d. Supportive care to maintain client's health
    e. Completion of any antibiotic therapy
    f. Continue with medical appointments for follow-up   *Stop here*
C. Client with lung abscess
    1. Localized area of lung destruction, necrosis, and pus formation
       a. Often follows aspiration pneumonia
       b. Follows staphylococcal, Klebsiella and Legionella pneumonias
    2. Risk Factors
       a. Decreased level of consciousness related to multiple causes
       b. Swallowing disorders, dental caries
       c. Debilitation secondary to cancer, chronic disease
    3. Pathophysiology
       a. Consolidated lung tissue of pneumonia becomes necrotic
       b. Necrotic process spreads and ruptures leaving a cavity of air and fluid
       c. If not expectorated, infection spreads
       d. Leads to diffuse pneumonia or acute respiratory distress syndrome (ARDS)
    4. Manifestations
       a. Onset about 2 weeks after pneumonia, aspiration
       b. Similar to pneumonia: fever, chills, pleurtic chest pain
       c. Post abscess rupture expectoration of large amounts of purulent blood-streaked sputum
    5. Diagnosis
       a. History and presentation
       b. Chest x-ray shows thick-walled solitary cavity with surrounding consolidation
    6. Treatment
       a. Antibiotic therapy
       b. Postural drainage

c. If pleural space involved, tube thoracostomy (chest tube) for drainage
    7. Nursing Care: similar to that of pneumonia
D. Client with tuberculosis (TB)
    1. Chronic recurrent infectious disease
       a. Usually affecting lungs but may affect any organ
       b. Caused by *Mycobacterium tuberculosis*
       c. Slow growing acid-fast organism, transmitted by droplet infection
    2. Incidence in U.S. fell steadily until 1980s when resurgence of multiple drug resistant strains related to HIV/AIDS epidemic; world wide health problem, in U.S. today tuberculosis mainly affecting immigrants, HIV-infected and disadvantaged
    3. Tuberculosis spreads by droplet infection; airborne droplets produced with coughing, sneezing, speaking, singing
    4. Risk for infection
       a. Characteristics of infectious person
       b. Extent of air contamination
       c. Duration of exposure
       d. Susceptibility of host (more common in homeless, injection drug users, alcoholics)
    5. Pathophysiology
       a. General pathophysiology
          1. Bacilli enter upper airway via droplet
          2. Implant in alveolus or bronchiole
          3. Local inflammation and develops into granulomatous lesion called tubercle
          4. Infected tissue dies within and forms caseation necrosis
          5. With adequate immune response, scar tissue develops, scar tissue calcifies (visible on x-ray)
          6. With inadequate immune response: disease develops with cavitation
       b. Forms of disease
          1. Respiratory
             a. Primary tuberculosis: granulomatous tissue erodes bronchus or blood vessel spreading disease throughout lungs, organs
             b. Reactivation tuberculosis: previously healed lesion ruptures when immune system is suppressed due to age, disease, immunosuppression

c. Chronic disease: infected person spreads disease continually by droplet infection into environment

2. Extrapulmonary tuberculosis: spreads through blood and lymph system to other organs; more prevalent in persons with HIV disease
   a. Military tuberculosis: hematogenous spread
   b. Genitourinary tuberculosis
   c. Tuberculosis meningitis
   d. Skeletal meningitis: painful warm joints

6. Manifestations
   a. Initial infection has few symptoms until tuberculosis test is positive or calcified lesions are visible on x-ray
   b. Primary progressive or reactivation tuberculosis
      1. Fatigue
      2. Anorexia and weight loss
      3. Low-grade afternoon fever and night sweats
      4. Dry cough that becomes productive (client usually seeks treatment at this point)
   c. Complications
      1. Tuberculosis empyema
      2. Bronchopleural fistula
      3. Pneumothorax

7. Collaborative Care
   a. Significant public health threat with development of drug-resistant strains; focus includes
      1. Early detection
      2. Accurate diagnosis
      3. Effective disease treatment
      4. Prevention of spread of tuberculosis
   b. Non-compliance with prescribed treatment is major problem
   c. Screening
      1. Cellular (delayed hypersensitivity) develops within 3–10 weeks after infection
      2. Detected by injection of small amount of purified protein derivative (PPD) of tuberculin which produces local inflammatory response: induration at injection site
      3. Methods
         a. Intradermal PPD (Mantoux) test: read within 48–72 hours; read by induration, not redness

1. 2-step method: if first step elicits negative response, second PPD given a week later, if negative person is free of infection or anergic (non-responsive to common antigens)
2. Recommended for health care workers and long-term care workers and residents
   b. Multiple-puncture (tine) test: puncture test, less accurate

4. Persons at risk
   a. Persons with or at risk for HIV infection
   b. Close contacts of persons diagnosed with infectious TB
   c. Medical risks: chronic disease, impaired immunity
   d. Persons born in countries with high TB rates
   e. Medically underserved
   f. Alcoholics and infectable drug users
   g. Residents and staff of long-term residential facilities (long-term care, correctional institutions)

8. Diagnostic Tests
   a. Active disease diagnosed by
      1. Sputum tests: Acid fast smear and culture
      2. Chest x-ray screening
      3. Polymerase chain reaction (PCR): rapid detection of DNA from *M. tuberculosis*
   b. Baseline testing prior to antituberculosis drug therapy
      1. Liver function tests before isoniazid (INH)
      2. Vision examination before ethambutol
      3. Audiometric testing before streptomycin therapy

9. Medications: Prevention and treatment of tuberculosis infection
   a. Prophylactic treatment to prevent active tuberculosis
      1. Clients with positive skin test conversion
      2. Close contacts of persons with positive sputum
      3. 6–12 months of isoniazid (INH) 300 mg orally
      4. Bacilli Calmette-Guerin (BCG) vaccine

a. Used in developing countries or where prophylaxis contraindicated
b. Persons will have positive skin tests, screening with chest x-ray

b. Treatment for active disease uses 2 or more medications to prevent TB organism from mutating into drug-resistant forms
1. Initial regimen is 2 months daily treatment with INH, rifampin, pyrazinamide; 4 more months of INH and rifampin
2. If drug resistant strain is suspected, therapy adjusted to resistance and includes 4 or 5 drugs
3. Adverse and toxic effects of antitubercular medications
   a. Hepatotoxicity: avoid alcohol and toxic drugs
   b. Audiometric monitoring (hearing)
4. Clients need to continue with medical follow-up where compliance is assessed
5. Twice weekly therapy administered under direct supervision of public health personnel for non-compliant
6. Effectiveness of therapy assessed by repeat sputum specimens and chest x-rays
7. With adherence to treatment, negative sputum specimens within 3 months; relapse rate with current treatment is < 5%; reason for relapse being non-compliance

10. Nursing Care: Health promotion
a. Public awareness of re-emerging threat, covering mouth and proper disposal of sputum
b. Public awareness of benefits of screening, early diagnosis appropriate treatment and prophylaxis

11. Nursing Diagnoses
a. Knowledge Deficit regarding disease management and prevention
b. Ineffective Therapeutic Regimen Management: intervention with homeless and other high-risk groups
c. Risk for Infection
   1. Isolation of clients: private room with air flow control: negative flow room in which air is diluted by at least 6 fresh-air exchanges

2. OSHA requires use of HEPA-filtered respirator for protection for health care workers delivering care
3. Appropriate masking for visitors and client outside room when disease is active

12. Home Care
a. Most persons with active disease managed in community with prescribed treatment, nutrition, screening and prophylaxis of close contacts, monitoring for complications
b. Appropriate referrals for smoking cessation, alcohol and drug treatment

E. Client with inhalation anthrax
1. Recent threat
   a. *Bacillus anthracis* is agent
   b. Spores can be aerosolized as biologic weapon
   c. No person-to-person contact
2. Manifestations
   a. Initial flulike symptoms: malaise, dry cough, fever
   b. Abrupt onset of severe dyspnea, stridor, cyanosis
   c. Lymph nodes in mediastinum and thorax become inflamed
   d. Septic shock or meningitis
   e. Death from hemorrhagic thoracic lymphadenitis or mediastinitis
3. Diagnostic Tests
   a. Blood cultures and chest x-ray are used
   b. Vaccine considered experimental
4. Treatment: Persons exposed to spores are treated prophylactically with ciprofloxacin (Cipro) or doxycycline (Vibramycin)

F. Client with fungal infection
1. Fungal spores present in air usually do not cause disease or infections
   a. Mild and self-limiting
   b. Most are opportunistic, i.e., develop in persons with compromised immune system
2. Course and manifestations similar to tuberculosis
   a. Lung lesions develop slowly and symptoms are mild
   b. Can disseminate from lungs to other organs
3. Types of fungal respiratory infections
   a. Histoplasmosis (agent: *Histoplasma capsulatum*)

1. Most common infection found in soil in U.S., associated with exposure to bird droppings and bats
2. Course: latent asymptomatic disease or primary acute, which is mild and self-limiting
3. Immunocompromised develop disseminated disease throughout body which is often fatal
   b. Coccidiomycosis (agent: *Coccidioides immitis*)
   1. Mold in soil of southwestern U.S.; usually self-limiting infection
   2. Immunocompromised develop disseminated disease; often high mortality rate from meningitis
   c. Blastomycosis (agent: *Blastomyces dermatitidis*)
   1. Occurs in south central and Midwest U.S.
   2. Lungs are primary site; untreated slowly develops into disseminated disease and progresses to fatal state
   d. Aspergillosis
   1. Rarely cause disease unless client immunocompromised
   2. Cause venous or arterial thrombosis or in lungs acute, diffuse self-limited pneumonitis
4. Collaborative Care
   a. Diagnosis by microscopic exam of sputum, blood cultures
   b. Typical changes on x-ray
5. Treatment
   a. Usually self-limiting with histoplasmosis, coccidioidomycosis
   b. Drug treatment includes oral itraconczole (Sporanox), intravenous amphotericin B
   c. Severe hemoptysis treated with lobectomy
6. Nursing Care/Home Care
   a. Education to limit risk by prevention of exposure to bird droppings
   b. General good health practice to promote immune system

III. Obstructive and Restrictive Lung Diseases
   A. Diseases are characterized by limited airflow related to
   1. Reduced lung elastic recoil
   2. Airway obstruction, which increases resistance
   3. Thickened airway walls
   4. Bronchoconstriction of smooth muscle of airways

5. Interstitial support needed for airway distention and patency is lost
6. Aging contributes to the overall process
   B. Client with asthma
   1. Chronic inflammatory disorder of airways characterized by recurrent episodes of wheezing, breathlessness, chest tightness, and coughing
   2. Risk factors (some persons develop without known risk)
      a. Allergies, especially in childhood asthma
      b. Genetic predisposition
      c. Environmental factors: air pollution, occupational exposure
      d. Respiratory viruses, exercise, emotional stress
   3. Pathophysiology
      a. Acute or early response: trigger occurs, mast cells in bronchial muscosa release histamine, prostaglandins, leukotrienes causing
         1. Bronchoconstriction
         2. Increased capillary permeability
         3. Mucosal edema and increased mucus production
      b. Late phase response: 4–12 hours later; inflammatory cells damage airway epithelium
         1. Adding to mucus production
         2. Limiting mucus clearance
         3. Prolonging bronchoconstriction
      c. Airway resistance is increased, limiting airflow and increasing work of breathing
      d. Limited expiratory airflow traps air distal to spastic airways
         1. Reduces gas exchange across alveolar-capillary membrane
         2. Hypoxemia develops which stimulates respiratory rate and leads to respiratory alkalosis
   4. Manifestations
      a. Subjective sensation of chest tightness, dyspnea, wheezing, cough
      b. Tachycardia, tachypnea, prolonged expiration
      c. Auscultation: diffuse wheezing
      d. Severe attacks: use of accessory muscles, intercostals retractions, fatigue, anxiety, apprehension, severe dyspnea
      e. Onset respiratory failure: inaudible breath sounds with reduced wheezing, ineffective cough

f. Degree and frequency of attacks vary with individual
5. Status asthmaticus
   a. Severe, prolonged asthma not responding to treatment
   b. Without effective treatment, leads to respiratory failure with hypoxemia, hypercapnea, acidosis
6. Collaborative Care
   a. Diagnosis made of history and manifestations
   b. Treatment goals are to control symptoms, prevent acute attacks
7. Diagnostic Tests: Determine degree of airway involvement during and between attacks, and identify causative factors
   a. Pulmonary function tests: evaluation of airway obstruction; severity of asthma attack gauged by measurement of forced expiratory volume and peak expiratory flow rate
   b. Challenge or bronchial provocation testing: confirm diagnosis of asthma by detecting airway hyperresponsiveness when given inhaled substance
   c. Arterial blood gases: evaluation of oxygenation and CO_2 elimination, acid-base status during acute attack
   d. Skin testing: identify allergic trigger for attacks
8. Disease Monitoring: Peak expiratory flow rate (PEF)
   a. Used on day-to-day basis
   b. Evaluates
      1. Severity of bronchial hyperresponsiveness
      2. Severity of airway obstruction
9. Preventative Measures: avoidance of allergens and triggers
   a. Modification of home environment (eliminate dust, install air filters)
   b. Removal of pets
   c. Elimination all tobacco smoke
   d. Wear mask during exercise in cold weather
   e. Early treatment of respiratory infections
10. Medications
    a. Anti-inflammatory agents
       1. Corticosteroids
          a. Block late response to inhaled allergens, reduce bronchial hyperresponsiveness
          b. Inhaled or systemic

2. Non-steroidal anti-inflammatory agents
   a. Inhibit release of mediator substances
   b. Cromolyn sodium, nedocromil
   b. Bronchodilators
      1. Adrenergic stimulants
         a. Relax smooth muscles, bronchodilation
         b. Oral or inhaled (metered dose inhaler); albuterol
      2. Methylxanthines
         a. Theophylline (oral), aminophylline (intravenous)
         b. Serum theophylline levels: therapeutic 10–20 ug/mL
      3. Anticholinergic agents: ipratropium bromide (metered dose inhaler)
   c. Leukotriene modifiers
      1. Reduce inflammatory response in asthma
      2. Oral medications: zafirlukast, zileuton
11. Complementary Therapies
    a. Herbal
    b. Biofeedback
    c. Yoga
    d. Breathing techniques
    e. Acupuncture
    f. Homeopathy
    g. Massage
12. Nursing Care: Health promotion encourage persons to stop and not start smoking
13. Nursing Diagnoses
    a. Ineffective Airway Clearance
    b. Ineffective Breathing Patterns
    c. Anxiety
    d. Therapeutic Regimen Management
14. Home Care: Educate client to
    a. Promote good health
    b. Manage acute episodes
    c. Eliminate triggers
    d. Use PEF meter
    e. Follow prescribed medications
C. Client with chronic obstructive pulmonary disease (COPD)
   1. Chronic air flow obstruction from chronic bronchitis and/or emphysema
      a. Fourth leading cause of death in U.S.
      b. Second leading cause of disability
      c. Affects middle-aged and older adults
   2. Causes and contributing factors
      a. Cigarette smoking
      b. Air pollution

c. Occupational exposure to dusts and gases
d. Airway infection
e. Genetic and familial factors

3. Pathophysiology
   a. Chronic bronchitis
      1. Excessive bronchial mucus secretion; major factor: cigarette smoking
      2. Characterized by productive cough lasting 3 or more months in 2 consecutive years
      3. Client develops narrowed airways, impaired ciliary function, recurrent infection, pulmonary HPT, right-sided heart failure
      4. Manifestations
         a. Productive cough with copious thick tenacious sputum, cyanosis
         b. Evidence of right-sided heart failure: neck vein distention, edema, liver engorgement, enlarged heart
         c. Auscultation: loud rhonchi, possible wheezes
   b. Emphysema
      1. Characterized by destruction of alveolar walls with enlargement of abnormal air spaces; major factor: cigarette smoking
      2. Enlarged air spaces causes loss of portions of pulmonary capillary bed decreasing gas exchange; loss of support tissue causes airways to collapse during expiration leading to trapped air
      3. Manifestations
         a. Insidious onset: initially dyspnea on exertion; progresses to severe dyspnea occurring at rest
         b. Anterior-posterior chest diameter increases due to air trapping, hyperinflation: barrel chest
         c. Client is often thin, tachypnic, uses accessory muscles to breath and leans forward while sitting to ease breathing
         d. Prolonged expiration; diminished breath sounds and percussion tone is hyperresonant

4. Collaborative Care
   a. Smoking abstinence is key to prevention and slowing progression
   b. Treatment focuses on symptom relief, minimizing obstruction, slowing disability

5. Diagnostic Tests
   a. Pulmonary function tests
   b. Ventilation/perfusion scan: determine level of ventilation-perfusion mismatch
   c. Serum alpha$_1$-antitrypsin level: screen for deficiency especially in persons with positive family history of obstructive airway disease (non-smoking women with early onset)
   d. Arterial blood gases
      1. Emphysema: mild hypoxemia with normal or low carbon dioxide tension
      2. Respiratory alkalosis due to increased respiratory rate
   e. Pulse oximetry
   f. Exhaled carbon dioxide (capnogram or ETCO$_2$)
      1. Measured to evaluate alveolar ventilation
      2. Increased with inadequate ventilation
      3. Decreased with impaired pulmonary perfusion
   g. CBC with differential
      1. Increased RBCs and hematocrit increased due to chronic hypoxia
      2. Increased WBC with infection
   h. Chest x-ray: shows flattening of diaphragm due to hyperinflation, presence of infection

6. Smoking cessation: only 6% successful long term

7. Medications
   a. Immunization against pneumococcal pneumonia
   b. Antibiotics for infections
   c. Bronchodilators: improve airflow and reduce air-trapping (adrenergic stimulants, anticholinergic, methylxanthine)
   d. Corticosteroids if asthma component of COPD
   e. Alpha$_1$-antitrypsin replacement therapy, if emphysema due to genetic defect; given intravenously on weekly basis

8. Treatment
   a. Remain inside during times of significant air pollution; air filters and air conditioning

   b. Pulmonary hygiene measures
      1. Hydration
      2. Effective cough: "huffing" between relaxed breathing
      3. Percussion and postural drainage
   c. Avoiding cough suppressants and sedation
   d. Regular exercise program
      1. Improve tolerance
      2. Improve ability for ADL's
      3. Prevent physical deterioration
   e. Breathing exercises to slow respiratory rate and relieve accessory muscle fatigue
      1. Pursed-lip breathing
      2. Abdominal breathing
9. Oxygen
   a. Long term therapy used for severe, progressive hypoxemia
   b. Intermittent or continuous, only at night
   c. If oxygen administered without intubation and mechanical ventilation, use with caution
      1. Clients have chronic elevated carbon dioxide levels and do not respond to that as stimulus to breathe
      2. Client only responds to low levels of oxygen as stimulus to breathe; giving high flow rates of oxygen will reduce all stimulus to breathe
10. Surgery: Lung transplantation may be only option if medical therapy not effective
11. Complementary Therapies
    a. Limit salt and dairy product intake
    b. Use of herbal teas
    c. Acupuncture
12. Nursing Care/Health Promotion: Stop or never start smoking
13. Nursing Diagnoses
    a. Ineffective Airway Clearance: prepare for intubation and mechanical ventilation, if client status is deteriorating
    b. Imbalanced Nutrition: Less than body requirements
       1. Diet high in protein and fats without excess carbohydrates to minimize carbon dioxide
       2. Specific oral supplements
    c. Compromised Family Coping
    d. Decisional Conflict: Smoking

14. Home Care: Education focuses on
    a. Effective coughing and breathing techniques
    b. Preventing exacerbations
    c. Managing prescribed therapies
D. Client with cystic fibrosis (CF)
   1. Autosomal recessive disorder that affects epithelial cells of respiratory, GI, reproductive tracts and leads to abnormal exocrine secretions
   2. Excess mucus production in respiratory tract with impaired ability to clear secretions and progressive COPD
      a. Viscous mucus plugs small airways leading to atelectasis, infection, bronchiectasis, dilation of distal airways
      b. Respiratory manifestations are cause of morbidity and death
   3. CF also involves pancreatic enzyme deficiency and impaired digestion; abnormal elevation of sodium and chloride concentrations in sweat
   4. Manifestations
      a. Recurrent pneumonia, exercise intolerance, chronic cough
      b. Clubbed fingers and toes
      c. Development of barrel chest, right-sided heart failure
      d. Abdominal pain and steatorrhea, stunted growth
   5. Diagnostic Tests
      a. Pilocarpine iontophoresis sweat chloride test
      b. Pulmonary function tests
      c. ABG and oxygen saturation levels
   6. Medications
      a. Immunizations against respiratory infections, influenza vaccine
      b. Bronchodilators
      c. Antibiotics
      d. Dornase alfa, as aerosol breaks down excess DNA in sputum
   7. Treatments
      a. Chest physiotherapy with percussion and postural drainage
      b. Oxygen therapy required for hypoxemia
      c. Genetic screening
      d. Lung transplantation
   8. Nursing Care: similar to care for other clients with COPD
   9. Home Care: extensive education and support for client and family in maintaining pulmonary function

E. Client with atelectasis
  1. Condition associated with respiratory disorders; state of partial or total lung collapse and airlessness
  2. Causes
    a. Obstruction of bronchus
    b. Compression of lung by pneumothorax, pleural effusion, tumor
    c. Loss of pulmonary surfactant
  3. Manifestations (depend on size)
    a. Diminished breath sounds
    b. Tachycardia, tachydypnea, dyspnea, fever
    c. Reduced chest expansion, absent breath sounds
  4. Diagnosis
    a. Chest x-ray shows area of airless lung
    b. CT scan may show the cause
  5. Treatment
    a. Prevention: vigorous chest physiotherapy, incentive spirometry
    b. Position client on unaffected side; frequent position change, ambulation, coughing and deep breathing
    c. Bronchoscopy to remove mucous plug
F. Client with bronchiectasis
  1. Permanent abnormal dilation of one or more large bronchi and destruction of bronchial walls
    a. Infection usually present
    b. Inflammation and airway obstruction common
    c. Occurs in clients with CF or chronic infections
  2. Manifestations
    a. Chronic cough productive with large amounts of sputum
    b. Hemoptysis, shortness of breath
    c. Malnutrition
    d. Right-sided heart failure
  3. Diagnosis
    a. History and physical examination
    b. Chest x-ray
    c. CT scan
    d. Bronchoscopy
  4. Treatment
    a. Antibiotics
    b. Bronchodilators
    c. Chest physiotherapy
    d. If unresponsive to conservative treatment, surgical lung resection
G. Client with occupational lung disease
  1. Groups of disorders related to inhalation of noxious substances in the work environment

  2. Classifications
    a. Pneumoconiosis: chronic fibrotic lung disease caused by inhalation and retention of dust and particulate matter
    b. Hypersensitivity pneumonitis: allergic pulmonary diseases in which client is allergic to organic dusts
  3. Diseases affect lung compliance
    a. Inhaled substances damage alveolar epithelium and interstitial tissue
    b. Replaced with fibrotic tissue
    c. Lungs are stiff and noncompliant
    d. Impaired alveolar–capillary diffusion and increased work of breathing
  4. Specific diseases
    a. Asbestosis: also increased risk of bronchogenic carcinoma, mesothelioma
    b. Silicosis
    c. Coal worker's pneumonconiosis ("black lung disease")
    d. Hypersensitive pneumonitis: exposure to organic dusts and gases
  5. Collaborative Care
    a. Prevention
    b. Use of personal protective devices
    c. Limiting exposure
  6. Diagnosis
    a. Chest x-ray
    b. Pulmonary function studies
    c. Bronchoscopy
  7. Home Care: education regarding pulmonary hygiene measures, vaccines, and medications
H. Client with sarcoidosis
  1. Chronic, multisystem disease in which body tissues develop granulomatous lesions which develop into fibrosis due to auto-immune response; lungs affected in 90% of cases
  2. Manifestations vary from no symptoms to all body systems being affected
  3. Diagnosis made by biopsy of granulomatous lesion; pulmonary involvement determined by chest x-ray, pulmonary function tests
  4. Treatment
    a. May resolve spontaneously
    b. Medications include corticosteroids
    c. Immunosuppressant therapy
  5. Clients with severe respiratory involvement need
    a. Supportive care
    b. Prevention of infection

c. Treatments and medications to maintain ventilation functioning
IV. Pulmonary Vascular Disorders
  A. Client with pulmonary embolism (PE)
    1. Obstruction of blood flow in pulmonary vascular system by embolus; embolus is most frequently a blood clot from deep venous thrombosis, heart, tumor, amniotic fluid, fat embolism, air, foreign substance
    2. Risk factors
      a. Prolonged immobility
      b. Trauma
      c. Myocardial infarction
      d. Obesity
      e. Advanced age
    3. Medical emergency; may be presenting manifestation of undiagnosed DVT
    4. Impact of PE depends on extent to which pulmonary blood flow is obstructed, size of embolus, secondary effects of obstruction
      a. Occlusion of large pulmonary artery: sudden death
      b. Lung tissue infarct
      c. Obstruction of small segment of pulmonary circulation: no permanent lung damage
      d. Chronic, recurrent small emboli
    5. Manifestations
      a. Asymptomatic, if very small
      b. Usually develops abruptly: dyspnea, pleuritic chest pain
      c. Anxiety, impending doom
      d. Diaphoresis, low-grade fever
      e. Hemoptysis
      f. Massive embolus results in syncope and cyanosis
    6. Collaborative Care
      a. Prevention is primary goal
      b. Measures to prevent DVT
      c. Supportive care if pulmonary embolism occurs
    7. Diagnostic Tests
      a. Plasma D-dimer levels: specific to presence of thrombus
      b. Lung scan, perfusion and ventilation
      c. Pulmonary angiography: confirm diagnosis
      d. Chest x-ray: shows pulmonary infiltration
      e. Electrocardiogram: to rule out MI; PE shows tachycardia and nonspecific T wave changes
      f. Arterial blood gases: hypoxemia (PO_2 < 80 mm Hg)
      g. Exhaled carbon dioxide ($ETCO_2$): evaluate alveolar perfusion
      h. Coagulation studies: PTT, PT (INR) to monitor response to anticoagulant therapy
    8. Medications and Treatments
      a. Anticoagulation
        1. Initially intravenous heparin; 5 days or until oral therapy is effective
        2. Oral anticoagulation with warfarin (Coumadin) for 2–3 months; long term if chronic disorder with DVT risk existing
      b. Thrombolytic therapy: may be used to treat massive pulmonary embolus with hypotension
      c. Surgery: insertion of filter into vena cava to stop emboli coming from legs
    9. Nursing Care
      a. Prevention
      b. Teach clients at high risk or history of previous DVT
        1. To stop and walk every 1–2 hours during automobile trips
        2. To do leg exercises during long flights
        3. To avoid tight hose or crossing legs
    10. Nursing Diagnoses
      a. Impaired Gas Exchange
      b. Decreased Cardiac Output
      c. Ineffective Protection: risk for bleeding with anticoagulant therapy
    11. Home Care: education regarding anticoagulant therapy, recognition of recurrent PE
  B. Client with pulmonary hypertension
    1. Abnormal elevation of pulmonary arterial pressure
    2. Occurs as primary disorder rarely in females in 30–40's, but commonly occurs as secondary (from another condition)
    3. Results from reduced size of pulmonary vascular bed due to vasoconstriction or widespread vessel obstruction of damage
    4. Possible causes
      a. Hypoxemia resulting from chronic lung diseases, sleep apnea, hypoventilation
      b. Alveolar wall destruction with emphysema
      c. Vessel obstruction from large or multiple PE
    5. Manifestations (may be masked by those of underlying condition)
      a. Dyspnea
      b. Retrosternal chest pain
      c. Fatigue and syncope on exertion

6. Corpulmonale
   a. Condition of right ventricular hypertrophy and failure resulting from long standing pulmonary hypertension
   b. Manifestations are related to pulmonary disorder and right-sided heart failure
   c. Chronic productive cough, progressive dyspnea, wheezing; skin is warm moist and cyanotic and ruddy (hypoxemia and increased RBCs)
7. Diagnostic Tests
   a. CBC: polycythemia
   b. ABG: hypoxemia
   c. ECG: changes consistent with right ventricular hypertrophy
   d. Echocardiogram: changes occurring with pulmonary HPT
   e. Doppler ultrasonography: estimate of pulmonary artery pressure
   f. Cardiac catheterization: definitive diagnosis
8. Treatment (none particularly effective to reverse or slow disease)
   a. Treatment of underlying disease process
   b. Calcium channel blockers: reduce pulmonary vascular resistance and improve cardiac output
   c. For acute episodes: short acting direct vasodilators: intravenous adenosine or prostacyclin or inhaled nitric oxide
   d. Surgery: bilateral lung or heart-lung transplant
9. Nursing Care/Home Care
   a. Largely supportive
   b. Teaching client and family to deal with
      1. Chronic condition
      2. Manifestations of hypoxemia and heart failure and associated complications
      3. Transplant or terminal diagnosis, depending on situation

V. Lung cancer
   A. Description
      1. Leading cause of cancer deaths in U.S.: 31% males and 25% females
      2. Causative factors
         a. Incidence increases with age (over 50)
         b. Cigarette smoking > 80% related to smoking
         c. Exposure to ionizing radiation, inhaled irritants (asbestos)
      3. Lung cancer usually well advanced at time of diagnosis with metastasis

      4. Most persons die within one year of initial diagnosis
      5. Five year survival rate is 15%
   B. Pathophysiology
      1. Primary lung lesions: bronchogenic carcinoma, tumor occurs in airway epithelium
      2. Aggressive, locally invasive, widespread metastasis
      3. Types
         a. Small-cell carcinomas
            1. 25% of lung cancers: grow rapidly, spread early
            2. Paraneoplastic properties: tumors produce ACTH, ADH, parathormone-like hormone, gastrin-releasing peptide
         b. Non-small-cell carcinomas
            1. Includes adenocarcinoma, squamous cell, large-cell carcinoma
            2. Account for 75% of lung cancers
   C. Manifestations: Related to location and spread of tumor
      1. Initial symptoms often attributed to smoking or chronic bronchitis: chronic cough, hemoptysis, wheezing, shortness of breath
      2. Dull, aching chest pain developing into pleuritic pain
      3. Hoarseness and dysphagia (pressure on trachea, esophagus)
      4. Systemic and paraneoplastic manifestations
         a. Weight loss, anorexia, fatigue, weakness
         b. Bone pain, tenderness, swelling
         c. Clubbing of fingers and toes
         d. Symptoms of endocrine, cardiovascular function
      5. Metastasis manifestations
         a. Brain: confusion, impaired gait and balance, headache, personality changes
         b. Bone: bone pain, pathologic fractures, spinal cord compression, thrombocytopenia and anemia
         c. Liver: jaundice, anorexia, RUQ pain
      6. Superior vena cava syndrome: partial or complete obstruction of superior vena cava
         a. Edema of neck and face
         b. Headache, dizziness, visual disturbances, syncope
         c. Veins of upper chest and neck are dilated
         d. Cerebral edema symptoms, laryngeal edema

D. Collaborative Care
1. Emphasis is on prevention: no smoking
2. Treatment decisions are based on tumor location, type and staging of tumor, client's overall state of health to tolerate treatment
3. Staging consists of tumor size, location, degree of invasion, presence of metastatic disease
E. Diagnostic Tests
1. Chest x-ray: often first evidence of lung cancer
2. Sputum specimen for cytologic examination: first morning sputum for presence of malignant cells
3. Bronchoscopy: visualize and obtain tissue for biopsy; bronchial washing to obtain cells if tumor not visualized
4. CT scan: evaluate and locate tumors (for needle biopsy); detect distant metastasis, evaluate tumor response to treatment
5. Cytologic examination and biopsy: aspiration of fluid from pleural effusion, percutaneous needle biopsy, lymph node biopsy
6. CBC, liver function studies, electrolytes including calcium: evidence of metastasis or paraneoplastic syndromes
F. Medications and Treatments
1. Combination chemotherapy
a. Treatment of choice for small cell lung cancer
b. 50% of persons in early stages achieve complete remission and improved survival
c. Used as adjunct to surgery and radiation therapy
2. Surgery
a. Most tumors are inoperable or only partially respectable
b. Goal is to remove as much involved tissue as much as possible and reserve functionable lung
3. Radiation therapy
a. Used alone or with surgery and/or chemotherapy
b. Goal is cure or symptom relief (palliative)
c. May be done prior to surgery to debulk tumors
d. May be used to lessen manifestations from bone or brain metastasis; superior vena cava syndrome
G. Nursing Diagnoses
1. Ineffective Breathing Pattern
2. Activity Intolerance
3. Pain

4. Anticipatory Grieving
H. Home Care
1. Client and family education regarding disease, expected prognosis, and planned treatment strategies
2. Referrals for home care, hospice, American Cancer Society
VI. Disorders of the Pleura
A. Pleuritis
1. Inflammation of pleura
a. Irritation of sensory fibers of parietal pleura causes characteristic pain
b. Often results from another condition such as pneumonia, rib injury
2. Manifestations
a. Onset is abrupt
b. Pain is unilateral and well-localized
c. Sharp and may be referred to neck, shoulder
d. Aggravated by breathing, coughing, movement
3. As a result, client breathes shallowly, rapid and limits chest movement; pleural friction rub may be heard over area
4. Diagnosis is by manifestations; chest x-ray and ECG may be done to rule out other causes of chest pain
5. Treatment is symptomatic: analgesics such as NSAID's (non-steroidal anti-inflammatory drugs) such as indomethacin, Codeine; splint chest while coughing, positioning
B. Client with a pleural effusion
1. Collection of excess fluid in pleural space, which normally contains 10–20 mL serous fluid
2. Occurs with local disease, such as lung cancer, pneumonia or systemic disease, such as heart failure, liver or renal disease
3. Pathophysiology
a. Pleural fluid may be transudate: formed when capillary pressure is high or plasma proteins are low
b. Pleural fluid may be exudate: result of increased capillary permeability
c. Collections of specific fluids in pleural cavity
1. Empyema: pus
2. Hemothorax: blood
3. Hemorrhagic pleural effusion: blood and pleural fluid
4. Manifestations
a. Dyspnea due to compressed lung tissue
b. Pleuritic pain relieved when effusion forms

c. Diminished or absent breath sounds, dull percussion tone over affected area; chest wall movement may be limited

5. Diagnostic Tests
   a. Chest x-ray: fluid collects at base of affected lung or lateral wall
   b. CT scan or ultrasounds may be used to localize
   c. Thoracentesis: invasive procedure where fluid is removed with needle and analyzed for content including abnormal cells or culture if indicated
      1. May be done to improve breathing if effusion is large and causes dyspnea
      2. Done under local anesthesia and can be done at bedside
      3. Usually remove only 1200–1500 mL at a time
      4. Potential complication: pneumothorax

6. Treatment
   a. Depends on cause
   b. Recurrent effusions, often due to cancer, may be treated by instillation of irritant such as doxycycline or talc

7. Nursing Care: Education of client, if prone to reoccurrence, to be aware of developing manifestations

C. Client with pneumothorax
   1. Accumulation of air in pleural space
   2. Pathophysiology
      a. When either visceral or parietal pleura are breached, air enters pleural space
      b. Lung expansion is impaired and lung collapses
   3. Spontaneous pneumothorax
      a. Develops when air-filled bleb or blister on lung surface ruptures; rupture allows air to enter pleural space
      b. Types
         1. Primary (simple)
            a. Occurs in healthy persons usually tall thin men 16–24
            b. Cause unknown
            c. Benign but reoccurrences are common
         2. Secondary
            a. Overdistention and rupture of alveolus
            b. Affects persons with COPD
            c. More serious and life threatening

c. Manifestations (dependent on size, extent of lung collapse, any underlying lung disease)
   1. Pleuritic chest pain, shortness of breath at rest
   2. Increased respiratory and heart rate
   3. Asymmetrical chest wall movement
   4. Absent lung sounds, hyperresonant to percussion

4. Traumatic pneumothorax
   a. Result of blunt or penetrating trauma
      1. Closed: often due to fractured ribs
      2. Open (sucking chest wound): penetrating chest trauma
      3. Iatrogenic cause (post thoracentesis or central line insertion, mechanical ventilation)
   b. Manifestations of pain and dyspnea may be attributed to other injuries; hemothorax often occurs with traumatic pneumothorax

5. Tension pneumothorax
   a. Injury to chest wall or lungs allows air to enter pleural space but prevents it from escaping making positive pressure in pleural space
   b. Lung on affected side collapses and pressure on mediastinum shifts thoracic organs to unaffected side
   c. Severely compromised ventilation, impaired venous return to heart: medical emergency requiring immediate intervention
   d. Manifestations
      1. Same as pneumothorax
      2. Plus
         a. Hypotension
         b. Neck vein distention
         c. Tracheal displacement

6. Diagnostic Tests
   a. Chest x-ray: diagnostic
   b. ABGs may be done to assess gas exchange

7. Treatment
   a. Dependent upon severity of problem
      1. Small ones: may involve serial x-rays to monitor resolution without intervention
      2. Symptomatic requires insertion of chest tubes (thoracostomy)
   b. Thoracostomy: placement of closed-chest catheter to allow lungs to re-expand
      1. Chest tube under "water seal" or closed drainage system; low suction

applied to re-establish negative
pressure in pleural space
2. Heimlich (one-way valve) may also
be inserted
3. Emergency treatment for tension
pneumothorax: insertion of large
bore needle to relieve pressure on
mediastinum
c. Pleurodesis
1. Creation of adhesions between
parietal and visceral pleura to
prevent recurrent pneumothorax
2. Instillation of chemical agent
(doxycycline) to cause
inflammation and scarring
d. Surgery: surgical creation of adhesions
or partially excise parietal pleura
8. Health Promotion: prevent smoking and
accidents
9. Nursing Diagnoses
a. Impaired Gas Exchange
b. Risk for Injury: maintenance of chest
tube keeping drainage system lower
than the chest; especially during
ambulation
10. Home Care
a. Risk of recurrence 40–50% after single
episode of spontaneous pneumothorax
b. May be advised to avoid change in
altitude
c. Avoid contact sports
d. Seek medical assistance if
manifestations occur
D. Client with hemothorax
1. Blood in pleural space resulting from
chest trauma, surgery, diagnostic
procedures
2. Blood collection results in impaired
ventilation and gas exchange, risk of
shock
3. Manifestations are similar to
pneumothorax; diminished lung sounds
and dull percussion tone
4. Diagnosis is made by chest x-ray
5. Treatment includes insertion of chest
tube; blood replacement if significant loss
(may be replaced by autotransfusion in
which blood collected in chest tube and
then reinfused within 4 hours as with
planned thoracic surgery)
VII. Chest and Lung Trauma
A. Client with a thoracic injury
1. Most thoracic trauma caused by motor
vehicle collisions or falls; most are either
acceleration/deceleration or crush injuries

2. Injuries depend on velocity at point of
impact, part of body involved, previous
health status of individual
3. Rib fracture
a. Simple rib fracture most common
chest wall injury
1. Resolves with supportive treatment
in healthy persons
2. May develop serious complications,
in older persons or those with
preexisting lung disease
b. Displaced fractured ribs may cause
pneumothorax or hemothorax
c. Particular rib fractures associated with
specific organ injuries
1. First and second ribs: torn
intrathoracic vessels
2. Ribs 7–10: liver, spleen injuries
d. Manifestations
1. Pain on inspiration, coughing
2. Voluntary splinting, rapid and
shallow breathing, inhibited
cough, diminished breath sounds
over area
3. Palpable crepitus over area, bruising
4. Flail chest
a. Multiple rib fracture in which 2 or
more consecutive ribs are fractured in
multiple places creating free-floating
segment of chest wall
b. Paradoxic chest movement: flail
segment sucked inward during
inspiration, outward during exhalation;
work of breathing increased
c. Associated with underlying pulmonary
contusion
d. Manifestations
1. Pain and dyspnea on inspiration
2. Paradoxic chest movement
3. Palpable crepitus
4. Diminished breath sounds
5. Pulmonary contusion (lung tissue injury)
a. Often results from abrupt chest
compression: rupture of alveoli and
pulmonary arterioles with
hemorrhage and interstitial and
bronchial edema
b. May result in airway obstruction,
atelectasis, impaired gas diffusion
impacting ability to clear secretions
and breathe
c. Manifestations:
1. Appear 12–24 hours after injury
2. Increasing shortness of breath,
restlessness, chest pain

3. Copious sputum, possibly blood tinged
4. May lead to ARDS, death
6. Diagnostic Test
   a. Chest x-ray used to identify most chest wall injuries
   b. ABG and oxygen saturation used to identify altered ventilation and gas exchange
7. Treatment
   a. Rib fracture: adequate analgesia, rib belt, binders, taping
   b. Flail chest and pulmonary contusion: often requires intubation and mechanical ventilation; intensive care management
8. Nursing Diagnoses
   a. Acute Pain
   b. Ineffective Airway Clearance
   c. Impaired Gas Exchange: hyperoxgenation prior to suctioning; fluid management to control pulmonary edema
9. Home Care
   a. Rib fractures are often managed at home
   b. Significant pulmonary contusion can result in long-term insufficiency requiring home health referral
   c. Client and family education regarding care of chronic respiratory problem
B. Client with inhalation injury
   1. Pulmonary injury due to inhalation of hot air, toxic gases, or particulate matter
      a. Leading cause of death in burn injury
      b. Suspected when fire occurs in closed space, burns of face, upper torso or singed nasal hairs
   2. Smoke inhalation affects normal respiration
      a. Thermal damage to airways (impaired ventilation)
      b. Carbon monoxide or cyanide poisoning (tissue hypoxia)
      c. Chemical damage (impaired gas exchange)
   3. Near-drowning
      a. Aspiration and asphyxiation primary problems
         1. Fluid aspiration leads to asphyxia and hypoxemia
         2. "Dry drowning" asphyxia due to laryngospasm
         3. Loss of consciousness in 3–5 minutes after total immersion; brain injury, death in 5–10 minutes

4. Immersion in very cold water body tolerates longer periods of hypoxemia: dive reflex: protective mechanism slows heart beat, constricts peripheral vessels shunting blood to brain and heart
      b. Fresh water near-drowning
         1. Water is hypotonic
         2. Leads to hypervolemia, hemodilution resulting in hemolysis (acute renal failure) and dilution of electrolytes (dysrhythmias)
      c. Salt water near-drowning
         1. Water is hypertonic
         2. Leads to hypovolemia and hemoconcentration
      d. Risk of pneumonia exists with both due to inhaled microorganisms and debris
      e. Manifestations
         1. Altered level of consciousness, restlessness, apprehension
         2. May develop pulmonary edema, shock
         3. Hypothermia may also be present
         4. Improved prognosis if no, or very short, loss of consciousness
   4. Collaborative Care
      a. Prevention: use of smoke detectors, safe boating and swimming; avoidance of alcohol with water activities
      b. Education to remove victim from area of fire or water and administer CPR
      c. If victim, hypothermic continue resuscitation until core temperature reaches 90°F
   5. Diagnostic Tests
      a. ABG's evaluate air exchange, level of hypoxemia
      b. Carboxyhemoglobin levels: suspected carbon monoxide poisoning
      c. Electrolytes, osmolality: near drowning
      d. Chest x-ray: changes occur > 12 hours; acute respiratory distress syndrome may develop 24–48 hours
      e. Bronchoscopy: inspection of lung tissue damage
   6. Treatments
      a. Supportive: supplemental oxygen and may require endotracheal intubation and mechanical ventilation
      b. Hyperbaric oxygen therapy for carbon monoxide poisoning
      c. Bronchodilator therapy, coughing and suctioning, chest physiotherapy

d. Careful fluid therapy, frequent assessment, monitor for complications
7. Nursing Diagnoses
   a. Ineffective Airway Clearance
   b. Impaired Gas Exchange
   c. Ineffective Tissue Perfusion: Cerebral
8. Home Care
   a. Education regarding signs of respiratory failure
   b. Home health referrals as indicated
   c. Significant hypoxia can result in long term neurological deficits interfering with client independence

VIII. Acute Respiratory Failure
A. Description
1. Consequence of severe respiratory dysfunction: lungs are unable to oxygenate blood and remove carbon dioxide
2. Definition in terms of arterial blood gas values
   a. Arterial oxygen level (Po_2) < 50–60 mm Hg
   b. Arterial carbon dioxide (Pco_2) > than 50 mm Hg
3. Clients with advanced COPD may be alert and functional with blood gas values indicating what would be failure in persons with normal respiratory function; failure in these clients is indicated by acute drop in oxygen levels and increased carbon dioxide levels
4. Common causes
   a. COPD most common cause
   b. Chest injury, inhalation trauma, neuromuscular disorders, cardiac conditions
B. Pathophysiology
1. Hypoxemia, without corresponding rise in carbon dioxide levels, indicates failure of oxygenation
2. Hypoxemia with hypercapnia result of lung hypoventilation
C. Prognosis varies with underlying cause, often worse for clients with underlying lung conditions
D. Manifestations
1. Hypoxemia
   a. Dyspnea and neurologic symptoms (restlessness, apprehension, impaired judgment, motor impairment)
   b. Initially tachycardia and HPT
   c. May progress to dysrhythmias, hypotension, decreased cardiac output

2. Hypercapnea
   a. Dyspnea and headache early
   b. Decreased level of consciousness, peripheral vasodilation, neuromuscular irritability
   c. As condition worsens: reduced dyspnea and slowed respirations
   d. Administration of oxygen to this client will eliminate any drive to breathe
E. Diagnostic Tests
1. Exhaled carbon dioxide: evaluate alveolar ventilation; normal $ETCO_2$: 35–45 mm Hg
2. Arterial blood gases:hypoxemia, carbon dioxide retention, pH and acidosis
F. Medications
1. Medications that promote bronchodilation
2. Corticosteroids to reduce airway edema
3. Antibiotics to treat infections
4. Medications used to control pain and anxiety associated with mechanical ventilation
   a. Benzodiazepines: diazepam (Valium), lorazepam (Ativan), midazolam (Versed)
   b. Intravenous morphine or fentanyl: analgesia and inhibit respiratory drive
   c. Neuromusclular blocking agents to induce paralysis and suppress ability to breathe if client is breathing against the ventilator
G. Oxygen Therapy
1. Goal: achieve oxygen saturation of 90% or > without oxygen toxicity
2. Po_2 of 60 mm Hg adequate to meet oxygen needs of body tissues
3. May require only small amounts of oxygen (1–3 L by cannula in advanced COPD)
4. High concentrations are limited to short periods to avoid oxygen toxicity
5. Continued high oxygen concentrations impair synthesis of surfactant, lead to reduced lung compliance and may lead to development of ARDS or absorption atelectasis
6. Continuous positive airway pressure (CPAP) may be used with hypoventilation
H. Airway Management
1. Intubation is necessary if upper airway is obstructed or positive pressure mechanical ventilation is necessary
2. Endoctracheal tube extends from mouth or nose to trachea and has cuff which when inflated obstructs airway,

preventing escape of air; cuffs are low pressure to decrease likelihood of tissue ischemia
3. If long-term ventilatory support is needed, tracheostomy is done; associated risks include cuff necrosis and infection
4. When client is able to breathe without ventilator, may be extubated, tube removed after cuff deflated
5. Risk of respiratory distress and laryngeal edema post extubation
6. Must have gag, cough, swallow reflexes to prevent aspiration

I. Indications for Mechanical Ventilation
1. Apnea or acute respiratory failure
2. Hypoxemia unresponsive to oxygen therapy alone
3. Increased work of breathing with progressive client fatigue

J. Nursing Care/Health Promotion
1. Client education to prevent respiratory failure, including hazards of smoking, fire prevention
2. Preventative measures for clients with chronic respiratory conditions

K. Nursing Diagnoses
1. Impaired Spontaneous Ventilation
2. Ineffective Airway Clearance
3. Risk for Injury
4. Anxiety
5. Impaired Communication (client is on ventilator)

L. Home Care: Education regarding factors leading to respiratory failure and measures to prevent reoccurrence

IX. Background information for caring for clients on mechanical ventilation
A. Types of ventilators
1. Negative pressure: creates subatmosheric pressure externally to draw chest outward and air into lungs mimicking normal breathing; Examples: iron lung, Curiass ventilator, PulmoWrap
2. Positive-pressure ventilator: pushes air into lungs
   a. Requires endotracheal tube or tracheostomy
   b. Commonly used, especially in acute respiratory failure
   c. Trigger: prompts ventilator to deliver breath
      1. Client's inspiratory effort: ventilator-assisted breath
      2. Preset time: ventilator-controlled breath
   d. Cycle: duration of inspiration
      1. Preset volume: delivered: volume controlled ventilator
      2. Preset pressure achieved in airway: pressure-cycled ventilator
      3. Preset inspiratory flow rate: flow-cycled ventilators
      4. Set time interval: time-cycled ventilators
   e. Airflow limited by airway pressure

B. Modes commonly used with positive-pressure ventilators
1. Assist-control mode ventilation (ACMV)
   a. Triggered by inspiratory effort but will deliver preset number of breaths per minute; all breaths are delivered at specific tidal volume or pressure and inspiratory flow rate
   b. Used to initiate mechanical ventilation and when client at risk for respiratory arrest
2. Synchronized intermittent mandatory ventilation (SIMV)
   a. Allows client to breathe spontaneously between preset rate of ventilator breaths (with preset rate, volume or pressure) that is coordinated with client's inspiratory efforts
   b. Used during weaning from ventilator
3. Continuous positive airway pressure (CPAP)
   a. Applies positive pressure to airways of spontaneously breathing client
   b. Used with either endotracheal intubation of tight-fitting face mask
   c. All breathing spontaneous and pressure controlled
   d. Used to help maintain open airways and alveoli: decreases work of breathing
4. Positive end-expiratory pressure (PEEP)
   a. Requires intubation and may be applied in addition to one of first 3 modes
   b. Positive pressure maintained in airways during exhalation and between breaths
   c. Improves ventilation-perfusion relationship and diffusion across alveolar-capillary membrane
   d. Reduces hypoxemia and allows lower percentage of inspired oxygen
   e. Useful in treating acute respiratory distress syndrome
   f. Causes decrease in cardiac output

5. Pressure support ventilation (PSV)
   a. Ventilator assisted breaths are delivered whenever client makes inspiratory effort; no mandatory breaths given by ventilator
   b. Cycle is flow-limited, inspiration terminated when inspiratory airflow falls below preset rate; decreases work of breathing
   c. Use in combination with SIMV when respiratory drive depressed
   d. Useful with weaning
6. Pressure-controlled ventilation (PCV)
   a. Controls pressure within airways to risk airway trauma
   b. All breaths are controlled by ventilator; client may require heavy sedation
7. Noninvasive ventilator (NIV)
   a. Ventilator support using tight-fitting facemask, no intubation
   b. Success depends on ability of client to tolerate mask while dyspneic
C. Ventilator settings
   1. Rate: number of respirations per minute; initially 12–15
      a. With ACMV or SIMV, client's rate usually higher than ventilator rate
      b. Rate changed according to ETCO$_2$, whether client is showing hypoventilation or hyperventilation
   2. Tidal volume: the amount of gas delivered with each ventilator breath
      a. Normal adult tidal volume at rest is 400–550 mL
      b. Ventilator normally set slightly higher
      c. Too high causes lung tissue trauma
   3. Percentage of oxygen (FiO$_2$): amount of oxygen delivered with ventilator breaths
      a. Sufficient to maintain oxygen saturation and PO$_2$ in acceptable ranges (oxygen saturation level usually > 90% except clients with long-standing COPD)
      b. Prolonged delivery of high oxygen increases risk of oxygen toxicity and pulmonary fibrosis
D. Complications of mechanical ventilation
   1. Improper endotracheal tube placement or advancement into mainstem bronchus which results in ventilation and overdistention of one lung while the other develops atelectasis
   2. Nonsocomial pneumonia: lower airways contaminated within 24 hours of intubation
3. Barotrauma: lung injury due to alveolar overdistention
   a. Alveoli rupture and results in subcutaneous emphysema, pneumonthorax or pneumomediastinum
   b. Subcutaneous emphysema (air in subcutaneous tissue) can be palpated under skin: chest, face, neck
   c. Pneumothorax requires immediate insertion of chest tube to avoid tension pneumothorax and cardiovascular compromise
4. Decreased cardiac output: decreased venous return to heart and ventricular filling, which can affect liver and kidney circulation
5. Effects on GI system
   a. Stress ulcers or erosive gastritis: treated with histamine H$_2$ receptor blockers
   b. Gastric distension: client usually has nasogastric tube
   c. Constipation
E. Care of client on ventilator
   1. Continuous monitoring of ventilator function by respiratory therapy
   2. Continuous oxygen saturation, frequent pulmonary assessment
   3. Client needs suctioning of respiratory secretions with sterile technique (inline suction catheters), hyperoxygenation before, no longer than 10 seconds
   4. Emotional support and sedation to client as necessary
   5. Means of communication for client if alert (writing tablet, picture board)
F. Weaning from the ventilator
   1. Process of removing ventilator support and reestablishing spontaneous respirations
   2. Underlying problem for respiratory failure must be corrected or stabilized
   3. Parameters used to determine if client ready for weaning
      a. Vital signs
      b. Respiratory rate
      c. Dyspnea, blood gas, and oxygen saturation
      d. Overall clinical status
   4. May use T-piece or CPAP for weaning if ventilator time is short
      a. With T-piece client removed off ventilator for short periods with oxygen delivered with T-piece

  b. Vital signs: oxygen saturation, $ETCO_2$, PO_2 monitored; when well-tolerated extubated
 5. SIMV and PSV are used when client has been on ventilator for longer time
  a. SIMV of 4 tolerated
  b. PSV gradually lowered
  c. May then use T-piece or CPAP
  d. When weaning process completed client is extubated
 6. Terminal weaning is gradual withdrawal of ventilation when survival without assisted ventilation is not expected
  a. Client and/or family participate in decision with physician
  b. May be given analgesia or sedation to provide comfort

X. Client with acute respiratory distress syndrome (ARDS)
 A. Characterized by noncardiac pulmonary edema and progressive refractory hypoxemia
 B. Severe form of respiratory failure with mortality rate around 50%
 C. Pathophysiology
  1. Acute lung injury resulting from an unregulated systemic inflammatory response, which damages the alveolar-capillary membrane
  2. Increased interstitial pressure and damage to alveolar membrane allow fluid to enter alveoli, which dilutes and deactivates surfactant
  3. Atelectasis occurs, lungs become less compliant and gas exchange impaired
  4. Hyaline membrane forms and lungs become fibrotic
  5. Hypoxemia becomes refractory and resistant to improvement even with supplemental oxygen
  6. Metabolic acidosis occurs leading to multiple organs system dysfunction

 D. ARDS develops about 24–48 hours post initial insult
  1. Early manifestations: dyspnea, tachypnea, anxiety
  2. Client increases respiratory rate and uses accessory muscles
  3. Client becomes cyanotic and client develops crackles
  4. Continued respiratory failure results in mental confusion
 E. Diagnostic Tests
  1. ABG: hypoxemia with $PO_2 < 60$ mmHg and respiratory acidosis
  2. Chest x-ray: after 24 hours of onset shows diffuse infiltrated and then white out period
  3. Pulmonary function tests show decreased lung compliance and reduced vital capacity
  4. Pulmonary artery pressure shows normal pressure in ARDS; differentiates ARDs from pulmonary edema
 F. Treatment
  1. Intubation and mechanical ventilation with oxygen set to maintain $PO_2 > 60$ mm HG and oxygen saturation is 90%
  2. Prone positioning
  3. Careful fluid balance
  4. Treat underlying problem
 G. Nursing Diagnoses
  1. Decreased cardiac output
  2. Dysfunctional ventilator weaning response
 H. Home Care
  1. Often long hospitalization including intensive care
  2. Extended recovery with referral for home health care for support

FOCUSED STUDY TIPS

- Contact the local chapter of the American Lung Society. Identify resources for clients who wish to quit smoking.
- In your clinical setting, identify clinical pathways for care of the client with active TB (tuberculosis). Observe precautions taken to prevent the spread of the disease.
- Interview a client utilizing home oxygen therapy. Describe safety precautions utilized to prevent accidents within the home setting.

CASE STUDY

J. T. is 2 hours post operative for bilateral knee replacements. He has a history of chronic bronchitis. What nursing interventions can be implemented to prevent postoperative pneumonia and atelectasis?

CARE PLAN CRITICAL THINKING ACTIVITY

A client presents to the clinic complaining of chest pain. He appears acutely ill, and you begin your assessment immediately. What manifestations will the client exhibit that will help to differentiate among a pulmonary embolus, myocardial infarction, and pneumonia? What necessary equipment and/or responses are necessary in each of these disorders? What diagnostic tests can you anticipate?

NCLEX TEST QUESTIONS

1. A client who is being treated for tuberculosis is at risk for which nutrient deficiencies?
   a. vitamins C and A
   b. vitamin B_6 and niacin
   c. all fat-soluble vitamins
   d. all water-soluble vitamins

2. A client is admitted to the unit after a traumatic encounter with a bull that speared his right chest wall. The client is admitted with a flail chest and is treated accordingly. The nurse should be aware of the sudden changes that may be evidence of which of the following complications?
   a. hypercapnia
   b. sepsis
   c. adult respiratory distress syndrome
   d. metabolic acidosis

3. In planning care for a client, the nurse understands that pulmonary hypertension is a more severe condition than essential hypertension because
   a. an underlying condition may be masking the symptoms of pulmonary hypertension.
   b. the low resistance in the pulmonary vascular system makes the diagnosis more difficult to detect.
   c. the pulmonary artery pressure rises significantly high before a systolic increase occurs.
   d. the pulmonary vasculature thins and can rupture in pulmonary hypertension.

4. A 42-year-old male is admitted to the unit with a diagnosis of pneumonia. After not responding well to treatment, he is later diagnosed with *pneumocystis carinii* pneumonia. The nurse should place him in isolation because he:
   a. is positive for human immunodeficiency virus (HIV).
   b. has acquired immunodeficiency syndrome (AIDS).
   c. has tuberculosis (TB).
   d. has an infection of unknown origin.

5. The child with cystic fibrosis should take pancrelipase (Pancrease) how often?
   a. three times daily
   b. after each loose stool
   c. as ordered
   d. with each meal and snack

6. The client with cystic fibrosis is currently being treated for pneumonia. The nurse caring for the client is attempting to decrease the viscosity of the respiratory secretions. What nursing intervention is the best for liquefying secretions?
   a. increase daily fluid intake
   b. chest physiotherapy
   c. tobramycin aerosol treatment
   d. albuterol aerosol treatment

7. CDC (Centers for Disease Control) guidelines are specific for clients with tuberculosis (TB). The major differences in providing care for the client with TB versus other clients requiring barrier nursing are that
   a. the staff must wear gowns, masks, and gloves.
   b. the client should be in a private room with a special ventilation system.
   c. the client may be placed in a room with other clients requiring barrier nursing protocol.
   d. the protocol of donning and removing isolation garb before entering or leaving the client's room is different.

8. A client has chronic respiratory acidosis caused by end-stage chronic obstructive pulmonary disease (COPD). Oxygen is delivered at 1 L/min per nasal cannula. The nurse teaches the family that the reason for this precaution is to avoid respiratory depression, based on which of the following as the best explanation?
   a. COPD clients depend on a low oxygen level.
   b. COPD clients depend on a low carbon dioxide level.
   c. COPD clients tend to retain hydrogen ions if they are given high doses of oxygen.
   d. COPD clients thrive on a high oxygen level.

9. When assessing a client with early impairment of oxygen perfusion, such as in pulmonary embolus, the nurse would expect to find anxiety,

apprehension, and which of the following symptoms?

  a. warm, dry skin

  b. bradycardia

  c. tachycardia

  d. eupnea

10. A client has a chest tube inserted for a pneumothorax. The nurse assesses the drainage system for adequacy. Which of the following signifies that the system is working correctly?

  a. There is no fluctuation in the water-seal compartment.

  b. Constant bubbles are noted in the water-seal compartment without fluctuation.

  c. There are no bubbles noted in the water-seal compartment.

  d. There is fluctuation in the water-seal compartment coinciding with respirations.

CHAPTER **37**

ASSESSING CLIENTS WITH MUSCULOSKELETAL DISORDERS

LEARNING OUTCOMES

After completing this chapter, you will be able to:

- Review the anatomy and physiology of the musculoskeletal system.
- Describe the normal movements allowed by synovial joints.
- Identify specific topics for consideration during a health history interview of the client with health problems involving the musculoskeletal system.
- Describe physical assessment techniques for musculoskeletal function.
- Identify abnormal findings that may indicate impairment of the musculoskeletal system.

KEY TOPICS

- Review of anatomy and physiology of the musculoskeletal system
- Assessing musculoskeletal functioning

LECTURE OUTLINE

I. Background of Anatomy and Physiology
   A. Human skeleton made up of 206 bones
      1. Axial skeleton includes
         a. Bones of skull
         b. Ribs and sternum
         c. Vertebral column
      2. Appendicular skeleton includes
         a. Bones of limbs
         b. Shoulder girdles
         c. Pelvic girdle

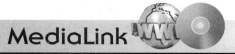
MediaLink

www.prenhall.com/lemone

Additional resources for this chapter can be found on the Student CD-ROM accompanying this textbook, and on the Companion Website at www.prenhall.com/lemone. Click on Chapter 37 to select the activities for this chapter.

CD-ROM
- Audio Glossary
- NCLEX Review

Animation
- Musculoskeletal A&P

Companion Website
- More NCLEX Review
- Functional Health Pattern Assessment
- Case Study
   Knee Pain

   B. Functions of bones
      1. Form structure and provide support for soft tissues
      2. Protect vital organs from injury
      3. Serve to move body parts by providing points of attachment for muscles

4. Store minerals
5. Serve as site for hematopoiesis
C. Bone cells include
  1. Osteoblasts: cells that form bone
  2. Osteocytes: cells that maintain bone matrix
  3. Osteoclasts: cells that resorb bone
D. Bone matrix: extracellular element of bone tissue
  1. Composed of
    a. Collagen fibers
    b. Minerals (mainly calcium and phosphate)
    c. Proteins, carbohydrates, ground substance
  2. Ground substance: gelatinous material that facilitates diffusion of nutrients, wastes, gases between blood vessels and bone tissue
  3. Periosteum: double-layered connective tissue that covers bones
    a. Outer layer: blood vessels and nerves
    b. Inner layer: anchored to bone
E. Bones are composed of rigid connective tissue: osseous tissue
  1. Compact bone is smooth and dense
    a. Haversian system (osteon): basic structural unit of compact bone
    b. Composed of
      1. Central canal (Haversian canal)
      2. Concentric layers of bone matrix (lamellae)
      3. Spaces between lamellae (lacunae)
      4. Osteocytes within lacunae
      5. Small channels (canaliculi)
  2. Spongy bones contains spaces between meshworks of bone
    a. Lamellae are arranged in concentric layers (trabeculae) that branch and join to form meshworks
    b. Red marrow cavities: spongy sections of long bones and flat bones contain tissue for hematopoesis (sternum, humerus, head of femur)
F. Bones classified according to shape
  1. Long bones are longer than they are wide
    a. Parts
      1. Diaphysis: midportion of shaft; composed of compact bone and contains marrow cavity, lined with endosteum
      2. Epiphyses (2 broad ends)
      3. Composed of spongy bone, covered by thin layer of compact bone
    b. Bones of arms, legs, fingers, toes

2. Short bones (cuboid bones)
  a. Composed of spongy bone covered by compact bone
  b. Bones of wrist and ankle
3. Flat bones: thin and flat, most are curved
  a. Consists of layer of spongy bone between 2 thin layers of compact bone
  b. Bones of skull, sternum, and the ribs
4. Irregular bones: various shapes and sizes
  a. Consists of layer of plates of compact bone with spongy bone between
  b. Vertebrae, scapulae, bones of pelvic girdle
G. Bone remodeling in adults
  1. Bones of adults do not normally increase in length and size but constant remodeling occurs
  2. Bone remodeling process: bone resorption and bone deposit occur at all periosteal and endosteal surfaces
    a. Involves combined action of osteocytes, osteoclasts, osteoblasts
      1. Bones in use (subjected to stress) increase osteoblastic activity to increase ossification (bone development)
      2. Inactive bones undergo increased osteoclast activity and bone resorption
    b. Hormonal stimulus controlled by negative feedback mechanism that regulates blood calcium levels
      1. When blood calcium decreases, parathyroid hormone (PTH) released: osteoclast activity stimulated and bone resorption so calcium released from bone matrix; calcium levels rise and PTH releases ends
      2. When blood calcium rise, secretion of calcitonin from thyroid gland, inhibit bone resorption, cause deposit of calcium salts in bone matrix
      3. Calcium ions required for
        a. Transmission of nerve impulses
        b. Muscle contraction
        c. Blood clotting
        d. Glandular secretion
        e. Cell division
      4. 99% of calcium in body present as bone minerals
    c. Bone remodeling regulated by gravitational pull and mechanical stress from pull of muscles

1. Bones that undergo increased stress are heavier and larger
2. Wolff's law: bone develops and remodels to resist stresses placed on it

H. Joints (articulations)
1. Regions where 2 or more bones meet, hold bones of skeleton together and allow movement
2. Types
   a. Fibrous: permit little or no movement e.g., sutures of skull
   b. Cartilaginous
      1. Composed of hyaline cartilage growths that fuse together articulating bone ends and are immobile, e.g., sternocostal joints of rib cage (immobile)
      2. Composed of hyaline cartilage growths that fuse to intervening plate of flexible fibrocartilage, e.g., intervertebral discs (allows for flexibility)
   c. Synovial
      1. Enclosed by cavity filled with synovial fluid (filtrate of blood plasma)
      2. Freely movable; e.g., limb joints
      3. Characteristics of synovial joints
         a. Articular surfaces covered with articular cartilage
         b. Joint cavity enclosed by tough, fibrous, double-layered articular capsule; internally cavity is lined with synovial membrane that covers surfaces not covered by articular cartilage
         c. Synovial fluid fills free spaces of joint capsule, enhancing smooth movement of articulating bones
         d. Allow many kinds of movements

I. Ligaments: dense band of connective tissue connecting bone to bone
1. Limit or enhance movement
2. Provide joint stability
3. Enhance joint strength

J. Tendons: fibrous connective tissue bands connecting muscles to periosteum of bones
1. Enable bones to move when skeletal muscles contract
2. When muscles contract, increased pressure causes tendon to pull, push, or rotate the bone when it is connected

K. Bursae
1. Small sacs of synovial fluid that cushion and protect bony areas at high risk for friction such as knee or shoulder
2. Tendon sheaths which are wrapped around tendons in high-friction areas are a form of bursae

L. Muscles: Skeletal muscle that allows musculoskeletal function
1. Thick bundles of parallel contractile cells called fibers; each fiber made up of myofibrils giving striated appearance containing myosin and actin
2. Functional properties
   a. Excitability
   b. Contractibility
   c. Extensibility
   d. Elasticity
3. Skeletal muscle movement
   a. Triggered when motor neurons release acetylcholine which alters permeability of muscle fiber; action potential causes muscle contraction
   b. More fibers that contract, stronger contraction of entire muscle
4. Prolonged strenuous activity
   a. Causes continuous nerve impulses
   b. Results in buildup of lactic acid, reduced energy in muscle, or muscle fatigue
   c. Regular exercise increases size and strength of muscles; lack of use results in muscle atrophy
5. Skeletal muscles
   a. Promote body movement
   b. Help maintain posture
   c. Produce body heat
   d. Are moved by conscious voluntary control or reflex activity
   e. 600 skeletal muscles in body

II. Assessing Musculoskeletal Function
A. Health assessment interview to collect subjective data
1. May involve neurologic system
2. Define health problem involving bones or muscles regarding
   a. Onset
   b. Characteristics and course
   c. Severity, precipitating, and relieving factors
   d. Associated manifestations including timing and circumstances
3. Altered function of musculoskeletal system: Pain and limited mobility

   a. Location and nature
   b. Associated manifestations: fever, fatigue, changes in weight, rash, swelling
   c. Lifestyle
      1. Type of employment
      2. Ability for ADL
      3. Exercise, participation in sports
      4. Use of alcohol, drugs, nutrition
      5. Past injuries
      6. Measures used in self-treatment
B. Physical assessment to collect objective data
   1. Gait and body posture assessment with abnormal findings
      a. Changes: joint stiffness, pain, deformities, muscle weakness
      b. Flattened lumbar curve, decreased spinal mobility: herniated lumbar discs
      c. Increased lumbar curve (lordosis): obesity or pregnancy
      d. Lateral, S-shaped curvature (scoliosis): functional scoliosis is compensatory response to painful paravertebral muscles, herniated discs, discrepancy in leg length
      e. Exaggerated thoracic curvature (kyphosis): common in older adults
   2. Joint assessment with abnormal findings
      a. Deformities such as tissue loss, tissue overgrowth, contractures, irreversible shortenings of muscles and tendons: joint disease
      b. Obvious bulging joint: edema in joint
      c. Redness, swelling pain: inflammation or infection in joint
      d. Joint pain: inflammation or injury
      e. Painful, hot joints: arthritis, bursitis, tendonitis, osteomyelitis
      f. Crepitation (grating sound) in joint: articulating surfaces have lost cartilage as with arthritis
   3. Range of motion (ROM) assessment of head, jaw, spine with abnormal findings
      a. Clicking or popping noises, decreased ROM, pain, swelling in temporomandibular joint: temporomandibular joint syndrome or osteoarthritis
      b. Neck pain and limited extension with lateral bending: herniated cervical discs and cervical spondylosis
      c. Immobile neck with head and neck thrust forward: ankylosing spondylitis
      d. Decreased movement or painful movement: abnormal spinal curvature, arthritis, herniated disc, spasm of paravertebral muscles
   4. Range of motion (ROM) assessment of hands, fingers with abnormal findings
      a. Decreased flexion and extension of fingers: arthritis
      b. Heberden's nodes and Bouchard's nodes on dorsolateral parts of distal and proximal interphalangeal joints are common in osteoarthritis
      c. Stiff, painful, swollen finger joints: acute rheumatoid arthritis
      d. Boutonniere and swan-neck deformities: chronic rheumatoid arthritis
      e. Swollen finger joints with white chalky discharge: chronic gout
      f. Bilateral chronic swelling in wrist: arthritis
   5. Range of motion (ROM) assessment of elbow, shoulder with abnormal findings
      a. Swollen tender inflamed elbows: gouty and rheumatoid arthritis
      b. Pain and tenderness at lateral epicondyle: tennis elbow
      c. Pain and tenderness over biceps tendon: tendonitis
      d. Limited arm abduction: rupture of supraspinatus tendon of shoulder
      e. Pain and limited abduction: bursitis, calcium deposits
   6. Range of motion (ROM) assessment of toes, ankles, knees, hips with abnormal findings
      a. Excessive abduction of great toe: hallux valgus
      b. Joint above great toe is swollen, inflamed, painful: gouty arthritis
      c. Hyperextension of metatarsophalangeal joint and flexion of proximal interphalangeal joint: hammer toes
      d. Contracture of achilles tendon: clients with rheumatoid arthritis following prolonged bed rest
      e. Swelling over suprapatellar pouch seen with inflammation and fluid in articular capsule of knee: synovitis with knee trauma
      f. Limited or painful hip movement: arthritis
   7. Special assessment with abnormal findings
      a. Numbness and burning in fingers during Phalen's test: carpel tunnel syndrome

b. Various amounts of fluid on knee: soft tissue swelling

c. Pain, locking (inability to fully extend knee) or popping sound: injury to meniscus in knee

d. Positive Thomas test: hip flexion contracture

FOCUSED STUDY TIPS

- Perform a ROM (range of motion) assessment on a young adult and an elderly client. Compare and contrast assessment findings. Identify implications of assessment findings on nursing care.
- Visit a pharmacy and identify equipment available to aid clients with musculoskeletal disorders. Describe the functioning of each piece of equipment identified.
- At a shopping mall, study gait patterns of different individuals. Compare and contrast differences. Speculate factors contributing to these differences.
- Visit the physical therapy department in your clinical setting. Observe treatment plans and therapies. Identify equipment and skills training that maximize independent functioning.

CASE STUDY

A client with right knee trauma presents to the clinic. The physician asks you to assess the knee for ROM and increased fluid. How will you carry out this instruction? Differentiate between health assessment interview techniques and physical assessment techniques.

CARE PLAN CRITICAL THINKING ACTIVITY

How will you assess a client diagnosed with temporomandibular joint syndrome? What are reportable assessment findings?

NCLEX TEST QUESTIONS

1. The nurse is assessing the capillary refill time of a client who has a leg cast. When compressing one of the client's toenails and releasing the compression, the nurse would expect the color to return to the nail within:
   a. 1 second.
   b. 3 seconds
   c. 10 seconds.
   d. 15 seconds.
2. For a client who has ataxia, which of the following tests would be performed to assess the ability to ambulate?
   a. Kernig's
   b. Romberg's.
   c. Riley-Day's.
   d. Hoffmann's.
3. After a fall from the bed, a client complains of loss of warmth in the foot. The assessment technique the nurse should perform following inspection of the foot would be to
   a. palpate the pedal pulses.
   b. palpate for sensation of touch.
   c. palpate for any bony deformities.
   d. percuss the bony prominence.
4. The nurse is assessing the client for signs of hypocalcemia. The nurse assesses for:
   a. a negative Chvostek's sign.
   b. a positive Trousseau's sign.
   c. a positive Kernig's sign.
   d. hypoactive bowel sounds.
5. The nurse concludes that decreased deep tendon reflexes found in a client are associated with which of the following conditions?
   a. diuresis from medication therapy
   b. increased magnesium level
   c. decreased magnesium level
   d. decreased sodium level
6. Which of the following occurs during the remodeling phase of bone healing?
   a. Callus formation occurs
   b. Callus is replaced with mature bone
   c. Osteoclasts resorb excess callus to return the bone to its original shape

d. Proliferation of osteoblast and fibroblasts occurs within the hematoma at the fracture site

7. The nurse observes that a female client has asymmetry of the shoulder, hips, and tail/hem of her dress. The nurse suspects that the client may be presenting with which of the following disorders?

a. congenital hip dislocation

b. scoliosis

c. a fractured tibia

d. degenerative disc disease

8. The nurse assessing a client with osteoarthritis notes finger deformities on the proximal and distal interphalangeal joints. The nurse documents this common finding as which of the following in the medical record?

a. interphalangeal drift and ulnar deviation

b. Boutonniere deformity

c. Heberden's and Bouchard nodes

d. Swan neck deformity

9. A client presents to the emergency department with multiple injuries caused by a motor vehicle accident. The nurse suspects that the client may have a right fractured hip after noting which of the following distinctive signs?

a. The client reports increased pain with movement of the limb.

b. There is bruising over the right hip.

c. The right leg is shorter than the left leg.

d. The right leg is longer than the left leg.

10. The nurse is assessing a client with hypercalcemia. The nurse expects a neuromuscular examination to show

a. tetany.

b. a positive Trousseau's sign.

c. muscle weakness.

d. hyperactive deep tendon reflexes.

CHAPTER 38

NURSING CARE OF CLIENTS WITH MUSCULOSKELETAL TRAUMA

LEARNING OUTCOMES

After completing this chapter, you will be able to:

- Apply knowledge of normal anatomy, physiology, and assessments when providing care for clients with musculoskeletal trauma (see Chapter 37).
- Explain the factors that lead to musculoskeletal trauma and amputations.
- Describe the pathophysiology, manifestations, complications, and collaborative care for clients with contusions, strains, sprains, fractures, amputations, and repetitive use injury.
- Describe the stages of bone healing.
- Explain the purposes and related nursing interventions for casts, traction, and stump care.
- Use the nursing process as a framework for providing individualized care for clients who have experienced musculoskeletal trauma.

KEY TOPICS

- Traumatic injury of the muscles, ligaments, and joints
- Traumatic injuries of the bones
- Repetitive use injuries
- Nursing care of clients with musculoskeletal trauma

LECTURE OUTLINE

I. Client with Contusion, Strain, Sprain (soft tissue trauma)
   A. Definitions
      1. Contusion: bleeding into soft tissue resulting from blunt force

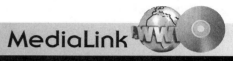

MediaLink

www.prenhall.com/lemone

Additional resources for this chapter can be found on the Student CD-ROM accompanying this textbook, and on the Companion Website at www.prenhall.com/lemone. Click on Chapter 38 to select the activities for this chapter.

CD-ROM
- Audio Glossary
- NCLEX Review

Animation
- Bone Healing
- Fracture Repair

Companion Website
- More NCLEX Review
- Case Study
   A Client with Fractures
- Care Plan Activity
   Below-the-Knee Amputation
- MediaLink Applications
   Preventing Musculoskeletal
   Injuries

      2. Hematoma: contusion with a large amount of bleeding
      3. Strain: stretching injury to a muscle or muscle-tendon unit caused by mechanical overloading

a. Most common sites: lower back and cervical region of spine

b. Manifestations: pain increasing with isometric contraction, swelling and stiffness

4. Sprain: injury to ligament surrounding a joint; overstretch and/or tear

 a. Most common: ankle and knee

 b. Manifestations: joint instability, pain, rapid swelling

B. Treatment

1. Rest, immobilization, ice for first 24–48 hours post injury

2. Compression dressing, elevation above level of heart

3. More severe injuries may require surgery, physical therapy

C. Diagnostic Tests

1. X-ray to rule out fracture

2. MRI to further assess if necessary

D. Medications: Analgesics and NSAIDs

E. Nursing Diagnoses

1. Acute pain

2. Impaired Physical Mobility

II. Client with Joint Dislocation

A. Loss of articulation of the bone ends in the joint capsule following severe trauma

1. Most common site: shoulder acromicoclavicular joints

2. Subluxation: partial dislocation

B. Pathophysiology: May be congenital, traumatic, or pathologic

C. Manifestations

1. Pain

2. Deformity

3. Limited motion

D. Diagnostic Tests

1. Physical examination

2. X-ray

E. Collaborative Care

1. Focus

 a. Pain relief

 b. Correction of dislocation

 c. Prevention of complications

2. Shoulder dislocation treatment includes immobilization with sling for several weeks followed by rehabilitation

3. Hip: usually requires immediate reduction in emergency room to prevent necrosis to head of femur and sciatic and femoral nerve damage

F. Nursing Diagnoses

1. Acute Pain

2. Impaired Physical Mobility

3. Risk for Injury

G. Home care usually involves prolonged immobilization and aggressive rehabilitation

III. Client with a Fracture

A. Fracture: Any break in continuity of bone

1. Occurs when bone is subjected to more kinetic energy than the bone can absorb

2. Mechanisms producing fracture

 a. Direct: energy applied at or near site of fracture

 b. Indirect: transmitted from point of impact to site where bone is weaker

3. Classifications of fractures

 a. Simple (closed) skin intact over fracture or compound (open) where skin is interrupted over injury and there is increased risk for infection

 b. Fracture line may be

  1. Oblique: at 45-degree angle to bone

  2. Spiral: curves around the bone

  3. Avulsed: occurs when fracture pulls bone and other tissues away from point of attachment

  4. Comminuted: bone breaks in many small pieces

  5. Compressed: bone is crushed

  6. Impacted: broken bone ends are forced into each other

  7. Depressed: broken bone is forced inward

 c. Complete fracture involves entire width of bone; incomplete fracture does not involve the entire width of bone

 d. Stable (nondisplaced) fracture is fracture in which bones maintain their anatomic alignment; unstable (displaced) fracture: fracture in which bones move out of correct anatomic alignment

 e. Description according to point of reference i.e., midshaft, intrarticular

4. Manifestations

 a. May be accompanied by soft tissue injuries involving muscles, arteries, veins, nerves, skin

 b. May be alteration in circulation, sensation, swelling, pain

 c. May be obvious deformity or fracture

 d. May have felt the breakage of bone during the injury event

5. Fracture healing

 a. Phases include

  1. Inflammatory phase

   a. Bleeding and inflammation develop at site of fracture

b. Hematoma forms around the bone surface

c. Necrosis of osteocytes leads to vasodilation and edema

d. Collagen forms and allows calcium to be deposited

2. Reparative phase

a. Callus begins to form

b. Osteoblasts promote formation of new bone

c. Osteoclasts destroy dead bone and assist in synthesis of new bone

3. Remodeling phase

a. Excess callus is removed

b. New bone is laid down along the fracture line

c. Eventually fracture site is calcified and bone is reunited

b. Healing of fracture influenced by

1. Age and physical condition of client

2. Type of fracture

c. Time

1. Uncomplicated fracture of arm or foot heals in 6–8 weeks

2. Fractured hip heals in 12–16 weeks

6. Emergency care involves

a. Immobilization of fracture

1. Immobilize above and below the deformity

2. Splint to maintain normal anatomical alignment and prevent further dislocation or damage

3. Use air splint or splint to body

b. Maintenance of tissue perfusion

1. Control obvious bleeding with pressure dressing

2. Assessment of pulses, movement, sensation; any alteration requires prompt medical evaluation

c. Prevention of infection: Cover open wounds with sterile dressing

7. Diagnostic Tests

a. History of incident and initial assessment

b. X-ray of bones involved in fracture

c. Additional tests as indicated: CBC, blood chemistries, coagulation studies to assess for blood loss, renal function, muscle breakdown, excessive bleeding or clotting

8. Medications

a. Pain relief according to degree of injury and client's assessment of pain (may require narcotics)

b. NSAID's for anti-inflammatory affect as well as analgesia

c. Medications to guard against ulcers

d. Stool softeners to prevent constipation

e. Antibiotics especially with open fractures

f. Anticoagulants, if client considered at risk for deep vein thrombosis

9. Treatments

a. Surgery

1. Indications

a. Requires direct visualization and repair

b. Fracture associated with long-term complications

c. Severely comminuted fracture, which threatens vascular supply

2. Types

a. External fixation: external fixator (frame connected to pins inserted into long axis of bone) maintains immobilization of fracture but increases independence of client

b. Internal fixation: surgical procedure open reduction internal fixation (ORIF); involves reducing fracture and applying hardware (pins, nails, screws, or plates) to hold bones in place

b. Traction: application of straightening or pulling force to maintain or return fractured bones in normal alignment; prevent muscle spasms

1. Weights are used to maintain necessary force

2. Types of traction

a. Manual: by hand

b. Straight: pulling force in straight line; Buck's traction: straight skin traction often used with fractured hip

c. Balanced suspension: involves more than one force of pull

d. Skeletal: application of pulling force through placement of pins into the bone; allows use of more weight to maintain alignment; increased risk of infection

c. Casting: rigid device applied to immobilize bones and promote healing

1. Extends above and below the fractured bone which must be relatively stable

2. Types include
   a. Plaster: 48 hours needed to dry
   b. Fiberglass: dries within one hour
d. Electrical bone stimulation: application of electrical current at the fracture site; used to treat fractures that are not healing properly
   1. Increases migration of osteoblasts and osteoclasts to fracture site
   2. May be accomplished invasively or noninvasively
   3. Contraindicated in presence of infection
10. Complications
   a. Compartment syndrome: excess pressure in limited space, constricting structures within and reducing circulation to muscles and nerves; normal pressure is 10–20 mm Hg
      1. Results from hemorrhage and edema following a fracture or crush injury or external compression of limb, if cast is too tight
      2. May result in cyclic ischemia and edema increasing risk for loss of limb or sepsis
      3. Usually develops within first 48 hours of injury
      4. Manifestations include progressive pain often distal to injury not responsive to analgesia, decreased sensation, loss of movement; pulses may remain normal
      5. Interventions
         a. Bivalve or removal of cast
         b. Internal pressure is treated by fasciotomy, surgical incision in which muscle fascia is cut to relieve pressure within that compartment
      6. Volkmann's contracture: occurs with elbow fracture; contracture and degeneration of muscle limiting mobility are from compartment syndrome
   b. Fat Embolism Syndrome (FES)
      1. Fat globules lodge in pulmonary vascular bed or peripheral circulation: occurs with long bone fracture, pressure within bone marrow rises, exceeds capillary pressure, and fat globules leave bone marrow and enter circulation
      2. Manifestations: characterized by neurologic dysfunction, pulmonary

insufficiency, petechial rash on chest, axilla, and upper arms within few hours or week after injury
      3. May result in pulmonary edema, atelectasis, ARDS
      4. Prevention: early stabilization of long-bone fractures
   c. Deep vein thrombosis (DVT): blood clot forms in lining of large vein; can lead to pulmonary embolism
      1. Prevention: early immobilization of fracture and early ambulation
      2. Prophylactic anticoagulation, antiembolism stocking, and compression boots
      3. Prompt diagnosis of DVT and adequate treatment
   d. Infection: any complication decreasing blood supply increases risk; may result from contamination at time of injury or during surgery
      1. Organisms include Pseudomonas, Staphylococcus or Clostridium
      2. May lead to osteomyelitis, infection within the bone
   e. Delayed union: prolonged healing of bones beyond usual time period
      1. Risk factors include
         a. Poor nutrition
         b. Inadequate immobilization
         c. Prolonged reduction time
         d. Infection, necrosis, age
         e. Immunosuppression
         f. Severe bone trauma
      2. Detected by serial x-rays (x-ray findings lag 1–2 weeks behind the healing process)
   f. Nonunion
      1. Persistent pain and movement at fracture site
      2. Treatments
         a. Surgery: internal fixation, bone grafting
         b. Debridement if infection present
         c. Electrical stimulation
   g. Reflex sympathetic dystrophy
      1. Poorly understood post-traumatic condition
      2. Manifestations of persistent pain, hyperesthesias, swelling, changes in skin color, texture, temperature, and decreased motion
      3. Treatment includes sympathetic nerve block

B. Fractures of specific bones or bony areas
  1. Fracture of skull: Displacement noted; depressed skull fracture
     a. May put pressure on brain causing neurologic deficit
     b. May require surgical intervention
  2. Fracture of facial bones
     a. Assure airway is not compromised
     b. Severely displaced fractures are treated with open reduction and internal fixation with wires or plates
  3. Fracture of spine
     a. Most severe complication is spinal cord injury
     b. Displaced cervical fracture reduced with manual or skeletal traction, brace application
     c. May require surgical stabilization
  4. Fracture of the clavicle
     a. Client often assumes a protective slumping position to immobilize arm and avoid shoulder movement
     b. Treatment includes application of clavicular strap or surgery
  5. Fracture of humerus: Location of the fracture within humerus determines type of treatment
  6. Fracture of elbow
     a. Complications include nerve or artery damage and hemarthrosis, collection of blood in elbow joint
     b. Volkmann's contracture
  7. Fracture of radius and/or ulna: Treatments include casting or surgery
  8. Fracture of wrist and hand
     a. Colles's fracture: distal radius fractures after a fall onto outstretched hand
     b. Often treated with closed reduction, cast application
  9. Fracture of rib
     a. Simple rib fracture treated with analgesia and instructions regarding coughing, deep breathing, and splinting
     b. More serious rib fracture causes flail chest, often requiring intubation and mechanical ventilation
  10. Fracture of pelvis
     a. Simple fracture: bed rest on a firm mattress
     b. More than 2 fracture sites usually requires surgery with application of external fixator
     c. Complications include hypovolemia, spinal injury, injury involving urinary or GI systems
  11. Fracture of shaft of femur
     a. Manifested by painful deformed edematous thigh with inability to move hip or knee
     b. Priority to assess circulation to extremity
     c. Complications include hypovolemia (may lose 10000–1500 mL of blood), fat embolism, hip or knee dislocation
     d. Treatment
        1. Initially skeletal traction
        2. Followed by external or internal fixation
  12. Fracture of hip
     a. Classifications
        1. Intracapsular: fractures of the head or neck of femur; greater risk of nonunion and avascular necrosis
        2. Extracapsular: fractures of trochanter region
     b. Cause greatest number of deaths and health problems; high risk for postmenopausal females who have greatest incidence of osteoporosis
     c. Most persons are hospitalized for 2 weeks post hip fracture and are unable to return home after the fracture (reside in a nursing home or assisted living facility)
     d. Risk is higher in older adults due to decrease in bone mass and increased tendency to fall
     e. Manifestations: pain, shortening of affected leg, external rotation
     f. Treatment often includes
        1. Traction (frequently Buck's traction) to decrease muscle spasms
        2. Surgery: ORIF using hardware to secure femur
        3. Fractures of femoral neck often disrupts blood supply to head of femur; surgery may be hemiarthroplasty (replacement of either femoral head or acetabulum with prosthesis)
  13. Fracture of tibia and/or fibula
     a. Common complications of fracture include
        1. Damage to peroneal nerve or tibial artery
        2. Compartment syndrome
        3. Hemarthroses
        4. Ligament damage
     b. Closed fracture: closed reduction with casting

14. Fracture of ankle and foot: most fractures treated by closed reduction and casting

C. Nursing Care involved with fractures includes management of
   1. Pain
   2. Impaired physical mobility
   3. Impaired tissue perfusion
   4. Neurovascular compromise
   5. Assessment of client's response to trauma

D. Health Promotion
   1. Emphasis is trauma prevention
   2. Maintain good bone health including weight-bearing exercise, avoiding obesity, adequate calcium intake

E. Nursing Diagnoses
   1. Acute Pain
   2. Risk for Peripheral Neurovascular Dysfunction
   3. Risk for Infection
   4. Impaired Physical Mobility
   5. Risk for Disturbed Sensory Perception: tactile

F. Home Care: Client and family teaching focuses on individualized needs
   1. Cast care
   2. Following physician's directions regarding weight bearing
   3. Home physical therapy referral
   4. Obtaining needed equipment

IV. Client with an Amputation
A. Partial or total removal of body part resulting from traumatic event or chronic condition

B. Causes of amputation
   1. PVD is major cause
   2. Trauma is major cause of upper extremity amputation
   3. Other traumatic events resulting in amputation include frostbite, burns, electrocution

C. Underlying cause of amputation is interruption in blood flow either acute or chronic

D. Levels of amputation
   1. Determined by local (ischemia and gangrene) and system factors (cardiovascular status, renal function, severity of diabetes mellitus)
   2. Goals
      a. Alleviate symptoms
      b. Maintain healthy tissue
      c. Increase functional outcome: joints are preserved whenever possible to allow for greater function

E. Types of amputation
   1. Open (guillotine): performed when infection is present and remains open to drain
   2. Closed (flap): wound is closed with flap of skin sutured in place over stump

F. Amputation site healing
   1. Immediate postoperative: assess circulation to stump
   2. Rigid or compression dressing is applied to prevent infection and minimize edema
   3. Stump is wrapped in Ace bandage to allow a conical shape to form and prevent edema applied from distal to the proximal extremity

G. Complications
   1. Infection:
      a. Local
         1. Drainage or odor
         2. Redness
         3. Positive wound culture
         4. Increased discomfort at suture line
      b. Systemic
         1. Fever, chills
         2. Increased heart rate or decreased blood pressure
         3. Positive wound or blood cultures
   2. Delayed healing
      a. Slower rate of healing than normal
      b. Factors include
         1. Poor or inadequate nutrition
         2. Poor blood flow, possibly related to smoking
         3. Decreased cardiac output limits circulation
   3. Chronic stump pain
      a. Results from neuroma formation causing severe burning pain
      b. Treatments include
         1. Medications
         2. Nerve blocks
         3. Transcutaneous electrical nerve stimulation (TENS)
         4. Surgical stump reconstruction
   4. Phantom limb pain/phantom limb sensation
      a. Majority of amputees have sensations such as tingling, numbness, cramping or itching in the phantom foot or hand, often self-limited
      b. Phantom limb pain is pain often difficult to treat; may be referred to pain clinic for comprehensive pain management

5. Contracture
   a. Abnormal flexion and fixation of joint caused by muscle atrophy and shortening
   b. Common complication associated with above the knee amputation
   c. Interventions include
      1. Lying prone for periods throughout day
      2. Active and passive range of motion
      3. Avoid prolonged sitting
6. Prosthesis
   a. Type depends on level of amputation, client's occupation and lifestyle
   b. Client with lower extremity amputation often fitted with early walking aids: pneumatic device that fits over stump and allows early ambulation, decreased postoperative swelling
7. Nursing Diagnoses
   a. Acute Pain
   b. Risk for Infection
   c. Impaired Skin Integrity
   d. Risk for Dysfunctional Grieving
   e. Disturbed Body Image
   f. Impaired Physical Mobility
8. Home Care: education and information for client and family regarding stump care, prosthesis fitting and care, assistive devices, exercises, rehabilitation, safety issues

V. Client with Repetitive Use Injury
   A. Carpal tunnel syndrome
      1. Compression of median nerve as result of inflammation and swelling of synovial lining of tendon sheaths
      2. Manifestations
         a. Numbness and tingling of thumb, index finger, lateral ventral surface of middle finger
         b. Pain interfering with sleep and relieved by massage and shaking hands and fingers
         c. Weakness and inability to hold items or perform precise activities
   B. Bursitis
      1. Inflammation of bursa: enclosed sac found between muscles, tendons, bony prominences especially in shoulder, hip, leg, and elbow
      2. Manifestations
         a. Involved joint is tender, hot, red, edematous
         b. Pain upon flexion or extension of joint
   C. Epicondylitis
      1. Inflammation of tendon at point of origin into the bone
      2. Common ailments include tennis elbow, golfer's elbow with point tenderness and pain radiating down the dorsal surface of forearm
   D. Collaborative Care
      1. Pain relief
      2. Increasing mobility
   E. Diagnostic Tests
      1. History and physical examination
      2. Phalen test for carpel tunnel syndrome
   F. Medications
      1. Often NSAID's
      2. Corticosteroid injections
   G. Treatments
      1. Conservative: immobilization with splinting, rest, ice or heat application; ergonomic evaluation of workplace
      2. Surgery
         a. Carpal tunnel syndrome: resection of carpal ligament to enlarge the tunnel
         b. Epicondylitis, bursitis: removal of calcium deposits from area surrounding tendon or bursa
   H. Nursing Diagnoses
      1. Acute Pain
      2. Impaired Physical Mobility
   I. Home Care
      1. Rehabilitation to return to state of independence
      2. Teaching client to avoid activities that increase risk of redeveloping injury

FOCUSED STUDY TIPS

▪ Interview a family member or friend who has experienced musculoskeletal trauma. Ask him or her to identify initial emergency care. Ask him or her to share information regarding pain control during initial emergency care. Share information with classmates.

▪ Practice adjusting crutches for different-size classmates. Demonstrate with accuracy weight-bearing and non-weight-bearing crutch gaits.

- Participate in the application of a cast. Identify measures taken to preserve skin integrity. Perform a circulatory assessment of the affected limb. Identify normal and abnormal findings.

CASE STUDY

T. C. has a long bone fracture, which places him at risk for FES (fat embolism syndrome). His caregiver asks what FES means. What do you tell her? What signs and symptoms do you ask her to monitor? What interventions should she make if any of those signs and symptoms occur? How can FES be prevented?

CARE PLAN CRITICAL THINKING ACTIVITY

Create plans of care to prevent contractures for a client with an above-the-knee amputation and a client with a below-the-knee amputation. Describe all nursing interventions and give a rationale for each.

NCLEX TEST QUESTIONS

1. A client on bed rest for the past 48 hours secondary to a fractured femur presents with tachycardia and a petechial rash. The nurse attributes these symptoms to
   a. deep vein thrombosis (DVT).
   b. fat emboli.
   c. hypovolemic shock.
   d. allergic reaction to medication.

2. An 86-year-old client has Buck's traction applied for a fractured hip. The nursing assessment is to ensure that there is adequate countertraction, which will include:
   a. weights hanging freely off the floor and bed.
   b. ropes knotted to prevent them from moving through the pulleys.
   c. checking that the client is pulled down on the bed, using the end board as a foot rest.
   d. checking that the foot of the bed is elevated to provide countertraction.

3. When wrapping the extremity of a client who has had an above-the-knee amputation, the nurse would start the bandage
   a. around the waist.
   b. on the thigh of the amputated leg.
   c. just above the level of the amputation, moving in a figure-eight fashion.
   d. on the thigh of the amputated leg, proceeding with a circular wrap.

4. A young male client has had a cast placed on his right leg. While caring for the client, the nurse identifies a hot spot or area on the cast that feels warm. The nurse reports to the physician the signs of:
   a. poor ci prculation.
   b. the cast being too tight.
   c. uneven cast drying.
   d. infection.

5. To determine if a client is experiencing compartment syndrome, which of the following is a priority area for nursing assessment?
   a. assessing for edema at the fracture site
   b. palpation of a pulse at the fracture site
   c. performing a pain assessment
   d. assessing for the presence of drainage on the cast

6. A 4-year-old child has been casted for a fractured radius. When evaluating circulation in the casted extremity, the finding that requires immediate notification of the physician is:
   a. a radial pulse of 100.
   b. complaints of pain in the affected arm.
   c. cold, pale fingers.
   d. increasing irritibility of the child.

7. The nurse is preparing to discharge a client who sustained a hip fracture. The nurse should teach the client to avoid which of the following groups of activities to prevent dislocation of the hip?
   a. crossing legs, bending at hips, and sitting on low toilet seats
   b. taking leisurely walks, using low chair seats, and bending at hips
   c. using reachers for applying shoes and socks and sitting in chairs with arms
   d. all exercises, bed rest, and using raised toilet seats

8. A 55-year-old client had a total hip replacement yesterday. In order to facilitate recovery, the nurse should
    a. elevate the client's legs on pillows and keep them in an adducted position.
    b. place the affected leg in traction and limit motion.
    c. position pillows or supports to maintain the hip in an abducted position.
    d. remove any braces, supports, or pillows while turning.

9. Which statement indicates that a client who is instructed to apply an ice pack to a sprained ankle requires further teaching?
    a. "I should keep the leg elevated whenever possible."
    b. "The pack should be padded with a towel or cloth."
    c. "The cold pack should be applied once per day."
    d. "I should expect some swelling even after the application."

10. A nurse on an orthopedic unit is planning care for a group of clients. When planning the prevention of complications, the nurse considers that the major cause of death after fracture of a long bone is:
    a. gas gangrene.
    b. tetanus.
    c. fat embolism.
    d. avascular necrosis.

CHAPTER 39

NURSING CARE OF CLIENTS WITH MUSCULOSKELETAL DISORDERS

LEARNING OUTCOMES

After completing this chapter, you will be able to:

- Apply knowledge of normal anatomy, physiology, and assessments when providing care for clients with musculoskeletal disorders (see Chapter 37).
- Explain the pathophysiology, manifestations, and complications of metabolic, degenerative, autoimmune, inflammatory, infectious, neoplastic, connective tissue, and structural musculoskeletal disorders.
- Describe the collaborative care, with related nursing care, of clients with musculoskeletal disorders.
- Provide appropriate nursing care for the client having musculoskeletal surgery.
- Use the nursing process as a framework for providing individualized care to clients with musculoskeletal disorders.

KEY TOPICS

- Metabolic disorders of the musculoskeletal system
- Degenerative disorders of the musculoskeletal system
- Autoimmune and inflammatory disorders of the musculoskeletal system
- Infectious disorders of the musculoskeletal system
- Neoplastic musculoskeletal disorders
- Connective tissue disorders of the musculoskeletal system
- Structural disorders of the musculoskeletal system
- Nursing care of clients with musculoskeletal disorders

MediaLink

www.prenhall.com/lemone

Additional resources for this chapter can be found on the Student CD-ROM accompanying this textbook, and on the Companion Website at www.prenhall.com/lemone. Click on Chapter 39 to select the activities for this chapter.

CD-ROM
- Audio Glossary
- NCLEX Review

Companion Website
- More NCLEX Review
- Case Study
    Rheumatoid Arthritis
- Care Plan Activity
    Lower Back Pain
- MediaLink Application
    Osteoporosis Prevention

LECTURE OUTLINE

I. Metabolic disorders
   A. Background
      1. Normal bone remodeling process involves sequence of bone reabsorption and formation
      2. Adults replace about 25% of trabecular bone (the porous type of bone found in the spine and all articulating joints) every 4 months through reabsorption of old bone by osteoclasts and formation of new bone by osteoblasts
   B. Client with osteoporosis
      1. Definition
         a. Disorder characterized by loss of bone mass, increased bone fragility, increased risk for fractures
         b. Imbalance of processes that influence bone growth and maintenance; associated with aging, but may result from endocrine disorder or malignancy
         c. Significant health threat for Americans: estimated 28 million persons; more common in aging women: half of women over 50 experience osteoporosis-related fracture in lifetime (hip, wrist, vertebrae)
      2. Risk Factors
         a. Risk of developing osteoporosis depends on amount of bone mass achieved between ages 25–35
         b. Unmodifiable risk factors
            1. Aging: decrease in osteoblastic and osteoclastic activity related to decreasing levels of hormones (estrogen in females; testosterone in males)
            2. Gender: women have 10–15% less peak bone mass than men; bone loss begins earlier (30's) and proceeds more rapidly (before menopause)
            3. European Americans and Asians have less bone density than African Americans
            4. Endocrine disorders affecting metabolism: hyperthyroidism, hyperparathyroidism, Cushing's syndrome, diabetes mellitus
         c. Modifiable risk factors
            1. Calcium deficiency: insufficient calcium in diet results in body removing calcium from bones; diets high in protein lead to acidosis, and high in diet soda are high in phosphate
            2. Menopause, decreasing estrogen levels: estrogen replacement therapy can reverse bone changes but may increase risk for other diseases
            3. Cigarette smoking: decreased blood supply to bones
            4. Excessive alcohol intake: toxic effect on osteoblastic activity; high alcohol intake frequently associated with nutritional deficiencies
            5. Sedentary lifestyle: weight-bearing exercise such as walking positively influences bone metabolism
            6. Use of specific medications: aluminum-containing antacids, corticosteroids, anticonvulsants, prolonged heparin therapy, antiretroviral
      3. Pathophysiology
         a. Diameter of bone increases, thinning outer supportive cortex
         b. Trabeculae (spongy tissue) lost and outer cortex thins
         c. Minimal stress leads to fracture
      4. Manifestations ("silent disease": bone loss occurs without symptoms)
         a. Loss of height
         b. Progressive curvature of spine (dorsal kyphosis, cervical lordosis, accounting for "dowager's hump")
         c. Low back pain
         d. Fractures of forearm, spine or hip
      5. Complications
         a. Fractures (> 1.5 million fractures yearly), many spontaneous or resulting from everyday activities
         b. Persistent pain and associated posture changes restrict client activities and ability to perform ADL
      6. Collaborative Care
         a. Stopping or slowing osteoporosis
         b. Alleviating symptoms
         c. Preventing complications
      7. Diagnostic Tests
         a. X-rays: picture of skeletal structures but osteoporotic changes not seen until > 30% of bone mass lost
         b. Quantitative computed tomography (QCT) of spine: measures trabecular bone within vertebral bodies

c. Dual-energy x-ray absorptiometry (DEXA): measures bone density in lumbar spine or hip; highly accurate
d. Alkaline phosphatase (AST): elevated post fracture
e. Serum bone Gla-protein (osteocalcin) marker of osteoclastic activity and is indicator of rate of bone turnover; used to evaluate effects of treatment

8. Medications
   a. Estrogen replacement therapy reduces bone loss, increases bone density in spine and hip, reducing risk of fractures in postmenopausal women
      1. Recommended for women who have undergone surgical menopause before age 50
      2. Associated risk for estrogen therapy alone is increased risk of endometrial cancer
      3. Hormone replacement therapy (estrogen and progestin) associated with increased risk for cardiovascular disease and breast cancer
   b. Raloxifene (Evista): selective estrogen receptor modulator (SERM) that prevents bone loss by mimicking estrogen effects on bone density; side effects are hot flashes; contraindicated for women with history of blood clots
   c. Biphosphonates: potent inhibitors of bone resorption used to prevent and treat osteoporosis
      1. Alendronate (Fosamax)
      2. Risedronate (Actonel)
      3. Etidronate (Didronel)
   d. Calcitonin (Miacalcin): hormone increases bone formation and decreases bone resorption; available as nasal spray or parenteral
   e. Sodium fluoride: stimulates osteoblast activity, decreases risk of spinal fractures but associated with increased risk of other fractures including hip

9. Nursing Care
   a. Emphasis is prevention and education of clients under age of 35
   b. Prevention of complications in those with osteoporosis

10. Health Promotion
    a. Calcium intake
       1. Maintain daily intake of calcium at recommended levels, in divided doses
          a. Age 19–50: 1000 mg
          b. Age 51–64: 1200 mg
          c. Age 65 and >: 1500 mg
       2. Optimal intake before age 30–35 increases peak bone mass
       3. Foods high in calcium include milk, milk products, salmon, sardines, clams, oysters, dark green leafy vegetables
       4. Supplementation: calcium carbonate (Tums); calcium combined with Vitamin D for older adults
    b. Exercise
       1. Physical activity that is weight bearing
       2. Walking 20 minutes, 4 or > times per week
    c. Health-related behaviors
       1. Include not smoking
       2. Avoid excessive alcohol
       3. Limit caffeine to 2–3 cups of coffee daily
       4. Limit diet soda

11. Nursing Diagnoses
    a. Health Seeking Behaviors
    b. Risk for Injury
    c. Imbalanced Nutrition: Less than body requirements
    d. Acute Pain

12. Home Care: Focus is on education including safety and fall prevention inside and outside the home

C. Client with Paget's Disease (osteitis deformans)
   1. Description
      a. Progressive skeletal disorder with excessive metabolic bone activity leading to affected bones becoming larger and softer
      b. Affects femur, pelvis, vertebrae, sacrum, sternum, skull
      c. Relatively rare
      d. Occurs more often in whites
      e. Slightly more common in males
      f. Familial tendency
   2. Pathophysiology
      a. Bones are initially soft and bowing occurs; then become hard and brittle leading to fractures
      b. Slow progression with 2-stage process
         1. Excessive osteoclastic bone resorption
         2. Excessive osteoblastic bone formation

3. Manifestations
   a. Most are asymptomatic
   b. Localized pain of long bones, spine, pelvis, cranium; pain is mild to moderate deep ache which is aggravated by pressure and weight bearing noticed at night and when resting
   c. Flushing and warmth over areas of bone involvement
4. Complications
   a. Degenerative osteoarthritis
   b. Pathological fractures
   c. Nerve palsy syndromes from involvement of upper extremities
   d. Compression of spinal cord causing tetraplegia
   e. Mental deterioration from skull involvement and brain compression
5. Collaborative Care
   a. Pain relief
   b. Suppression of bone cell activity
   c. Complication prevention
6. Diagnostic Test
   a. X-ray (often incidental) slow localized areas of demineralization in early phase; later enlargement of bones with tiny cracks in long bones or bowing in weight-bearing bones
   b. Bone scan: active Paget's disease
   c. CT scans and MRI: show degenerative problems, spinal stenosis, nerve root impingement
   d. Serum alkaline phosphatase: steady rise as disease progresses
   e. Urinary collagen pyridinoline testing: indicator of rate of bone resorption
7. Medications
   a. Mild symptoms relieved by aspirin or NSAIDs
   b. Bone resorption retarded by
      1. Biphosphonates: calcium supplements are prescribed in addition
         a. Alendronate (Fosamax)
         b. Pamidronate (Aredia)
         c. Tiludronate (Skelid)
      2. Calcitonic: works as analgesic for bone pain
         a. Salmon calcitonin (Calcimar)
         b. Human calcitonin (Cibacalcin)
8. Surgery
   a. Total hip or knee replacement is usually required when client with Paget's disease develops degenerative arthritis of hip or knee

      b. May require surgery for spinal stenosis, nerve root compression
9. Nursing Diagnoses
   a. Chronic Pain
      1. May involve wearing a back brace for relief of back pain
      2. Heat therapy and massage
   b. Impaired Physical Mobility
10. Home Care: manifestations often relieved by treatment

D. Client with gout
   1. Definition
      a. Syndrome occurs from inflammatory response to production or excretion of uric acid resulting in high levels of uric acid in blood and other body fluids such as synovial fluid
      b. Metabolic disorder characterized by deposits of urates in connective tissues of body
      c. Primary gout: characterized by elevated serum uric acid levels from inborn error of purine metabolism or decrease in renal uric acid excretion due to unknown cause
      d. Secondary gout: hyperuricemia occurs as a result of other disorders or treatments
         1. Malignancies (leukemia)
         2. Chronic renal failure
         3. Certain medications, such as some diuretics
   2. Pathophysiology
      a. Uric acid is a breakdown product of purine metabolism and is normally excreted through urine and feces
      b. Levels > 7.0 mg/dL (normal: 3.4–7.0 mg/dL in males; 2.4–6.0 mg/dL in females) lead to formation of urate crystals in peripheral tissues (synovial membranes, cartilage, heart, earlobe, kidneys) and perpetuate inflammation
   3. Manifestations: 3 stages in untreated gout
      a. Hyperuricemia
         1. Uric acid levels average 9–10 mg/dL
         2. Recurrent attacks of inflammation of single joint
         3. Tophi in and around the joint
         4. Renal disease and renal stones
         5. Many persons do not progress beyond this level
      b. Acute gouty arthritis
         1. Acute attack usually affecting a single joint

2. May be triggered by trauma, alcohol ingestion, dietary excess, stressor, such as surgery or hospitalization
3. Affected joint is red, hot, swollen, very painful and tender; often first metatarsophalangeal joint (great toe)
4. Accompanied by fever, elevated WBC and ESR (sedimentation rate)
5. Episode last hours to weeks followed by asymptomatic period
   c. Tophaceous (chronic) gout
1. Occurs when hyperuricemia not treated
2. Tophi develop in cartilage, synovial membranes, tendons, soft tissues
3. Skin over tophi may ulcerate exude chalky material and urate crystals
4. Leads to joint deformities and nerve compression
5. May lead to kidney disease (uric acid stones and can lead to ARF)
4. Collaborative Care
   a. Treatment directed towards ending acute attack
   b. Treatment directed towards preventing recurrent attacks and complications
5. Diagnostic Tests
   a. Diagnosis with classic presentation: by history and physical examination
   b. Uric acid: usually elevated above 7.5 mg/dL
   c. WBC: elevation as high as 20,000/mm^3 during acute attack
   d. Erythrocyte sedimentation rate (ESR): elevated from acute inflammation process
   e. 24-hour urine collection to determine uric acid production and excretion
   f. Fluid aspirated from acutely inflamed joints shows urate crystals
6. Medications
   a. Used to terminate acute attack and prevent future ones
   b. Reduce serum uric acid levels
   c. Treatment of acute gout attack
1. NSAIDs, specifically indomethacin (Indocin)
2. Colchicine: interrupts cycle of urate crystal deposits and inflammation
   a. Anti-inflammatory use limited to gout
   b. Use limited by significant side effects: with oral administration:

abdominal cramping, diarrhea, nausea, vomiting
3. Corticosteroids, including intra-articular route
4. Analgesia, including narcotics
   d. Prophylactic therapy
1. Clients who do not eliminate uric acid adequately are treated with colchicines and uricosuric drugs, such as probenecid (Benemid) and sulfinpyrazone (Aprazone, Anturane, Zynol)
2. Clients who produce excessive amounts of uric acid are treated with allopurinol (Zyloprim), which lowers serum uric acid levels
7. Dietary Management
   a. Dietary purines contribute only slightly to uric acid levels; if low-purine diet recommended, client must avoid all meats, seafood, yeast, beans, oatmeal, spinach, mushrooms
   b. Client may be advised to lose weight, but fasting not advised
   c. Avoid alcohol, foods known to precipitate gout attack
8. Other Treatments
   a. During acute attack of gouty arthritis, bed rest until 24 hours post attack, elevate joint with hot or cold compresses
   b. Liberal fluid intake (2000 mL) to increase urate excretion; urinary alkalinizing agents (sodium bicarbonate and potassium citrate) to minimize risk of uric acid stones
9. Nursing Diagnoses
   a. Acute Pain
   b. Impaired Physical Mobility
10. Home Care
   a. Education regarding prescribed medications
   b. Education on maintaining high fluid intake of fluid and avoiding alcohol
E. Client with osteomalacia (adult rickets)
1. Metabolic bone disorder characterized by inadequate or delayed mineralization of bone matrix leading to marked deformities of weight bearing bone and pathologic fractures
2. Pathophysiology
   a. Primary causes are vitamin D deficiency and hypophosphatemia
1. Vitamin D deficiency
   a. Present in

1. Older adults
2. Very-low-birth weight infants
3. Strict vegetarians
   b. Caused by
   1. Diet low in vitamin D
   2. Impaired intestinal absorption of fats
   3. Inadequate sun exposure
   4. Some types of renal failure
   2. Hypophosphatemia: most commonly caused by alcohol abuse
   b. Other causes
   1. Insufficient calcium absorption in intestines, due to lack of calcium or resistance to action of Vitamin D
   2. Increase loss of phosphorus through urine
3. Manifestations
   a. Bone pain and tenderness
   b. Common fractures are distal radius and proximal femur
4. Collaborative Care: requires differential diagnosis from osteoporosis
5. Diagnostic Tests
   a. X-ray demonstrates generalized bone demineralization
   b. Serum calcium levels are normal or low
   c. Serum parathyroid hormone is frequently elevated as compensatory response
   d. Alkaline phosphatase level usually elevated
6. Medications
   a. Treatment of underlying condition
   b. Vitamin D therapy with calcium and phosphate supplements
   c. Radiologic evidence of healing apparent within weeks of therapy
7. Nursing Care
   a. Assessment of dietary intake of Vitamin D, calcium, phosphorus, exposure to ultraviolet light
   b. Management of client responses to bone pain and tenderness, fractures, muscle weakness
   c. Vitamin D sources include dairy products fortified with Vitamin D and cod liver oil
   d. If client takes supplements, must be aware of potential for toxicity with fat soluble vitamins
   e. Fall prevention

II. Degenerative Disorders
   A. Client with osteoarthritis (OA): degenerative joint disease

1. Description
   a. Most common of all forms of arthritis
   b. Characterized by loss of articular cartilage in articulating joints and hypertrophy of bones at articular margins
   c. Causes are idiopathic or secondary (post injury)
   d. Affects more than 60 million adult Americans
   e. Males more often than females, until age 55 when incidence twice as high in females
   f. Men more likely to have OA in the hips, women in the hands
2. Risk Factors
   a. Age, but may be inherited as autosomal recessive trait
   b. Excessive weight especially in hip and knee
   c. Inactivity
   d. Strenuous, repetitive exercise as with sports participants increased risk for secondary OA
   e. Hormonal factors such as decreased estrogen in menopausal women
3. Pathophysiology
   a. Cartilage lining joints degenerates and loses tensile strength; loss of articular cartilage results in bone thickening, reducing the ability to absorb energy in joint loading
   b. Osteophytes (bony outgrowths) form, change anatomy of joint; these spurs enlarge, break off and lead to mild synovitis
4. Manifestations
   a. Onset is gradual, insidious, slowly progressive
   b. Pain and stiffness in one or more joints; pain is a deep ache aggravated by use of motion and relieved by rest but may be persistent with time
   c. Pain may be referred to other places
   d. Periods of immobility are followed by stiffness
   e. Decreased range of motion of joint and grating or crepitus during movement
   f. Bony overgrowth causes joint enlargement
   1. Herberden's nodes: terminal, interphalangeal joints
   2. Bouchard's nodes: proximal, interphalangeal joints
   g. Flexion contractures occur with joint instability

5. Complications: Spondylosis, a degenerative disk disease, which may lead to herniated disk
6. Collaborative Care
   a. Relieve pain
   b. Maintain client's function and mobility
7. Diagnostic Tests
   a. Based on client's history and physical examination
   b. Characteristic changes seen on x-ray
8. Medications
   a. Pain management with aspirin, acetaminophen, NSAID's
   b. Capsaicin cream topically to reduce joint pain and tenderness
   c. NSAID COX-2 inhibitors
      1. Results similar to conventional NSAIDs with fewer GI and renal systems side effects
      2. Meloxicam (Mobic), celecoxib (Celebrex), rofecoxib (Vioxx)
   d. Corticosteroid injection of joints, but this may hasten rate of cartilage breakdown
9. Conservative Treatment
   a. Physical therapy
   b. Rest of involved joint
   c. Using ambulation devices
   d. Weight loss
   e. Analgesic and anti-inflammatory medications
10. Surgery
    a. Arthroscopy
       1. Arthroscopic debridement and lavage of involved joints
       2. Unclear about effectiveness long term
    b. Osteotomy
       1. Incision into or transection of bone to realign affected joint
       2. Shifts joint load toward areas of less cartilage damage
       3. Delays joint replacement for several years
    c. Joint arthroplasty
       1. Reconstruction or replacement of joint indicated when client has severely restricted joint mobility and pain at rest
       2. Total joint replacement is procedure done for most OA clients, which involves replacing both surfaces of affected joint with prosthetic parts
       3. Most prosthetic joints are uncemented; made of porous ceramic and metal components

inserted to fit tightly into existing bone; implant secured by new bone growth in about 6 weeks; requires longer non-weight-bearing period but implant has longer useful life span
4. Cemented joint replacement uses methyl methacrylate to secure prosthesis to existing bone; client able to resume normal activities sooner but inflammation eventually loosens joint
5. Potential complications
   a. Infection is major complication
   b. Dislocation of joint
   c. Loosening of prosthesis
   d. Impaired circulation
   e. Thromboembolism
6. Specific joint replacements
   a. Total hip replacement (THR)
      1. Articular surfaces of acetabulum and femoral head are replaced
      2. Success rate > 90%
   b. Total knee replacement
      1. > 80% clients obtain significant or total relief
      2. Vigorous rehabilitation program required
      3. Joint failure rate higher than with THR: due to loosened joint components on tibial side
   c. Total shoulder replacement
      1. Indicated for unremitting pain and limited ROM
      2. Joint immobilized in sling of abduction splint for 2–3 weeks post arthroplasty
   d. Total elbow replacement
11. Complementary Therapies
    a. Bioelectromagnetic therapy
    b. Elimination of nightshade foods
    c. Nutritional supplements, herbal therapies, vitamins
    d. Osteopathic manipulation
    e. Yoga
12. Nursing Care
    a. Promote comfort
    b. Maintain mobility
    c. Assist with adaptation of lifestyle
13. Health Promotion
    a. Maintenance of normal weight
    b. Program of regular, moderate exercise
    c. Use of glucosamine and chrondroitin

14. Nursing Diagnoses
    a. Chronic Pain
    b. Impaired Physical Mobility
    c. Self-care Deficit
15. Home Care
    a. Education regarding avoiding overuse or stress on affected joints
    b. Education regarding pharmacological and other forms of pain relief
    c. Clients post TJR (total joint replacement) activity: restrictions and assistive devices
B. Client with Muscular Dystrophy
    1. MD is a group of inherited muscle diseases with progressive muscle degeneration and wasting; most cases have a positive family history
    2. Duchenne's muscular dystrophy
       a. Most common form
       b. Inherited as sex-linked recessive disorder (mother to male children)
       c. Manifestations appear in early childhood, with lifespan of 15 years post onset
    3. Pathophysiology: Defect unknown, but theories are
       a. Altered blood or nervous supply to muscle
       b. Altered cell membranes of muscles
       c. Deficiency in amount of muscle membrane protein
    4. Manifestations
       a. Progressive muscle weakness with cardiac and endocrine abnormalities
       b. Mental retardation may also be involved
    5. Collaborative Care
       a. Preserving and promoting mobility
       b. Supporting client and family
    6. Diagnostic Tests
       a. Creatine kinase (CK-MM): elevated levels
       b. Muscle biopsy: muscle fibers are replaced with fibrous connective tissue and fatty deposits
       c. Electromyelogram (EMG): decrease in amplitude
    7. Nursing Care
       a. Promotion of independence and mobility
       b. Psychological support to client and family
       c. Interventions to deal with client's self-care deficit
    8. Home Care
       a. Education to maintain functioning, prevent deformities, deal with chronic disease

    b. Immunizations against pneumonia and influenza
    c. Referral to Muscular Dystrophy Association
III. Autoimmune and Inflammatory Disorders
    A. Rheumatoid arthritis (RA)
       1. Definition
          a. Chronic systemic autoimmune disease causing inflammation of connective tissue primarily in joints
             1. Three times more likely to affect females than males
             2. Onset is between 20–40 years
          b. Course and severity are variable; clients exhibit pattern of symmetrical multiple peripheral joints involvement with periods of remission and exacerbation
          c. Cause is unknown; combination of genetic, environmental, hormonal, reproductive factors; infectious agents, especially Epstein-Barr, thought to play role
       2. Pathophysiology
          a. Normal antibodies become autoantibodies (rheumatoid factors–RF) and attack host tissues, which bind with target antigens in blood and with synovial membranes forming immune complexes
          b. Synovial membrane damaged from inflammatory and immune processes; leads to erosion of articular cartilage and inflammation of ligaments and tendons
          c. Granulation tissue (pannus) forms over denuded areas of synovial membrane and scar tissue forms immobilizing joint
       3. Joint manifestations
          a. Onset is usually insidious but may be acute after stressor, such as infection
          b. Systemic manifestations: fatigue, anorexia, weight loss and non-specific aching and stiffness precedes joint involvement
          c. Joint swelling with stiffness, warmth, tenderness and pain; usually multiple joints and symmetric involvement
          d. Proximal interphalangeal and metacarpophalangeal joints of fingers, wrists, knees, ankles, and toes are frequently involved
          e. Joint deformity of fingers include swan-neck deformity and boutonniere deformity; wrist deformity leads to

carpal tunnel syndrome; knee deformity leads to disability and feet and toes develop typical deformities
4. Extra-articular manifestations
   a. While disease is active: fatigue, weakness, anorexia, weight loss, low-grade fever
   b. Anemia develops as does skeletal muscle atrophy
   c. Rheumatoid nodules develop in subcutaneous tissue in areas subject to pressure on forearm, olecranon bursa, over metacarpophalangeal joints
   d. Pleural effusion, pericarditis, splenomegaly may occur
5. Collaborative Care
   a. Relief of pain and reduction of inflammation
   b. Slow or stop joint damage
   c. Improve well-being and ability to function
   d. Relief of manifestations
6. Diagnostic Tests
   a. Client history and physical assessment
   b. Rheumatoid factors (RF), autoantibodies to IgG present in 75% of persons with RA
   c. Elevation of ESR; indicator of disease and inflammatory activity; used to evaluate effectiveness of treatment
   d. Examination of synovial fluid: signs associated with inflammation
   e. X-rays of affected joints: show diagnostic changes
   f. CBC: shows moderate anemia with elevated platelet count
7. Medications
   a. Aspirin and NSAID's, mild analgesics to relieve manifestations, but have little effect on disease progression
      1. Aspirin
         a. Often first prescribed in high doses just under toxic dose, which produces tinnitus and hearing loss
         b. GI side effects and interference with platelet function are hazards associated with aspirin therapy
         c. May use enteric-coated forms of aspirin or nonacetylated salicylate compounds
      2. NSAID's
         a. Different, specific NSAID's are tried to determine the most effective drug for individual clients

      b. Have GI side effects and can be toxic to kidneys
   b. Low dose oral corticosteroids
      1. To reduce pain and inflammation
      2. To slow development and progression of disease
      3. Often have dramatic effects, but long-term use results in multiple side effects
   c. Diverse group of drugs, disease-modifying or slow-acting antirheumatic drugs
      1. Gold compounds: weekly IM injection is initial therapy
         a. Toxic reactions include stomatitis, dermatitis, bone marrow depression, proteinuria
         b. CBC and urinalysis are monitored
      2. D-penicillinamine: potential for severe toxic reactions: bone marrow suppression, proteinuria, nephrosis
      3. Antimalarial agents: hydroxychloroquine (Plaquenil); clients need vision exam every 6 months since can cause pigmentary retinitis and vision loss
      4. Sulfasalazine: may be used
      5. Leflunomide (Arava): inhibits enzyme in autoimmune process
      6. Etanercept (Enbrel): inhibits binding of tumor necrosis factor to receptor sites
      7. Immunosuppressive and cytotoxic drugs
         a. Methotrexate treatment of choice for aggressive RA
         b. May also use cyclosporine, azathioprine, monoclonal antibodies
   d. Intra-articular corticosteroids
8. Treatments
   a. Balanced program of rest and exercise
      1. Rest with exacerbation and may utilize splinting
      2. Exercise to maintain ROM, muscle strength
      3. Low-impact exercise such as swimming or walking
   b. Physical and occupational therapy
   c. Heat and cold: analgesia and muscle relaxation
   d. Assistive devices and splints which help rest joints and prevent contractures

e. Diet: well-balanced; some benefit from omega-3 fatty acids found in fish oils
f. Surgery: variety of procedures may be done: synovectomy, arthrodesis, joint fusion, arthroplasty or total joint replacement
g. Other therapies
   1. Experimental therapies
   2. Plasmapheresis
9. Nursing Care: assist client to deal effectively with physical manifestations and psychosocial effects
10. Health Promotion
   a. Support client in becoming arthritis self-managers: prevent deformities and effects of arthritis by balance of exercise and rest, weight management, posture, and positioning
   b. Referral: Arthritis Foundation
11. Nursing Diagnoses
   a. Chronic Pain: increasing pain requires need to decrease activity level
   b. Fatigue
   c. Ineffective Role Performance
   d. Disturbed Body Image
12. Home Care: support for client and family to become active in disease management
B. Client with ankylosing spondylitis
   1. Chronic inflammatory arthritis primarily affecting axial skeleton leading to pain and progressive stiffening and fusion of the spine
   2. Occurs more often in males with more severe disease
   3. Cause is unknown but strong genetic component
   4. Pathophysiology
      a. Early inflammation occurs in sacroiliac joints: cartilage erodes, joint margins ossify and are replaced with scar tissue
      b. Joints of spine become involved, gradual calcification leading to ankylosis: joint consolidation and immobility
      c. Involvement may include eyes, lungs, heart, kidneys
   5. Manifestations
      a. Gradual and insidious onset
      b. Bouts of low back pain worse at night, followed by morning stiffness relieved by activity
      c. Back motion becomes limited, lumbar curve is lost, thoracic curve is accentuated and entire spine becomes fused

d. Systemic manifestations: anorexia, weight loss, fever, fatigue
e. Uveitis
f. Usually occurs intermittently with mild to moderate acute episodes
6. Collaborative Care
   a. Management includes physical therapy and daily exercise
   b. Medications include NSAIDs, especially indomethacin (Indocin), sulfasalazine (Azulfidine), topical or intra-articular corticosteroids
7. Nursing Care: supportive care and education, especially for maintenance of exercise program
C. Client with reactive arthritis (Reiter's syndrome)
   1. Acute nonpurulent inflammatory arthritis
      a. Complicating bacterial infection of GU or GI tract that typically is self-limited
      b. More common in young males
      c. Affects some clients with HIV infection
   2. Manifestations
      a. Usually begins with nonbacterial urethritis, in females urethritis/cervicitis is asymptomatic
      b. Conjunctivitis and arthritis follow
      c. Arthritis usually is asymmetric affecting knees, ankles, sacroiliac joints or spine; may be followed by mouth ulcers or skin lesions
   3. No specific diagnostic tests but client may have cultures done to rule out sexually transmitted disease
   4. Treatment is symptomatic, usually with NSAID's
D. Client with Systemic Lupus Erythematosus (SLE)
   1. Definition
      a. SLE is chronic inflammatory immune complex connective tissue disease affecting multiple body systems; can range from mild episodic disorder to rapidly fatal disease process
      b. Affects mostly females in childbearing age; more common in African Americans, Hispanics, Asians
      c. Cause is unknown; causative factors are genetic, environmental, and hormonal
      d. Most clients have mild chronic case with periods of remissions and exacerbations; those with virulent disease often develop renal and CNS

involvement and death is related to infection

2. Pathophysiology
   a. Production of large variety of autoantibodies against the normal components of body especially the nucleic acids; leads to development of immune complexes which leads to tissue damage in multiple organs
   b. Reaction to some medications (procainamide, hydralazine) causes a syndrome similar to lupus, which usually resolves when medication is discontinued

3. Manifestations
   a. Early manifestations: fever, anorexia, malaise, weight loss, multiple arthralgias and symmetric non-deforming polyarthritis
   b. Skin manifestations usually occur: red butterfly rash across the cheeks and bridge of the nose; accompanied by photosensitivity (maculopapular rash upon sun exposure); alopecia is common
   c. 50% of persons have renal involvement including proteinuria, cellular casts, and nephrotic syndrome; 10% develop renal failure
   d. Hematologic manifestations: anemia, leukopenia, thrombocytopenia
   e. Cardiovascular system: pericarditis, vasculitis, Raynaud's phenomenon, endocarditis
   f. Pulmonary system: pleurisy, pleural effusion
   g. Neurologic involvement: organic brain syndrome, psychosis, seizures
   h. Ocular system: conjunctivitis, photophobia, retinal vasculitis
   i. GI symptoms: anorexia, nausea, abdominal pain, diarrhea

4. Collaborative Care
   a. Diagnosis is often difficult due to the diversity of manifestations in individual clients
   b. Effective management has improved survival rate

5. Diagnostic Tests
   a. Clinical history, physical examination
   b. Anti-DNA: of various antibodies, this antibody is more specific for SLE; rarely found in any other disorder
   c. ESR: typically elevated, especially during exacerbations
   d. Serum complement levels: levels are low (used in development of antigen-antibody complexes)
   e. CBC: severe anemia, leukopenia with lymphcytopenia, thrombocytopenia
   f. Urinalysis: mild proteinuria, hematuria, blood cell casts
   g. BUN and creatinine: determine renal function
   h. Kidney biopsy: obtain accurate diagnosis of kidney lesion and plan definitive treatment with renal insufficiency

6. Medications
   a. Mild cases of SLE may be treated with supportive care and possible aspirin and NSAIDs
   b. Skin and arthritic manifestations are treated with anti-malarial drugs
   c. Severe cases are often treated with high-dose corticosteroid therapy tapered as client's disease allows; treatment may also include immunosuppressive agents (cyclophosphamide or azathioprine) alone or with the steroids

7. Other treatments
   a. Avoid sun exposure: use of sunscreens
   b. Clients with ESRD (end stage renal disease) require dialysis and kidney transplantation

8. Nursing Care: client with severe disease has needs related to system involvement and similar to client with RA

9. Nursing Diagnoses
   a. Impaired Skin Integrity
   b. Ineffective Protection
      1. Teach client to follow aseptic techniques
      2. Monitor closely for signs of infection, which are often suppressed
   c. Impaired Health Maintenance: client often has involved physical and psychological needs

10. Home Care
    a. Teaching regarding skin care, avoiding sun, following treatment plan including medications
    b. Wearing medical identification
    c. Family planning
    d. Referral to home nursing care, resources and support groups

E. Client with polymyositis
   1. Systemic connective-tissue disorder with inflammation of connective tissue and

muscles leading to muscle weakness and atrophy; if accompanied by skin involvement know as dermatomyositis

2. Autoimmune disease affecting females more than males usually between ages of 40–60

3. Manifestations
   a. Initial manifestations
      1. Muscle pain, tenderness, weakness
      2. Rash
      3. Arthralgias
      4. Fatigue, fever, and weight loss
   b. Later manifestations
      1. Development of increased muscle weakness
      2. Dysphagia
      3. Cough
      4. Increased risk of malignancy with dermatomyositis

4. No specific diagnostic tests
   a. Autoantibodies are found and elevated levels of muscle enzymes (creatine kinase–CK, aldolase)
   b. Muscle biopsies show patchy muscle fiber necrosis and inflammatory cells

5. Treatment consists of rest and corticosteroids, and possibly, immunosuppressive agents

6. Nursing care is largely supportive
   a. Promotion of comfort
   b. Dealing with muscle weakness regarding nutrition and communication
   c. Skin care
   d. Management of medications
   e. Maintenance of mobility

F. Client with Lyme disease
   1. Inflammatory disorder caused by a spirochete *Borrelia burgdorferi* and transmitted by ticks carried by deer and mice; prevalent in mid-Atlantic, northeastern and north central areas of U.S.
   2. Manifestations
      a. Initial manifestations
         1. Flu-like symptoms and skin rash
         2. "Bull's eye" skin lesion at site of tick bite
         3. Followed by fatigue, malaise, fever, chills, myalgias
         4. Later more skin lesions and muscle and joint pain
      b. Weeks to months later
         1. Bell's palsy and meningitis
         2. Headache and neck stiffness
      c. Months to years later: chronic recurrent arthritis often affecting the knee

d. Progression is highly individualized; may result in permanent disability with neurologic and cardiac involvement

3. Diagnostic Tests: Manifestations and laboratory studies
   a. Antibodies to *B. burgdorferi* detected by ELISA or Western blot methods within 2–4 weeks of initial skin lesion
   b. Organism is difficult and slow to culture from tissues or body fluids

4. Treatment is important to prevent development of complications
   a. Antibiotics such as doxycycline, tetracycline, amoxicillin, cefuroxime axetil, or erythromycin for up to a month
   b. Arthritic manifestations are treated with aspirin or NSAIDs

5. Nursing Care: Focus on prevention
   a. Avoid tick-infested areas
   b. If going outdoors in areas with ticks, dress appropriately and use insect repellents containing DEET
   c. Inspect skin afterward, remove ticks
   d. Seek specific treatment for Lyme disease, if manifestations of disease occur (especially site of tick bite)

IV. Infectious Disorders
   A. Client with osteomyelitis
      1. Infection of the bone, may occur as acute, subacute, or chronic
      2. Consequence of bacteremia, invasion from contiguous focus of infection, skin breakdown; more prevalent in adults over age of 50
      3. Pathophysiology
         a. Usually bacterial in nature: most commonly *Staphylococcus aureus*
         b. Sources of infection
            1. Direct contamination of bone from open wounds (trauma)
            2. Complication of surgery
            3. Extension of chronic ulcers including venous, arterial, diabetic
         c. Infection develops in bone, which may interfere with vascular supply to bone, and necrosis occurs; difficult for antibiotics to reach the bacteria within the bone
      4. Specific incidents of osteomyelitis
         a. Hematogenous osteomyelitis
            1. Pathogens carried by blood, primarily occur in older adults, persons with sickle cell anemia, intravenous drug users

2. Site of infection is usually the spine, commonly lumbar
  b. Osteomyelitis from a contiguous infection
    1. Infection results from deep penetrating wounds, TJR, decubitus ulcers, neurosurgery
    2. Diagnosis often not made until infection has become chronic because acute signs are masked by chronic inflammation; non-healing wound or fracture
  c. Osteomyelitis associated with vascular insufficiency
    1. Clients with PVD and diabetic neuropathy at risk
    2. Infection often diagnosed when client seeks treatment for nonhealing wound, swollen toe, acute cellulitis
5. Collaborative Care
  a. Pain relief
  b. Infection elimination or prevention
  c. Early diagnosis to prevent bone necrosis by early antibiotic therapy
  d. Often requires bone debridement and long course of antibiotics
6. Diagnostic Tests
  a. MRI and CT scans: show abscesses and soft tissue changes
  b. Radionucleotides bone scans: determine whether infectious or inflammatory changes in bone
  c. CBC and ESR: WBC and ESR are elevated
  d. Blood and tissue cultures: identify infectious organism and determine appropriate antibiotic therapy
7. Medications
  a. Antibiotics mandatory to prevent acute case from becoming chronic osteomyelitis
  b. Initially treated as staph infection until results of culture are obtained
  c. Definitive antibiotics prescribed according to culture results
  d. Continued at least 4–6 weeks with intravenous or oral antibiotics
8. Surgery
  a. Needle aspiration or percutaneous needle biopsy performed to obtain specimen; specimen may also be obtained during debridement procedure
    b. Surgical debridement is primary treatment for chronic cases: wound is opened, irrigated; drainage tubes may be inserted for irrigation, suction, and antibiotic instillation
9. Nursing Care
  a. Persons with chronic osteomyelitis face frequent and lengthy treatments
  b. Client needs to be aware of manifestations of recurrent infection (inflammation in area, temperature elevation)
  c. Prognosis is uncertain and client must be maintained under care to prevent amputation or functional deficits
10. Nursing Diagnoses
  a. Risk for Infection
  b. Hyperthermia: interventions include maintenance of adequate fluid intake
  c. Acute Pain: splinting or use of immobilizer may limit swelling and improve pain
  d. Anxiety
11. Home Care
  a. Often vital part of treatment of osteomyelitis
  b. Referral to home care agency for support with wound treatment, antibiotic administration, obtaining supplies, nutritional teaching
B. Client with septic arthritis
  1. Occurs when joint space invaded by pathogen
  2. Risk Factors
    a. Persistent bacteremia (use of intravenous recreational drugs, endocarditis)
    b. Previous joint damage (trauma, RA)
    c. Arthroscopic surgery and TJR
  3. Pathophysiology
    a. Common bacteria: gonococci, *Staphylococcus aureus, streptococci; E. coli* and *Pseudomonas* in intravenous drug users or those immunocompromised
    b. Infection of joint leads to synovitis and joint effusion; knee often affected
  4. Manifestations
    a. Onset: abrupt with pain and stiffness of affected joint which is red, swollen, hot and tender to touch
    b. Systemic infection: chills and fever

5. Collaborative Care
   a. Requires prompt treatment to preserve joint function
   b. Joint is aspirated and fluid sent for gram stain and culture; fluid usually cloudy due to high WBC count
   c. X-ray will eventually show demineralization, bony erosion, joint space narrowing
6. Treatment
   a. Rest, joint immobilization and elevation
   b. Systemic antibiotic therapy; continued for at least 2 weeks after inflammation has subsided
   c. Recurrent joint aspiration and re-culture
   d. Physical therapy implemented during recovery to maintain joint function
7. Nursing Care
   a. Supportive and educative to relieve client pain and inflammation
   b. Education to prevent problem including stopping use of injected drugs, preventing sexually transmitted diseases

V. Neoplastic Disorders: Bone Tumors
   A. Description
      1. Tumors may be malignant or benign
         a. Benign tumors grow slowly and do not invade surrounding tissues
         b. Malignant tumors grow rapidly and metastasize
      2. Tumors can be primary (rare) or metastatic lesions originating from primary tumors of prostate, breast, kidney, thyroid, lung
   B. Pathophysiology
      1. Cause unknown, but connection exists between bone activity and development of primary bone tumors
      2. Primary tumors cause osteolysis, bone breakdown, which weakens bone and leads to bone fractures
      3. Malignant bone tumors invade and destroy adjacent bone tissue
   C. Manifestations: often history of fall or blow to extremity brings mass to attention
      1. Pain
      2. Mass
      3. Impaired function
   D. Diagnostic Tests
      1. X-ray: shows location of tumors and extent of bone involvement
         a. Benign tumors show sharp margins separating from normal bones

      b. Metastatic bone destruction: characteristic "moth-eaten" pattern
      2. CT scan: evaluation of extent of tumor invasion into bone, soft tissues, neurovascular structures
      3. MRI: determine extent of tumor invasion, response of bone tumors to radiation and chemotherapy, recurrent disease
      4. Needle biopsy to determine exact type of bone tumor
      5. Serum alkaline phosphatase: elevated with malignant bone tumors
      6. elevated RBC's
      7. Serum calcium: elevated with massive bone destruction
   E. Treatments
      1. Chemotherapy
         a. Used to shrink tumor before surgery
         b. Control reoccurrence
         c. Treat metastasis
      2. Radiation
         a. Often combined with chemotherapy
         b. Used for pain control with metastatic carcinomas
         c. Eliminate tumor remains after surgery
      3. Surgery
         a. Eliminate primary bone tumors to eliminate tumors completely; may involve excise tumor or amputate affected limb
         b. With some surgeries, cadaver allografts or metal prostheses used to replace missing bone to avoid amputation
   F. Nursing Diagnoses
      1. Risk for Injury (pathologic fractures)
      2. Acute and Chronic Pain
      3. Impaired Physical Mobility
      4. Decisional Conflict: assist client in gaining information for informed decisions regarding treatment options
   G. Home Care
      1. Client education regarding treatment plan, wound care, activity and weight-bearing restrictions
      2. Support with referral to prosthetic specialist or hospice as case indicates

VI. Connective Tissue Disorders
   A. Client with systemic sclerosis (scleroderma)
      1. Chronic disease characterized by formation of excess fibrous connective tissue and diffuse fibrosis of skin and internal organs
      2. Cause is unknown but higher incidence in females, persons exposed to certain chemicals; onset between 30–50

3. Prognosis
   a. Localized and limited scleroderma: good
   b. Diffuse systemic scleroderma: highly variable; disease is usually progressive and complete remission is rare
4. Pathophysiology
   a. Abnormalities in cellular immune function; fibrosis occurs in tissue involving skin, blood vessels, lungs, kidneys
   b. May be localized (skin only) or generalized with both skin and organ involvement
5. Manifestations
   a. Initially marked thickening of skin, diffuse non-pitting swelling
   b. Eventually skin atrophies, becoming taut and hyperpigmented
   c. Arthralgias and Raynaud's phenomenon
   d. Visceral organ involvement
      1. Dysphagia related to esophageal motility
      2. Pulmonary hypertension
      3. Pericarditis, cardiac dysrhythmias
      4. GI problems including malabsorption
      5. Proteinuria, HPT, renal failure
6. Diagnostic Tests
   a. ESR elevated due to chronic inflammatory process
   b. CBC: anemia
   c. Gammaglobulin levels are high; may be low levels of antinuclear antibodies
   d. Diagnosis confirmed by skin biopsy
7. Medications: Treatment is aimed at the specific visceral involvement
   a. Immunosuppressive therapy and corticosteroids used with pulmonary fibrosis
   b. Calcium channel blockers and alpha-adrenergic blocking agents to treat Raynaud's phenomenon
   c. H_2 receptor blockers to treat esophagitis
   d. Antibiotics for intestinal malabsorption
   e. ACE-inhibitors to treat HPT and renal involvement
8. Physical Therapy: treatment to maintain mobility of affected tissues especially in hands and face pertaining to ability to eat
9. Nursing Care
   a. Maintaining skin integrity and flexibility
   b. Maintaining nutritional status
   c. Dealing with chronic restrictive respiratory disorder
   d. Dealing with psychological effects of dermatologic effects and chronic illness
10. Home care
   a. Supportive and client education regarding care involved
   b. Referral to Scleroderma Foundation
B. Client with Sjogren's syndrome
   1. Autoimmune disorder
      a. Causes inflammation and dysfunction of exocrine glands throughout body
      b. Affects mainly females between ages of 40–60
   2. Occurs as primary disorder, but also associated with rheumatic diseases and other disorders
   3. Pathophysiology: Exocrine glands are destroyed by infiltration of lymphocytes and deposition of immune complexes
   4. Manifestations
      a. Salivary and lacrimal glands are affected, leading to dry eyes (xerophthalmia) and dry mouth (xerostomia)
      b. Excessive dryness of all mucous membranes
      c. Systemic effects include arthritis and other systems
      d. Increased risk of developing malignant lymphoma
   5. Diagnostic Tests: Diagnosis often made on client history and clinical presentation
      a. Schirmer's Test: measurement of quality of tears in 5-minute period in response to irritation and slit-lamp eye exam
      b. Biopsy of lacrimal or salivary glands
   6. Treatment/Nursing Care
      a. Supportive measures to maintain moisture of eyes (artificial tears)
      b. Ample fluid intake
      c. Frequent oral hygiene
C. Client with fibromyalgia
   1. Common rheumatic syndrome characterized by musculoskeletal pain, stiffness, tenderness; most commonly in females ages 20–50
   2. Cause unknown but associated etiologies include sleep disorders, depression, infections
   3. No inflammatory, structural or physiologic muscle changes demonstrated with disease

4. Manifestations
   a. Gradual onset of chronic, achy muscle pain, which may be localized (neck, spine, shoulders, hips) or entire body; tightness or muscle spasms
   b. Pain can be produced by palpating localized tender points
   c. Fatigue, sleep disruption, headache, irritable bowel
5. Diagnosis
   a. Based on history and physical assessment
   b. May occur with hypothyroidism so thyroid studies are performed
6. Treatment
   a. May resolve spontaneously or become chronic and recurrent
   b. Therapeutic measures for relief
      1. Heat application
      2. Massage
      3. Stretching exercises
      4. Sleep improvement
      5. Stress-reduction
      6. Anti-depressant therapy
7. Nursing Care
   a. Supportive and educational; syndrome is recognizable and manageable
   b. Referral to support groups
VII. Structural Disorders
   A. Client with spinal deformities
      1. Scoliosis: lateral curvature of spine
         a. Evident in thoracic, lumbar, or thoracolumbar regions of spine; vertebral bodies are rotated as well as curved to one side; muscles and ligaments shorten the concave of curvature; progresses into deformities of vertebral column and ribs
         b. If curvature is < 40 degrees when client reaches maturity, risk for further progression is small; if curvature is > 50 degrees or spine becomes unstable curvature continues to worsen
         c. Manifestations
            1. Curvature noted along with one shoulder higher than other; one prominent hip, projecting scapula
            2. Severe cases may result in pain in lumbar region, shortness of breath and gastrointestinal disturbances related to crowding of lungs and abdominal organs
      2. Kyphosis: excessive angulation of normal posterior curve of thoracic spine

   a. Caused by slumping posture; as adult occurs with vertebral tuberculosis, Paget's disease, osteoporosis, osteomalacia, spinal pathology
   b. Manifestations include back pain, increased thoracic spinal curvature ("hunchback"), which may impair mobility and respiratory function
3. Collaborative Care: screening procedures and diagnosis by upright and lateral x-rays
4. Treatment
   a. Conservative: braces, electrical stimulation, traction, weight reduction, active and passive exercises
   b. Surgery: depending on degree of curvature and client's overall health; procedures include attaching metal reinforcing rods to vertebrae by anterior or anterior and posterior approach
5. Nursing Care
   a. Postoperative care, which often includes log-rolling techniques in turning client
   b. Dependent upon client condition and mode of treatment
6. Nursing Diagnoses
   a. Risk for Injury
   b. Risk for Peripheral Neurovascular Dysfunction
7. Home Care
   a. Education and support
   b. Clients should be encouraged not to smoke and take actions to prevent respiratory infections
   B. Client with low back pain
      1. Most often due to strain of muscles and tendons of back caused by abnormal stress or overuse; need to rule out degenerative disc disease and herniated vertebral disc
      2. Pathophysiology
         a. Local pain due to compression or irritation of sensory nerves related to fractures, strains, sprains
         b. Referred pain from abdominal or pelvic viscera
         c. Spinal origin associated with disc disease or arthritis
         d. Radicular back pain along nerve root; aggravated by movement, coughing, sitting
         e. Muscle spasm pain

3. Collaborative Care
   a. Pain relief
   b. Correct underlying condition, if possible
   c. Prevent complications
   d. Client education
4. Diagnostic Tests
   a. Conservative treatment is tried for four weeks
   b. X-rays, CT scans, and MRI used when potentially serious condition is considered
5. Medications
   a. NSAID's, analgesics, muscle relaxants
   b. Epidural steroid injection for intense, intractable pain
6. Conservative Treatment
   a. Limited rest, appropriate exercise (early mobilization) and education
   b. Applications of ice or heat
   c. Exercise programs
   d. Physical therapy, including diathermy (deep heat therapy), ultrasonography, hydrotherapy, TENS units
7. Health Promotion
   a. Regular exercise program
   b. Lose weight if obese or overweight
   c. Using appropriate body mechanics
   d. Ergonomically appropriate work places
8. Nursing Diagnoses
   a. Acute Pain
   b. Limited Knowledge: regarding activity, use of heat or ice (limit to 15 minutes use at one time), prescribed back exercises

   c. Risk for Impaired Adjustment: modification of environment and lifestyle habits to limit exacerbations of back pain
9. Home Care: education regarding proper body mechanics, exercise, adequate support, proper weight

C. Client with common foot disorders
1. Foot disorders: cause pain and interfere with ability to walk
   a. Hallux valgus (bunion)
   b. Hammertoe
   c. Morton's neuroma
2. Collaborative Care
   a. Pain relief
   b. Correct structural deformity
   c. Prevent recurrence
3. Conservative Treatment: use of corrective shoes, orthotic devices, analgesics
4. Surgery
   a. Bunionectomy to correct hallux valgus
   b. Shortening or lengthening of ligaments
   c. Placement of pins to correct toe positioning
   d. Casting
5. Nursing Diagnoses
   a. Chronic Pain
   b. Risk for Infection
6. Home Care
   a. Education regarding well-fitting footwear, feet inspection
   b. Injury and fall prevention

FOCUSED STUDY TIPS

- Design a children's health fair. Describe information that could be presented age appropriate (NSAID's) for the prevention of osteoporosis in later life.
- Detail disadvantages of long-term use of aspirin and nonsteroidal anti-inflammatory drugs. Identify assessments needed to monitor the development of complications related to their use.
- As often as possible, review X-rays with physicians while working in the clinical setting. Identify bones and tissues. Ask questions about what you see. Share this information with classmates.

CASE STUDY

A client with systemic sclerosis presents with a BP of 188/104. She also complains of esophagitis and shortness of breath. She has a history of Raynaud's phenomenon. Her laboratory tests return with an elevated serum BUN and creatinine. What complication may be occurring with this client? What nursing interventions are implemented as soon as possible? What are the medications that will most likely be prescribed for this client? What is the purpose of each in the treatment of this client's disease?

CARE PLAN CRITICAL THINKING ACTIVITY

What nursing care would be appropriate for the client experiencing bone disease?

NCLEX TEST QUESTIONS

1. A 48-year-old female client is concerned about getting osteoporosis as she ages and states that she has "heard a lot about osteoporosis and calcium" but doesn't understand exactly what the relationship is. How would you best respond to the client's concerns?
   a. Tell the client that there is an established health claim between calcium and osteoporosis.
   b. Tell the client that calcium intake should be maintained throughout one's life in order to prevent the effects of osteoporosis.
   c. Tell the client that calcium supplementation is advisable because most women do not eat enough calcium in the diet.
   d. Tell the client that calcium is needed to support bone density but that many other factors (genetic makeup, diet, and lifestyle) play a part in the development of osteoporosis.

2. An elderly female client with newly diagnosed osteoporosis requires counseling prior to discharge. The most important component of the discharge plan is
   a. instruction in safety factors to prevent injury.
   b. monitoring medications.
   c. instruction in regular exercise and diet.
   d. appropriate use of body mechanics.

3. Which of the following statements made by the parents of a child diagnosed with Duchenne's muscular dystrophy (MD) verifies to the nurse that they understand teaching regarding the disease process?
   a. "Any child from future pregnancies is at risk for inheriting the disease."
   b. "The disease occurred because my child has a defective immune system."
   c. "The disease is genetically transmitted from mother to son."
   d. "The disease relates to a genetic disorder on the father's side."

4. A client presents to the clinic with Paget's disease. The client's chief complaint is skeletal pain. The nurse interprets this symptom as which of the following?
   a. a characteristic of the disease process

   b. an ominous sign that should be reported to the physician immediately
   c. caused by bony deformities
   d. caused by poor calcium uptake by the bones

5. The nurse provides teaching about managing symptoms associated with chronic low back pain to a 35-year-old client who is a construction worker. The nurse determines that the teaching objective was met when the client makes which of the following statements?
   a. "I will wear a brace at work."
   b. "I plan to start a regular exercise program."
   c. "I will not carry objects more than 10 pounds."
   d. "I will try to exercise whenever I can."

6. A client with an open fracture is at risk for developing osteomyelitis. Which of the following classic symptoms would the nurse assess for to detect development of this complication?
   a. low bone density
   b. elevated temperature
   c. acute respiratory distress
   d. shortening of the affected extremity

7. The nurse provides teaching to a 50-year-old male Caucasian client with chronic low back pain. The client weighs 200 pounds, works as a truck driver, sits for prolonged periods, and seldom participates in exercise activities. The client smokes one pack of cigarettes and drinks six cans of beer per day. What risk factors should the nurse include in the discussion?
   a. lack of exercise, obesity, sitting for long periods, smoking, sedentary occupation
   b. degenerative disk disease, gender, race, smoking
   c. degenerative disk disease, race, alcohol use, smoking, inactivity
   d. age, obesity, lack of exercise, genetic factors

8. Which of the following lab data would be most significant in the client with Paget's disease?
   a. elevated white blood cells (WBC)
   b. elevated eosinophil sedimentation rate (ESR)
   c. positive tissue biopsy for *Staphylococcus*
   d. elevated serum alkaline phosphatase

9. A client has been diagnosed with a metastatic bone tumor. Which of the following interventions would be most effective in preventing a pathological fracture?

   a. Restricting activities to complete bedrest.

   b. Instructing the client on pivot transfers.

   c. Gently supporting limbs during position changes.

   d. Providing a calcium supplement.

10. A young client, age 14, will receive a Milwaukee brace for scoliosis. Reviewing her discharge instructions, the nurse will know the client understands the teaching when she states she will

   a. wear the brace all day and remove it only to bathe.

   b. wear the brace after school and at night.

   c. put the brace on a minimum of 1 hour 3 times per day.

   d. take off the brace if her skin gets sore or starts to break down.

CHAPTER 40

ASSESSING CLIENTS WITH NEUROLOGIC DISORDERS

LEARNING OUTCOMES

After completing this chapter, you will be able to:

- Review the anatomy and physiology of the nervous system.
- Identify specific topics for consideration during a health history assessment interview of the client with neurologic disorders.
- Describe assessment of neurologic function, including examinations of mental status, cranial nerves, sensory nerves, motor nerves, cerebellar function, and reflexes.
- Describe special neurologic examinations for clients with suspected meningeal irritation and for comatose clients.
- Identify abnormal findings that may indicate impairment of neurologic function.

KEY TOPICS

- Review of anatomy and physiology of the neurological system
- Assessing clients with neurological disorders

LECTURE OUTLINE

I. Background of anatomy and physiology
  A. Nervous system divided into 2 regions
    1. Central nervous system (CNS): brain and spinal cord
    2. Peripheral nervous system (PNS) cranial nerves, spinal nerves and autonomic nervous system
  B. Cells of nervous system
    1. Neurons: which receive and send impulses
      a. Types
        1. Dendrite: short process from cell body that conducts impulses toward (afferent) cell body

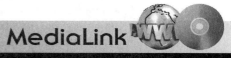

MediaLink

www.prenhall.com/lemone

Additional resources for this chapter can be found on the Student CD-ROM accompanying this textbook, and on the Companion Website at www.prenhall.com/lemone. Click on Chapter 40 to select the activities for this chapter.

CD-ROM
- Audio Glossary
- NCLEX Review

Animation
- Nervous System A&P

Video
- Extrapyramidal Signs

Companion Website
- More NCLEX Review
- Functional Health Pattern Assessment
- Case Study
  Assessing an Unconscious Client

    2. Cell body: clustered together in ganglia or nuclei
    3. Axon: long process that conducts impulses away (efferent) from cell body
      b. Grey matter: cell bodies and dendrites
      c. White matter: myelinated nerve fibers

1. Many axons covered with myelin sheath (white lipid substance): increases speeds of nerve impulse conduction in axons; essential for survival of large nerve processes
2. Myelin sheath interrupted at intervals by unmyelinated areas called nodes of Ranvier which allow movement of ions between axons and extracellular fluid

2. Neuroglia: protect and nourish neurons

C. Action Potentials
1. Impulses that allow neurons to communicate with other neurons and body cells
2. Impulses to and from CNS require
   a. Afferent (sensory) neurons which have receptors in skin, muscles, and other impulses and relay impulses to CNS
   b. Efferent (motor) neurons transmit impulses from CNS to cause some type of action
3. Impulses occur when stimulus reaches a point great enough to generate change in the electrical charge across cell membrane of neuron
4. Chief regulators of membrane potential: sodium (positive ion in extracellular fluid) and potassium (positive ion in intracellular fluid)
5. Action potential generated only at point of stimulus but once generated propagates along entire length of axon whether stimulus continues
6. Conduction is rapid in myelinated fibers; conduction is slower in unmyelinated fibers

D. Neurotransmitters
1. Chemical messengers of nervous system: neurotransmitter is released when action potential reaches end of axon at presynaptic terminal
2. Neurotransmitter travels across synapse to bind with receptors in the postsynaptic neuron dendrite or cell body
3. Neurotransmitters
   a. Inhibitory or excitatory
   b. Specific neurotransmitters
      1. Acetylcholine (ACh): excitatory, rapidly degraded by enzyme acetylcholinesterase
      2. Norepinephrine (NE): may be inhibitory or excitatory
   c. Cholinergic: nerves that transmit impulses through release of ACh

1. Receptors found in viscera, skeletal muscle cells, adrenal medulla (where release of epinephrine occurs)
2. May be excitatory or inhibitory

d. Adrenergic: nerves that transmit impulses through release of NE
1. Found in heart, lungs, kidneys, blood vessels, all target organs stimulated by sympathetic division except heart
2. Adrenergic receptors are 2 types
   a. Alpha-adrenergic receptors: binding to alpha receptors stimulates a response; functions include arterial vasoconstriction
   b. Beta-adrenergic receptors: binding to beta receptors inhibits a response; 2 types
      1. Beta-1: receptors in heart, regulate rate and force of contraction
      2. Beta-2: receptor cells of lungs, arteries, liver, uterus (regulate bronchial diameter, arterial diameter, glycogenesis)

e. Other neurotransmitters
1. Gamma aminobutyric acid (GABA): inhibits CNS function
2. Dopamine: inhibitory or excitatory and controls fine movement and emotions
3. Serotonin: usually inhibitory; controls sleep, hunger, behavior, affects consciousness

E. Central Nervous System
1. Brain: control center of nervous system
   a. Surrounded by skull which provides support and protection
   b. Composed of 2 hemispheres and has 4 major regions:
      1. Cerebrum
      2. Diencephalon
      3. Brain stem
      4. Cerebellum
   c. Surface of cerebrum
      1. Folded into elevated ridges of tissue called gyri
      2. Separated by shallow grooves called sulci
      3. Cerebral surface divide by deep grooves called fissures
         a. Longitudinal fissure: separates hemispheres

b. Transverse fissure: separates cerebrum from cerebellum
d. Each cerebral hemisphere divided into 4 lobes
   1. Frontal
   2. Parietal
   3. Temporal
   4. Occipital
e. Cerebral hemispheres connected by corpus callosum, thick band of nerve fibers that allows communication between hemispheres
   1. Each hemisphere receives sensory and motor impulses from opposite side of body
   2. One of hemisphere is more developed than other
      a. Left usually more developed and controls language development
      b. Right has greater control over nonverbal perceptual functions
f. Diencephalon: embedded in cerebrum superior to brain stem
   1. Thalamus: serves as sorting, processing, and relaying station for inputs into cortical region
   2. Hypothalamus: regulation of temperature, water metabolism, appetite, emotional expression, part of sleep-wake cycle, thirst
   3. Epithalamus: includes pineal body part of endocrine system affecting growth and development
g. Brainstem
   1. Midbrain: center for auditory and visual reflexes; nerve pathway between cerebral hemispheres and lower brain
   2. Pons: contains nuclei that control respiration
   3. Medulla oblongata: continuous with superior portion of spinal cord; plays role in controlling heart rate, blood pressure, respiration, swallowing
h. Cerebellum: functions include coordination of skeletal muscle activity, maintenance of balance, control of fine movements
i. Ventricles
   1. Chambers filled with cerebrospinal fluid (CSF), linked by ducts that allow CSF to circulate
   2. One lateral ventricle located within each hemisphere which

communicates with third ventricle through foramen of Monro; third ventricle communicates with fourth ventricle through cerebral aqueduct that runs through midbrain
   3. Cerebral aqueduct is continuous with central canal of spinal cord
j. Cerebrospinal fluid (CSF)
   1. Clear, colorless liquid formed by choroid plexus located in brain ventricles
   2. Cushions brain tissue, protects brain and spinal cord from trauma, provides nourishment to brain, removes waster of cerebrospinal cellular metabolism
   3. Amount is 150 mL, replaced several times per day
   4. Circulation: lateral ventricles to third ventricle through midbrain into fourth ventricle; some CSF circulates through spinal cord and circulates into subarachnoid space and returns to blood through arachnoid villi
k. Meninges: Covering of CNS composed of 3 connective tissue membranes
   1. Dura mater: outermost, double layer
   2. Arachnoid layer: middle layer forms space that contains CSF, site of all major cerebral blood vessels
   3. Pia mater: innermost layer and clings to brain, filled with many small blood vessels
l. Cerebral circulation
   1. Cerebral hemispheres supplied by anterior and middle cerebral arteries, branches of common carotid arteries
   2. Brain stem and cerebellum supplied by basilar artery
   3. Posterior cerebrum supplied by posterior cerebral arteries
   4. Major arteries connected by small arteries and for circle of connected blood vessels called circle of Willis, which provides alternative routes for circulation to brain
   5. Brain receives 750 mL of blood per minute; uses 20% of body's total oxygen uptake (needed for glucose metabolism, brain's sole source of energy)

m. Blood-brain barrier
1. Brain protected from many harmful substances in blood because capillaries of brain have low permeability
2. Allows lipids, glucose, some amino acids, water, carbon dioxide, oxygen to pass through
3. Usually blocks, urea, creatinine, some toxins, proteins, most antibiotics
n. Limbic system
1. Tissue in medial side of each hemisphere
2. Integrates and modulates affective part of brain
3. Provides emotional and behavioral responses to environmental stimuli
o. Reticular formation
1. Relays sensory input from all body systems to all levels of brain
2. Reticular activating system (RAS): stimulating system for cerebral cortex keeping it alert and responsive to stimuli
3. Sleep center
4. Area that maintains motor tone and coordinated movements
5. Vasomotor and cardiovascular regulatory centers
2. Spinal cord
a. Surrounded and protected by 33 vertebrae
1. Types of vertebrae
a. 7 cervical
b. 12 thoracic
c. 5 lumbar
d. 5 sacral
e. Coccyx (4 fused vertebrae)
2. Vertebra consists of bone with body and vertebral arch; vertebral foramina form vertebral canal through which spinal cord passes
3. Intervertebral discs are located between each of moveable vertebrae; composed of thick capsule surrounding gelatinous core called nucleus pulposus
b. Extends from medulla to level of first lumbar vertebra
c. Serves as center for conducting messages to and from brain and as a reflex center
d. Protected by vertebrae, meninges, CSF (cerebro-spinal fluid)

e. Gray matter of cord on inside; white matter on outside
3. Spinal nerves
a. 31 pairs divided into cervical thoracic and lumbar nerves; each nerve has
1. Posterior (sensory): damage causes loss of sensation
2. Anterior (motor) root: damage causes flaccid paralysis
b. Messages to and from brain travel via
1. Ascending (sensory) pathways
a. Major ascending tracts are lateral and anterior spinothalamic tracts
b. Carry sensations for pain, temperature, crude touch
2. Descending (motor) pathways
a. Fasciculus gracilis, fasciculus cuneatus: carry sensations for fine touch, position, and vibration
b. Pyramidal tracts: mediate purposeful movement, stimulate and inhibit certain muscle actions; carry fibers that inhibit muscle tone
c. Extrapyrimaidal tracts: maintain muscle tone and gross body movements
4. Upper motor neurons (UMN): corticospinal and extrapyrimidal tract
a. Carry impulses from cerebral cortex to anterior gray column of spinal cord
b. Damage results in increased muscle tone, decreased muscle strength, decreased coordination and hyperactive reflexes
5. Lower motor neurons (LMN): peripheral and cranial nerves
a. Begin in anterior gray column of spinal cord and end in muscle "final common pathways"
b. Damage results in decreased muscle tone and loss of reflexes
F. Peripheral Nervous System
1. Links CNS and rest of body; responsible for receiving and transmitting information from and about external environment
2. Composed of nerves, ganglia (groups of nerve cells), sensory receptors outside CNS (i.e., peripheral)
3. Divided into sensory (afferent) division and motor (efferent) division; most PNS nerves contain fibers of both divisions
a. Spinal nerves

1. Each contains both sensory and motor fibers
2. Main spinal nerve plexuses (complex nerve clusters) innervate skin and underlying muscles of arms and legs, e.g., cervical, brachial, lumbar, sacral plexuses
3. Dermatome: area innervated by cutaneous branches of a single spinal nerve; provide anatomical landmarks that can be used to locate neurologic lesions
   b. Cranial nerves
      1. Twelve pairs of cranial nerves originate in forebrain and brain stem
      2. Vagus nerve extends into ventral body cavity; other 11 innervate head and neck regions
      3. Most cranial nerves are both sensory and motor
      4. Reflexes
         a. Rapid, involuntary, predictable motor response to a stimulus
            1. Somatic reflexes result in skeletal muscle contraction
            2. Autonomic reflexes: activate cardiac and smooth muscle and glands
         b. Reflex conducted over a pathway called a reflex arc; composed of
            1. Receptor
            2. Sensory neuron to carry afferent impulses to CNS
            3. Integration center in spinal cord or brain
            4. Motor neuron to carry efferent impulses
            5. Effector (tissue responding by contracting or secreting)
         c. Spinal reflexes: somatic reflexes mediated by spinal cord
            1. Many occur without impulses traveling back and forth to brain; cord serves as integration center
            2. Some require brain activity and modulation
         d. Deep tendon reflexes (DTR)
            1. Occur in response to muscle contraction causing muscle to relax and lengthen
            2. Abnormal DTR can indicate variety of pathology

including lesion of a spinal nerve
      e. DTR depend on
         1. Intact sensory and motor nerve root
         2. Functional synapses in spinal cord
         3. Functional neuromuscular junction
         4. Competent muscle
4. Autonomic Nervous System (ANS)
   a. Regulates internal environment of body; general visceral motor system; regulates cardiac muscle, smooth muscle, glands
   b. Reticular formation in brain stem primary controller of ANS; centers in medullar initiates reflexes that regulate
      1. Cardiac rate
      2. Blood vessel diameter
      3. GI function
   c. Divisions of ANS are sympathetic and parasympathetic
      1. Affect same structures with opposing effects
      2. Neurotransmitters
         a. Acetylcholine: parasympathetic
         b. Norepinephrine: sympathetic
      3. Stimulation of sympathetic nervous system: prepares body to handle situations perceived as stressful or harmful "fright or flight"; reactions include
         a. Dilated pupils, increased mental alertness
         b. Inhibited secretions (dry mouth), diaphoresis
         c. Coronary arteries dilate; rate and force of heartbeat increases; arteries vasoconstrict
         d. Bronchioles dilate
         e. Increased release of glucose by liver; increased metabolic rate, decreased digestion
         f. Vasoconstriction of abdominal and skin blood vessels
         g. Increased blood clotting
         h. Decreased urine output
      4. Parasympathetic division operates during nonstressful situations, more or less the body's normal day to day functioning; reactions include
         a. Constriction of pupils
         b. Stimulation of glandular secretions

c. Constriction of bronchioles

d. Increased peristalsis and secretion of GI fluid

II. Assessing Neurologic Function

A. Health assessment interview to collect subjective data

1. If client's ability to communicate is challenged by altered level of consciousness, interviewer may discuss with family member or close friend

2. If client has a health problem involving neurologic function, determine

a. Onset

b. Characteristics and course

c. Severity

d. Precipitating and relieving factors

e. Associated symptoms noting timing and circumstances

3. Questions about present health status include

a. Numbness or tingling sensations

b. Tremors, problems with coordination or balance

c. Loss of movement of any part of the body

d. Difficulty with speaking or senses

e. Information about memory

f. Feeling state, e.g., anxious, depressed

g. Changes in sleep patterns

h. Ability to perform self-care and ADL

i. Sexual activity

j. Weight changes

k. Prescribed and over the counter medications, frequency of use and duration

4. Determine history of

a. Seizures, fainting, dizziness, headaches

b. Trauma, tumors, surgery involving brain, spinal cord, nerves

c. Diseases that might affect neurologic function

1. Cardiac disease

2. Strokes

3. Pernicious anemia

4. Sinus infections

5. Liver dysfunctions

6. Diabetes mellitus

7. HPT

8. Mental health problems

5. Determine if client is exposed to any occupational hazards

a. Exposure to toxic chemicals or materials

b. Use of protective headgear

c. Time spent in performing repetitive motions

6. Assessment of

a. Usual diet

b. Use of tobacco, drugs, alcohol

c. Following safety precautions; risk-taking behaviors, e.g., wearing helmets while bicycling

B. Physical assessment to collect objective data

1. Mental status assessment with abnormal findings

a. Unilateral neglect: strokes involving middle cerebral artery

b. Poor hygiene and grooming: dementing disorders

c. Abnormal gait and posture: transient ischemic attacks (TIAs), strokes, Parkinson's disease

d. Emotional swings, personality changes: strokes of anterior cerebral artery

e. Masklike appearance on face: Parkinson's disease

f. Apathy: dementing disease

g. Aphasia (defective or absent language function): TIAs, strokes; strokes involving posterior or anterior artery involve receptive aphasia

h. Dysphonia (change in tone of voice): strokes of posterior inferior cerebral artery, paralysis of vocal cords, cranial nerve X

i. Dysarthria (difficulty in speaking): strokes involving anterior, inferior, and superior cerebral arteries, lesions involving UMN, LMN, cerebellum, extrapyramidal tract

j. Decreased level of consciousness: brain trauma, infections, TIAs, stroke, brain tumors

k. Confusion, coma: strokes affecting vertebralbasilar arteries

2. Cognitive function assessment with abnormal findings

a. Disorientation to time and place: stroke of right cerebral hemisphere

b. Memory deficits: anterior cerebral artery and vertebralbasilar artery

c. Perceptual deficits: strokes of middle cerebral artery, brain trauma, dementing conditions

d. Impaired cognition: strokes of middle cerebral artery, cerebral trauma, brain tumors

3. Cranial nerve assessments with abnormal findings
   a. CN (cranial nerve) I (olfactory): Anosmia (inability to smell)
      1. Lesions of frontal lobe
      2. Impaired blood flow to middle cerebral artery
   b. CN II (optic)
      1. Blindness in one eye: strokes of internal carotid artery, TIA's
      2. Homonymous hemianopia (impaired vision/blindness in one side of both eyes): blockage of posterior cerebral artery
      3. Impaired vision: strokes of anterior cerebral artery, brain tumors
      4. Blindness, double vision: involvement of vertebralbasilar arteries; double or blurred vision may occur with TIA's
      5. Papilledema (swelling of optic nerve): increased intracranial pressure
   c. CN III, IV, VI (oculomotor, trochlear, abducens)
      1. Nystagmus (involuntary eye movement): strokes of anterior, inferior, superior cerebellar arteries
      2. Constricted pupils: may signify impaired blood flow to vertebral basilar arteries
      3. Ptosis: strokes posterior inferior cerebellar artery, myasthenia gravis, palsy of CN III
   d. CN V (trigeminal): Changes in facial sensations; impaired blood flow to carotid artery
      1. Decreased sensation to face and cornea on same side of body: strokes of posterior inferior cerebral artery
      2. Lip and mouth numbness: strokes of vertebral basilar artery
      3. Loss of facial sensation, contraction of masseter and temporal muscles: lesions CN V
      4. Severe facial pain: trigeminal neuralgia (tic douloureux)
   e. CN VII (facial)
      1. Loss of ability to taste: brain tumors, nerve impairment
      2. Decreased movement of facial muscles: lesions of UMN, LMN
      3. Inability to close eyes, flat nasolabial fold, paralysis of lower face, inability to wrinkle forehead: paralysis of LMN
      4. Eyelid weakness, paralysis of lower face: paralysis of upper motor neuron
      5. Pain, paralysis, sagging of facial muscles: affected side in Bell's palsy
   f. CN VIII (acoustic): Decreased hearing or deafness: strokes of vertebral basilar arteries or tumors of CN VIII
   g. CN IX and X (glossopharyngeal, vagus)
      1. Dysphagia (difficulty in swallowing): impaired blood flow to vertebralbasilar arteries, posterior or anterior, inferior, or superior cerebellar arteries
      2. Unilateral loss of gag reflex: lesions of CN IX and X
   h. CN XI (spinal accessory)
      1. Muscle weakness: LMN disease
      2. Contralateral hemiparesis: strokes affecting middle cerebral artery and internal carotid artery
   i. CN XII (hypoglossal)
      1. Atrophy, fasciculations (twitches): LMN disease
      2. Tongue deviation toward involved side of body
4. Sensory function assessment with abnormal findings
   a. Altered sensation occurs with variety of neurologic pathology
      1. Decreased pain sensation: spinothalamic tract injury
      2. Decreased vibratory sensation: posterior column tract injuries
      3. Transient numbness of upper extremity: TIA's
      4. Sensory loss of one side of body: lesions involving higher pathways to spinal cord
      5. Bilateral sensory loss: polyneuropathy
      6. Impaired sensations: stroke, brain tumor, spinal cord compression or trauma
   b. Altered sense of position: lesions of posterior column of spinal cord
   c. Inability to discriminate fine touch: injury to posterior columns or sensory cortex
5. Motor function assessments with abnormal findings

a. Muscle atrophy: LMN diseases
b. Tremors: activity seen with multiple sclerosis, cerebellar disease
c. Tremors occurring at rest and abating with movement commonly occur with Parkinson's disease
d. Fasciculations: disease or trauma to LMN, side effects of medications, fever, sodium deficiency, uremia
e. Flaccidity (decreased muscle tone): disease or trauma to LMN and early stroke
f. Spasticity (increased muscle tone): disease of corticospinal motor tract
g. Muscle rigidity: disease of extrapyramidal motor tract
h. Cogwheel rigidity (muscular movement with small regular jerky movement): Parkinson's disease
i. Muscle weakness in arms, legs, hands: TIA's
j. Hemiplegia (paralysis of half of body vertically): strokes involving internal carotid artery and posterior cerebral artery
k. Weakness of extremities: strokes involving vertebralbasilar arteries
l. Flaccid paralysis: strokes of anterior spinal artery
m. Paralysis, decreased movement: multiple sclerosis or myasthenia gravis
n. Total loss of motor function below level of injury: complete spinal cord transaction, injuries to anterior portion of spinal cord
o. Spasticity of muscles: incomplete spinal cord injuries

6. Cerebellar function assessment with abnormal findings
   a. Ataxia (lack of coordination and clumsiness of movement; staggering, wide-based and unbalanced gait): anterior strokes, cerebellar tumors
   b. Swaying and falling: cerebellar ataxia
   c. Inability to walk on toes, then heels: UMN disease
   d. Spastic hemiparesis: strokes or UMN disease
   e. Steppage gait (client drags or lifts foot high, then slaps foot onto floor; inability to walk on heels): disease of LMN

f. Sensory ataxia (client walks on heels before bringing down toes and feet are held wide apart; gait worsens with eyes closed): polyneuropathy, damage to posterior columns
g. Parkinsonian gait (stooped over position while walking with shuffling gait with arms held close to the side): Parkinson's disease
h. Positive Romberg test: cerebellar ataxia

7. Reflex assessment with abnormal findings
   a. Hyperactive reflexes: lesions affecting UMN
   b. Decreased reflexes: LMN involvement
   c. Clonus of foot (hyperactive, rhythmic dorsiflexion and plantar flexion of foot): UMN disease
   d. Superficial reflexes (such as abdominal) and cremasteric reflex may be absent with LMN and UMN diseases
   e. Positive Babinski reflex (dorsiflexion of big toe with fanning of other toes): UMN diseases of pyramidal tract

8. Special neurologic assessment with abnormal findings
   a. Positive Brudzinski's sign (pain, resistance, flexion of hips and knees when head flexed to chest with client supine) indicates meningeal irritation
   b. Positive Kernig's sign (excessive pain and/or resistance when examiner attempts to straighten knees with client supine and knees and hips flexed) indicates meningeal irritation
   c. Decorticate posturing (upper arms close to sides, elbows, wrists and fingers flexed, legs extended with internal rotation, feet are flexed: body parts pulled into core of body): lesions of corticospinal tracts
   d. Decerebrate posturing (neck extended with jaw clenched, arms pronated, extended, close to sides, legs are extended straight out and feet plantar flexed): lesions of midbrain, pons, diencephalon

FOCUSED STUDY TIPS

- Practice assessing reflexes at home. As you are assessing, explain each reflex and describe normal and abnormal findings.
- Compare and contrast the functioning of the CNS (central nervous system) and the PNS (peripheral nervous system). Identify two drugs that affect the functioning of each system. Make drug cards for these drugs and share them with classmates.
- Describe how an external stimulus such as a pin prick is processed and interpreted by the neurological system. Identify sensory and motor responses.

CASE STUDY

During morning report, a client is described as being diagnosed with ataxia. What can the nurse anticipate when caring for this client? What nursing interventions will be utilized in the care of this client? What test can the nurse perform to confirm the diagnosis?

CARE PLAN CRITICAL THINKING ACTIVITY

Describe the purpose of each and how they will be utilized. For each, detail an abnormal assessment finding. How will peceberate posturing impact a nursing care for a client with a neurological disorder? Anticipate and describe nursing interventions that may be implemented.

NCLEX TEST QUESTIONS

1. If a client with increased intracranial pressure (ICP) demonstrates decorticate posturing, the nurse will observe:
   a. flexion of both upper and lower extremities.
   b. extension of elbows and knees, plantar flexion of feet, and flexion of the wrists.
   c. flexion of elbows, extension of the knees, and plantar flexion of the feet.
   d. extension of upper extremities, flexion of lower extremities.

2. A client is admitted following a head injury sustained in an auto accident. The nurse assessing the client's level of consciousness understands that maintenance of an awake and alert status is dependent on the proper functioning of which two cerebral structures?
   a. reticular activating system and both cerebral hemispheres
   b. parietal and occipital lobes
   c. pons and basal ganglia
   d. thalamus and hypothalamus

3. The nurse is caring for a 37-year-old female admitted with an intracerebral bleed. The nurse on the preceding shift reports that a neurological examination was performed on the client and that she had an abnormal "doll's eyes" test. Which of

the following descriptions best describes an abnormal oculocephalic response to the "doll's eyes" test?
   a. Bright light in one eye causes a constriction of the opposite pupil.
   b. The eyes follow the direction of a quick turn of the head.
   c. The eyes tend to remain opposite to the direction of the head turn.
   d. The eyes develop nystagmus following instillation of cold water into the ear.

4. When assessing a client on the neurological unit, the nurse knows that decerebrate posturing is characterized by
   a. abnormal extension response.
   b. abnormal flexion response.
   c. hyperflexion of the lower extremities.
   d. absent motor response.

5. Which of the following best describes Kernig's sign?
   a. muscle spasms in the arm upon occlusion with a blood pressure cuff
   b. twitching of the face upon tapping the cheek
   c. inability to flex the neck
   d. inability to extend the leg when the thigh is flexed to the abdomen

6. To assess third cranial nerve function, the nurse would test the client's
   a. pupillary light reflexes.
   b. eye movement.
   c. smell.
   d. hearing.

7. Gentamycin is prescribed for a client with urinary tract infection. The nurse will observe for cranial nerve VIII toxicity indicated by:
   a. vertigo.
   b. dilated pupils
   c. tinnitus.
   d. facial tremors.

8. The telephone triage nurse tells the client who is complaining of fever, nausea, chills, and malaise to come immediately to the emergency department when he relates he also has a:
   a. bad headache.
   b. stiff, sore neck.
   c. heart rate of 106.
   d. roommate with the same symptoms.

9. Chvostek's sign, which may be positive in the presence of hypomagnesemia, would be noted if the client had which of the following responses to stimulation?
   a. twitch of nose or lip
   b. blink
   c. lacrimation
   d. pain

10. A client has just been admitted to the unit following an accident in which he sustained an injury to the temporal lobe. The nurse's assessment will focus on disturbances in the client's:
    a. sight.
    b. hearing.
    c. spatial orientation.
    d. taste.

CHAPTER 41

NURSING CARE OF CLIENTS WITH CEREBROVASCULAR AND SPINAL CORD DISORDERS

LEARNING OUTCOMES

After completing this chapter, you will be able to:

- Apply knowledge of normal neurologic anatomy and physiology and assessments when providing nursing care for clients with cerebrovascular and spinal cord disorders (see Chapter 40).
- Identify factors responsible for disorders in cerebral blood flow.
- Explain the pathophysiologic effects, manifestations, and complications of alterations in cerebral blood flow due to thrombi, emboli, hemorrhage, aneurysm, and arteriovenous malformation.
- Identify factors responsible for spinal cord injuries.
- Discuss the pathophysiologic effects of injuries of the spinal cord by level of injury.
- Describe the causes and manifestations of cervical and lumbar herniated intervertebral disks.
- Discuss the types and manifestations of spinal cord tumors.
- Explain the collaborative care of clients with cerebrovascular and spinal cord disorders.
- Use the nursing process as a framework for providing individualized care to clients with cerebrovascular and spinal cord disorders.

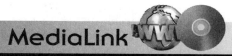

MediaLink

www.prenhall.com/lemone

Additional resources for this chapter can be found on the Student CD-ROM accompanying this textbook, and on the Companion Website at www.prenhall.com/lemone. Click on Chapter 41 to select the activities for this chapter.

CD-ROM
- Audio Glossary
- NCLEX Review

Companion Website
- More NCLEX Review
- Case Study
  Spinal Cord Injury
- Care Plan Activity
  Hemorrhagic Stroke

KEY TOPICS

- Cerebral vascular disorders
- Spinal cord disorders
- Nursing care of clients with cerebrovascular and spinal cord disorders

LECTURE OUTLINE

I. Client with a stroke
  A. General Description and Physiology
    1. Stroke (cerebral vascular accident or CVA): condition in which neurologic deficits result from decreased blood flow to localized area of brain
    2. Categories
      a. Ischemic: blood supply to part of brain suddenly interrupted by thrombus or embolus
      b. Hemorrhagic: when blood vessel breaks open, spilling blood into brain
    3. Neurologic deficits determined by the area of brain involved, size of affected area, length of time blood flow is decreased or stopped
    4. Major loss of blood supply to brain can cause severe disability or death; if short or small area involved client may not be aware
    5. Third leading cause of death in North America
      a. Many clients survive and are left with some type of functional impairment
      b. Highest incidence in age > 65
      c. More frequently males than females
    6. Risk Factors
      a. HPT
      b. Diabetes mellitus
      c. Sickle cell disease
      d. Substance abuse including alcohol, nicotine, heroin, amphetamines, cocaine
      e. Atherosclerosis
    7. Additional Factors
      a. Obesity, sedentary life-style, hyperlipidemia, atrial fibrillation, cardiac disease, cigarette smoking, previous transient ischemic attacks
      b. Women: oral contraceptive use, pregnancy, menopause
    8. Pathophysiology
      a. Characterized by gradual, rapid onset of neurologic deficits due to compromised cerebral blood flow
      b. Blood flow and oxygenation of cerebral neurons decreased or interrupted; changes occur in 4–5 minutes
      c. Cells swell and cerebral blood vessels swell decreasing blood flow; vasospasm and increased blood viscosity further impede blood flow

    d. Penumbra: central core of dead or dying cells surrounded by band of minimally perfused cells; these cells may survive if adequate circulation is re-established; use of thrombolytic agents in early treatment of ischemic stroke
    e. Neurologic deficits occur on opposite side where stroke occurred in brain: contralateral deficit
  B. Ischemic Strokes
    1. Transient Ischemic Attack (TIA)
      a. Brief period of localized cerebral ischemia causing neurologic deficits lasting < 24 hours; usually 1–2 hours
      b. Warning signal of ischemic thrombotic stroke
      c. Etiology: inflammatory artery disorders, sickle cell anemia, atherosclerotic changes in cerebral vessels, thrombosis, emboli, subclavian steal syndrome
      d. Neurological manifestation:
        1. According to location and size of cerebral vessel involved
        2. Sudden onset with disappearance within minutes or hours
        3. Common occurring deficits
          a. Contralateral numbness or weakness of hand, forearm, corner of mouth (middle cerebral artery)
          b. Aphasia (due to ischemia of left hemisphere)
          c. Visual disturbances such as blurring (posterior cerebral artery)
    2. Thrombotic CVA
      a. Occlusion of a large cerebral vessel by thrombus; often in older persons who are resting or sleeping when blood pressure is lower
      b. Thrombi tend to form in large arteries that bifurcate; narrowed lumens as result of atherosclerotic plaque
      c. Common locations of thrombi are internal carotid artery, vertebral arteries, junction of vertebral and basilar arteries
      d. Lacunar strokes: thrombotic strokes affecting smaller cerebral vessels; leave small cavity or "lake"

e. Occurs rapidly, progresses slowly; begins as TIA and worsens over 1–2 day period: stroke-in-evolution; when maximum neurologic deficit has been reached (3 days), called completed stroke; damaged area is edematous, necrotic

3. Embolic CVA
   a. Occurs when blood clot or clump of matter traveling through cerebral blood vessels lodges in vessel
   b. Most frequent site of cerebral emboli at bifurcation of vessels (carotid and middle cerebral arteries)
   c. Client usually younger and occurs when client is awake and active; most embolic strokes originate from thrombus in left chambers of heart during atrial fibrillation: cardiac embolic CVAs
   d. Other sources of emboli: carotid artery atherosclerotic plaque, bacterial endocarditis, recent myocardial infarction, rheumatic heart disease, ventricular aneurysm

4. Hemorrhagic Stroke (intracranial hemorrhage)
   a. Occurs when cerebral blood vessel ruptures; occurring most often in persons with sustained increase in systolic-diastolic pressure
   b. Causative factors: hypertension main cause
   c. Other factors: ruptured intracranial aneurysms, trauma, erosion of blood vessels by tumors, arteriovenous malformations, anticoagulant therapy, blood disorders
   d. Most fatal form of stroke
   e. Pathophysiology: blood vessel ruptures and blood enters blood tissue, cerebral ventricles or subarachnoid space; this compresses adjacent tissues causing blood vessel spasm and cerebral edema
   f. Blood in ventricles or subarachnoid space irritates meninges and brain tissue causing inflammatory reaction and impairing absorption and circulation of cerebrospinal fluid (CSF)
   g. Onset of manifestations is rapid
      1. Depends on location of hemorrhage
      2. Vomiting, headache, seizures, hemiplegia, loss of consciousness

C. Manifestations
   1. Sudden onset, focal, usually one-sided
   2. Most common: weakness of face and arm, sometimes leg
   3. Numbness on one side, loss of vision in one eye or to one side
   4. Speech difficulties
   5. Difficulties with balance
D. Complications
   1. Motor Deficits
      a. Affects connections involving motor areas of cerebral cortex, basal ganglia, cerebellum, peripheral nerves
      b. Produce effects in contralateral side ranging from mild weakness to severe limitation
      c. Hemiplegia: paralysis of half of body
      d. Hemiparesis: weakness of half of body
      e. Flaccidity: absence of muscle tone (hypotonia)
      f. Spasticity: increased muscle tone usually with some degree of weakness
      g. Affected arm and leg are initially flaccid and become spastic in 6–8 weeks, causes characteristic body positioning:
         1. Adduction of shoulder
         2. Pronation of forearm
         3. Flexion of fingers
         4. Extension of hip and knee
         5. Foot drop, outward rotation of leg, with dependent edema
      h. Complications of immobility associated with stroke
         1. Orthostatic hypotension
         2. Increased thrombus formation
         3. Decreased cardiac output
         4. Impaired respiratory function
         5. Osteoporosis
         6. Formation of renal calculi
         7. Contractures
         8. Decubitus ulcer formation
   2. Elimination Disorders
      a. Partial loss of sensation that triggers bladder elimination: urinary frequency, urgency incontinence
      b. May also relate to cognitive deficits
      c. Bowel elimination changes result from LOC (level of conciousness) changes, immobility, dehydration
   3. Sensory-perceptual Deficits
      a. Hemianopia: loss of half of visual field on one or both eyes; homonymous hemianopia: same half missing in each eye

b. Agnosia: inability to recognize one or more subjects that were previously familiar: includes visual, tactile, auditory
c. Apraxia: inability to carry out some motor pattern even when strength and coordination is adequate (e.g., getting dressed)
d. Neglect syndrome (unilateral neglect): attention disorder in which client ignores affected part of body; client cannot integrate or use perceptions from affected side of body or from environment on affected side

4. Communication Disorders
   a. Usually result of stroke affecting dominant hemisphere (left hemisphere dominant in 95% right-handed persons; 70% left-handed persons)
   b. Aphasia: inability to use or understand language
      1. Expressive: motor speech problem; client understands what is said but can only respond verbally in short phases: Broca's aphasia
      2. Receptive aphasia: sensory speech problem in which one cannot understand spoken or written word; speech may be fluent but with inappropriate content: Wernicke's aphasia
      3. Mixed or global aphasia: language dysfunction in both understand and expression
   c. Dysarthria: any disturbance in muscular control of speech

5. Cognitive and Behavioral Changes
   a. Ranges from mild confusion to coma
   b. May result from actual tissue damage from stroke, cerebral edema, or increased intracranial pressure
   c. Manifestations
      1. Emotional lability: laughing or crying inappropriately
      2. Loss of self-control (i.e., swearing, refusing to cooperate)
      3. Decreased tolerance for stress (anger, depression)
      4. Intellectual changes: memory loss, decreased attention span, poor judgment, inability to think abstractly

E. Diagnostic Tests
   1. CT scan without contrast: determine hemorrhage, tumors, aneurysms, ischemia, edema, tissue necrosis, shifting in intracranial contents
   2. Arteriography of cerebral vessels: reveals abnormal vessel structures, vasospasm, stenosis of arteries
   3. Transcranial ultrasound Doppler: velocity of blood flow through intracranial arteries, degree of occlusion
   4. MRI: detect shifting of brain tissues resulting from hemorrhage or edema
   5. Positron emission tomography (PET), single-photon emission computed tomography (SPECT): examine cerebral blood flow distribution and metabolic activity of brain
   6. Lumbar puncture: obtain CSF for examination, if there is no danger of increased intracranial pressure; hemorrhagic stroke shows frank blood in CSF

F. Medications: Preventative drugs: antiplatelet agents
   1. Aspirin
   2. Clopidrogrel (Plavix)
   3. Dipyridamole (Persantine)
   4. Pentoxifylline (Trental)
   5. Ticlopidine (Ticlid)

G. Acute Stroke
   1. Anticoagulant therapy
      a. Ordered for thrombotic stroke during stroke-in-evolution
      b. Contraindicated in completed stroke
      c. Never used in hemorrhagic stroke
      d. Prevent further extension of clot; Heparin, warfarin sodium (Coumadin)
   2. Thrombolytic therapy: must be given within 3 hours of onset of manifestations and will dissolve clot; recombinant altephase (Activase rt-pa)
   3. Antithrombotic: inhibit platelet phase of clot formation; contraindicated with hemorrhagic stroke (aspirin, dipyridamole)
   4. Calcium channel blockers: reduce ischemic deficits, death (Nimodipine (Nimotop))
   5. Corticosteroids: used to treat cerebral edema
   6. Diuretics: reduce increased intracranial pressure: mannitol, furosemide
   7. Anticonvulsants: phenytoin (Dilantin)

H. Treatments
   1. Surgery
      a. Carotid endarectomy: in clients who have had TIAs
      b. Extracranial-intracranial bypass

2. Physical therapy: prevents contractures, improves muscle strength and coordination
3. Occupational therapy: provides assistive devices and plans for regaining lost motor skills
4. Speech therapy: improves communication disorder
I. Nursing Care
1. Promote full recovery, reduce disabilities
2. Provide care during acute and rehabilitative phases of care
3. Facilitate changes in role within family
J. Health Promotion
1. Stop smoking, lower all risks for heart disease, hypertension
2. Increase public awareness of signs of TIA and stroke and the need to call 911 immediately and seek medical care
K. Nursing Diagnoses
1. Ineffective Tissue Perfusion: Cerebral; frequent monitoring of neurologic status, cardiac status
2. Impaired Physical Mobility
3. Self-care Deficit
4. Impaired Verbal Communication
5. Impaired Urinary Elimination and Risk for Constipation
6. Impaired Swallowing
L. Home Care
1. Encourage self-care as much as possible with family involvement
2. Referrals to home health care and rehabilitative sources
II. Client with Intracranial Aneurysm
A. Description
1. Saccular outpouching of cerebral artery occurs at site of weakness in vessel wall
2. Results from atherosclerosis, congenital defect, trauma to head, aging, HPT
3. Most common cause of hemorrhagic stroke
4. Most common in adults 30–60
B. Pathophysiology
1. Occur at bifurcation and branches of carotid arteries and vertebrobasilar arteries
2. Types of aneurysms
a. Berry: probably result of congenital abnormality of tunica media of artery
b. Saccular: saccular outpouching, commonly results from trauma
c. Fusiform: entire circumference of blood vessel forms elongated tube; results from arteriosclerosis, and are space occupying lesions

d. Dissecting: tunica intima pulls away from tunica media; blood is forced between 2 layers; results from atherosclerosis, inflammation, trauma
3. Aneurysms rupture from dome rather than base forcing blood into subarachnoid space at base of brain; blood forced into brain tissue, ventricles, subdural space
C. Manifestations
1. Usually asymptomatic until it ruptures
2. May cause headache and/or neurologic deficits due to pressure on adjacent structures: headache, nausea, vomiting, pain in neck and back
3. Prodromal manifestations before rupture: headache, eye pain, visual deficits, dilated pupil
4. Ruptured intracranial aneurysm and subsequent subarachnoid hemorrhage
a. Sudden explosive headache
b. Loss of consciousness
c. Nausea and vomiting
d. Stiff neck and photophobia (meningeal irritation)
e. Cranial nerve deficits
f. Stroke syndrome and pituitary manifestations
5. Subarachnoid hemorrhage is graded according to manifestations
a. Grade I: no symptoms or slight headache, neck stiffness
b. Grade V: deep coma with decerebrate posturing
D. Complications
1. Rebleeding: sudden severe headache, nausea and vomiting, decreasing level of consciousness, new neurologic deficits
2. Vasospasm
a. Occurs between 3 and 10 days post subarachnoid hemorrhage causing ischemia and infarction of tissue supplied by blood vessels
b. Results include focal deficits or global alterations: loss of consciousness
3. Hydrocephalus
a. Abnormal accumulation of CSF within cranial vault
b. Dilation of ventricles due to obstruction of reabsorption of CSF by arachnoid villi
c. Signs of increased intracranial pressure
E. Collaborative Care
1. Determine location of aneurysm
2. Treat manifestation of hemorrhage
3. Prevent rebleeding and vasospasm

F. Diagnostic Tests
  1. CT scan of brain: demonstrates blood in subarachnoid space within 24–48 hours after rupture
  2. Lumbar puncture: confirmation of subarachnoid hemorrhage; risks include risk of rebleeding, brain herniation
  3. Bilateral carotid and vertebral cerebral angiography: determine site and size of aneurysm
G. Treatments
  1. Medications
    a. Aminocaroic acid (Amicar, Epsikapron) fibrinolysis inhibitor used to treat excessive bleeding in acute life threatening situations; used in first 2 weeks after the event to reduce risk of rebleeding (given IV, then orally)
    b. Calcium channel blockers such as nimodipine to improve neurologic deficits due to vasospasm; administered orally for 3 weeks after hemorrhage; reduces ischemic deficits from arterial spasm
    c. Anticonvulsants to prevent seizures if increased intracranial pressure
    d. Stool softeners to prevent constipation and straining with bowel movement
    e. Analgesics for headache
  2. Surgery
    a. Done to prevent rupture or isolate vessel to prevent further bleeding
    b. Clients in good neurologic status may have surgery soon after rupture; for those with significant deficits surgery is delayed until clients are more stable
    c. Surgeries include repair ruptured intracranial aneurysm including clipping, insertion of endovascular coils
H. Nursing Diagnosis: Ineffective Tissue Perfusion: Cerebral
  1. Maintain head of bed at least 30 degrees to promote venous return from brain
  2. Quiet environment and limited stress
  3. Monitoring vital signs and neurologic status
  4. Measures to avoid increased intracranial pressure including seizure precautions, avoiding coughing, vomiting, straining, Valsalva maneuver
III. Client with an Arteriovenous Malformation
  A. Description
    1. Congenital intracranial lesion formed by tangled collection of dilated arteries and veins

  2. 90% occur in cerebral hemispheres
  3. Accounts for 2% of strokes
  4. Occurs before age of 40 years of age
B. Pathophysiology
  Shunting of arterial blood directly into venous system, which is likely to cause spontaneous bleeding or progressive expansion and rupture of blood vessel; adjacent areas may be ischemic due to diversion of blood flow
C. Manifestations
  1. Seizure activity with large malformations
  2. Recurrent headaches not responsive to treatment
D. Diagnostic Tests
  1. CT scan
  2. MRI
  3. Angiography
E. Treatment
  1. Surgery
    a. Excision of malformation and removal of any hematoma
    b. Embolization: with Gelfoam or metallic pellets introduced into area of malformation
  2. Radiation therapy or laser therapy to coagulate blood in malformation
IV. Client with Spinal Cord Injury (SCI)
  A. Background
    1. Usually due to trauma
    2. Most common in the 16–30 age group
    3. Causes
      a. Motor vehicle accidents
      b. Falls, violence, sport injuries (diving)
    4. Physical Description
      a. Concussion, contusion, laceration, transection, hemorrhage, damage to blood vessels supplying spinal cord
      b. Fractured vertebrae damage cord
      c. Injuries are identified by vertebral level
  B. Risk Factors
    1. Age
      a. Youth (take risks)
      b. Older adults (age-related vertebral degeneration)
    2. Gender: males more than females
    3. Alcohol or drug use
  C. Pathophysiology
    1. Primary injury causes microscopic hemorrhages in gray matter of cord and edema of white matter of cord
    2. Microcirculation of cord is impaired by edema and hemorrhage; further impaired by vasospasm

3. Necrosis of gray and white matter occurs and function of nerves through injured area is lost
4. Acceleration and deceleration as occurs in motor vehicle accidents and falls and is most common cause of abnormal spinal column movements
   a. Hyperflexion: forcible forward bending, compression of vertebral bodies and disrupt ligaments and intervertebral disks
   b. Hyperextension: forcible backward bending, disrupts ligaments and causes vertebral fracture
   c. Axial loading: form of compression applying vertical force as with falling and landing on feet or buttocks; diving into shallow water
   d. Excessive rotation: head excessively turned causing compression fractures
5. Other causes include penetration by bullets or foreign objects
D. Sites of Pathology: Most common areas of involvement
   1. Cervical (C1, C2, C4–C6)
   2. T11 to L2
E. Classifications
   1. Completeness
      a. Complete SCI: motor and sensory neural pathways are completely transected resulting in total loss of motor and sensory function below level of injury
      b. Incomplete SCI: motor and sensory neural pathways are only partially interrupted resulting with variable loss of function below level of injury
   2. Cause of injury: specific as to trauma
   3. Level of injury: area of spinal cord affected
F. Manifestations
   1. General
      a. Depend upon degree and level spinal cord is injured
      b. Affects every body system
   2. Spinal Shock
      a. Temporary loss of reflex function (areflexia) below level of injury beginning immediately after complete transection of spinal cord
      b. Normal activity of spinal cord depends on constant impulses from higher centers of brain; with SCI impulses stop, spinal shock follows

   c. Manifestations
      1. Bradycardia and hypotension
      2. Flaccid paralysis of skeletal muscles distal to injury
      3. Loss of all sensation distal to injury
      4. Absence of visceral and somatic sensations
      5. Bladder and bowel dysfunction
      6. Loss of ability to perspire
   d. Spinal shock begins within hour of injury and lasts from few minutes up to several months; ends with return of reflex activity: hyperreflexia, muscle spasticity, reflex bladder emptying
   e. Client with cervical cord injuries may have persistent cardiovascular changes after spinal shock resolves
      1. Orthostatic hypotension, bradycardia
      2. Decreased peripheral resistance and loss of muscle tone leading to sluggish circulation and decreased venous return
      3. Client at risk for thrombophlebitis
3. Motor Neuron Involvement
   a. Upper motor neuron involvement includes spastic paralysis, hyperreflexia, inability to carry out skilled movement
   b. Lower motor neuron involvement: flaccid muscle and extensive muscle atrophy, loss of voluntary and involuntary movement
   c. Partial motor neuron movement: partial paralysis
   d. All motor neurons affected: complete paralysis
   e. Client may be treated with antispasmodics such as baclofen (Lioresal) or diazepam (Valium)
4. Paraplegia
   a. Paralysis of lower portion of body involving injury to thoracic, lumbar, or sacral portion of spinal cord
   b. Impairment of sensory and/or motor function
5. Tetraplegia (formerly quadriplegia)
   a. Injuries affecting the cervical segments of cord
   b. Impairment of upper extremities as well
6. Autonomic Dysreflexia (autonomic hyperreflexia)
   a. Exaggerated sympathetic response occurring in clients with cord injuries at T6 or higher and after resolution of spinal shock

b. Because of lack of control of autonomic nervous system by higher centers, a stimuli such as full bladder results in mass reflex stimulation of sympathetic nerves below level of injury

c. Client develops bradycardia and severe HPT, flushed, warm skin with profuse sweating above the lesion and dry skin below and anxiety; if sustained could result in stroke, myocardial infarction or seizures

d. Stimuli include
   1. Abdominal discomfort: full bladder
   2. Stimulation of pain receptors: pressure ulcers
   3. Visceral contractions: fecal impaction

e. Prompt intervention is required
   1. Elevate client's head and remove any support hose: this will immediately decrease the blood pressure since client has orthostatic hypotension
   2. Monitor blood pressure while assessing for causative factor: relief of full bladder, impacted stool, skin pressure
   3. If there is a history of autonomic dysreflexia, client may be able to warn of occurrence
   4. Notification of physician and administration of medication to lower blood pressure

G. Collaborative Care
   1. Care at the scene
      a. Care must start at scene of injury to reduce injury, preserve function
      b. Rapid assessment of ABC (airway, breathing, circulation)
      c. Immobilize and stabilize head and neck
         1. Use cervical collar before moving onto backboard
         2. Secure head and maintain client in supine position
      d. Care with all transfers not to complicate original injury
      e. Fractures at C1–C4 levels result in respiratory paralysis but advances in trauma care allow clients to survive (will require ventilator assistance)
      f. Address other injuries that may necessitate immediate care
   2. Care in emergency department
      a. Assessment of level of injury

   1. Manifestations of injury at cervical level
      a. Paralysis or weakness of all extremities
      b. Respiratory distress
      c. Pulse < 60; blood pressure < 80
      d. Decreased peristalsis
   2. Manifestations of injury at thoracic or lumbar level: Paralysis or weakness of lower extremities
   3. Findings indicative of spinal shock
      a. Loss of skin sensation
      b. Areflexia, flaccid paralysis
      c. Absent bowel sounds
      d. Bladder distention
      e. Decreasing blood pressure
      f. Loss of cremasteric reflex in male

   b. Interventions
      1. Address respiratory status
         a. Oxygen administration
         b. Ventilator support to those in distress
      2. Continuous monitoring of cardiovascular status
      3. Monitor fluid status and prevent bladder overdistention; insert indwelling urinary catheter
      4. Paralytic ileus: insertion of nasogastric tube and connect to suction
      5. Administration of high-dose corticosteroid to prevent secondary cord damage from edema and ischemia (within 8 hours of injury and continued for 23 hours)

H. Diagnostic Tests: maintain position during testing
   1. X-rays of cervical spine to establish level and extent of vertebral injury
   2. CT scan and MRI: changes in vertebrae, spinal cord, tissues around cord
   3. Arterial blood gases to establish baseline

I. Medications
   1. Corticosteroids
   2. Vasopressors to treat bradycardia and hypotension
   3. Histamine H_2 receptor antagonists to prevent stress ulcers
   4. Anticoagulation if not contraindicated

J. Treatments
   1. Surgery may be indicated early, if there is evidence of spinal cord compression by bone fragments or hematoma; surgeries

include decompression laminectomy, spinal fusion, insertion of metal rods
  2. Stabilization and immobilization
    a. Application of traction (Gardner-Wells tongs)
    b. External fixation (halo external fixation device): allows for greater mobility, self-care, participation in rehabilitation program
K. Health Promotion: Education regarding prevention of injuries including use of seat belts
L. Nursing Diagnoses
  1. Impaired Physical Mobility
    a. Intervention to maintain joint mobility, prevent contractures
    b. Maintain skin integrity; use of special beds
    c. Prevention of deep venous thrombosis
  2. Impaired Gas Exchange
    a. Ventilator support often indicated in cervical injuries
    b. T1–T7 injuries impair intercostal muscles
    c. Assist client to cough by splinting lower chest region
  3. Ineffective Breathing Pattern
  4. Dysreflexia
  5. Altered Urinary Elimination and Constipation
    a. Long-term client usually requires intermittent catheterization procedure
    b. Use of stool softeners and bowel training program
  6. Sexual Dysfunction
    a. Males have different abilities to have erections (reflexogenic or psychogenic) depending on injuries
    b. Females usually do not have sensation but pregnancy is possible
    c. Discuss client concern, referral for counseling
  7. Low Self-esteem
    a. Client has sustained threat to body image, self-esteem, role performance
    b. Promotion of self-care, independent decision making
M. Home Care
  1. Client moves from intensive care, intermediate care to rehabilitation to home care
  2. Client needs continued support home health agency, physical therapy, support groups for client and family
V. Client with Herniated Intervertebral Disk

A. Definition
  1. Rupture of cartilage surrounding inteverteberal disk with protrusion of nucleus pulposus
  2. Occurs more often as persons enter middle age and affects males more than females
  3. Site most commonly affected: L4, L5, S1; if herniated disk occurs in cervical region C6, C7 are affected
B. Pathophysiology
  1. Protrusion occurs spontaneously or as result of trauma; pressure on adjacent spinal nerves causes manifestations
  2. Abrupt herniation causes intense pain and muscle spasms
  3. Gradual herniation occurs with degenerative changes, osteoarthritis and develops as slow onset of pain and neurologic deficits
C. Manifestations
  1. Herniated disk in lumbar disk
    a. Recurrent episodes of pain in lower back with radiation across buttock
    b. Sciatica: lumbar pain following sciatic nerve down posterior leg
    c. Motor deficits: weakness, difficulties with sexual function and urinary elimination
    d. Sensory deficits: paresthesia and numbness
  2. Herniated disk in cervical area
    a. Pain in shoulder, arm, neck
    b. Paresthesias, muscle spasms
D. Diagnostic Tests
  1. X-ray: lumbosacral and cervical area to identify deformities and narrowing of disk spaces
  2. CT scan and MRI
  3. Myelography: used to rule out tumors
  4. Electromyography (EMG): measures electrical activity of skeletal muscles at rest; identification of muscles affected by pressure of herniated disk
E. Medications
  1. Management of pain with analgesics, NSAID's
  2. Management of muscle spasms with muscle relaxants
F. Treatment
  1. Conservative treatment is utilized for 2–6 weeks
    a. Decrease activity level
    b. Avoid flexion of spine

     c. Adequate support (corset, cervical collar)

     d. Firm mattress

     e. Prescribed exercise program

     f. Take analgesics, NSAID's, muscle relaxants

     g. TENS units

  2. Surgery (may be combination of different procedures

     a. Laminectomy: removal of part of vertebral lamina to relieve pressure on nerve

     b. Diskectomy: removal of nucleus pulposus of intervertbral disk

     c. Microdiskectomy: use of microscopic procedure through very small incision

     d. Spinal fusion: insertion of wedge-shaped piece of bone or bone chips between vertebrae to stabilize them; results in limited movement

G. Nursing Care: Emphasis on prevention: proper body mechanics, proper lifting techniques

H. Nursing Diagnoses

  1. Acute Pain

  2. Chronic Pain

  3. Constipation

I. Home Care

  1. Adequate pain control to enable client to be able to participate in ADL

  2. Utilization of nonpharmacological methods

VI. Client with spinal cord tumor

A. Definition

  1. Tumors may be benign or malignant, primary or metastatic

  2. Occur most often in thoracic area; also cervical and lumbarsacral areas

  3. Affect clients in age group 20–60

B. Classifications

  1. Intramedullary tumors arise from tissues of spinal cord

  2. Extramedullary tumors develop from tissues outside spinal cord

C. Pathophysiology: As tumors grow neural deficits result from further compression, invasion, or ischemia, secondary to vascular obstruction

D. Manifestations

  1. Depend on area of tumor and anatomic level of involvement

  2. Pain

     a. Locally at site of tumor

     b. Radicular pain: involving nerve that is compressed

  3. Motor deficits: paresis, paralysis, hyperactive reflexes

  4. Sensory deficits

  5. Changes in bowel and bladder elimination, sexual function

E. Diagnostic Tests

  1. Flat plate x-ray of spine

  2. CT scan, MRI: site of cord compression

  3. Myelogram: clarify area of tumor involvement

  4. Lumbar puncture: CSF when tumors are present is often xanthochromic (yellow in color)

F. Medications

  1. Analgesics and NSAID's to control pain

  2. Steroids (dexamethasome (Decadron): to decrease tumor size and inflammation

G. Treatment

  1. Surgery: procedures include microsurgery, laser surgery for excision; then laminectomy and fusion to stabilize spine

  2. Radiation therapy: used to treat metastatic tumors reduce pain, stop progression of neurologic deficits

H. Nursing Care: similar in aspects to care of client with SCI

FOCUSED STUDY TIPS

- Rehabilitation for stroke clients begins the day the client is admitted to the hospital. Identify initial nursing interventions that contribute to the rehabilitation process in the early stages of stroke.

- Visit the OT (occupational therapy) department in your clinical facility. Identify different aids available to achieve optimal functioning for clients experiencing stroke or spinal cord disorders.

- Identify goals and interventions aimed at minimizing impatience and frustration occurring as a result of stroke. Discuss and share ideas with classmates.

CASE STUDY

When assessing a client with SCI (spinal cord injury) above the T-6 level, he complains of a pounding headache. You note his pulse rate is very slow, his blood pressure is high, and he appears anxious and flushed. You also note that his lower extremities are pale and cold. What do these symptoms indicate? What nursing interventions are implemented immediately? What potential complications can occur as a result of these symptoms?

CARE PLAN CRITICAL THINKING ACTIVITY

Impaired urinary elimination is a nursing diagnosis associated with many neurological disorders. Describe the psychological impact this diagnosis may have on the client. What interventions can the nurse implement to relieve stress associated with this diagnosis?

NCLEX TEST QUESTIONS

1. Which of the following nutritional interventions would be most effective for a client who has recently suffered a cerebrovascular accident (CVA)?
   a. Have the client eat bite-size portions of foods to facilitate digestion.
   b. Place the client on a full liquid diet.
   c. Use thickening agents to minimize the risk of aspiration and monitor the client closely during all feedings.
   d. Allow the client to eat alone as post-CVA clients are often self-conscious about their residual deficits.

2. The nurse provides care for a 13-year-old in a halo brace because of a spinal cord injury. Which of the following is the first priority?
   a. Tighten any loose connections on the vest.
   b. Assess the pin sites.
   c. Turn the client every hour.
   d. Provide range of motion to extremities.

3. A young client was hit by a car, however, the level of his injury did not interrupt his respiratory function. Cord injury to which level or above results in interruption of respiratory function?
   a. thoracic level 5
   b. thoracic level 2
   c. cervical level 7
   d. cervical level 3

4. A quadriplegic client tells the nurse that he believes he is experiencing an episode of autonomic hyperreflexia (dysreflexia). The first nursing intervention is to:
   a. ask him what he thinks has precipitated this episode.
   b. assess his blood pressure and pulse.
   c. elevate his head as high as possible.
   d. assist him in emptying his bladder.

5. When a client suffers a left-sided CVA (cerebrovascular accident), he or she will often demonstrate the signs and symptoms of:
   a. confusion.
   b. aphasia.
   c. left-sided hemiplegia.
   d. neglect syndrome.

6. When a male client returns from the recovery room following a lumbar laminectomy, the most important postoperative assessment is to
   a. check for sensation in the lower extremities.
   b. observe the dressing for any drainage.
   c. check the client's temperature for signs of infection.
   d. determine client's level of pain.

7. A 16-year-old girl has a known arteriovenous malformation of the middle cerebral artery. In talking to the school nurse, she complains of a headache and stiff neck. The nurse would take which of the following actions?
   a. Call her mother and have her picked up from school to see the physician.
   b. Send her home right away to rest.
   c. Make preparations for emergency transfer to an acute care setting.
   d. Have the client rest for 2 hours, then reevaluate the situation.

8. The R.N. is observing a nursing assistant ambulating a client with hemiplegia. Which of the following activities would indicate unsafe practice?

a. standing next to the client's affected side and supporting the client by grasping the safety belt in the middle of the client's back or placing one arm around the client's waist and the other arm around the inferior aspect of the client's upper arm

b. standing next to the client's unaffected side and supporting the client by placing one arm around the client's waist and the other arm around the inferior aspect of the client's upper arm

c. taking a few steps forward with the client to assess for strength and balance

d. standing on the client's affected side while the client moves with a cane

9. A client has just returned from a myelogram when he complains of a headache and stiff neck. The first intervention is to

   a. encourage fluids and administer analgesics.

   b. administer oxygen at 6 liters/minute

   c. call the physician.

   d. start an IV with normal saline.

10. A client has a Swan-Ganz catheter inserted before undergoing spinal fusion surgery. The nurse will use this catheter to monitor the client's:

   a. intracranial pressure.

   b. spinal cord perfusion.

   c. renal function.

   d. hemodynamic status.

CHAPTER 42

NURSING CARE OF CLIENTS WITH INTRACRANIAL DISORDERS

LEARNING OUTCOMES

After completing this chapter, you will be able to:

- Apply knowledge of normal anatomy, physiology, and assessments when providing nursing care for clients with intracranial disorders (see Chapter 40).
- Explain the pathophysiology, manifestations, collaborative care, and nursing care of altered level of consciousness and increased intracranial pressure.
- Describe the pathophysiology and manifestations of seizures, headaches, traumatic brain injury, intracranial infections, and brain tumors.
- Identify diagnostic tests used to identify and manage intracranial disorders.
- Discuss nursing implications for medications used to treat intracranial disorders.
- Explain collaborative care for clients with intracranial disorders.
- Describe nursing interventions in the preoperative and postoperative care of the client having intracranial surgery.
- Use the nursing process as a framework for providing individualized care to clients with intracranial disorders.

KEY TOPICS

- Altered cerebral functioning
- Traumatic brain injury
- Central nervous system infections
- Brain tumors
- Nursing care of clients with intracranial disorders

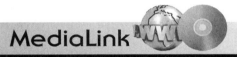

MediaLink

www.prenhall.com/lemone

Additional resources for this chapter can be found on the Student CD-ROM accompanying this textbook, and on the Companion Website at www.prenhall.com/lemone. Click on Chapter 42 to select the activities for this chapter.

CD-ROM
- Audio Glossary
- NCLEX Review

Animation
- Coup-Contrecoup Injury

Companion Website
- More NCLEX Review
- Care Plan Activity
    Subdural Hematoma
- MediaLink Application
    Meningitis Prevention

387

LECTURE OUTLINE

I. Altered Cerebral Function: (color) occurs with illness and injury
   A. Brain Function Deterioration
      1. Follows a predictable rostral to caudal progression
      2. Higher levels of function progress to more primitive function
   B. Altered Level of Consciousness (LOC)
      1. Consciousness
         a. Condition in which person is aware of self and environment and able to respond to stimuli appropriately
         b. Requires
            1. Arousal: alertness; dependent upon reticular activating system (RAS); system of neurons in thalamus and upper brain stem
            2. Cognition: complex process involving all mental activities; controlled by cerebral hemispheres
         c. Components depend on normal physiologic function and connection between 2 systems
      2. Pathophysiology
         a. Lesions or injuries affecting cerebral hemisphere directly or that compress or destroy neurons in RAS
         b. Metabolic disorders
      3. Arousal affected by
         a. Destruction of RAS: stroke, demyelinating diseases
         b. Compression of brain stem producing edema and ischemia: tumors, increased intracranial pressure, hematomas or hemorrhage, aneurysm
         c. Cerebral hemisphere function depends on continuous supply of oxygen and glucose
            1. Most common impairment caused by global ischemia, hypoglycemia
            2. Localized masses: hematoma, cerebral edema
      4. Processes within brain that destroy or compress structures affect LOC
         a. Increased intracranial pressure
         b. Stroke, hematoma, intracranial hemorrhage
         c. Tumors
         d. Infections
         e. Demyelinating disorders
      5. Systemic conditions affecting brain function
         a. Hypoglycemia

      b. Fluid and electrolyte imbalances
         1. Hyponatremia
         2. Hyperosmolality
         3. Acid-base alterations: hypercapnia
         4. Accumulated waste products from liver or renal failure
         5. Drugs affecting CNS: alcohol, analgesics, anesthetics
      c. Seizure activity: exhausts energy metabolites
      6. Client assessment results with decreasing LOC
         a. Increased stimulation required to elicit response from client
         b. More difficult to rouse; client agitated and confused when awakened
         c. Orientation changes: loses orientation to time first; then place; finally person
         d. Continuous stimulation required to maintain wakefulness
         e. Client has no response, even to painful stimuli
   C. Patterns of breathing
      1. As respiratory center are affected: predictable changes in breathing patterns
      2. Types of respirations and brain involvement
         a. Diencephalon: Cheyne-Stokes respirations (as with acidosis)
         b. Midbrain: neurogenic hyperventilation; may exceed 40/minute; due to uninhibited stimulation of respiratory centers
         c. Pons: apneustic respirations: sighing on mid inspiration or prolonged inhalation and exhalation; excessive stimulation of respiratory centers
         d. Medulla: ataxic/apneic respirations (totally uncoordinated and irregular); loss of response to CO_2
   D. Pupillary and oculomotor responses: Predictable progression
      1. Localized lesion effects ipsilateral pupil (same side as lesion)
      2. Generalized or systemic processes pupils affected equally
      3. Compression of cranial nerve III at midbrain, pupils become oval and eccentric (off center); progress to pupils become fixed (no response to light); progress to dilation
      4. With deteriorating LOC, spontaneous eye movement is lost and reflexive ocular movements are altered

a. Loss of simultaneous eye movement
b. Loss of normal reflex functioning:
   1. Doll's eye movements: eye movement in opposite direction of head rotation (normal function of brain stem)
   2. Oculocephalic reflex: eyes move upward with passive flexion of neck; downward with passive neck extension (normal function)
   3. Oculovestibular response (cold caloric testing): instillation of cold water in ear canal cause nystagmus (lateral tonic deviation of eyes) toward stimulus (normal function)

E. Motor Function
   1. Predictable progression
   2. Assessment of level of brain dysfunction and side of brain affected
      a. Client follows verbal commands
      b. Pushes away purposely from noxious stimulus
      c. Movements are more generalized and less purposeful (withdrawal, grimacing)
      d. Reflexive motor responses:
         1. Decorticate movement: flexion of upper extremities accompanied by extension of lower extremities
         2. Decerebrate posturing: adduction and rigid extension of upper and lower extremities
      e. Flaccid with little or no motor response

F. Coma States
   1. Outcome of altered LOC
   2. Comas range from full recovery, without any residual effects, to persistent vegetative state (cerebral death) or brain death
   3. Stages
      a. Irreversible coma (vegetative state)
         1. Permanent condition of complete unawareness of self and environment; death of cerebral hemispheres with continued function of brain stem and cerebellum
         2. Client does not respond meaningfully to environment but has sleep-wake cycles and retains ability to chew, swallow, and cough
         3. Eyes may wander but cannot track object
         4. Minimally conscious state: client aware of environment, can follow simple commands, indicate yes/no

responses; make meaningful movements (blink, smile)
         5. Often results from severe head injury or global anoxia
      b. Locked-in syndrome
         1. Client is alert and fully aware of environment; intact cognitive abilities but unable to communicate through speech or movement because of blocked efferent pathways from brain
         2. Motor paralysis but cranial nerves may be intact allowing client to communicate through eye movement and blinking
         3. Occurs with hemorrhage or infarction of pons; disorders of lower motor neurons or muscles (polyneuritis, myasthenia gravis, amyotrophic lateral sclerosis (ALS)
      c. Brain death
         1. Cessation and irreversibility of all brain functions
         2. General criteria
            a. Absent motor and reflex movements
            b. Apnea
            c. Fixed and dilated pupils
            d. No ocular responses to head turning and caloric stimulation
            e. Flat EEG

G. Prognosis
   1. Outcome varies according to underlying cause and pathologic process
   2. Young adults can recover from deep coma
   3. Recovery within 2 weeks associated with favorable outcome

H. Collaborative Care
   1. Management includes identifying cause, preserve function and prevent deterioration
   2. Involves total system maintenance in many cases

I. Diagnostic Tests
   1. Blood glucose: cerebral function declines rapidly when < 40–50 mg/dL
   2. Serum electrolytes: hyponatremia: coma and convulsions when Na < 115 mEq/L
   3. ABG's: hypoxemia frequent cause of altered LOC; increased levels CO_2 especially if acute
   4. BUN and creatinine: renal function
   5. Liver function tests: tests determine liver function; high ammonia levels interfere with cerebral metabolism

6. Toxicology screening of blood and urine (acute drug or alcohol)
7. CBC: anemia or infectious cause of coma
8. CT, MRI: identification of neurologic damage
9. EEG: evaluate electrical activity of brain, unrecognized seizure activity
10. Radioisotope brain scan: identify abnormal brain lesions
11. Cerebral angiography: visualization of cerebral vascular system including aneurysms, occluded vessels, tumors
12. Transcranial Doppler: assess cerebral blood flow
13. Lumbar puncture: CSF to assess infection, possible meningitis

J. Medications
1. IV fluids normal saline, lactated Ringer's
2. Specific medications to address specific problems
   a. 50% glucose: hypoglycemia
   b. Naloxone for narcotic overdose
   c. Thiamine: Wernicke's encephalopathy
   d. Regulation of osmolality with diuretics
   e. Antibiotics: infections

K. Surgery: May be indicated if cause of coma is tumor, hemorrhage, hematoma

L. Other Measures (as indicated)
1. Airway support and mechanical ventilation if indicated; controlled hyperventilation to promote vasoconstriction to reduce cerebral edema
2. Maintenance of nutritional status with enteral feedings

M. Nursing Diagnoses
1. Ineffective Airway Clearance: limit suctioning to < 10–15 seconds; hyperoxygenate before
2. Risk for Aspiration
3. Risk for Impaired Skin Integrity: preventative measures, continual inspection
4. Impaired Physical Mobility: maintain functionality of joints, physical therapy
5. Risk for Imbalanced Nutrition: Less than body requirements
6. Anxiety (of family)
   a. Extremely stressful time
   b. Reinforce information from physician
   c. Encourage to speak with client who is in coma

II. Increased Intracranial Pressure
A. Intracranial Pressure (ICP)
1. Pressure within cranial cavity measured within lateral ventricles

2. Transient increases occur with normal activities coughing, sneezing, straining, bending forward
3. Sustained increases associated with
   a. Cerebral edema
   b. Head trauma
   c. Tumors
   d. Abscesses
   e. Stroke
   f. Inflammation
   g. Hemorrhage

B. Monro-Lellie hypothesis
1. Within skull there are 3 components that maintain state of dynamic equilibrium
   a. Brain (80%)
   b. Cerebrospinal fluid (10%)
   c. Blood (10%)
2. If volume of any one increases the volume of others must decrease to maintain normal pressure

C. Normal intracranial pressure
1. 5–15 mm Hg, with pressure transducer with head elevated 30 degrees
2. 60–180 cm water, water manometer with client lateral recumbent

D. Background regarding regulation of ICP
1. Cerebral blood flow and perfusion account for twice the amount of increase as CSF does
   a. Cerebral blood vessels respond to changes in arterial oxygen and carbon dioxide
   b. Cerebral perfusion pressure (CPP) is pressure needed to perfuse brain cells
      1. Difference between mean arterial pressure (MAP) and ICP
      2. Normal pressure is 80–100 Hg; to maintain blood flow CPP must be 50 mm Hg
2. Autoregulation: compensatory mechanisms in which cerebral arterioles change diameter to maintain cerebral blood flow when ICP increases
   a. Pressure autoregulation: receptors within small vessels respond to changes in arterial pressure
      1. Vasodilation: in response to elevated blood pressure
      2. Vasoconstriction: in response to low blood pressure
   b. Chemical (metabolic) autoregulation
      1. Vasodilation: carbon dioxide, increased hydrogen ion concentration, low oxygen

2. Vasoconstriction: fall in carbon dioxide
3. There is limited ability of brain to respond to ICP; ability for autoregulation is severely limited

E. Increased ICP
1. Increased ICP must be recognized early when interventions can be instituted to stop its progress
2. Medical emergency requiring intensive nursing care
3. Manifestations
   a. Changes in LOC: initially behavior and personality changes and progresses in predictable pattern to coma and responsiveness
   b. Pressure affects motor functioning: initially hemiparesis on contralateral side and if not effectively treated progresses to decorticate and decerebrate positioning
   c. Altered vision (blurred vision, diplopia, decreased acuity) pupillary response (gradual dilation, sluggish response)
   d. Headache on rising; common with slowly developing increased ICP
   e. Papilledema noted on fundoscopic exam
   f. Projectile vomiting
   g. CNS ischemic response: occurs late in course of increased ICP; Cushing's response (triad): increased MAP, increased pulse pressure, bradycardia
   h. Changes in respiratory pattern and dramatic rise in temperature
4. Causes
   a. Space occupying lesions
   b. Cerebral edema: increase in volume of brain tissue due to abnormal accumulation of fluid; local process or affecting entire brain
   c. Hydrocephalus: increase in volume of CSF within ventricular system, which becomes dilated
      1. Noncommunicating: obstruction in CSF drainage from ventricular system
      2. Communicating: CSF is not effectively reabsorbed through arachnoid villi
      3. Normal pressure hydrocephalus: occurs in persons > 60 in which ventricles enlarge causing cerebral tissue compression

4. Manifestations depend on rate of onset: progressive cognitive dysfunction, gait disruptions, urinary incontinence
   d. Intracranial hemorrhage

F. Brain herniation
1. Cerebral tissue can be displaced to more compliant area, if ICP is not treated
2. Displacement of brain tissue results in further increased ICP and brain damage including lethal brain damage
3. Brain herniation syndromes are categorized according to location
   a. Cingulate herniation
   b. Central or transtentorial herniation
   c. Uncal or latral transtentorial herniation
   d. Infratentorial herniation

G. Collaborative Care
1. Identify and treat underlying condition
2. Control ICP to prevent herniation syndromes

H. Diagnostic Tests
1. Diagnosis is made on observation and neurological assessment
2. Measures to control pressure are instituted while identifying underlying cause
3. Tests for underlying cause
   a. CT scan and MRI: identify possible cause and evaluate therapeutic options
   b. Serum osmolality: used as indicator of hydration status; usually maintained slightly elevated to draw excess fluid into vascular system from brain tissue
   c. Arterial blood gases: monitor pH, CO_2, Po_2 levels and effect on cerebral circulation; hydrogen ions and carbon dioxide are potent vasodilators; hypoxemia also causes vasodilation but to lesser degree

I. Medications
1. Diuretics
   a. Osmotic diuretics increase osmolarity of blood and draw fluid from edematous brain tissue into vascular bed where it can be eliminated by kidneys
   b. Mannitol is commonly used
   c. Loop diuretics such as furosemide are used, in addition, to further promote diuresis
   d. Serum electrolytes and osmolality are monitored
   e. Urine specific gravity may also be monitored at intervals

2. Antipyretics or hypothermia blanket: used to control hyperthermia, which increases cerebral metabolic rate
3. Anticonvulsants to manage seizure activity
4. Histamine H_2 receptors blockers to decrease risk of stress ulcers
5. Barbiturates: may be given as continuous infusion to induce coma and decrease metabolic demands of injured brain; controversial
6. Vasoactive medications may be given to maintain blood pressure to support cerebral perfusion

J. Surgery
1. May be indicated to treat underlying cause of increased ICP
2. Include removal of brain tumors, burr holes, insertion of drainage catheter or shunt to drain excessive CSF

K. ICP Monitoring
1. Continuous intracranial pressure monitor is used for continual assessment of ICP and to monitor effects of medical therapy and nursing interventions
2. Allows for more precise manipulation of therapeutic measures to maintain adequate cerebral perfusion while controlling ICP
3. Systems include intraventricular catheter, subarachnoid bolt or screw and epidural catheters; can be used to drain CSF and measure ICP
4. Risk for infection exists with invasive procedure

L. Mechanical Ventilation: Involves airway management and prevention of hypoxemia and hypercapnia, which both increase intracranial pressure

M. Nursing Care
1. Protect client from sudden increases in ICP and decrease in cerebral blood flow
2. Clients are often critically ill and are in special neurological intensive care unit for constant observation and continuous treatment

N. Nursing Diagnoses
1. Ineffective Tissue Perfusion: Cerebral
   a. Frequent neurologic assessment based on client baseline and changing status
   b. Early signs are LOC and breathing patterns
   c. Measures in place to limit increases in intracranial pressure; limit stimulation
2. Risk for Infection: open head wounds and intracranial monitoring device require meticulous aseptic technique

3. Anxiety (of family): need for teaching to maintain restful environment, emotional support

III. Client with a Headache
A. Pain within cranial vault and occuring commonly
   1. May be due to benign or pathological condition
   2. Majority are mild
B. Pathophysiology: Multiple pain-sensitive structures within cranial vault, face, and scalp
C. Types of Headaches
   1. Tension
      a. Most common
      b. Characterized by sensation of tightness around head and may have specific localized painful areas
      c. Caused by sustained contraction of muscles of head and neck
      d. Precipitated by stress and anxiety
   2. Migraine
      a. Recurring vascular headache often initiated by triggering event and accompanied by neurologic dysfunction
      b. More common in females between ages 25–55
      c. Cause not understood but related to abnormalities in cerebrovascular blood flow, reduction in brain activity, or increase release of sensory substances (e.g., serotonin)
      d. Stages include
         1. Aura: visual disturbances; lasts 5–60 minutes
         2. Headache: throbbing pain often with nausea and vomiting; hypersensitive to light and sound; lasts hours to 1–2 days
         3. Postheadache: area of headache is sensitive; client exhausted
      e. Triggers include stress, fluctuating glucose levels, fatigue, hormones, bright lights
   3. Cluster
      a. Common with middle-aged men
      b. Typically awakens client with unilateral pain around eye accompanied by rhinorrhea, lacrimation, flushing
      c. Attacks occur in clusters of 1–8 days for weeks
D. Collaborative Care: identification of underlying cause and therapeutic management

E. Diagnostic Tests: may involve neurodiagnostic testing depending on client history and assessment

F. Medications: According to type of headache
  1. Migraine headache may require prophylactic therapy including serotonin antagonist or beta blocker
  2. Management of migraine may include
    a. Ergotamine tartrate (Cafergot)
    b. Sumatriptan (Imitrex)
    c. Zolmitriptan (Zomig)
    d. Narcotic analgesic and anti-emetics
  3. Cluster headaches are often treated with same medications as migraines
  4. Tension headaches are treated with aspirin, acetaminophen

G. Complementary Therapies
  1. Supplements
  2. Relaxation techniques
  3. Herbal therapy
  4. Osteopathic manipulation

H. Nursing Care
  1. Teach client to manage discomfort effectively, identify any triggers (headache diary), stress management
  2. Use of medications, and effective use of heat and cold

IV. Client with Seizure Disorder
A. Seizures: paroxysmal motor, sensory, or cognitive manifestations of spontaneous abnormal discharges from neurons in cerebral cortex
  1. May involve all or part of brain: consciousness, autonomic function, motor function, and sensation
  2. Epilepsy: any disorder characterized by recurrent seizures
  3. Affects 2.3 million Americans; increased incidence in children and elderly

B. Cause may be idiopathic or associated with birth injuries, infection, vascular abnormalities, trauma, tumors
  1. Theories propose causes related to altered permeability of ions, neuron excitability, imbalances of neurotransmitters
  2. When seizure threshold exceeded, a seizure may result; neurons that initiate seizure activity are called epileptogenic focus
  3. Unprovoked seizures have no known cause; provoked seizures are related to another condition such as fever, rapid withdrawal from alcohol, electrolyte imbalance, brain pathology

C. Affects of seizure on brain tissue
  1. Increased metabolic demand: fourfold requirement of additional glucose and oxygen, resulting in increased cerebral blood flow
  2. If unmet, cellular destruction can result

D. Categorization of seizures
  1. Partial seizures: activation of part of one cerebral hemisphere
    a. Simple partial seizure: no altered consciousness; recurrent muscle contraction; motor portion of cortex affected
    b. Complex partial seizure: impaired consciousness; may engage in automatisms (repetitive nonpurposeful activity such as lip smacking); preceded by aura, originates in temporal lobe
  2. Generalized seizures: involves both brain hemispheres; consciousness always impaired
    a. Absence seizures (petit mal): characterized by sudden brief cessation of all motor activity, blank stare and unresponsiveness often with eye fluttering
    b. Tonic-clonic seizures
      1. Most common type in adults
      2. Preceded by aura, sudden loss of consciousness
      3. Tonic phase: rigid muscles, incontinence
      4. Clonic phase: altered contraction, relaxation; eyes roll back, froths at mouth
      5. Postictal phase: unconscious and unresponsive to stimuli

E. Status epilepticus
  1. Continuous seizure activity, generally tonic-clonic type
  2. Client at risk to develop hypoxia, acidosis, hypoglycemia, hyperthermia, exhaustion
  3. Life threatening medical emergency requiring immediate treatment
    a. Establish and maintain airway
    b. Diazepam (Valium) and lorazepam (Ativan) intravenously at 10-minute intervals
    c. 50% Dextose intravenously
    d. Phenytoin (Dilantin) intravenously
    e. Possibly Phenobarbital

F. Collaborative Care
  1. Control seizure
  2. Establish cause
  3. Prevent further seizures

G. Diagnostic Tests
   1. Neurologic exam
   2. EEG to confirm diagnosis and locate lesion
   3. X-ray, MRI, CT scan identify any neurologic abnormalities
   4. Lumbar puncture may be done if infection suspected
   5. CBC, electrolytes, BUN, blood glucose
   6. ECG to determine cardiac dysrhythmias
H. Medications
   1. Anticonvulsants
      a. Manage but do not cure seizure
      b. Actions
         1. Raise seizure threshold
         2. Limit spread of abnormal activity within brain
      c. Try to use lowest dose of single medication to control seizures if possible; may need to try different medications and use combinations
   2. Medications
      a. Carbamazepine (Tegretol)
      b. Phenytoin (Dilantin)
      c. Valproic acid (Depakote)
      d. Tiagabine (Gabitril)
I. Surgery: if all attempts to control seizures are not successful
   1. May attempt to excise tissue involved in seizure activity
   2. EEG done during surgery to identify epileptogenic focus
J. Care of client during a seizure
   1. Protect client from injury and maintain airway
   2. Do not force anything into client's mouth
   3. Loosen clothing around neck
K. Health Promotion: Stress the following to clients
   1. Importance of medical follow-up, taking prescribed medications
   2. Driving privileges are prohibited in clients with seizure disorders; driver's licenses are reinstated after seizure free period and statement from health care practitioner
   3. Client needs proper identification
   4. Family members need to be educated in preventing injury if seizure occurs
L. Nursing Diagnoses
   1. Risk for Ineffective Airway Clearance
   2. Anxiety
M. Home Care
   1. Education of client and family regarding seizure disorder; safety measures, avoidance of alcohol and caffeine
   2. Referral to support group, national organizations
V. Client with traumatic brain injury
   A. Traumatic brain injury: a leading cause of death and disability; any traumatic insult to brain causing physical, intellectual, emotional, social, or vocational changes
      1. Includes penetrating head injury (open) and closed head injury
      2. Estimates of 1 million persons are treated and released with head injuries yearly in U.S.
      3. Risk Factors
         a. Motor vehicle accidents
         b. Elevated blood alcohol levels
         c. Greatest risk: males aged 15–30 and those over 75
   B. Mechanisms of trauma
      1. Acceleration injury: head struck by moving object
      2. Deceleration injury: head hits stationary object
      3. Acceleration-deceleration (coup-contrecoup phenomenon): head hits object and brain rebounds within skull
      4. Deformation: force deforms and disrupts body integrity: skull fracture
   C. Types of injuries
      1. Skull fracture: break in continuity of skull usually resulting in brain trauma
      2. Classifications
         a. Linear: dura remains intact; subdural or epidural hematoma may occur underneath
         b. Comminuted and depressed skull fractures: increase risk for direct injury to brain tissue from contusion (bruise) and bone fragments; risk for infection
         c. Basilar
            1. Involves base of skull and usually involve extension of adjacent fractures
            2. If dura disrupted may have leakage of CSF occurring as
               a. Rhinorrhea: through nose
               b. Otorrhea: through ear
            3. May appear on x-ray; signs of basilar skull fracture
               a. Hemotympanum: blood behind tympanic membrane
               b. Battle's sign: blood over mastoid process
               c. "Raccoon eyes": bilateral periorbital ecchymosis

4. Test clear fluid from ear or nose for glucose by using glucose reagent strip: if positive indicates CSF
5. CSF leakage: increased risk of infection
   a. Keep nasopharnyx and external ear clean
   b. No blowing nose, coughing or hard sneezing
   c. Prophylactic antibiotic
D. Collaborative Care
   1. All require minimal bed rest and observation of underlying injury
   2. Depressed skull fractures require surgical intervention to debride wound and remove bone fragments embedded in brain tissue
   3. Basilar fractures with CSF leakage may require surgery
E. Nursing Care/Home Care
   1. Client must be monitored for signs of increased intracranial pressure
   2. Observe in hospital
   3. Educate family regarding changes in LOC: wake up every 2 hours during first 24 hours home
   4. Follow-up care
VI. Client with focal or diffuse brain injury
   A. Primary and secondary mechanism occur with brain injury
      1. Primary: impact of injury
      2. Progression of initial injury affecting perfusion and oxygenation of brain cells: intracranial edema, hematoma, infection, hypoxia, ischemia
   B. Focal brain injuries
      1. Specific observable brain lesion confined to one area of brain; includes epidural hemorrhage, subdural and intracerebral hematoma
      2. Depending on site and rate of bleeding, manifestations may occur within hours to weeks
      3. Client may develop increased ICP with altered level of consciousness and potential for brain herniation
   C. Specific types of brain injuries
      1. Contusion: bruise of surface of brain; manifestations and degree of impairment depend on size and location of injury; slow recovery of consciousness
      2. Epidural hematoma (extradural hematoma): blood collects in potential space between dura and skull

a. Occurs more often in young to middle aged adults
b. Occurs with skull fracture from torn artery, tend to occur rapidly
c. May have brief lucid period after injury and then rapid decline from drowsiness to coma with neurological deficits
d. Require rapid treatment to prevent complications
3. Subdural hematoma
   a. Localized mass of blood collects between dura mater and arachnoid mater
   b. More common than epidural hematoma
   c. Types
      1. Acute subdural hematomas develop within 48 hours of injury
      2. Chronic subdural hematomas develop over weeks to months
   d. Manifestations of neurologic deficits develop at the same rate of the hematomas
4. Intracerebral hematomas: occur more often in older clients because cerebral blood vessels are more fragile and easily torn
5. Diffuse brain injury (DBI): affects entire brain and is caused by shaking motion with twisting movement
   a. Mild concussion
      1. Momentary interruption of brain function with or without loss of consciousness
      2. Manifestations
         a. Retrograde and antegrade amnesia
         b. Headache
         c. Drowsiness, confusion, dizziness
         d. Visual disturbances
   b. Classic cerebral concussion
      1. Diffuse cerebral disconnection from brain stem RAS
      2. Has manifestations as with mild concussion but immediate period of loss of consciousness is less than 6 hours; client may have exhibited seizure and respiratory arrest with bradycardia and hypotension
      3. May have postconcussion syndrome
   c. Diffuse axonal injury: high speed acceleration-deceleration injury causing widespread disruption of

axons in white matter; Poor prognosis: death or persistent vegetative state

D. Treatment
1. Concussion
   a. Client should be observed for 1–2 hours in emergency department
   b. Discharged home with instruction for observations, if loss of consciousness only a few minutes
   c. Longer period of unconsciousness, admit to hospital for observation
2. Acute DBI
   a. Recognition and management begins at scene with transport to emergency department
   b. Hospitalization with critical care and specific neurologic observation and interventions as indicated

E. Diagnostic Tests: same tests as increased ICP

F. Treatments
1. Management of increased ICP
2. Surgery: epidural and subdural hematomas; surgical evacuation of clot through burr holes

G. Health Promotion: Injury prevention: use of seat belts, bicycle and motorcycle helmets, gun safety

VII. Client CNS infection
A. CNS infections
1. Most common is bacterial meningitis
2. Mortality rate 25% in adults
3. Meningococcal occurs in epidemics with people living in close contact
4. Pneumococcal affects very young and very old

B. Risk Factors
1. High risk for old and young
2. High risk for clients with debilitating diseases, or immunosuppressed

C. Pathophysiology
1. Pathogens enter CNS and meninges causing inflammatory process, which leads to inflammation and increased ICP
2. May result in brain damage and life-threatening complications

D. Meningitis
1. Inflammation of pia mater, arachnoid, and subarachnoid space
2. Spreads rapidly through CNS because of circulation of CSF around brain and spinal cord
3. May be bacterial, viral, fungal, parasitic in origin
4. Infection enters CNS though invasive procedure or through bloodstream, secondary to another infection in body

E. Bacterial meningitis
1. Causative organisms: *Neisseria meningitis,* meningococcus, *Streptococcus pneumoniae, Haemophilus influenzae, E. coli*
2. Risk factors: head trauma with basilar skull fracture, otitis media, sinusitis, immunocompromised, neurosurgery, systemic sepsis
3. Manifestations
   a. Fever, chills
   b. Headache, back and abdominal pain
   c. Nausea and vomiting
   d. Meningeal irritation: nuchal rigidity, positive Brudzinski's sign, Kernig's sign, photophobia
   e. Meningococcal meningitis: rapidly spreading petechial rash of skin and mucous membranes
   f. Increased ICP: decreased LOC, papilledema
4. Complications
   a. Arthritis
   b. Cranial nerve damage (deafness)
   c. Hydrocephalus

F. Viral meningitis
1. Less severe, benign course with short duration
2. Intense headache with malaise, nausea, vomiting, lethargy
3. Signs of meningeal irritation

G. Encephalitis
1. Acute inflammation of parenchyma of brain or spinal cord
2. Usually caused by virus
3. Inflammation occurs with manifestations similar to meningitis
4. LOC deteriorates and client may become comatose
5. Arboviruses are agents including West Nile virus

H. Brain abscess
1. Infection with a collection of purulent material within brain tissue usually in cerebrum
2. Causes include open trauma and neurosurgery; infections of ear, sinuses
3. Common pathogens are streptococci, staphylococci, bacteroids
4. Becomes space-occupying lesion
5. At risk for infection and increased ICP
6. Manifestations
   a. General symptoms associated with acute infectious process
   b. Client develops seizures, altered LOC, signs of increased ICP

c. Specific neurologic symptoms are related to location
7. May be drained surgically, if considered feasible
I. Collaborative Care
1. Bacterial meningitis: requires immediate treatment and isolation of client
2. Viral meningitis: supportive treatment and management of client symptoms
3. Brain abscess treatment focuses on antibiotic therapy
J. Diagnostic Tests
1. Lumbar puncture: definitive test for bacterial meningitis demonstrating infection: turbid cloudy appearance, increased WBC, gram stain, culture
2. CT scan, MRI
K. Medications
1. Meningitis: immediate treatment with effective antibiotics for 7–21 days; according to culture results; dexamethasone to suppress inflammation
2. Encephalitis: viral treated with anti-viral medications
3. Brain abscess: antibiotic therapy, which may include intraventricular administration; anticonvulsant medications, antipyretics
L. Health Promotion
1. Vaccinations for meningococcal, pneumococcal, hemophilic meningitis
2. Prophylactic rifampin for persons exposed to meningococcal meningitis
3. Mosquito control
4. Prompt diagnosis and treatment of clients with infections
5. Asepsis care for clients with open head injury or neurosurgery
M. Nursing Diagnoses
1. Ineffective Protection
2. Risk for Deficient Fluid Volume
N. Home Care
1. Client education for future prevention
2. Complete medications and treatment plan

VIII. Client with a brain tumor
A. Description
1. Growths within cranium including tumors of brain tissue, meninges, pituitary gland, blood vessels
2. May be benign or malignant, primary or metastatic
3. May be lethal, due to location (inaccessible to treatment) and capacity to impinge on CNS structures

4. In adults most common tumor is glioblastoma followed by meningioma and cytoma
5. Cause is unknown: factors associated include heredity, cranial irradiation, exposure to some chemicals
6. Tumors within brain
a. Compress or destroy brain tissue
b. Cause edema in adjacent tissues
c. Cause hemorrhage
d. Obstruct circulation of CSF, causing hydrocephalus
7. Estimated 25% persons with cancer develop brain metastasis, often multiple sites throughout the brain
B. Manifestations: Multiple depending on location of lesion and rate of growth
1. Changes in cognition and LOC
2. Headache usually worse in morning
3. Seizures
4. Vomiting
5. Manifestations associated with cerebral edema, increased ICP, cerebral ischemia leading to brain herniation syndromes
C. Collaborative Care
1. Effective treatment includes chemotherapy, radiation therapy, and/or surgery
2. Treatment depends on size and location of tumor, type of tumor, neurologic deficits, and client's over all condition
D. Diagnostic Tests
1. CT scan or MRI: determine tumor location and extent
2. Arteriography
3. EEG: information about cerebral function, seizure data
4. Endocrine studies if pituitary tumor suspected
E. Treatment
1. Medications: Chemotherapy, corticosteroids, anticonvulsants
2. Surgery
a. Purposes include tumor excision, reduction, or for symptom relief
b. Craniotomy: location according to approach to tumor
3. Radiation: Alone or as adjunctive therapy
4. Specialty procedures: Stereotaxic techniques and use of laser beam
F. Nursing Care
1. Support during diagnosis and management through selected treatment
2. Nursing care involves interventions to deal with altered LOC, increased ICP, and seizures

G. Nursing Diagnoses
   1. Anxiety
   2. Risk for Infection
   3. Ineffective Protection
   4. Acute Pain
   5. Disturbed Self-esteem

H. Home Care
   1. Education, support to client and family
   2. Instructions for treatment plan and follow-up care
   3. Referral to home care agencies
   4. Referrals to therapies, community resources, support groups as appropriate

FOCUSED STUDY TIPS

- Practice each of the assessments necessary to implement the physician's order "neuro checks q1h." Describe normal and abnormal parameters for each.
- Compare and contrast nursing care for a client hospitalized with viral meningitis and a client hospitalized with bacterial meningitis. Identify public health issues associated with both.
- When caring for clients with brain tumors, the nursing diagnosis *"Disturbed self-esteem"* is often utilized. Discuss with classmates goals and interventions the nurse may implement when using this diagnosis.

CASE STUDY

When reviewing the care plan of a client with a CNS (central nervous system) infection, you notice he is at risk for fluid volume deficit. Why? How do you assess for the presence or worsening of fluid volume deficit?

CARE PLAN CRITICAL THINKING ACTIVITY

What are the major classifications of medications and most commonly used drugs in the treatment of ICP (increased intracranial pressure)?

NCLEX TEST QUESTIONS

1. Upon return of the closed-head injury client from CT scan, the head of the bed is maintained at 30 degrees and the client is positioned on his side with a towel roll placed vertically under the pillow. This unique positioning facilitates
   a. prevention of pulmonary embolism.
   b. venous drainage from the brain.
   c. airway management.
   d. intracranial pressure (ICP) readings.

2. The nurse is providing discharge instructions to a client hospitalized for meningitis. Which of the following instructions will be of the highest priority?
   a. Take all of the antibiotics as directed until completely gone.
   b. Eat a high-protein, high-calorie diet.
   c. Exercise daily beginning with active range-of-motion exercises.
   d. Get at least 8 hours of sleep per night with frequent rest periods.

3. In providing for the safety of the client during a grand mal seizure, the nurse performs which of the following?

   a. positions the client on his back
   b. gently places a padded tongue blade between the teeth
   c. protects the client from injury with padded bedrails
   d. applies oxygen immediately per mask

4. The physician orders dexamethasone (Decadron) to be administered to a client with a head injury. Based on nursing knowledge of this medication, the nurse would question the physician if he did not order which of the following additional medications?
   a. morphine sulfate
   b. sodium bicarbonate
   c. cimetidine
   d. levophed

5. A client is admitted to the trauma unit with a suspected arterial bleed following a head injury. He lost consciousness at the time of the injury and has since experienced a period of lucidity followed by a rapid decline in level of consciousness. As the nurse assesses his status, she recognizes these are signs indicative of:

a. subdural hematoma.

b. increased intracranial pressure.

c. epidural hematoma.

d. increased blood pressure.

6. A client with increased ICP is receiving mannitol. The nurse recognizes that mannitol is exerting the desired effect when the client demonstrates

a. decreased pupillary response.

b. increased decorticate posturing.

c. decreased seizure activity.

d. increased diuresis.

7. A 30-year-old male client with a suspected brain tumor is admitted to the hospital with rapidly progressing symptoms. The assessment finding that is the most reliable index of cerebral status is a/an:

a. unilateral pupillary dilatation.

b. increased systolic blood pressure.

c. decreased pulse pressure.

d. altered level of consciousness.

8. When concerned about increasing intracranial pressure, the nurse recalls that the client presenting with increasing intracranial pressure (ICP) and Cushing's triad presents with

a. increased pulse pressure, decreased mean arterial pressure, and tachycardia.

b. decreased pulse pressure, increased mean arterial pressure, and tachycardia.

c. decreased pulse pressure, decreased mean arterial pressure, and bradycardia.

d. increased pulse pressure, increased mean arterial pressure, and bradycardia.

9. A 28-year-old male is admitted to the intensive care unit with a diagnosis of closed head injury. The nurse should monitor for the potential complication of

a. hypotension.

b. respiratory alkalosis.

c. tremors.

d. cerebral edema.

10. Which of the following questions would the nurse use to collect data about the aura experienced by a seizure client?

a. "Do you have any indications that a seizure is coming on?"

b. "Do you have difficulty breathing during the seizure?"

c. "Are you able to awaken without problems after the seizure?"

d. "Can you describe how the seizure occurs from beginning to end?"

CHAPTER 43

NURSING CARE OF CLIENTS WITH NEUROLOGIC DISORDERS

LEARNING OUTCOMES

After completing this chapter, you will be able to:

- Apply knowledge of normal anatomy, physiology, and assessments when providing nursing care for clients with neurologic disorders (see Chapter 40).
- Explain the pathophysiology of neurologic disorders.
- Identify diagnostic tests used to diagnose selected neurologic disorders.
- Discuss the nursing implications of medications used to treat clients experiencing neurologic disorders.
- Discuss collaborative care for clients with neurologic disorders.
- Provide appropriate nursing care to clients undergoing neurologic surgery.
- Use the nursing process as a framework for providing individualized care to clients with neurologic disorders.

KEY TOPICS

- Degenerative neurological disorders
- PNS (peripheral nervous system) disorders
- Cranial nerve disorders
- Neurological disorders resulting from viral infections and neurotoxins
- Nursing care of clients with neurological disorders

MediaLink

www.prenhall.com/lemone

Additional resources for this chapter can be found on the Student CD-ROM accompanying this textbook, and on the Companion Website at www.prenhall.com/lemone. Click on Chapter 43 to select the activities for this chapter.

CD-ROM
- Audio Glossary
- NCLEX Review

Animations
- Multiple Sclerosis
- Dopamine
- Levodopa

Videos
- Akinesia
- Bradykinesia

Companion Website
- More NCLEX Review
- Case Study
    Parkinson's Disease
- Care Plan Activity
    Guillain-Barré Syndrome
- MediaLink Application
    Alzheimer's Disease

LECTURE OUTLINE

I. Client with Alzheimer's Disease (AD)
  A. Form of dementia characterized by progressive, irreversible deterioration of general intellectual functioning
    1. Begins with memory loss, initially subtle until progresses to being more noticeable; course includes deteriorating cognition and judgment with eventual physical decline and total inability to perform ADL
    2. Accounts for majority of dementia in America, affecting adults in middle to late life
    3. Risk factors include older age, female, family history
    4. Warning signs include
      a. Memory loss affecting ability to function in job
      b. Difficulty with familiar tasks
      c. Problems with language, abstract thinking
      d. Disorientation, changes in mood and personality
  B. Cause
    1. Exact cause is unknown; theories include loss of transmitter stimulation, genetic defects, viral and autoimmune cases
    2. Types
      a. Familial (follows inheritance pattern) and sporadic
      b. Early-onset (< 65)
      c. Older-onset (> 65)
    3. Changes in brain
      a. Loss of nerve cells and presence of neurofibrillary tangles and amyloid plaques
      b. Progressive brain atrophy
  C. Manifestations
    1. Stage I
      a. Appears healthy and alert
      b. Cognitive deficits are undetected
      c. Subtle memory lapses, personality changes
      d. Seems restless, forgetful, uncoordinated
    2. Stage II
      a. Memory deficits more apparent
      b. Less able to behave spontaneously
      c. Wandering behavior, deterioration in orientation to time and place
      d. Changes in sleeping patterns, agitation, stress
      e. Trouble with simple decisions
      f. Sundowning: increased agitation, wandering, disorientation in afternoon and evening hours
      g. Echolalia, scanning speech, total aphasia at times, apraxia, astereognosis, inability to write
      h. Becomes frustrated and depressed
    3. Stage III
      a. Increasing dependence with inability to communicate, loss of continence
      b. Progressive loss of cognitive abilities, falls, delusion, paranoid reactions
    4. Average life expectancy is 7 years from diagnosis to death, often from pneumonia, secondary to aspiration
  D. Collaborative Care
    1. No cure
    2. Supportive care for client and family
  E. Diagnostic Tests
    1. Diagnosis by ruling out other conditions including depression, hypothyroidism, infection, stroke
    2. EEG shows slow pattern in later stages of disease
    3. MRI and CT scan: shrinkage of hippocanthus
    4. Positron emission tomography (PET): visualizes brain activity and interactions
    5. Folstein Mini-Mental Status: instrument reflecting loss of memory and cognitive skills
  F. Medications
    1. Cholinesterase inhibitors used to treat mild to moderate dementia
      a. Tacrine hydrochloride (Cognex)
      b. Donepezil hydrochloride (Aricept)
      c. Rivastigmine (Exelon)
    2. Medications to treat depressions
    3. Tranquilizers for severe agitation
      a. Thioridazine (Mellaril)
      b. Haloperidol (Haldol)
    4. Antioxidants: vitamin E, anti-inflammatory agents, estrogen replacement therapy in women
  G. Complementary Therapy
    1. Massage, herbs, gingko biloba, Coenzyme Q10
    2. Art therapy, music, dance
  H. Nursing Care: Intensive, supportive nursing interventions directed at physical and psychosocial responses to illness

I. Health Promotion
1. Maintain functional abilities
2. Maintain safety of client and caregiver
J. Nursing Diagnoses
1. Impaired Memory
a. Include written or verbal reminders
b. Use cues to deal with memory loss
2. Chronic Confusion
3. Anxiety
4. Hopelessness
5. Caregiver Role Strain
K. Home Care
1. Education regarding disease, anticipation of needs, use of memory cues, support groups and peer counseling
2. Refer to home health agencies, family support, group support

II. Client with Multiple Sclerosis
A. Description
1. Chronic demyelinating disease of CNS associated with abnormal immune response to environmental factor
2. Initial onset followed by total remission making diagnosis difficult
3. Most persons have disease with periods of exacerbations and remissions
4. Progression of disease with increasing loss of function
5. Incidence is highest in young adults (20–40); onset between 20–50
6. Affects females more than males
7. More common in temperate climates
8. Occurs mainly in Caucasians
B. Pathophysiology
1. Believed to be autoimmune response to prior viral infection
2. Inflammation destroys myelin leading to axon dysfunction
a. Myelin sheaths of white matter of spinal cord, brain, optic nerve destroyed in patches called plaques
b. Demyelination slows and distorts nerve conduction resulting in absence of impulse transmission
c. Neurons in spinal cord, brain stem, cerebrum, cerebellum, and optic nerve affected
3. Recurrent demyelination and plaque formation result in scarring of glia and degeneration of axons
4. Disease follows different courses, most common is the relapsing-remitting type
5. Stressors trigger MS: febrile states, pregnancy, physical exertion and fatigue; and these also can trigger relapses

C. Manifestations: some systemic and some associated with area of demyelination
1. Fatigue
2. Optic nerve involvement: blurred vision, haziness
3. Brain stem involvement: nystagmus, dysarthria (scanning speech), cognitive dysfunctions, vertigo, deafness
4. Weakness, numbness in leg(s), spastic paresis, bladder and bowel dysfunction
5. Cerebellar: nystagmus, ataxia, hyoptonia
6. Blindness
D. Collaborative Care: Focus is on retaining optimum functioning, limiting disability
E. Diagnostic Tests
1. Neurological exam, careful history
2. Lumbar puncture with CSF analysis: increased number of T lymphocytes; elevated level of immunoglobulin G (IgG)
3. Cerebral, spinal optic nerve MRI: shows multifocal lesions
4. CT scan of brain: changes
5. PET: measures brain activity
6. Evoked response testing of visual, auditory, somatosensory impulses show delayed conduction
F. Medications: slow progression and decrease number of attacks
1. ACTH
2. Glucocorticosteroids
3. Immunosuppressants: azathioprine (Imuran), cyclophosphamide (Cytoxan)
4. Cyclophosphamide
5. Antispasmodics to treat muscle spasms
6. Medications to deal with bladder problems: anticholinergics or cholinergics depending on problem experienced by client
G. Rehabilitation: Physical therapy to maintain abilities and deal with spasticity
H. Nursing Care: Education and support of client dealing with chronic disease with unpredictable course
I. Health Promotion
1. Client needs to develop strategies to deal with fatigue, exacerbations
2. Prevention of respiratory and urinary tract infections
J. Nursing Diagnoses
1. Fatigue
2. Self Care Deficits
K. Home Care
1. Education
2. Referral to support group and resources
3. Referral to home health agencies when condition requires

III. Client with Parkinson's Disease
   A. Progressive, degenerative neurological disease characterized by tremor at rest, muscle rigidity and akinesia (poor movement); cause unknown
      1. Affects older adults mostly, mean age 60 with males more often than females
      2. Parkinson-like syndrome can occur with some medications, encephalitis, toxins; these are usually reversible
   B. Pathophysiology
      1. Neurons in cerebral cortex atrophy and dopamine receptors in basal ganglia decrease
      2. Decrease in dopamine, which is neurotransmitter involved with motor function
      3. Disturbance between balance of dopamine and acetylcholine
      4. Balance needed for smooth coordinated movement
   C. Manifestations
      1. Tremor at rest with pill rolling motion of thumb and fingers
         a. Lessens with purposeful movement
         b. Worsens with stress and anxiety
         c. Progressive impairment affecting ability to write and eat
      2. Rigidity
         a. Involuntary contraction of skeletal muscles
         b. Cogwheel rigidity: jerky motion
      3. Akinesia
         a. Slowed or delayed movement that affects chewing, speaking, eating
         b. May freeze: loss of voluntary movement
         c. Bradykinesia: slowed movement
      4. Abnormal posture
         a. Involuntary flexion of head and shoulders, stooped leaning forward position
         b. Equilibrium problems causing falls, and short, accelerated steps
      5. Autonomic nervous system
         a. Constipation and urinary hesitation or frequency
         b. Orthostatic hypotension, dizziness with position change
         c. Eczema, seborrhea
      6. Depression and dementia; confusion, disorientation, memory loss, slowed thinking
      7. Inability to change position while sleeping, sleep disturbance

   D. Complications
      1. Oculogyric crisis (fixed lateral and upward gaze)
      2. Impaired communication
      3. Falls
      4. Infection related to immobility and pneumonia
      5. Malnutrition related to dysphagia
      6. Skin breakdown
      7. Depression and isolation
   E. Prognosis
      1. Slow progressive degeneration
      2. Eventual debilitation
   F. Diagnostic Tests: No specific test for disease
      1. Drug screens to determine medications or toxins causing parkinsonism
      2. EEG: slowed and disorganized pattern
   G. Medications
      1. Initially selegiline (Carbex), amantadine (Symmetrel), anticholinergics
      2. Combination carbidopa-levodopa (Sinemet)
      3. Bromocriptine (Parlodel) pergolide (Permax) inhibit dopamine breakdown
      4. Medications may lose their efficacy; response to drugs fluctuates: "on-off" effect
   H. Treatments
      1. Electrical stimulation for tremor suppression
      2. Surgery has sometimes been done
         a. Pallidotomy: destruction of involved tissue
         b. Stereotaxic thalamotomy: destroys specific tissue involved in tremor
         c. Autologous adrenal medullary transplant
   I. Rehabilitation
      1. Physical therapy
      2. Occupational therapy
      3. Speech therapy
   J. Nursing Care
      1. Education and support to client and family
      2. Maintain functioning
      3. Referral to home care, community resources
   K. Health Promotion: Fall, malnutrition, aspiration prevention
   L. Nursing Diagnoses
      1. Impaired Physical Mobility
      2. Impaired Verbal Communication
      3. Impaired Nutrition: Less than body requirements
      4. Disturbed Sleep Patterns

M. Home Care
  1. Medication education
  2. Adaptation of home environment
  3. Gait training and exercises
  4. Nutritional teaching
IV. Client with Huntington's Disease (chorea)
  A. Progressive, degenerative inherited neurologic disease characterized by increasing dementia and chorea (rapid, jerky involuntary movements)
    1. Cause unknown
    2. No cure
    3. Usually asymptomatic until age of 30–40
  B. Pathophysiology: involves destruction of cells in basal ganglia and other brain areas, decrease in acetylcholine
  C. Manifestations
    1. Abnormal movement and progressive dementia
    2. Early signs are personality change with severe depression, memory loss; mood swings, signs of dementia
    3. Increasing restlessness, worsened by environmental stimuli and emotional stress; arms and face and entire body develops choreiform movements, lurching gait; difficulty swallowing, chewing, speaking
    4. Slow progressive debilitation and total dependence
    5. Death usually results from aspiration pneumonia or another infectious process
  D. Collaborative Care: almost always requires long-term care
  E. Diagnostic Tests: genetic testing of blood
  F. Medications
    1. Antipsychotic (phenothiazines and butyrophenones) to restore neurotransmitters
    2. Antidepressants
  G. Nursing Care
    1. Very challenging: physiological, psychosocial and ethical problems
    2. Genetic counseling
  H. Nursing Diagnoses
    1. Risk for Aspiration
    2. Imbalanced Nutrition: Less than body requirements
    3. Impaired Skin Integrity
    4. Impaired Verbal Communication
  I. Home Care: Referral to agencies to assist client and family, support group and organization
V. Client with Amyotrophic Lateral Sclerosis (ALS)
  A. Description

  1. Progressive, degenerative neurologic disease characterized by weakness and wasting of muscles without sensory or cognitive changes
  2. Several types of disease including a familial type; onset is usually between age of 40–60; higher incidence in males at earlier ages but equally post menopause
  3. Physiologic problems involve swallowing, managing secretions, communication, respiratory muscle dysfunction
  4. Death usually occurs in 2–5 years due to respiratory failure
  B. Pathophysiology
    1. Degeneration and demyelination of motor neurons in anterior horn of spinal cord, brain stem and cerebral cortex
    2. Involves upper and lower motor neurons
    3. Reinnervation occurs in the early course of disease, but fails as disease progresses
  C. Manifestations
    1. Initial: spastic, weak muscles with increased DTRs (UMN involvement); muscle flaccidity, paresis, paralysis, atrophy (LMN involvement); clients note muscle weakness and fasciculations (twitching of involved muscles); muscles weaken, atrophy; client complains of progressive fatigue; usually involves hands, shoulders, upper arms, and then legs
    2. Atrophy of tongue and facial muscles result in dysphagia and dysarthria; emotional lability and loss of control occur
    3. 50% of clients die within 2–5 years of diagnosis, often from respiratory failure or aspiration pneumonia
  D. Collaborative Care
    1. Evaluation to make the diagnosis
    2. Referrals for home health support
    3. Client needs to make decisions regarding gastrostomy tube, ventilator support
  E. Diagnostic Test
    1. Testing rules out other conditions that may mimic early ALS such as hyperthyroidism, compression of spinal cord, infections, neoplasms
    2. EMG to differentiate neuropathy from myopathy
    3. Muscle biopsy shows atrophy and loss of muscle fiber
    4. Serum creatine kinase if elevated (non-specific)

5. Pulmonary function tests: to determine degree of respiratory involvement
F. Medications: Rilutek (Riluzole) antiglutamate
   1. Prescribed to slow muscle degeneration
   2. Requires monitoring of liver function, blood count, chemistries, alkaline phosphatase
G. Nursing Care
   1. Help client and family deal with current health problems
   2. Plan for future needs including inability to communicate
H. Nursing Diagnoses
   1. Risk for Disuse Syndrome
   2. Ineffective Breathing Pattern: may require mechanical ventilation and tracheostomy
I. Home Care: Education regarding disease, community resources for health care assistance and dealing with disabilities

VI. Client with Creutzfeldt-Jakob disease (CJD, spongiform encephalopathy)
A. Description
   1. Rapid progressive degenerative neurologic disease causing brain degeneration without inflammation
   2. Transmissible and progressively fatal
   3. Caused by prion protein: transmission of prion is through direct contamination with infected neural tissue
   4. Rare in U.S. affecting persons 55–74
   5. Variant form of CJD is "mad cow disease": believed transmitted by consumption of beef contaminated with bovine form of disease; none identified in U.S. as of yet
   6. Pathophysiology: spongiform degeneration of gray matter of brain
B. Manifestations
   1. Onset: memory changes, exaggerated startle reflex, sleep disturbances
   2. Rapid deterioration in motor, sensory, language function
   3. Confusion progresses to dementia
   4. Terminal states: clients are comatose with decorticate and decerebrate posturing
C. Diagnostic Tests
   1. Clinical pictures, suggestive changes on EEG and CT scan
   2. Similar to Alzheimers in early stages
   3. Final diagnosis made on postmortem exam
D. Nursing Care
   1. Use of standard precautions with blood and body fluids

2. Support and assistance to client and family

VII. Client with Myasthenia gravis (MG)
A. Description
   1. Chronic neuromuscular disorder characterized by fatigue and severe weakness of skeletal muscles
   2. Occurs with remissions and exacerbations
   3. Believed to be autoimmune in origin
   4. Occurs more frequently in females, with onset between ages 20–30
B. Pathophysiology
   1. Antibodies destroy or block neuromuscular junction receptor sites, resulting in decreased number of acetylcholine receptors
   2. Causes decrease in muscle's ability to contract, despite sufficient acetylcholine
   3. Majority of clients have hyperplasia of thymus gland which is usually inactive after puberty; believed that thymus is source of autoantigen causing MG
   4. Associated in some clients with other autoimmune conditions
C. Manifestations
   1. Seen in the muscles that are affected
      a. Ptosis (drooping of eyelids), diplopia (double vision)
      b. Weakness in mouth muscles resulting in dysarthria and dysplagia
      c. Weak voice, smile appears as snarl
      d. Head juts forward
   2. Muscles are weak but DTRs are normal
   3. Weakness and fatigue exacerbated by stress, fever, overexertion, exposure to heat; improved with rest
D. Complications
   1. Pneumonia
   2. Myasthenic Crisis
      a. Sudden exacerbation of motor weakness putting client at risk for respiratory failure and aspiration
      b. Manifestations: tachycardia, tachypnea, respiratory distress, dysphasia
   3. Cholinergic Crisis
      a. Occurs with overdosage of medications (anticholinesterase drugs) used to treat MG
      b. Develops GI symptoms, severe muscle weakness, vertigo and respiratory distress
   4. Both crises often require ventilation assistance

5. Differentiation is by administration of Tensilon (edrophonium chloride), which will improve the muscle weakness in myasthenic crisis and be ineffective with cholinergic crisis

E. Diagnostic Tests
   1. Physical examination and history
   2. Tensilon Test: edrophonium chloride (Tensilon) administered and client with myasthenia will show significant improvement lasting 5 minutes
   3. EMG: reduced action potential
   4. Antiacetylcholine receptor antibody serum levels: increased in 80% MG clients; used to follow course of treatment
   5. Serum assay of circulating acetylcholine receptor antibodies: if increased is diagnostic of MG

F. Medications
   1. Anticholinesterase medications, which act at neuromuscular junction, allowing acetylcholine to concentrate at receptor sites and promote muscle contraction; most commonly used medication is pyridostigmine (Mestinon)
   2. Immunosuppression medications including glucocorticoids
   3. Cyclosporineor azathioprine (Imuran)

G. Surgery
   1. Thymectomy is recommended in clients < 60
   2. Remission occurs in 40% of clients, but may take several years to occur

H. Plasmapheresis
   1. Used to remove antibodies
   2. Often done before planned surgery, or when respiratory involvement has occurred

I. Nursing Care
   1. Teaching interventions to deal with fatigue
   2. Importance of following medication therapy

J. Nursing Diagnoses
   1. Ineffective Airway Clearance
   2. Impaired Swallowing: plan to take medication to assist with chewing activity

K. Home Care
   1. Avoid fatigue and stress
   2. Plan for future with treatment options
   3. Keep medications available
   4. Carry medical identification
   5. Referral to support group, community resources

VIII. Client with Guillain-Barre Syndrome
   A. Description
      1. Acute inflammatory demyelinating disorder of peripheral nervous system characterized by acute onset of motor paralysis (usually ascending)
      2. Cause is unknown but precipitating events include GI or respiratory infection prior, surgery, or viral immunizations
      3. 80–90% of clients have spontaneous recovery with little or no disabilities
      4. 4–6% mortality rate, and up to 10% have permanent disabling weakness
      5. Characterized by progressive ascending flaccid paralysis of extremities with paresthesia and numbness
      6. 20% require mechanical ventilation due to respiratory involvement
   B. Pathophysiology
      1. Destruction of myelin sheath covering peripheral nerves as result of immunologic response
      2. Demyelinization causes sudden muscle weakness and loss of reflex response
   C. Manifestations
      1. Most clients have symmetric weakness beginning in lower extremities
      2. Ascends body to include upper extremities, torso, and cranial nerves
      3. Sensory involvement causes severe pain, paresthesia and numbness
      4. Client cannot close eyes
      5. Paralysis of intercostals and diaphragmatic muscle can result in respiratory failure
      6. Autonomic nervous system involvement: blood pressure fluctuations, cardiac dysrhythmias, paralytic illness, SIADH, urinary retention
      7. Weakness usually plateaus or starts to improve in the fourth week with slow return of muscle strength
   D. Collaborative Care
      1. Ensuring adequate respiration and oxygenation
      2. Preventing complications due to immobility
   E. Diagnostic Tests: diagnosis made through history and clinical examination; there is no specific test
      1. CSF analysis: increased protein
      2. EMG: decrease nerve conduction
      3. Pulmonary function tests reflect degree of respiratory involvement
   F. Medications: supportive and prophylactic care
      1. Antibiotics

2. Morphine for pain control
3. Anticoagulation to prevent thromboembolic complications
4. Vasopressors as needed
G. Surgery: may need tracheostomy, if prolonged ventilator support necessary
H. Plasmapheresis: may be helpful, if used early in the course of disease
I. Dietary Management: usually requires enteral feeding or total parenteral nutrition
J. Physical and Occupational Therapy: usually require long-term rehabilitation to regain maximum muscle strength
K. Nursing Care: involves acute neurological and critical care nursing and rehabilitation
L. Nursing Diagnoses
   1. Acute Pain
   2. Risk for Impaired Skin Integrity
   3. Impaired Communication
M. Home Care
   1. Clients will usually require hospitalization, rehabilitation, and eventually discharge to home
   2. Client and family will need support; support groups
IX. Trigeminal neuralgia (tic douloureux)
A. Description
   1. Chronic disease of trigeminal nerve (cranial nerve V) causing severe facial pain
   2. The maxillary and mandibular divisions of nerve are affected
   3. Occurs more often in middle and older adults, females more than males
   4. Cause is unknown
B. Manifestations
   1. Severe facial pain occurring for brief seconds to minutes hundreds of times a day, several times a year
   2. Usually occurs unilaterally in area of mouth and rises toward ear and eye
   3. Wincing or grimacing in response to the pain
   4. Trigger areas on the face may initiate the pain
   5. Sensory contact or eating, swallowing, talking may set off the pain
   6. Often there is spontaneous remission after years, and then condition recurs with dull ache in between pain episodes
C. Diagnosis: by physical assessment
D. Medications: Anticonvulsants; carbamazepine (Tegretol), phenytoin (Dilantin), or gabapentin (Neurotin)
E. Surgery

1. Intractable pain may be treated by severing the nerve root: rhizotomy
2. Client may have lost facial sensation and have loss of corneal reflex
F. Nursing Care
   1. Teaching client self-management of pain
   2. Maintaining nutrition
   3. Preventing injury
X. Bell's Palsy
A. Description
   1. Disorder of seventh cranial nerve and causes unilateral facial paralysis
   2. Occurs between age of 20–60 equally in males and females
   3. Cause unknown, but thought to be related to herpes virus
B. Manifestations
   1. Numbness, stiffness noticed first
   2. Later face appears asymmetric: side of face droops; unable to close eye, wrinkle forehead or pucker lips on one side
   3. Lower facial muscles are pulled to one side; appears as if a stroke
C. Prognosis
   1. Majority of people recover fully in few weeks to months
   2. Some people have residual paralysis
D. Diagnosis: based on physical examination
E. Collaborative Care
   1. Corticosteroids are prescribed in some cases but use has been questioned
   2. Treatment is supportive
F. Nursing Care
   1. Teaching client self-care: prevent injury and maintain nutrition
   2. Use of artificial tears, wearing eye patch or taping eye shut at night; wearing sunglasses
   3. Soft diet that can be chewed easily, small frequent meals
XI. Neurologic Diseases that result from viral infections or neurotoxins
A. Postpoliomyelitis Syndrome
   1. Complication of previous poliomyelitis virus (epidemic occurred in U.S. during 1940s and 1950s); persons who recovered are re-experiencing manifestation of acute illness in their advanced age
   2. Pathophysiology: Process is unknown
   3. Manifestations: Fatigue, muscle and joint weakness, loss of muscle mass, respiratory difficulties, and pain
   4. Diagnosis: By history and physical examination

5. Treatment: Involves physical therapy and pulmonary rehabilitation
6. Nursing Care: Involves emotional support and interventions to deal with dysfunction; ADL, safety are included in interventions

B. Rabies
1. Rhabovirus infection of CNS transmitted by infected saliva that enters the body through bite or open wound
   a. Critical illness almost always fatal
   b. Source often is bite of infected domestic or wild animal
   c. Incubation is 10 days to years
2. Manifestations occur in stages
   a. Prodromal: wound is painful, various paresthesias, general signs of infection; increased sensitivity to light, sound, and skin temperature changes
   b. Excitement stage: periods of excitement and quiet; develops laryngospasm and is afraid to drink (hydrophobia), convulsions, muscle spasms and death usually due to respiratory failure
3. Collaborative Care
   a. Animal that bit person is held under observation for 7–10 days to detect rabies
   b. Sick animals are killed and their brains are tested for presence of rabies virus
   c. Blood of client may be tested for rabies antibodies
4. Post-exposure treatment
   a. Rabies immune globulin (RIG) is administered for passive immunization
   b. Client often has local and mild systemic reaction; treatment is over 30 days
5. Treatment of client with rabies: involves intensive care treatment
6. Health Promotion
   a. Vaccination of pets
   b. Avoid wild animals, especially those appearing ill
   c. Follow up care for any bites

C. Tetanus (lockjaw)
1. Disorder of nervous system caused by neurotoxin from *Clostridium tetani,* anaerobic bacillus present in the soil
   a. Contract disease from open wound contaminated with dirt, debris
   b. Has high mortality rate
2. Incubation is usually 8–12 days

3. Manifestations
   a. Stiffness of jaw and neck and dysphagia
   b. Spasms of jaw and facial muscles
   c. Develops generalized seizures and painful body muscle spasms
   d. Death occurs from respiratory and cardiac complications
4. Diagnosis is made on clinical manifestations
5. Clients with disease are treated in intensive care with antibiotics, chlorpromazine (Thorazine) and diazepam (Valium) for muscle spasms
6. Health Promotion
   a. Active immunization with boosters given at time of exposure
   b. Passive immunization is given to persons who are not adequately immunized

D. Botulism
1. Food poisoning caused by ingestion of food contaminated with toxin from *Clostridium botulinum,* anaerobic bacteria found in soil
   a. Contracted by eating contaminated foods usually improperly canned or cooked
   b. Untreated death rate is high
2. Pathophysiology: Bacteria produce a toxin, which blocks release of acetylcholine from nerve endings causing respiratory failure by paralysis of muscles
3. Manifestations
   a. Visual disturbances
   b. Gastrointestinal symptoms
   c. Paralysis of all muscle groups
   d. Effecting respiration
4. Diagnosis
   a. Based on clinical picture
   b. Verified by laboratory analysis of client's serum and stool
   c. Testing the suspected food
5. Treatment
   a. Administration of antitoxin
   b. Supportive treatment including mechanical ventilation and systemic support in intensive care unit
6. Health Promotion
   a. Teaching clients to process foods properly when home canning
   b. Boiling foods for 10 minutes which destroys the toxin
   c. Not eating spoiled foods

FOCUSED STUDY TIPS

- Visit an Alzheimer's unit. Identify environmental safety measures utilized. Interview a client. Observe manifestations of the disease. Share your experience with classmates.
- Describe how MS (multiple sclerosis) is diagnosed. Identify resources in your community that are available for MS clients. Discuss how referrals to these resources are made.
- Care for a client with MS in the clinical setting. Assess and interview the client. Observe manifestations of the disease. Identify social services utilized by the client. Evaluate the effectiveness of home care.

CASE STUDY

Clients with myasthenia gravis can develop two life-threatening emergencies: myasthenic crisis and cholinergic crisis. Describe the etiology of each, the signs and symptoms of each, and how your nursing assessment would differentiate between the two. What medical intervention would confirm diagnosis of one or the other? How?

CARE PLAN CRITICAL THINKING ACTIVITY

Managing pain in clients with Guillain-Barre syndrome is a difficult nursing task. The intense pain combined with altered sensations leads to increased anxiety that in turn causes more pain. What nursing interventions can make a difference in breaking the cycle of increasing pain?

NCLEX TEST QUESTIONS

1. The nurse formulates a diagnosis of altered nutrition: less than body requirements due to chronic fatigue for a client with myasthenia gravis (MG). Which of the following interventions would be appropriate in helping the client to meet nutritional needs?
   a. Encourage the client to eat every 2 hours in order to increase caloric intake.
   b. Have the client eat the largest meal in the morning and drink fluids for the rest of the day.
   c. Coincide medication therapy for relief of clinical symptoms with feeding times to maximize client's ability to eat.
   d. Discuss with the physician and dietician that the client should be switched to enteral feedings due to client fatigue level.

2. A collaborative plan of care is being developed for a 52-year-old client who has recently been diagnosed with Parkinson disease. Which of the following actions would be appropriate at this time?
   a. Refer client to a speech pathologist.
   b. Begin active and passive ROM exercises three times a day.
   c. Have the client return in a month to talk with the physician about nutritional needs.
   d. Discuss with the client concerns related to the diagnosis, nutritional therapy, and effects of medications.

3. The client presents to the emergency department complaining of weakness that has been progressing upward in both legs for a few days. The nurse, suspecting Guillain-Barré syndrome, begins by
   a. taking medical history, noting recent viral influenza.
   b. giving the client orange juice for fatigue and low blood sugar.
   c. instructing on testing for myasthenia gravis.
   d. evaluating for petit mal seizures.

4. The client with Parkinson disease finds the resting tremor he is experiencing in his right hand very frustrating. The nurse advises him to:
   a. practice deep breathing.
   b. take a warm bath.
   c. hold an object in that hand.
   d. take diazepam (Valium) as needed.

5. Why should a client with Huntington disease be given thickened soups, mashed potatoes, stews, or casseroles?
   a. The client is at risk for dehydration.
   b. The client is at risk for aspiration.
   c. The client may have difficulty chewing.
   d. The client may have pain on swallowing.

6. While obtaining the health history from the elderly client with Parkinson disease, the client's

daughter continually answers all questions directed to the client. The nurse

a. accepts this as helpful because the client's voice is low, monotone, and difficult to understand.

b. stops the interview and resumes it later when the daughter is not there.

c. allows the daughter to complete the interview form.

d. respectfully tells the daughter, "I need to hear what your father has to say."

7. The nurse caring for a client newly diagnosed with botulism plans client care according to the fact that:

a. it is caused by a *Staphylococcus* bacteria.

b. neurotoxins produced by the bacteria cause paralysis.

c. it is a resident bacterium in the intestinal flora.

d. it produces a toxin that leads to necrosis of epithelial cells.

8. The spouse of a client with Parkinson disease wants to know how to best assist her husband during feeding as he is having "increasing problems with drooling and swallowing." What instruction could you provide to this family member?

a. "Use thickened liquids along with upright positioning during feeding."

b. "It might be time to switch to enteral feedings if you are afraid that your husband may choke."

c. "Increase the amount of fluids he receives to decrease saliva formation and improve swallowing."

d. "Use a straw during feedings to facilitate swallowing."

9. The client with a positive gene marker for Huntington disease asks the nurse what symptom indicates that the disease is progressing. The correct response is

a. headaches.

b. dizziness.

c. chorea (uncontrollable movements).

d. seizures.

10. Which of the following medications would the nurse prepare to administer when evaluating a client suspected of having myasthenia gravis?

a. benztropine (Cogentin)

b. diazepam (Valium)

c. edrophonium (Tensilon)

d. radioactive iodine (I131)

CHAPTER **44**

ASSESSING CLIENTS WITH EYE AND EAR DISORDERS

LEARNING OUTCOMES

After completing this chapter, you will be able to:

- Review the anatomy and physiology of the eye and the ear.
- Explain the physiologic processes involved in vision, hearing, and equilibrium.
- Identify specific topics for consideration during a health history interview of the client with health problems of the eye or ear.
- Describe techniques for assessing the structure and function of the eye and ear.
- Identify abnormal findings that may indicate impairment in the function of the eye and the ear.

KEY TOPICS

- Review of anatomy and physiology of the eye and vision
- Review of anatomy and physiology of the ear and hearing
- Assessing the eye and vision
- Assessing the ear and hearing

LECTURE OUTLINE

I. Review of Anatomy and Physiology of the Eyes
  A. Primary function of eye: encode patterns of light from environment from eyes to brain which gives meaning to coded information
  B. Extraocular structures: vital to protecting internal structures
    1. Eyebrows: shade eyes and protect from perspiration

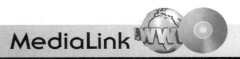

MediaLink

www.prenhall.com/lemone

Additional resources for this chapter can be found on the Student CD-ROM accompanying this textbook, and on the Companion Website at www.prenhall.com/lemone. Click on Chapter 44 to select the activities for this chapter.

CD-ROM
- Audio Glossary
- NCLEX Review

Animations
- Ear Anatomy
- Eye Anatomy

Companion Website
- More NCLEX Review
- Functional Health Pattern Assessment
- Case Study
   Otitis Media

2. Eyelids
  a. Protect from foreign bodies
  b. Regulate entry of light into eye
  c. Distribute tears through blinking
3. Eyelashes: blinking reflex protects eyes from foreign objects
4. Conjunctiva: lubricates eyes

411

5. Lacrimal gland, puncta, lacrimal sac, nasolacrimal duct: secrete, distribute, and drain tears to cleanse and moisten eye's surface
6. Six extrinsic eye muscles
   a. Control movement of eye
   b. Maintain shape of eyeball
C. Intraocular Structures: Transmit visual images and maintain homeostasis of the inner eye
   1. Anterior portion
      a. Sclera
         1. White in color and lines outside of eyeball
         2. Protects it and gives shape
      b. Cornea
         1. Transparent, avascular, very sensitive to touch
         2. Forms a window allowing light to enter eye; bends light
         3. Corneal reflex; when cornea is touched the eyelids blink
      c. Iris
         1. Disc of muscular tissue surrounding pupil and lies between cornea and lens
         2. Gives eye its color
         3. Regulates entry of light by controlling size of pupil
            a. Constricts with bright light
            b. Dilates to light is dim and for far vision
            c. Pupillary light reflex: pupil constricts rapidly in intense light
      d. Anterior Chamber
         1. Space between cornea and iris
         2. Filled with aqueous humor
            a. Nourishes and provides oxygen to lens and cornea
            b. Constantly formed and drained to maintain pressure of 15 and 20 mm Hg in eye
            c. Fluid moves between anterior and posterior chamber through canal of Schlemm
   2. Posterior cavity: Lies behind lens and is filled with clear gelatinous substance called vitreous humor
      a. Vitreous humor
         1. Supports posterior surface of lens
         2. Maintains position of retina
         3. Transmits light
      b. Lens
         1. Biconvex, avascular, transparent structure located directly behind pupil

2. Changes shape to focus and refract light onto retina
   c. Uvea (vascular tunic)
      1. Middle layer of eyeball
      2. Three components
         a. Iris
         b. Ciliary body: encircles lens and with iris controls shape of lens
         c. Choroid: pigmented and vascular; blood vessels nourish layer of eyeball; pigmented areas absorb light preventing it from shattering within eyeball
   d. Retina: innermost lining of eyeball
      1. Outer pigmented layer next to choroid links visual stimuli and brain
      2. Inner transparent layer composed of millions of light receptors in structures called rods and cones
         a. Rods: enable peripheral vision and vision in dim light
         b. Cones: enable vision in bright light, color perception
      3. Optic disc: cream colored oval area within retina where optic nerve enters eye
         a. Physiologic cup: slight depression in center of optic disc
         b. Macula: lateral to optic disc; darker area with no visible blood vessels; contains primarily cones
         c. Fovea centralis: light depression in center of macula contains only cones and is main receptor of detailed color vision
D. Visual Pathway
   1. Optic nerves are cranial nerves formed of axons of ganglion cells
   2. Two optic nerves meet at the optic chiasma, anterior to pituitary gland in brains; axons from medial half of each retina cross to opposite side and form pairs of axons from each eye
      a. Left optic tract carries visual information from lateral half of retina of left eye and medial half of retina of right eye
      b. Right optic tract carries visual information from lateral half of retina of right eye and medial half of retina of left eye
      c. Visual fields of each eye overlap and each eye sees slightly different view
      d. Brain fuses overlap of visual fields and visual view from optic tracts and fuses

the images into one image; this allows for depth perception (but also requires both eyes to focus well)

E. Refraction

    1. Bending of light rays; light is refracted when entering cornea, aqueous humor, lens and vitreous humor

    2. At lens, light is bent and converges at single point on retina; focusing of image is called accommodation

    3. For persons with emmetropic (normal) vision

        a. Far point of vision: distance from viewed object at which eyes require no accommodation; 20 feet

        b. Near point of vision: closest point on which person can focus; usually 8–10 inches

II. Assessment of the Eye

A. Health assessment interview to collect subjective data

    1. If problem involving one or both eyes is identified, collect information regarding

        a. Onset

        b. Characteristics and course

        c. Severity

        d. Precipitating or relieving factors

        e. Associated symptoms, including timing and circumstances

    2. During interview, note nonverbal behaviors such as squinting or abnormal eye movements

    3. Explore watery, irritated eyes, or changes in vision

    4. Use of eyewear, care of eyeglasses or contact lenses

    5. Use of eye medications: type and purpose

    6. History includes

        a. Eye trauma, surgery or infection

        b. Date and results of last eye exam

        c. Medical history of diabetes, HPT, thyroid disorders, glaucoma, cataracts, eye infections

        d. Family history of nearsightedness or farsightedness, cancer of retina, color blindness, eye or vision disorders

    7. Environmental or work exposure to irritating chemicals; activities that pose risk of eye injury, use of protective eyewear during potentially hazardous activities

B. Physical assessment to collect objective data

    1. Vision assessment with abnormal findings

        a. Vision acuity is assessed with Snellen chart or E chart for testing distance

vision; Rosenbaum chart for testing near vision

        b. Myopia or nearsightedness

            1. Reading of 20/100 using Snellen or E chart

            2. Impaired ability with near vision

            3. Presbyopia in clients' age > 45; loss of elasticity of lens

            4. Hyperopia in clients younger than 45

    2. Eye movement and alignment with abnormal findings

        a. Failure of eyes to converge equally on an approaching object may indicate neuromuscular disorder or improper eye alignment

        b. Failure of one or both eyes to follow an object in any given direction may indicate extraocular muscle weakness or cranial nerve dysfunction

        c. Involuntary rhythmic movement of eyes (nystagmus): associated with use of medications

        d. Unequal corneal light reflex reveals improper alignment

    3. Pupillary assessment with abnormal findings

        a. Pupils with unequal size may indicate severe neurologic problems including increased intracranial pressure

        b. Failure of pupils to respond to light may indicate retinal degeneration or destruction of optic nerve

        c. Client who has one dilated and one unresponsive pupil may have paralysis of one oculomotor nerve

        d. Unequal dilation, constriction or inequality of pupil size may be caused by some eye medications

            1. Morphine and narcotics: small, unresponsive pupils

            2. Anticholinergic drugs: dilated unresponsive pupils

        e. Failure of eyes to accommodate with lack of papillary response to light may indicate neurologic problem

        f. Pupils that do not respond to light but accommodate properly is seen in clients with diabetes

    4. External eye assessment with abnormal findings

        a. Unusual redness or discharge indicates inflammatory state due to trauma, allergies, or infection

b. Drooping of one eyelid, ptosis, may result from stroke, neuromuscular disorder, or congenital

c. Unusual widening of lids may be due to exophthalmos (protrusion of eyeball due to increase in intraocular volume) is often associated with hyperthyroid conditions

d. Yellow plaques noted on lid margins (xanthelasma) may indicate high lipid levels

e. Acute localized inflammation of hair follicle known as hordeolum (sty) often caused by staphylococcal organisms

f. Chalazion is infection or retention cyst of meibomian glands

g. Significant redness or discharge from puncta indicates inflammation due to trauma, infection, or allergies

h. Conjunctiva

1. Increased erythema, presence of exudates indicates acute conjunctivitis

2. Cobblestone appearance associated with allergies

3. Fold in conjunctiva (pterygium) is clouded area that is seen as clouded area over cornea (may interfere with vision if covering pupil)

i. Sclera

1. Unusual redness indicates inflammatory state resulting from trauma, allergies, or infection

2. Yellow discoloration occurs with jaundice involving liver conditions

3. Bright red areas are subconjunctival hemorrhages and may indicate trauma or bleeding disorders; may occur spontaneously

j. Cornea

1. Dullness, opacities, irregularities

2. Absence of blink reflex may indicate neurologic disorder

k. Iris

1. Lack of clarity may indicate cloudiness in cornea

2. Constriction of pupil accompanied by pain and circumcorneal redness indicates acute iritis

5. Internal eye assessment with abnormal findings: Ophthalmoscopic examination

a. Absence of red reflex may indicate total opacity of pupil by cataract or hemorrhage into vitreous humor

b. Dark shadow visualized is cataract (opacity of lens) due to aging, trauma, diabetes, or congenital defect

c. On retinal exam, areas of hemorrhage, exudates, white patches are found with diabetes or long-standing HPT

d. Loss of optic disc as well as increase in size of physiologic cup results from papilledema that occurs with increased intracranial pressure

e. Blood vessels of retina

1. Displacement of blood vessels from center of optic disc occurs with increased intraocular pressure as with glaucoma

2. Apparent narrowing of vein where an arteriole crosses over occurs with HPT

3. Engorged veins occur with diabetes, atherosclerosis, blood disorders

f. Variations in color of pale color in retinal background indicates disease

g. Upon inspection of macula, absence of fovea centralis may indicate macular degeneration

h. Tenderness over lacrimal glands, puncta, nasolacrimal duct or drainage may indicate infection

i. Excessive tearing may indicate blockage of nasolacrimal duct

III. Review of Anatomy and Physiology of the Ears

A. Functions of Ear

1. Hearing

2. Maintaining equilibrium

B. Anatomical Area of Ear

1. External Ear

a. Auricle (pinna)

1. Composed of elastic cartilage covered with thin skin

2. Contains sebaceous and sweat glands and hair

3. Directs sound waves to ear

b. External auditory canal

1. Extends from auricle to tympanic membrane

2. Lined with skin containing hair, sebaceous glands, and ceruminous glands

3. Serves as resonator for range of sound waves of human speech; increases pressure sound waves in frequency range on tympanic

4. Ceruminous glands secrete waxy substance cerumen which traps

foreign bodies, has bacteriostatic properties

c. Tympanic membrane: between external and middle ear
1. Thin semitransparent, fibrous structure covered with skin on external side, mucosa on inner side
2. Vibrates as sound waves strike it and are transferred as sound waves to middle ear

2. Middle Ear
a. Air-filled cavity in temporal bone
b. Contains 3 auditory ossicles
1. Malleus: attaches to tympanic membrane and articulates with incus
2. Incus: articulates with stapes
3. Stapes: fits into oval window
c. Median side of middle ear is bony wall containing two membrane-covered openings
1. Oval window
2. Round window
d. Communicates with mastoid sinuses helping middle ear to adjust to changes in pressure
e. Opens into eustachian tube (connects with nasopharynx)
1. Helps equalize air pressure in middle ear
2. Ensures vibrations of tympanic membrane remain adequate
f. If sudden loud noise occurs; 2 small muscles attached to ossicles contract reflexively to decrease vibrations and protect inner ear

3. Inner Ear (Labyrinth)
a. Maze of bony chambers located deep within temporal bone, behind eye socket
b. Two parts
1. Bony labyrinth: system of open channels containing 3 parts
a. Vestibule
1. Central portion of inner ear
2. Contains 2 sacs called saccule and utricle
3. Sacs contain receptors for equilibrium that respond to changes in gravity and changes in head position
b. Semicircular canals (3)
1. Each canal contains a semicircular duct that communicates with utricle of vestibule

2. Each duct contains equilibrium receptor that responds to angular movements of head
c. Cochlea
1. Tiny bony chamber that houses organ of Corti, the receptor organ for hearing
2. Series of sensory hair cells innervated by sensory fibers from cranial nerve VIII
2. Membranous labyrinth which contains fluid called endolymph

C. Sound Conduction
1. When molecules of medium are compressed, resulting in a pressure disturbance (sound wave), sound is produced
a. Loudness or intensity determined by amplitude (height) of sound wave (greater amplitudes = louder sounds)
b. Frequency of sound wave in vibrations per second determines pitch or tone of sound (higher frequencies = higher tone)
2. Transmission of sound
a. Sound waves enter external auditory canal
b. Tympanic membrane vibrates
c. Ossicles amplify energy of sound wave and transmit the motion of tympanic membrane to oval window
d. Perilymph in vestibule transmits motion
e. Increased pressure of perilymph transmitted to fibers of basilar membrane and then to organ of Corti
f. Hairs in organ of Corti generate action potentials that are transmitted to cranial nerve VIII and then to brain for interpretation
g. Brain stem auditory nuclei transmit impulses to cerebral cortex
h. Auditory processing finely tunes wide variety of sounds of different pitch and loudness; also sounds can be localized
3. Maintenance of equilibrium
a. Inner ear provides information about position of head, which is used to coordinate body movements to maintain equilibrium and balance
b. Types of balance
1. Static
a. Affected by changes in head position

  b. Receptors, called maculae, in utricle and saccule of vestibule detect changes
  2. Dynamic
    a. Affected by movement of head
    b. Receptor is in crista, a crest in the membrane lining ampulla of each semicircular canal, which responds to changes in endolymph and hair cell movement

IV. Assessment of the Ear
  A. Health assessment interview to collect subjective data
    1. If client has problem involving one or both ears, analyze
      a. Onset
      b. Character and course
      c. Severity
      d. Precipitating and relieving factors
      e. Associated symptoms including timing and circumstances
    2. Be aware of nonverbal behaviors (inappropriate answers, asking for statements to be repeated suggest altered hearing function)
    3. Explore with client
      a. Changes in hearing
      b. Ringing in ears (tinnitus)
      c. Ear pain
      d. Drainage from ears
      e. Use of hearing aids
    4. Determine history
      a. Trauma, surgery, infections of ear, date of last ear examination
      b. Medical history of infectious diseases such as meningitis or mumps
      c. Use of medication that affect hearing
      d. Family history of hearing loss, ear problems, diseases
      e. Type and care for hearing aid
  B. Physical assessment of ear and hearing
    1. Hearing test with abnormal findings
      a. Weber test
        1. Tuning fork placed on midline vertex of head
        2. If sound is heard in or lateralized to one ear, indicative of conductive hearing loss in that ear or sensorineural loss in other

  b. Rinne test
    1. Vibrating tuning fork placed on client's mastoid bone and client identifies when sound no longer heard
    2. Fork moved in front of client's ear close to ear canal, and client identifies when sound no longer heard
    3. Sound should be heard twice as long by air conduction than by bone conduction
    4. Bone conduction is greater than air conduction with a conductive hearing loss
  c. Whisper test: rough estimate that hearing loss exists
  2. External ear assessment with abnormal findings
    a. Unusual redness or drainage around auricle indicates inflammatory response to infection or trauma
    b. Scales or skin lesions around the rim may indicate skin cancer
    c. Small, raised lesions around rim of ear are tophi and indicate gout
    d. Unusual redness, lesion, or purulent drainage of external auditory canal indicates infection
    e. Hardened, dry, or foul-smelling cerumen in ear canal indicates infection or impaction of cerumen
    f. Inspection of tympanic membrane
      1. Inconsistent texture and color occur with scarring from previous perforation caused by infection, allergies, or trauma
      2. Bulging membranes (loss of bony landmarks, distorted light reflex) indicate otitis media or malfunctioning of auditory tubes
      3. Retracted membranes with accentuated bony landmarks and distorted light reflex occurs with obstructed auditory tube
    g. Tenderness, swelling or nodules over auricles and mastoid process indicate inflammation of external auditory canal or mastoiditis

FOCUSED STUDY TIPS

- Describe vision assessment for the culturally diverse client who does not read or speak English.
- Describe to a family member or friend how sound is conducted.
- Care for a client with a hearing aid. Become familiar with the device's use and care.

CASE STUDY

When asked to assess visual acuity for distant vision and near vision of a non-English-speaking client, which charts will the nurse utilize? Describe these charts in detail, as well as instruction for the client. How will the results of these tests be interpreted and reported?

CARE PLAN CRITICAL THINKING ACTIVITY

When assessing a client's pupils, the nurse notes one pupil is a different size and does not respond to light or accommodation. What assessment should follow this finding? How will this finding affect the nursing care plan for this client?

NCLEX TEST QUESTIONS

1. The nurse notes a cloudy appearance to the lens of an 80-year-old client's eye. Which of the following additional assessment findings would help confirm the diagnosis of cataracts?
   a. sense of a curtain falling over the visual field
   b. persistent, dull eye pain
   c. loss of red reflex
   d. double vision

2. A 75-year-old client reports to the nurse during the admission process that she was recently diagnosed with age-related hearing loss. The client is most likely describing
   a. otalgia.
   b. Ménière's disease.
   c. presbycusis.
   d. otitis externa.

3. Which of the following clients is at highest risk for macular degeneration?
   a. a biochemist exposed to various toxins
   b. an elderly client
   c. a youth hit in the eye with a baseball
   d. a young adult with multiple allergies

4. The pediatric health nurse explains to parents that acute otitis media is more common in infants and children than adults because a child's eustachian tubes
   a. are longer and curved.
   b. are undeveloped.
   c. are shorter and straighter.
   d. have fewer cilia.

5. The nurse observes another nurse enter the room of a blind client without announcing herself. The appropriate intervention is to
   a. inform the head nurse so that he can intervene.
   b. tell the nurse that she had always learned to announce herself when entering the room of a blind person.
   c. tell the client she is sorry the other nurse may have frightened her.
   d. do nothing, as there is no intervention required.

6. When educating the client with primary hypertension, the nurse instructs the client to
   a. take anti-hypertensive medications when blood pressure is elevated.
   b. monitor blood pressure annually.
   c. avoid foods with concentrated sugars.
   d. have regular eye exams.

7. A client seen in the neighborhood clinic complains of "eye problems" and generalized weakness that became markedly worse after visiting with a friend and frequently using the hot tub. The client is going into considerably long, detailed answers as you take the history. Your response is
   a. "This is important information, but there's just not enough staffing now."
   b. "You'll feel better after getting this all off your mind."

c. "Please be brief in your answers so I can get you through this."

d. "Tell me more about the eye problems."

8. Which of the following tests would the nurse employ when evaluating the hearing of a client?

a. Trendelenburg test

b. Weber test

c. Snellen test

d. Allen test

9. A client has begun taking acetylsalicylic acid (aspirin) 2.6 grams per day in divided doses every 6 hours. Which one of the following signs or symptoms is most likely to indicate an early stage of toxicity?

a. gastritis

b. hematuria

c. tinnitus

d. fever

10. A client with Ménière's disease would probably complain of which of the following?

a. bilateral hearing impairment

b. vertigo and nausea

c. pain when the tragus is touched

d. tenderness over the mastoid area

CHAPTER 45

NURSING CARE OF CLIENTS WITH EYE AND EAR DISORDERS

LEARNING OUTCOMES

After completing this chapter, you will be able to:

- Use knowledge of normal anatomy and physiology of the eye and ear and assessments to provide care for clients with disorders of the eyes and ears (see Chapter 44).
- Describe the pathophysiology of commonly occurring disorders of the eyes and ears, relating their manifestations to the pathophysiologic process.
- Identify diagnostic tests used to diagnose eye and ear disorders.
- Discuss the nursing implications for medications prescribed for clients with eye and ear disorders.
- Provide appropriate care for the client having eye or ear surgery.
- Use the nursing process as a framework for providing care to clients with impaired vision or hearing.

KEY TOPICS

- Infectious and inflammatory eye disorders
- Age-related visual changes
- Refractive disorders of the eye
- Eye trauma
- Structural disorders of the eye
- The blind client
- Ear disorders

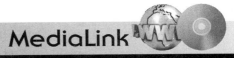

MediaLink

www.prenhall.com/lemone

Additional resources for this chapter can be found on the Student CD-ROM accompanying this textbook, and on the Companion Website at www.prenhall.com/lemone. Click on Chapter 45 to select the activities for this chapter.

CD-ROM
- Audio Glossary
- NCLEX Review

Animations
- Ear Abnormalities
- Middle Ear Dynamics
- Pilocarpine

Companion Website
- More NCLEX Review
- Case Study
  Retinal Detachment
- Care Plan Activity
  Hearing Aid

LECTURE OUTLINE

I. Vision and hearing provide primary means of input from the environment
  A. Enables persons to have ability to receive and organize information surrounding them
  B. Allows for communication
  C. Gains access to information
  D. Derives pleasure from sights and sounds of the world

II. Eye Disorders
  A. Client with age-related changes in vision
    1. Pupil decreases in size and does not dilate as readily, reducing the amount of light reaching the retina
    2. Night vision is diminished requiring increased light intensity for reading and close work
    3. Lens is less elastic causing difficulty in focusing for near vision
    4. Lens discolors causing decrease in color perception
    5. Changes in vitreous humor, choroids atrophy, thinning of retina, and changes in optic nerve diminishes depth perception and ability to see lines of demarcation
    6. Vision upward and to sides may be affected by loss of subcutaneous tissue and the recession of eyes further into sockets
  B. Client with infectious or inflammatory eye disorder
    1. Eyelid conditions
      a. Marginal blepharitis: inflammation of glands and lash follicles on eyelid margins
      b. Seborrheic, usually associated with dandruff
        1. May be red-rimmed with mucus discharge with crusting of eye lid margins
        2. Manifestations: irritated, burning, or itching eyelid margins
      c. Staphylococcal infections
        1. Hordeolum (sty): abscess occurring on external or internal margin of lid
        2. Manifestations: acute pain, redness, swelling
      d. Chalazion
        1. Granulomatous cyst of lid
        2. Chronic inflammation of meibomian gland presents as painless hard swelling
        3. May resolve within several months
    2. Conjunctivitis

      a. Most common eye disease and is usually bacterial or viral in origin
      b. Transmission: direct contact (hands, tissues, towels); allergens, chemical irritants, exposure to radiant energy
      c. Severity ranges from mild irritation with redness and tearing to conjunctival edema, hemorrhage or a severe necrotizing process
      d. Specific conditions
        1. Acute conjunctivitis
          a. Bacterial, viral, fungal in origin
          b. Bacterial
            1. "Pink eye": very contagious and caused by staphylococcus or haemophilus
            2. Gonococcal conjunctivitis: contact with contaminated genital secretions during birth process; may lead to corneal perforation
          c. Viral: include adenovirus, leading cause in adults: systemic herpes simplex infection
          d. Manifestations
            1. Eye redness and itching
            2. Scratchy or burning sensation, not usually pain
            3. Photophobia
            4. Tearing and discharge
        2. Trachoma
          a. Chronic conjunctivitis caused by *Chlamydia trachomatis*
          b. Significant preventable cause of blindness worldwide; seldom found in U.S. except infrequently found in Native American population in southwestern U.S.
          c. Contagious, transmitted by close contact
          d. Early manifestations: redness, eyelid edema; inflammation leads to corneal scarring and ulceration and loss of vision
    3. Corneal infections and inflammations
      a. Keratitis: inflammation of cornea
        1. Causes: pathogens, hypersensitivity, ischemia, tearing defects, trauma interrupted sensory innervation of cornea
        2. Types
          a. Nonulcerative: involvement of only epithelial layer of cornea;

does not destroy cornea or affect visual acuity
    b. Ulcerative: results in altered visual acuity
  b. Corneal ulcer: local necrosis of cornea
    1. Caused by infection, exposure trauma, misuse of contact lenses
    2. Infections include bacterial or viral including herpes simplex and zoster
    3. Immunosuppressed clients are at risk of developing corneal ulcers secondary to infection
    4. Pathophysiology
      a. Portion of epithelium and/or stroma are destroyed
      b. Deep ulceration may result in perforation and deeper infection or extrusion of eye contents
      c. Superficial ulceration can result in scarring and opacity of cornea
    5. Manifestations
      a. Tearing
      b. Discomfort (gritty sensation to severe eye pain)
      c. Decreased visual acuity
      d. Blepharospasm (spasm of eyelid and inability to open eye)
    6. Ulceration may be visible on direct examination
4. Uveitis (which includes inflammation of the iris)
  a. Uveitis involves the middle vascular layer of the eye
  b. Inflammation is usually limited to the eye
  c. 40% of cases are linked to systemic diseases including arthritis or autoimmune disorders
  d. Manifestations include papillary constriction, erythema around the limbus, severe eye pain, and photophobia
5. Collaborative Care
  a. Focus is to establish diagnosis and ensure prompt treatment
    1. Accurate history and physical assessment
    2. Reddened eye must be taken seriously because it could also occur with acute uveitis or acute angle-closure glaucoma
    3. Corneal ulcers are considered medical emergencies and need the attention of an ophthalmologist as soon as possible

  b. Diagnostic Tests
    1. Fluorescein stain with slit lamp examination: allows visualization of any corneal ulcerations or abrasions
    2. Conjunctival or ulcer scrapings are examined microscopically or cultured to identify causative organisms
6. Medications
  a. Infectious processes
    1. Topical anti-infectives, such as eye drops or ointments, are used, including antibiotics and antiviral therapy
    2. Severe infections, central ulcers, cellulitis may be treated with anti-infectives administered subconjunctivally or systemically by intravenous infusion
  b. Antihistamines to minimize allergic responses
  c. Corticosteroids are used for keratitis related to systemic disorders or trauma, but avoided with local infections; immunosuppressive therapy may be used to treat severe uveitis
  d. Atropine is sometimes ordered for clients with inflammation of iris
  e. Pain management is achieved with analgesics such as acetaminophen and/or codeine
7. Corneal transplant
  a. An opaque cornea cannot be restored to clarity
  b. Option is corneal transplant utilizing corneas from cadavers of uninfected adults < age 65, dying of acute trauma or illness
  c. Harvested corneas may be stored up to 4 weeks
  d. Corneal transplantation is usually an elective surgery
  e. Emergency transplantation may be required for perforation of the cornea
  f. Types of procedures
    1. Lamellar keratoplasty: superficial layer of cornea is removed and replaced with a graft; anterior chamber remains intact
    2. Penetrating keratoplasty: button or full thickness of cornea is removed and replaced with donated tissue
    3. Since the cornea is avascular, sutures are left in for a year to ensure healing

4. Most corneal transplants are done on outpatient basis; eye is patched for 24 hours post surgery and narcotic analgesia is prescribed; post-operative eye drops include corticosteroids and antibiotics

5. High success rate for transplants (> 90%); rejection usually occurs within 3 weeks of transplant

8. Complementary therapies for marginal blepharitis
   a. Careful cleansing of lids with non-irritating to eyes baby shampoo
   b. Soaking lids with warm saline compresses
   c. Frequent eye irrigations
   d. Local heat applications may be used with hordeolum or excision and drainage procedures

9. Health Promotion: Teaching prevention of infectious and inflammatory eye disorders
   a. Avoid sharing anything that touches other persons' eyes
   b. Avoid rubbing or scratching the eyes
   c. Prevention of eye trauma
   d. Correct techniques in wearing and cleaning contact lenses

10. Nursing Diagnoses
    a. Risk for Disturbed Sensory Perception: Visual
       1. Signs of corneal perforation are sudden severe eye pain and photophobia
       2. With suspected perforation, place client in supine position, close the eye and cover with dry sterile dressing and seek care of ophthalmologist or emergency department
    b. Acute Pain (cornea of eye is extremely sensitive)
    c. Risk for Injury (wearing eye shield at night post surgical procedures)

11. Home Care: Many clients are treated on outpatient basis and education of client and family is important to achieve and maintain health of eye; education includes
    a. Instillation of prescribed eye drops and ointments
    b. Avoidance of activities that increase intraocular pressure such as straining, coughing, sneezing, bending over, lifting heavy objects

C. Client with eye trauma

1. All eye injuries should be considered medical emergencies requiring immediate evaluation and intervention
2. Pathophysiology
   a. Common types include foreign bodies, abrasions, lacerations
   b. Other injuries include burns, penetrating objects, blunt force
3. Corneal abrasion
   a. Disruption of superficial epithelium of cornea
   b. Objects include contact lenses, eyelashes, small foreign bodies (dirt, dust, fingernails)
   c. Drying of eye surface and chemical irritants also are causative factors
4. Burns
   a. Chemical burns are the most common
      1. Acid substances: cause rapid eye damage, but less damage than alkali substances
      2. Alkaline substances: serious because tiny particles of chemicals remain in conjunctival sac causing progressive damage
   b. Explosions and flash burn injuries pose greatest risk for thermal burns of eye; burns also occur from ultraviolet light
   c. Manifestations
      1. Client complains of eye pain and decreased vision
      2. Eyelids are swollen; burns present on face and lids
      3. Eye appearance: reddened, edematous conjunctiva, possibly apparent sloughing; cornea is cloudy, hazy; ulcerations may be evident
5. Penetrating trauma
   a. Causes include metal flakes from drilling, gunshots, arrows
   b. Penetrating injuries may be hidden due to tissue swelling; whenever wound to eyelid, underlying eye tissue must be closely examined
   c. Manifestations include eye pain, vision impairment, bleeding, or extrusion of eye contents
6. Blunt trauma
   a. Sources include sports, motor vehicle accidents, falls, physical assaults
   b. Minor injury: lid ecchymosis (black eye) or subconjunctival hemorrhage (well-defined bright red area of erythema appears under conjunctiva);

no pain or discomfort is associated and blood is reabsorbed in 2–3 weeks
  c. Hyphema
   1. Bleeding into anterior chamber of eye; highly vascular uveal tract is disrupted by blunt force and hemorrhage fills anterior chamber
   2. Manifestations: eye pain, decreased visual acuity, seeing reddish tint; blood visible in anterior chamber
  d. Orbital blow-out fracture: ethmoid bone on orbital floor often site of fracture
   1. Orbital contents (fat, muscles, and eye itself) may be herniated through fracture into underlying maxillary sinus
   2. Manifestations: diplopia, pain with upward movement of affected eye, decreased sensation of affected cheek, sunken appearance of eye (enophthalmos)
 7. Collaborative Care
  a. With known or suspected eye trauma thorough exam
   1. Assessment of vision, evaluation of eye movement, inspection of lid and conjunctiva for laceration
    a. Strong light with magnification
    b. Use of topical anesthesia since pain and photophobia may interfere with exam
    c. Use of fluorescein staining
    d. Identification of hemorrhage, red reflex
   2. Ophthalmoscopic exam to detect injury in interior chamber
   3. Facial x-rays and CT scans to identify orbital fractures or presence of foreign bodies in the globe
  b. Treatment measures
   1. Removal of foreign bodies
    a. Use of irrigation
    b. Sterile cotton-tipped applicator, sterile needle or instrument
    c. Application of antibiotic ointment afterward
    d. Eyes with corneal abrasions and large foreign bodies are patched for 24 hours
   2. Chemical burns
    a. Require immediate flushing of affected eye with copious amounts of fluid; normal saline or water if saline is unavailable

    b. Topical anesthetic is used to relieve pain and ease the irrigation and inspection procedures for the client
    c. Irrigation continued until pH of eye is normal (7.2–7.4)
    d. Application of antibiotic ointment
   3. Penetrating wounds of eye
    a. Generally require surgical intervention by ophthalmic surgeon
    b. Immediate first aid includes gently covering eye with sterile gauze or eye pad
    c. Foreign objected embedded or sticking out should be left in and immobilized
    d. Care usually involves patching unaffected eye to decrease ocular movement
    e. Narcotic analgesics, sedation, antiemetics, intravenous antibiotics
 8. Health Promotion
  a. Teaching regarding prevention of eye injuries and first-aid measures
  b. Identification of hazardous occupations and activities
  c. Available facilities to flush eyes in areas where risks for chemical splashes exist
 9. Nursing Diagnosis: Impaired Tissue Integrity: Ocular
 10. Home Care
  a. Education for client and family regarding prescribed medications
  b. Application of eye pad or shield
  c. Avoidance of activities that increase intra-ocular pressure, activity restrictions
  d. Treatment plan including follow-up care
D. Client with refraction errors
 1. Causes
  a. Alteration in shape of eyeball
  b. Abnormal curvature of cornea
  c. Change in the lens focusing power
 2. Conditions
  a. Myopia (nearsightedness): eyeball is elongated and image focuses in front of retina instead of on it
  b. Hyperopia (farsightedness): eyeball is short and image focuses behind the retina
  c. Presbyopia: due to age, elasticity of lens decreases and leads to loss of

accommodation; client cannot see close objects without reading glasses
  d. Astigmatism: develops with abnormal curvature of cornea or eyeball and causes image to focus at multiple points on retina
3. Treatment
  a. Nonsurgical: correction of refraction errors with eyeglasses or contact lenses
  b. Surgical: reshaping cornea through series of radial incisions
    1. Involves outpatient surgery
    2. Preoperatively: limitations of correction and risks for postoperative infection and corneal scarring
    3. Postoperatively: education regarding antibiotics and analgesics, self-care instructions and follow-up care
E. Client with cataracts
  1. Cataract is opacification (clouding) of lens of eye which interferes with light transmission to retina and ability to perceive images clearly
  2. Pathophysiology
    a. 50–70% of persons > 65 have some degree of cataract formation; over 1.35 million cataract surgeries done yearly in U.S.
    b. With normal aging process, fibers and proteins change and degenerate; begins at periphery and involve central portion; entire lens may become opaque; when portion of lens involved, cataract is immature; if entire lens is opaque, cataract is mature
  3. Risk factors for senile cataracts (associated with aging)
    a. Long-term exposure to sunlight (UV-B rays)
    b. Cigarette smoking
    c. Heavy alcohol consumption
  4. Risk factors for acquired cataracts
    a. Eye trauma
    b. Diabetes mellitus especially with poorly controlled glucose levels
    c. Use of medications: corticosteroids, chlorpromazine (Thorazine), busulfan (Myleran)
  5. Manifestations
    a. Tend to occur bilaterally but development is usually not symmetric
    b. Decreased vision acuity, both close and distance vision, related to glare;

difficulty adjusting between light and dark environments
    c. Difficulty distinguishing between color hues
    d. With mature cataract, pupil appears cloudy gray or white, not black
  6. Diagnosis
    a. Based on client history and eye examination with Snellen vision test
    b. Ophthalmoscopic exam identifies location and extent of cataract
  7. Treatment
    a. Surgical removal of lens and implantation of intraocular lens
    b. Even with bilateral cataracts, only one eye is treated at a time
    c. Surgery indicated when cataract interferes with vision and ADL; or mature cataract may cause secondary condition such as glaucoma or uveitis
    d. Surgery usually done on outpatient basis under local anesthesia
    e. Intraocular lens is implanted at time of surgery and is made of plexiglas; rapidly restores binocular vision and depth perception
    f. Surgical procedures
      1. Intracapsular extraction: removal of entire lens and surrounding capsule and anterior chamber; implant of intraocular lens
      2. Extracapsular extraction: removal of lens but leaves posterior capsule intact which supports the lens implant and protects the retina; intraocular lens is implanted in posterior chamber
    g. Complications are unusual and occur with less than 1% of surgeries
  8. Nursing Care
    a. Involves client advocacy
    b. Psychologic and emotional support (fear of blindness)
    c. Teaching/learning needs
  9. Nursing Diagnoses
    a. Disturbed Sensory Perception
    b. Risk for Injury (altered vision, depth perception)
    c. Knowledge Deficit about cataracts, treatment options, post-operative care
    d. Risk for Ineffective Therapeutic Regimen Management
  10. Home Care: for client and family members

a. Instillation of eye drops, dressings, eye shield instructions

b. Post-operative limitations on reading, lifting, strenuous activity, and sleeping on operative side

c. Manifestations of postoperative complications

1. Eye pain
2. Decreased vision acuity, vision change
3. Headache, nausea
4. Itching or redness of affected eye

F. Client with glaucoma

1. Condition characterized by increased intraocular pressure of eye and a gradual loss of vision; "thief in the night," i.e., narrowing of vision field is so gradual that it is not noticed until late in disease process

2. Affects 3 million persons > age 40 in U.S. with 25% of cases undetected

3. Primary glaucoma exists without identified precipitating cause; can occur secondarily as result of infection, cataract, tumor hemorrhage, eye trauma

4. Pathophysiology

a. Aqueous humor is fluid within the eye: produced in ciliary's body, flows through pupil from posterior to anterior chamber of eye, and is absorbed through orbicular meshwork and canal of Schema (outflow); maintains a normal intraocular pressure of 15–20 mm Hg

b. Glaucoma: increase in intraocular pressure due to decrease in absorption of fluid, which usually causes ischemia of neurons within the eye and degeneration of optic nerve

c. Results in painless progressive narrowing of visual field and eventually blindness

5. Forms of primary glaucoma

a. Open-angle glaucoma (chronic simple glaucoma)

1. Accounts for 90% of cases; thought to have hereditary component, occurs more often and earlier with African Americans

2. Anterior chamber angle between iris and cornea is normal; flow through orbicular meshwork and canal so Schema is obstructed; increasing amount of aqueous humor and intraocular pressure

3. Usually affects both eyes although not symmetrically

4. Manifestations

a. Vague, and client is unaware of loss of peripheral vision

b. Mild headache, difficulty adapting to darkness, seeing halos around lights, and having difficulty focusing on near objects

b. Angle-closure glaucoma (narrow-angle or closed angle)

1. Accounts for 5–10% of glaucoma cases

2. Angle of anterior chamber narrows due to corneal flattening or bulging of iris into anterior chamber; pupil dilates and closure of angle blocks flow of aqueous humor; abrupt increase in intraocular pressure damages neurons of retina and optic nerve and leads to rapid, permanent loss of vision without prompt treatment

3. Manifestations

a. Episodes usually involve one eye; but other eye is at increased risk for angle-closure glaucoma in future

b. Episodes occur in association with factors that cause pupil dilation: darkness, emotional upset, etc.

c. Severe eye and face pain

d. Nausea and vomiting

e. Seeing colored halos around light

f. Abrupt decrease in visual acuitiy

g. Conjunctiva of affected eye is reddened and cornea clouded with corneal edema

h. Pupil may be fixed at midpoint

6. Collaborative Care

a. Cannot be prevented or cured

b. Can be controlled and vision preserved with early diagnosis and treatment

c. Routine eye exams for early detection

7. Diagnostic Tests

a. Tonometry: indirect measurement of intraocular pressure recommended for person > 60

1. Contact: eye is anesthetized, force needed to produce indentation in cornea; measured using Schiotz tonometer or Goldmann applanation tonometer

2. Noncontact: measures time required to flatten cornea with a puff of air; no anesthesia needed
   b. Fundoscopy: identifies pallor and increase in size and depth of optic cup of optic disk (changes related to glaucoma)
   c. Gonioscopy: uses goniscope to measure depth of anterior chamber; differentiates open-angle from angle-closure glaucoma
   d. Visual field testing: identifies degree of central visual field narrowing and peripheral vision loss
8. Medications: Clients with open-angle glaucoma control pressure and preserve vision indefinitely with drug therapy
   a. Cholinergics (miotics): facilitate outflow of aqueous humor; papillary constriction, e.g., pilocarpine, carbachol
   b. Adrenergics (mydriatics): used with miotics to counteract that effect; decreased production of aqueous humor, e.g., epinephrine, dipivefrin
   c. Beta-adrenergic blocking agents: decrease production of aqueous humor; may produce side effects of systemic beta-blockers, e.g., Timolol (Timoptic)
   d. Carbonic anhydrase inhibitors: decreases production of aqueous humor reducing pressure, e.g., dorzolamide (Trusopt); systemic drug: acetazolamide (Diamox)
   e. Prostaglandin analogs: increase outflow of aqueous humor, e.g., lantanoprost (Xalatan)
9. Treatment for acute angle-closure glaucoma: Diuretics (carbonic anyhydrase inhibitor or osmotic diuretics) may be administered intravenously to achieve rapid decrease in intraocular pressure prior to surgical treatment
10. Surgical Interventions
    a. Treatment for chronic open-angle glaucoma not responding to medication
       1. Laser trabeculoplasty: laser creates scars which stretch and open meshwork; outpatient procedure
       2. Trabeculectomy: surgery in which permanent fistula created to drain aqueous humor from anterior chamber of eye (requires general anesthesia)
    b. Treatment for acute angle-closure glaucoma (usually done in both eyes)
       1. Gonioplasty: scarring of iris at periphery to widen the chamber
       2. Laser iridotomy: multiple perforations of iris created with laser
       3. Peripheral iridectomy: small segment of iris removed surgically
11. Health Promotion: Encourage persons over age 40 to have eye examinations every 2–4 years including tonometry screening
12. Nursing Diagnoses
    a. Risk for Disturbed Sensory Perception: Visual; orient clients to their environment adequately
    b. Risk for Injury
    c. Anxiety
13. Home Care
    a. Education of client regarding need for lifetime therapy and continuing of physician care
    b. Avoiding all medications prescribed or over the counter unless approved by physician cognizant of client's glaucoma diagnosis
G. Client with a retinal detachment
   1. Disruption of retinal layer of eye by trauma or disease that interferes with light perception and image transmission and potentially results in blindness; separation of retina from choroid
   2. Pathophysiology
      a. Shrinkage of vitreous humor may pull retina away from choroids
      b. Break or tear in retina allows fluid from vitreous cavity to enter defect
      c. Detachment rapidly enlarges, increasing size of vision loss without prompt treatment
      d. Medical emergency
   3. Risk Factors
      a. Age
      b. Myopia
      c. Aphakia (absence of lens)
   4. Manifestations
      a. Seeing floaters or spots, lines, flashes of light in visual field
      b. Sensation of curtain drawn across vision
      c. No pain, eye appears normal to visual inspection

5. Collaborative Care
   a. Diagnosis is established by clinical manifestations and ophthalmoscopic exam of ocular fundus
   b. Early intervention is vital to prevent detached part from becoming necrotic
   c. If ophthalmologist is not readily available, the client's head is positioned so that gravity pulls detached portion in closer contact with choroids
6. Interventions
   a. Purpose: resume contact of retina and choroids to reestablish blood and nutrient supply to retina
   b. Creation of adhesion in area by use of cryotherapy or laser photocoagulation
   c. Scleral buckling: surgical procedure involving folding the sclera to regain contact between choroids and retina; uses implant or encircling strap on sclera or air bubble to hold the retina into contact with choroids
   d. If a tear in the retina excises, there is more involved surgery to manipulate the detached retina into place
7. Nursing Care
   a. Focus is on early identification and treatment to preserve sight
   b. Treatment is often on outpatient basis in ophthalmologist's office
8. Nursing Diagnoses
   a. Altered Tissue Perfusion: Retinal
   b. Anxiety
9. Home Care: Education of client and family
   a. Limiting position changes of head
   b. Following activity restrictions (avoiding increased intraocular pressure)
   c. Use of eye shield
   d. Promptly seek immediate treatment, if manifestations reoccur
   e. Follow-up care with ophthalmologist
H. Client with macular degeneration
   1. Macula, area of retina that receives light from center of visual field, and has highest visual acuity, gradually fails causing decreased vision progressing to blindness
   2. Leading cause of blindness in persons > age 65, affecting males and females equally
   3. Risk Factors
      a. Aging
      b. Smoking
      c. Hypertension
      d. Hypercholesterolemia
4. Pathophysiology
   a. Gradual failure of outer pigmented layer of retina (adjacent to choroid) resulting in loss of photoreceptor cells and damage to outer layer
   b. Serous fluid may enter subretinal space leading to retinal detachment
   c. Usually occurs in both eyes
5. Forms
   a. Atrophic degeneration (dry): Gradual and progressive vision loss
   b. Exudative degeneration (wet)
      1. Vision loss more rapid and severe
      2. Proliferation of new blood vessels (neovascularization) that form in subretinal space and leak fluid and blood into retina
      3. Accounts for 90% of cases of persons who are legally blind
6. Manifestations
   a. Central vision becomes blurred and distorted: straight lines appear wavy
   b. Peripheral vision remains intact
   c. Client experiences difficulty in activities requiring close central vision such as reading
7. Treatment
   a. No effective treatment; laser photocoagulation is used to slow exudative form and seal leaking capillaries
   b. Teach clients and family to adapt to gradual decline in vision by using visual aids (large print books, improved lighting)
8. Nursing Care: educate and refer clients with new and rapid onset of manifestations of macular degeneration for ophthalmologic evaluation
I. Client with retinitis pigmentosa
   1. Hereditary degenerative disease
      a. Characterized by atrophy of retina and loss of retinal function
      b. Progresses from peripheral to central vision
      c. May be associated with other genetic defects
   2. Pathophysiology
      a. Defect causes production of unstable form of rhodopsin, the receptor protein of rod cells in retina
      b. Progressive degeneration of rod cells starting at periphery of retina and

eventually including central vision as well

3. Manifestations
   a. Difficulty with night vision, often starting in childhood
   b. Slow loss of visual fields, photophobia, disrupted color vision
   c. Progression to tunnel vision and blindness gradually
4. Nursing Care
   a. Education about low-vision aids, planning for total loss of sight
   b. Educate client regarding referral for genetic counseling

J. Client with diabetic retinopathy
   1. Vascular disorder affecting retinal capillaries which become sclerotic in persons with diabetes; 85% of diabetics have some degree of retinopathy, not all resulting in blindness
   2. Affects both Type 1 and 2 diabetics and is reflective of the length or time client has been diabetic and their degree of glucose control
   3. Leading cause of new blindness of persons aged 20–74 in U.S.
   4. Major forms
      a. Nonproliferative (background retinopathy)
         1. Initial type in which venous capillaries develop microaneurysms, that leak and cause retinal edema, or rupture and cause small hemorrhages
         2. Ophthalmoscopic exam shows yellow exudates, cotton-wool patches (retinal ischemia) and red-dot hemorrhages
         3. Manifestations
            a. Light glare if peripheral retinal involved
            b. Macula involvement may cause vision loss
      b. Proliferative
         1. Progresses to large areas of retinal ischemia and formation of new blood vessels spreading over inner surface of retina and into the vitreous body
         2. Vessels are fragile and rupture easily adding to retinal edema and hemorrhage into vitreous body
         3. Vessels become fibrous and increase risk of retinal detachment

5. Nursing Care
   a. Education of client on the importance of achieving good control
   b. Education of client on the need to have yearly eye exams by ophthalmologist
6. Treatment
   a. Slows progression of disorder, but is not curative
   b. Both forms of retinopathy treated with laser photocoagulation which seals leaking microaneurysms and destroys proliferating blood vessels
   c. Vitrectomy may be done to treat vitreous hemorrhage
   d. Retinal detachments are treated
7. Health Promotion: Education of diabetic clients
   a. Maintain diabetes under good control
   b. Have regular eye exams by ophthalmologist
   c. Report promptly any new visual manifestations
      1. Blurred vision
      2. Blackspots (floaters)
      3. Seeing cobwebs or flashing lights in visual field
      4. Sudden loss of vision in one or both eyes

K. Client with HIV infection
   1. > 50% infected with HIV develop infectious and noninfectious ocular condition generally as a late manifestation of disease
   2. Conditions include
      a. HIV retinopathy: manifests as cotton-wool spots around optic nerve; is most common noninfectious eye lesion in clients with AIDS
      b. Neoplasms: Kaposi's sarcoma affects surface of eye or eyelids with lesions with varying colors (red, brown, purple) in various sizes, shapes, and locations; ptosis
      c. Cytomegalovirus (CMV) retinitis
         1. Opportunistic eye infection in which virus invades retinal directly producing exudates, hemorrhages, and necrosis
         2. Begins with one eye and progresses to other and may lead to blindness
      d. Corneal ulcerations occur secondary to opportunistic bacterial, fungal, protozoan, or viral infections
   3. Treatments
      a. Treatments directed toward pathogen

b. Medications used to treat HIV infection, retroviral medications
1. Zidovudine (AZT)
2. Didanosine (DDI)
3. Ganciclovir (Cytovene)
4. Foscarnet sodium (Foscavir)
L. Client with enucleation
1. Surgical removal of eye is sometimes necessary due to trauma, infection, glaucoma, intractable pain, or malignancy
2. Surgery done under local or general anesthesia; globe removed and conjunctiva and eye muscles are sutured to an implant to maintain shape of orbit; temporary prosthesis (conformer) is fitted within a week
3. Permanent prosthesis is fitted one–two months post surgery and is designed to closely resemble the client's other eye
4. Nursing care involves monitoring for complications of hemorrhage and infection, teaching, and psychological support
M. Client who is blind
1. Legal definition: visual acuity no greater than 20/200 in the better eye with optimal correction or visual field less than 20 degrees (normal = 180 degrees)
2. In practical terms, persons with visual deficits that require assistive devices or aid from other people for normal ADL are considered blind
3. More than 500,000 Americans are considered legally blind
4. Most common causes include
a. Glaucoma
b. Cataracts
c. Retinal disorders including diabetic retinopathy, macular degeneration, and congenital disorders
5. Nursing Care
a. Focus is on helping blind client cope with loss and deal effectively with societal attitudes that encourage feelings of inferiority, helplessness, and inadequacy
b. Foster independence in the hospitalized client by
1. Adequate orientation to environment physically and verbally
2. Verbalize about activities occurring around the client
3. Provide additional sensory stimuli (radio, television)
4. Assist with meals and describe position of foods according to face of clock
5. Assist with ambulation by allowing client to hold onto nurse's arm; describe environment
6. Refer to available community resources for mobility training, self-care activities, education, rehabilitation as the client needs
6. Nursing Diagnoses
a. Disturbed Sensory Perception: Visual
b. Self-care Deficit
c. Grieving
d. Risk for Situational Low Self-esteem
III. Ear Disorders
A. Client with external otitis
1. Common inflammation of ear canal, "swimmer's ear"
2. Occurs with persons spending significant time in water, also persons wearing hearing aids or ear plugs which hold moisture in ear canal
3. Causative organism is commonly *Pseudomonas aeruginosa,* may be fungal or due to mechanical trauma or local hypersensitivity
4. Manifestations
a. Feeling of fullness in ear
b. Ear pain increased by manipulation of the auricle
c. Odorless watery or purulent drainage
d. Ear canal appears inflamed and edematous
5. Treatment
a. Thorough cleansing of ear canal
b. Treatment of infection, if present, with antibiotics
c. Medication for pain and itching control (steroids)
d. Teaching regarding prevention: do not clean ear canal with any implement; wash external ear with soap and water
6. Cortisporin Otic
a. Combination of antibiotic and corticosteroid that is often prescribed
b. Client needs instruction regarding proper instillation of ear drops
7. Complication includes cellulites so client should seek medical care if pain, swelling, or redness of surrounding tissue occurs with fever or malaise
B. Client with impacted cerumen and foreign bodies
1. Increased incidence with aging

a. Less cerumen produced and prone to becoming hard and dry

b. Accumulation aggravated by attempts to remove it with items such as cotton-tipped applicators

2. As ear canal becomes occluded with cerumen and foreign bodies, client experiences conductive hearing loss

3. Manifestations
   a. Loss of hearing
   b. Sensation of fullness
   c. Coughing
   d. Possible tinnitus

4. Treatment focuses on clearing canal
   a. Irrigation of canal, if there is no evidence of tympanic membrane perforation
   b. Physical removal may be used to remove impacted wax, objects and insects after they are killed

5. Education regarding prevention: clients prone to cerumen impaction may benefit from commercial products to soften wax and irrigation to remove it

C. Client with otitis media
1. Inflammation or infection of middle ear associated with URI and auditory (Eustachian) tube dysfunction which occurs with allergies

2. Primary forms
   a. Serous ototis media
      1. Auditory is obstructed for prolonged time
         a. Impaired equalization of air pressure in middle ear
         b. Negative pressure results causing serous fluid to move from capillaries into middle ear
      2. Barotitis media
         a. Middle ear cannot adjust to rapid changes in barometric pressure (as with air travel or underwater diving)
         b. Acute pain, hemorrhage into middle ear, rupture of tympanic membrane
      3. Manifestations
         a. Decreased hearing in affected ear
         b. Snapping or popping in ear
         c. Tympanic membrane demonstrates decreased mobility, and may appear retracted or bulging
   b. Acute or suppurative otitis media

1. Typically follows URI; serous fluid is ideal environment for bacteria

2. Causative organisms in adult infections include *Streptococcus pneumoniae* and *pyogenes,* and *Haemophilus influenzae*; leads to pus formation increasing pressure in middle ear causing
   a. Rupture of tympanic membrane
   b. More serious complications include mastoiditis, brain abscess, bacterial meningitis

3. Manifestations
   a. Mild to severe pain in affected ear
   b. Temperature elevation
   c. Diminished hearing, dizziness, vertigo, tinnitus
   d. Otoscopic exam: tympanic membrane appears red, inflamed, or dull and bulging; spontaneous rupture of membrane releases purulent discharge

4. Myringotomy: incision into tympanic membrane may be performed to relieve pressure

3. Collaborative Care
   a. Diagnosis is based on client's history and physical examination
   b. Otoscopic exam: tympanic membrane moves poorly with air instillation or Valsalva maneuver

4. Diagnostic Tests
   a. Impedance audiometry (tympanometry); tone is delivered to tympanic membrane and compliance of tympanic membrane and middle ear system is measured
   b. CBC reveals elevation of WBC's
   c. Culture of drainage from ruptured tympanic membrane or with myringotomy reveals causative organism

5. Medication
   a. Auditory tube dysfunction and serous otitis media treated with
      1. Decongestants (reduce mucosal edema of tube)
      2. Autoinflation of middle ear: client performs Valsalva maneuver or forcibly exhaling against closed nostrils
   b. Acute otitis media

1. Antibiotic therapy: Amoxicillin, trimethoprimsulfamethoxazole, cefaclor, azithromycin for 5–10 days
2. Symptomatic relief: Analgesics, antipyretics, local heat application

6. Surgery
   a. Myringotomy or tympanocentesis to relieve excess pressure in middle ear and prevent spontaneous rupture of eardrum; obtain culture specimen
   b. Insertion of ventilation (tympanostomy) tubes: small tubes that provide ventilation and drainage of middle ear when healing; client must avoid getting water into ear canal

7. Health Promotion: Education of clients to seek medical care for prolonged severe ear pain and completing treatment to avoid complications

8. Home Care
   a. Education of client in pain relief, use of analgesia, local heat application
   b. Completion of prescribed antibiotics and completing follow-up care
   c. If client has had ventilation tubes inserted, avoid getting water into ears

D. Client with acute mastoiditis
   1. Infection of acute otitis media always extends to mastoid air cells (mastoid sinuses) in the portion of temporal skull bone
   2. Effective treatment of otitis media will effectively treat the mastoid air cells; with ineffective or no treatment, acute mastoiditis occurs
   3. Pathophysiology
      a. Complication of otitis media; rare due to advent of antibiotic therapy
      b. With acute mastoiditis, portions of mastoid process are eroded
      c. With chronic infection, abscess may form which increases risk of meningitis
   4. Manifestations: occur 2–3 weeks after an episode of acute otitis media
      a. Recurrent earache: persistent and throbbing pain
      b. Hearing loss on affected side
      c. Tenderness, redness, and inflammation over mastoid process behind the ear
      d. Fever, tinnitus, headache; profuse drainage from ear may be present
   5. Diagnostic Tests: Clinical manifestations and changes noted on radiologic examination

6. Medications: Aggressive antibiotic therapy, continued at least 14 days
7. Surgical Treatment
   a. Mastoidectomy: removal of the infected mastoid air cells necessitated by infections that do not respond to antibiotics
   b. Radical mastoidectomy with tympanoplasty (surgical reconstruction of middle ear): severe; done to remove infection and restore or preserve hearing
   c. Postoperative care
      1. Monitor dressing for infection and administer antibiotics
      2. Assist client to communicate, if hearing impaired
      3. Assist client with ambulation since dizziness and vertigo may occur post surgery

8. Home Care: Education of client and family to
   a. Complete antibiotics and continue for follow-up care
   b. Dressing changes
   c. Referral to community agencies to assist with dealing with hearing loss

E. Client with chronic otitis media
   1. Involves permanent perforation of tympanic membrane accompanied by changes in mucosal and bony structure of middle ear
   2. Marginal perforations can lead to migration of squamous epithelium from ear canal to middle ear
   3. Cholesteatoma (cyst or mass filled with epithelial cell debris)
      a. Forms and destroys adjacent bone leading to conductive hearing loss
      b. Tumor is benign and slow growing but will take over middle ear and can erode into inner ear causing profound hearing loss
      c. Removing tumor may require radical mastoidectomy and possible hearing loss
   4. Health Promotion: Otitis media and perforated tympanic membrane needs effective treatment to avoid complications associated with chronic condition

F. Client with otosclerosis
   1. Common cause of conductive hearing loss
   2. Abnormal bone formation in osseous labyrinth of temporal bone causes footplate of stapes to become fixed or immobile in oval window

3. Hereditary disorder with an autosomal dominant pattern of inheritance, occurring commonly in Caucasians and females; begins in adolescence and is accelerated by pregnancy
4. Manifestations
   a. Both ears are affected but rate of hearing loss is asymmetric; bone conduction of sound is retained
   b. Tympanic membrane appears reddish or pinkish-orange due to increased vascularity
5. Treatment
   a. Conservative
      1. Hearing aid
      2. Learning to deal with hearing impairment
      3. Sodium fluoride may slow bone resorption and overgrowth
   b. Surgical
      1. Stapedectomy removing diseased stapes
      2. Insertion of prosthesis to regain ability to hear
G. Client with inner ear (labyrinth) disorder
   1. Pathophysiology: Inflammatory process or excess endolymph in semicircular canals cause alterations in balance and permanent hearing loss
   2. Specific conditions
      a. Labyrinthitis: inflammation of inner ear
         1. May be due to bacteria or viruses
         2. Manifestations
            a. Vertigo: severe sense of motion, often accompanied by nausea and vomiting
            b. Sensorineural hearing deficit
            c. Nystagmus: involuntary rhythmic eye movements, usually horizontal
      b. Ménière's Disease (endolymphatic hydrops)
         1. Chronic disorder characterized by recurrent attacks of vertigo, tinnitis, and progressive unilateral hearing loss
         2. Affects males and females equally, ages 35–60; familial history for increased risk
         3. Due to over accumulation of endolymph in membranous labyrinth of inner ear
         4. Acute or gradual onset of manifestations lasting minutes to

hours; episodes are linked to increased sodium intake, stress, allergies, premenstrual fluid retention
         5. Progressive hearing loss and severe vertigo causing nausea, vomiting, and immobility
      c. Vertigo
         1. Disorder of equilibrium; sensation of whirling, rotation
            a. Subjective: client in motion, environment stable
            b. Objective: environment moving; client stable
         2. Results in falls, difficulty walking; attacks are accompanied by nausea, vomiting, nystagmus, and autonomic symptoms: pallor, sweating, hypotension, salivation
   3. Collaborative Care/Diagnostic Testing: To differentiate diagnosis
      a. Electronystagmography: evaluation of vestibular-ocular reflex by identifying nystagmus in response to caloric test (water instilled in ear canal)
      b. Rinne and Weber test: decreased air and bone conduction on affected side with sensorineural hearing loss
      c. X-rays and CT scans: evaluation of internal auditory canal
      d. Glycerol test: oral glycerol administered which decreases fluid pressure in inner ear: temporary hearing improvement with Ménière's disease
   4. Treatment
      a. Hospitalization may be necessary to manage vertigo and effects
      b. Medications to depress parasympathetic nervous system: Atropine, diazepam (Valium), lorazepam (Ativan)
      c. Droperidol (Inapsine) for sedation and antiemetic effect
      d. Antivertigo/antiemetic medications: meclizine (Antivert), prochlorperazine (Compazine), hydroxyzine hydrochloride (Vistaril)
      e. Intravenous fluids to maintain fluid and electrolyte imbalance
      f. Darkened room to decrease sensory stimuli and minimize movement
      g. Antibiotics are prescribed if labyrinthitis is bacterial in origin
      h. Prevention of further attacks in Ménière's disease

1. Low sodium diet
2. Oral diuretics
3. Furstenberg diet: salt-free neutral ash diet if increased sodium restrictions are needed
4. Avoid smoking, alcohol, caffeine

5. Surgical Interventions: Utilized if medical treatments are ineffective in controlling vertigo
   a. Surgical endolymphatic decompression: shunt excess endolymph away from labyrinths
   b. Vestibular neurectomy: portion of cranial nerve VIII is destroyed; may involve increased hearing loss
   c. Labryinthectomy: removal of labyrinth destroying cochlear function (hearing loss was already severe and is totally destroyed in affected ear)

6. Nursing Diagnoses
   a. Risk for Trauma: assist client to develop strategies to deal with vertigo
   b. Sleep Pattern Disturbance

7. Home Care: Teaching safety, including identifying hazards in home environment

H. Client with an acoustic neuroma (schwannoma)
1. Benign tumor of cranial nerve VIII
   a. Occurs adults aged 40–50
   b. Occurs in internal auditory meatus
   c. If continues to grow, destroys labyrinth and may impinge on parts of the brain
   d. May involve facial and trigeminal nerves as well

2. Early Manifestations
   a. Tinnitus
   b. Unilateral hearing loss
   c. Nystagmus

3. Progresses to dizziness or vertigo; other neurologic involvement depending on location of the tumor

4. Treatment
   a. Surgical excision; efforts are made to preserve the function of the cranial nerve(s) involved
   b. Large tumors may involve craniotomy, and facial nerve paralysis may result from the surgery

I. Client with a hearing loss
1. 10 million persons in U.S. are hearing impaired
2. Manifestations displayed by persons with hearing losses
   a. Increases voice volume
   b. Positions head with better ear toward speaker

   c. Difficulty hearing and communicating effectively

3. Types of hearing losses
   a. Conductive hearing loss
      1. Disruption of sound from external auditory meatus to inner ear; most common cause: obstruction of ear canal
      2. Equal hearing loss at all sound frequencies
      3. Benefits from amplification by a hearing aid
   b. Sensorineural hearing loss
      1. Disorders affecting inner ear, auditory nerve, or auditory pathways of brain; sound waves are transmitted to ear effectively but change within the inner ear; decrease or distort ability to receive and interpret stimuli
      2. Significant cause is damage to hair cells of organ of Corti related to noise exposure; causes include
         a. Exposure to high level of noise (rock concert)
         b. Ototoxic medications such as aspirin, furosemide (Lasix), aminoglycoside antibiotics, anti-malarial drugs, and some chemotherapy
         c. Prenatal exposure to rubella, viral infections, meningitis, trauma, Ménière's disease, aging
      3. Affect perception of high-frequency tones more than low tones; interferes with speech discrimination especially in noisy environments
      4. Hearing aids are generally not very useful
   c. Presbycusis
      1. Aging causes hair cells of cochlea to degenerate: progressive sensorineural hearing loss; higher pitched tones and conversational speech lost initially
      2. Hearing aids and other amplification devices are useful
      3. Hearing impaired older adults may appear: depressed, confused, inattentive, tense, negative, withdrawing from social interaction
   d. Tinnitus
      1. Perception of sound or noise in ears without stimulus from environment;

sound may be steady, intermittent, pulsatile; clients often describe as a buzz, roar, or ringing
2. Usually associated with conductive or sensorineural hearing loss; mechanism is not well understood
3. Sign of toxicity with aspirin, quinine, or quinidine therapy
4. Most is chronic and without pathologic importance
5. May prove to be significant stressor and interfere with ADL and sleep
4. Collaborative Care
   a. Prevention is best treatment for hearing loss
   b. Education regarding effects of noise exposure and ototoxic effects of medications
5. Diagnostic Tests: Hearing evaluation
   a. Rinne and Weber tests
   b. Audiometry: identifies type and pattern of hearing loss
   c. Speech audiometry: identifies intensity at which speech is recognized and interpreted
   d. Tympanometry: indirect measurement of compliance and impedance of middle ear to sound transmission
6. Treatments
   a. Amplification
      1. Devices do not treat hearing loss, but amplify sound presented to hearing apparatus of ear; less helpful with distorted hearing since distortion is amplified
      2. Less than one fifth of persons with hearing deficits have hearing aids
      3. Different styles of hearing aids may be more helpful to clients with particular problems
   b. Surgery
      1. Conductive hearing losses may be helped by reconstructive surgeries involving middle ear

2. Sensorineural hearing loss, only hope is cochlear implant to restore sound perception
3. Two types of cochlear implants available
   a. Electrode implanted in cochlea to stimulate remaining, intact, excitable auditory neurons; small processor carried outside body receives sound through microphone and sends signal to transmitter mounted behind ear; transmitter sends signal to receiver implanted under skin which transmits it to electrode implanted in cochlea
   b. If no auditory nerve fibers are available, external microphone-transmitter sends signal to implanted receiver which transits stimulus via electode implanted in brain stem over cochlear nucleus
4. Client is able to recognize warning sounds and can receive perception of sound but not normal hearing; client needs to learn to interpret perceived sounds as words
7. Health Promotion
   a. Prevention of hearing loss through education
   b. Environmental noise control and use of ear protection, especially in the work place
8. Nursing Diagnoses
   a. Disturbed Sensory Perception: Auditory
   b. Impaired Verbal Communication
   c. Social Isolation
9. Home Care: Appropriate referrals for clients with permanent hearing loss to manage deficits and develop coping strategies; community and national resources

FOCUSED STUDY TIPS

- Identify resources available for blind clients and for deaf clients in your community. Share what you learn with classmates.
- Ask to be involved in client care involving a deaf interpreter. Observe and evaluate the effectiveness of communication.
- Identify a TDD (telecommunication device for the deaf) in your clinical setting. Become familiar with its use.

CASE STUDY

What information would help a client understand the different procedures available for the surgical treatment of a cataract?

CARE PLAN CRITICAL THINKING ACTIVITY

The best treatment for hearing loss is prevention. Describe how the nurse teaches clients to prevent hearing loss.

NCLEX TEST QUESTIONS

1. A client is diagnosed with conductive hearing loss and asks how this occurred. The nurse should respond by stating that conductive hearing loss
   a. has an unknown etiology.
   b. occurs as a result of damage to the hair cells of the inner ear.
   c. usually results from chronic exposure to loud noise.
   d. occurs as a result of damage to the ear structures.

2. A 70-year-old client comes to the outpatient clinic complaining of increasing difficulty with close work such as knitting. She indicates she does not have difficulty seeing objects on either side but does state that straight lines appear distorted or wavy. The nurse suspects which of the following disorders that is consistent with the client's reported symptoms?
   a. cataracts
   b. macular degeneration
   c. glaucoma
   d. subconjunctival hemorrhage

3. After surgery for cataract removal, the nurse teaches the client about home care. Which of the following activities would be contraindicated?
   a. walking down the hall unassisted
   b. lying in bed on the nonoperative side
   c. bending over to pick up newspapers from the floor
   d. performing simple isometric exercises

4. The initial nursing intervention for a client in the emergency department who suffered a chemical burn to the eyes is to
   a. administer analgesics as prescribed.
   b. evaluate vision with and without prescription eyeglasses.
   c. administer antibiotics as prescribed.
   d. irrigate the eyes with normal saline or water.

5. When applying drops to the ear of an adult client, the nurse should carefully straighten the ear canal by pulling the pinna
   a. downward and outward.
   b. upward and outward.
   c. downward and back.
   d. upward and back.

6. A client with a right-side retinal detachment is admitted to the hospital and scheduled for surgery later that day. The most important nursing intervention in the preoperative hours is to position the client
   a. with the head of his bed flat.
   b. on his left side.
   c. so that the area of the detachment is dependent.
   d. with the head of his bed elevated.

7. A 72-year-old client diagnosed with Ménière's disease has been admitted to the medical–surgical unit. He asks the nurse if he can get up and go to the bathroom any time he needs to. The most appropriate response is
   a. "Yes, whenever you wish, you may go."
   b. "No, you are on strict bed rest."
   c. "Please ring for assistance when you wish to get out of bed."
   d. "We will have to check with the physician."

8. The priority nursing measure for the client with a penetrating eye injury from a visible foreign body is to
   a. patch both eyes.
   b. immobilize the foreign body and cover the eye.
   c. irrigate the eye with copious amounts of water.
   d. administer carbonic anhydrase inhibitors as prescribed.

9. In order to improve communication with the client having a diagnosis of sensorineural hearing loss, the nurse should instruct the client's family to
   a. use one-word answers.
   b. exaggerate pronunciation of words.
   c. speak loudly to get the client's attention.
   d. face the client directly when speaking

10. The nurse explaining the use of medication therapy for a client diagnosed with glaucoma would state that miotics are useful because they work by
    a. dilating the pupil.
    b. constricting intraocular vessels.
    c. constricting the pupil.
    d. relaxing the ciliary muscles.

CHAPTER 46

ASSESSING CLIENTS WITH REPRODUCTIVE DISORDERS

LEARNING OUTCOMES

After completing this chapter, you will be able to:

- Review the anatomy and physiology of the male and female reproductive systems.
- Explain the functions of the male and female sex hormones.
- Identify specific topics for consideration during a health history interview of the client with health problems involving reproductive function.
- Describe techniques for physical assessment of male and female reproductive function.
- Identify abnormal findings that may indicate impairment in reproductive function in men and women.

KEY TOPICS

- Review of anatomy and physiology of the male reproductive system
- Review of anatomy and physiology of the female reproductive system
- Assessing male reproductive functioning
- Assessing female reproductive functioning

LECTURE OUTLINE

I. Functions of Reproductive Systems
   A. Enabling sexual pleasure
   B. Reproduction
   C. Production of hormone important in biological development and sexual behavior
II. Review of Anatomy and Physiology of Male Reproductive System
   A. Testes

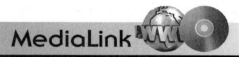

MediaLink

www.prenhall.com/lemone

Additional resources for this chapter can be found on the Student CD-ROM accompanying this textbook, and on the Companion Website at www.prenhall.com/lemone. Click on Chapter 46 to select the activities for this chapter.

CD-ROM
- Audio Glossary
- NCLEX Review

Animations
- Female Reproductive System
- Male Reproductive System

Companion Website
- More NCLEX Review
- Functional Health Pattern Assessment
- Case Study
   Irregular Menstrual Cycle

1. Develop in abdominal cavity of fetus and descend through inguinal canal into scrotum
2. Produce sperm and testosterone
   a. Seminiferous tubules: sperm production
   b. Leydig's cells (interstitial cells): testosterone production

3. Epididymis: final area for storage and maturation of sperm
4. Seminal vesicles at base of bladder produce 60% of volume of seminal fluid; remainder is secretions from epididymis, prostate gland and Cowper's glands
5. Seminal fluid nourishes sperm, provides bulk, and increases alkalinity, which is necessary for sperm to be mobile and able to fertilize the ova
6. Sperm and seminal fluid make up semen
7. During ejaculation, seminal fluid mixes with sperm at ejaculatory duct and enters urethra for expulsion; usual amount of semen is 2–4 ml containing 100–400 million sperm

B. Scrotum
1. Hangs at the base of penis and regulates the temperature of testes
2. Optimum temperature for sperm production is 2–3 degrees below body temperature
   a. When testicular temperature is too low, scrotum contracts to bring testes up against the body
   b. When testicular temperature is too high, scrotum relaxes to allow testes to move away from the body

C. Prostate Gland
1. Encircles the urethra just below the urinary bladder, surrounded by smooth muscle
2. Secretions make up a third of volume of semen and enter urethra during ejaculation

D. Penis
1. Genital organ that encloses urethra
2. Composed of shaft and glans (tip), which is covered by foreskin (prepuce) in uncircumcised males
3. Shaft contains 3 columns of erectile tissue: 2 lateral columns called corpora cavernosa and central mass called corpus spongiosum
4. Erection occurs when penile masses are filled with blood; in response to reflex that triggers parasympathetic nervous system to stimulate arteriolar dilation
5. Erection reflex: initiated by touch, pressure, sights, sounds, smells or thoughts of a sexual encounter
6. Post ejaculation, arterioles constrict and penis becomes flaccid

E. Spermatogenesis
1. Process of sperm generation in seminiferous tubules beginning with

puberty and continuing throughout a male's life span; several million sperm are produced daily
2. Spermatogenesis takes 64–72 days

F. Male sex hormones (androgens)
1. Most androgens are produced in testes; small amount produced by adrenal cortex
2. Testosterone is primary androgen
   a. Essential for development and maintenance of sexual organs and secondary sex characteristics; spermatogenesis
   b. Promotes metabolism, growth of muscles and bones, libido

III. Assessment of Male Reproductive Function
A. Health Assessment Strategies
1. Consideration of psychological, social, and cultural factors that affect sexual activity and sexuality
2. Strategies to make interview less threatening include
   a. Begin with generalized questions and progress to specific questions
   b. Ask questions in a way that gives client permission to report behaviors and manifestations

B. Health assessment interview to collect subjective data
1. Often part of assessment of urinary system
2. If problem is identified, collect information regarding
   a. Onset
   b. Characteristics
   c. Duration
   d. Frequency
   e. Precipitating or relieving factors
   f. Treat and/or self-care
   g. Outcome
3. Determine whether client has significant history that affects sexual functioning, i.e., impotence
   a. Chronic illness: diabetes, chronic renal failure, cardiovascular disease, multiple sclerosis, spinal cord tumors or trauma, thyroid disease
   b. Medication use: antihypertensives, antidepressants, antispasmodics, tranquilizers, sedatives, histamine$_2$ receptor antagonists
4. Determine whether mother was treated during pregnancy with client (1940–50's) with diethylstilbesterol (DES); client may have congenital deformities of urinary tract/decreased semen levels

5. History of mumps as child (possible sterility)
6. Determine risk for testicular cancer
   a. History of undescended testicle
   b. Inguinal hernia
   c. Testicular swelling with mumps
   d. Maternal use of DES or oral contraceptives
   e. Family history of testicular cancer
7. Determine life-style and social history
   a. Use of alcohol, cigarettes, street drugs
   b. Risk for sexually transmitted disease including HIV (number of sexual partners, use of condoms)
   c. Satisfaction with sexual function, sexual problems
C. Physical assessment with abnormal findings to collect objective data
   1. Breast and lymph node assessment
      a. Gynecomastia: smooth firm mobile tender area of breast tissue behind areola: requires investigation as to cause
      b. Hard, irregular nodule in nipple area could indicate carcinoma
      c. Enlargement of axillary lymph nodes could occur with infections of arm or hand, or cancer
      d. Enlargement of supraclavicular nodes could indicate metastasis
   2. External assessment
      a. Bulges in inguinal or femoral area with client bearing down or coughing suggests a hernia
      b. Inspection of penis
         1. In uncircumsized male
            a. Inability to retract foreskin: phimosis
            b. Narrow or inflamed foreskin causing painful swelling of glans found with paraphimosis retraction of foreskin
            c. Inflammation of glans may indicate bacterial or fungal infection
            d. Presence of ulcers, vesicles, warts could suggest sexually transmitted infection
            e. Nodules or sores in uncircumcised male could indicate cancer
         2. Urinary meatus: erythema or discharge indicates inflammatory disease

3. Skin around base of penis: excoriation or inflammation suggestive of lice or scabies
4. Induration with tenderness along ventral surface of shaft suggests urethral stricture with inflammation
5. Scrotum
   a. Unilateral or bilateral poorly developed scrotum: suggests cryptorchidism (failure of one or both testicles to descend into scrotum)
   b. Swelling occurs with indirect inguinal hernia, hydrocele (fluid in scrotum), scrotal edema
6. Testes and epididymis
   a. Tender, painful scrotal swelling occurs with acute epididymitis, acute orchitis, torsion of spermatic cord, strangulated hernia
   b. Painless nodule in testis associated with testicular cancer
3. Prostate
   a. Assessment by digital rectal examination
   b. Enlargement > 1 cm protrusion into rectum indicates benign prostatic hypertrophy
   c. Enlargement with asymmetry and tenderness indicates prostatitis
   d. Hard irregular nodule occurs with carcinoma
IV. Review of Anatomy and Physiology of Female Reproductive System
   A. Vagina
      1. Fibromuscular tube located posterior to bladder and urethra and anterior to rectum; upper end contains uterine cervix; walls of vagina form folds called rugae which is composed of mucus-secreting cells
      2. Serves as route for excretion of secretions including menstrual fluid and is organ of sexual response; birth canal
      3. pH of vagina is 3.8–4.2 normally and moist; pH is bacteriostatic, maintained by estrogen and normal vaginal flora
         a. Mucosal cells stimulated by estrogen to thicken and have increased glycogen content
         b. Normal bacterial flora, Doderlein's bacilli, lactobacilli: ferment glycogen to lactic acid

B. Uterus
1. Pear-shaped hollow organ located between bladder and rectum
2. Parts of uterus
   a. Fundus
   b. Body
   c. Cervix
      1. Pathway between uterus and vagina, projects into vagina
      2. Softens during pregnancy in response to hormones
      3. Protected by mucus
      4. Internal os: uterine opening of cervix
      5. External os: vaginal opening
3. Supported in abdominal cavity by broad ligaments, round ligaments, uterosacral ligaments, and transverse cervical ligaments
4. Uterus receives the fertilized ovum and is site for growth and development of fetus
5. Uterine wall has 3 layers
   a. Perimetrium: outer serous layer that merges with peritoneum
   b. Myometrium: middle layers of muscle fibers that run in various directions allowing for contraction
   c. Endometrium: uterus lining; outermost layer is shed during menstruation
C. Fallopian Tubes
1. Thin cylindrical structures attached to uterus on one end and supported by broad ligaments
2. Lateral ends are open and have projections called fimbriae that drape over each ovary
3. Fimbriae pick up ovum after it is discharged during ovulation
4. Composed of smooth muscle and contain cilia
5. Cilia act together to move ovum through tubes toward uterus
6. Fertilization occurs in outer portion of tube
D. Ovaries
1. Located on either side of uterus and below ends of Fallopian tubes
2. Attached to uterus by a ligament and attached to broad ligament
3. Store female germ cells (total number of ova present at birth)
4. Produce female hormones estrogen and progesterone
5. Contains small structures called ovarian follicles

a. Each follicle is immature ovum or oocyte
b. Each month several follicles are stimulated to maturity by follicle stimulating hormone (FSH) and luteinizing hormone (LH)
c. Developing follicles surrounded by mature follicles called graafian follicles which produce estrogen
d. Estrogen stimulates development of endometrium
e. Each month 1 or 2 of mature follicles eject oocytes: ovulation
f. Ruptured follicle then is called corpus luteum and produces estrogen and progesterone to support endometrium until conception occurs or cycle begins again
g. Corpus luteum slowly degenerates and leaves scar on surface of ovary
E. External Structures (collectively called vulva)
1. Mons pubis: pad of adipose tissue anterior to symphysis pubis; covered with pubic hair after puberty
2. Labia
   a. Labia majora: folds of skin and adipose tissue covered with hair from base of mons pubis and to the end of anus
   b. Labia minora: skin, adipose tissue, erectile tissue; enclosed by labia majora
3. Clitoris: formed by joining of labia minora; erectile organ, highly sensitive and distends during sexual arousal
4. Vestibule is area between labia that contains
   a. Introitus: opening of vagina
   b. Bartholin and Skene's glands: secrete lubricating fluid during sexual response cycle
   c. Urinary meatus (urethral opening)
5. Vaginal and urethral openings and glands
F. Breasts
1. Mammary glands located between third and seventh ribs on anterior chest wall
2. Have rich supply of nerves, blood, and lymph
3. Areola: pigmented area located near center containing sebaceous glands and nipple which becomes erect in response to cold and stimulation
4. Composed of adipose tissue, fibrous connective tissue, glandular tissue

5. Cooper's ligaments support breasts and extend from outer breast tissue to nipple
6. Lobes are composed of alveolar glands connected by ducts which open to nipple
G. Female Sex Hormones
1. Ovaries produce estrogens, progesterone, and androgens in cyclic pattern
2. Estrogen
   a. Essential for development and maintenance of secondary sex characteristics
   b. With other hormones, stimulates female reproductive organs to prepare for growth of fetus
   c. Responsible for normal structure of skin and blood vessels
   d. Decreases rate of bone resorption, promotes increased high-density lipoproteins, reduces cholesterol, enhances clotting of blood, promotes retention of sodium and water
3. Progesterone
   a. Primarily affects development of breast glandular tissue and endometrium
   b. During pregnancy relaxes smooth muscle to decrease uterine contractions
4. Androgens
   a. Responsible for normal hair growth patterns at puberty
   b. Have metabolic effects
H. Oogenesis and ovarian cycle
1. Ovarian cycle
   a. Has 3 consecutive phases that occur over 28 days (usual time)
   1. Follicular phase: day 1–10
      a. Follicle develops and oocyte matures
      b. Controlled by interaction of FSH (follicle stimulating hormone) and LH (luteinizing hormone)
      c. Always follicles at different stages of development; one follicle becomes dominant and matures to ovulation; others then degenerate
   2. Ovulatory phase: day 11–14
      a. Begins when estrogen levels are high enough to stimulate anterior pituitary and surge of LH is produced
      b. LH stimulates meiosis in developing oocyte; eventually

ovulation (release of mature ovarian follicle)
   c. Ends with ovulation
   3. Luteal phase: day 14–28
      a. Surge of LH stimulates ruptured follicle to change into corpus luteum, which produces progesterone and estrogen
      b. These hormone levels produce negative feedback which stops production of LH and stops further growth and development of other follicles
      c. If no pregnancy occurs, corpus luteum degenerates and declining levels of estrogen and progesterone stimulate the increased secretion of FSH and LH and the cycle continues
2. Menstrual cycle
   a. Endometrium of uterus prepares for implantation of a fertilized embryo under influence of estrogen and progesterone
   b. Phases of cycle
   1. Menstrual phase: day 1–5; inner endometrial layer detaches and is expelled as menstrual fluid for 3–5 days
   2. Proliferative phase: day 6–14; endometrial layer is repaired and thickens; cervical mucus changes, thins into crystalline substance improving sperm mobility into uterus
   3. Secretory phase: day 14–28; rising levels of progesterone from corpus luteum act on endometrium causing increased vascularity and thickening of cervical mucous; if no fertilization occurs hormone levels fall and the endometrial layer sloughs off
V. Assessment of Female Reproductive Function
A. Health Assessment Strategies
1. Consideration of psychological, social, and cultural factors that affect sexual activity and sexuality
2. Strategies to make interview less threatening include
   a. Begin with generalized questions and progress to specific questions
   b. Ask questions in a way that gives client permission to report behaviors and manifestations

B. Health assessment interview to collect subjective data
   1. Interview usually extensive
   2. If problem is identified, collect information regarding
      a. Onset
      b. Characteristics
      c. Duration
      d. Frequency
      e. Precipitating or relieving factors
      f. Treat and/or self-care
      g. Outcome
   3. Interview should cover
      a. Menstrual history
      b. Obstetric history
      c. Use of contraception
      d. Sexual history
      e. Use of medications
      f. Frequency of reproductive examinations
      g. Risk for sexually transmitted disease, including HIV infection (number of sexual partners, condom use)
      h. Smoking especially for females taking oral contraceptives
   4. Determine whether client has significant history that affects function of reproductive system
      a. Chronic diseases: diabetes, chronic heavy menstrual flow (risk for anemia), thyroid and adrenal disorders
      b. Family history of cancer especially history of breast, endometrial, ovarian, or colon cancer
      c. Exposure to DES in utero (increased risk for cancer of cervix and vagina)
      d. Exposure to asbestos (increased risk for cancer of ovary)
      e. History of fibrocystic breast disease (increased risk for cancer of breast)
   5. History of vaginal bleeding and/or vaginal discharge
   6. Sexuality
      a. Level of satisfaction
      b. Use of contraception
      c. Anorgasmia (absence of orgasm)
      d. Dyspareunia (painful intercourse)
C. Physical assessment with abnormal findings to collect objective data
   1. Breast assessment
      a. Retractions, dimpling, abnormal contours occur with benign or malignant lesions
      b. Thickened, dimpled skin with enlarged pores (peau d'orange, orange peel, pig

skin) and unilateral venous patterns associated with malignancy
      c. Redness occurs with infection or carcinoma
      d. Peau d'orange noted in areola, recent unilateral inversion of nipple or asymmetry in directions in which nipples point suggests cancer
      e. Tenderness upon palpation occurs; may be associated with premenstrual fullness, fibrocystic disease, inflammation, or cancer
      f. Nodules in tail of breast occurs with enlarged lymph nodes
      g. Hard irregular fixed unilateral masses that are poorly delineated suggest carcinoma
      h. Bilateral, single, or multiple round mobile masses that are well-delineated, occur with fibrocystic breast disease of fibroadenoma
      i. Swelling, tenderness, erythema, and heat occur with mastitis
      j. Loss of nipple elasticity occurs with cancer
      k. Bloody or serous discharge from nipples is associated with intraductal papilloma
      l. Milky discharge from both nipples and not associated with pregnancy suggests galactorrhea, which may occur with pituitary tumor
      m. Unilateral discharge from one or two ducts occurs with fibrocystic breast disease, intraductal papilloma, or carcinoma
   2. Axillary assessment
      a. Rash may be associated with allergy
      b. Signs of inflammation and infection associated with infection of sweat glands
      c. Enlarged axillary nodes occur with infection of hand and/or arm or with malignancy
      d. Enlarged supraclavicular nodes are associated with lymphatic metastases from abdominal or thoracic carcinoma
   3. External assessment
      a. Excoriation, rashes, lesions suggest inflammatory or infective processes
      b. Bulging of the labia with straining suggests hernia
      c. Presence of varicosities
      d. Inflammation, irritation, excoriation, caking of discharge in labial folds

occurs with vaginal infection or poor hygiene

e. Presence of ulcers or vesicles may occur with sexually transmitted infection

f. Palpable small firm round cystic nodules in labia suggest sebaceous cysts

g. Wartlike lesions in labias suggest condylomata acuminata (genital warts)

h. Firm painless ulcers suggest chancre or primary syphilis

i. Shallow painful ulcers suggest herpes infection

j. Ulcerations and red raised lesions in older women suggest vulvar carcinoma

k. Enlargement of clitoris is manifestation of masculinizing condition

l. Vaginal opening
   1. Swelling or discoloration may be caused by trauma
   2. Discharge or lesions occur with infection
   3. Fissures or fistulas occur with injury, infection, malignancy, trauma

m. Discharge or tenderness of Skene's glands suggests infection

n. Nontender mass in posterolateral position of labia suggests cyst of Bartholin's glands; swelling, redness, or tenderness in area suggests an abscess of Bartholin's glands

o. Vaginal orifice while client is straining or bearing down
   1. Bulging of anterior vaginal wall and incontinence: suggests cystocele
   2. Bulging of posterior vaginal wall: suggests rectocele
   3. Protrusion of cervix or uterus into vagina indicates uterine prolapse

p. Perineum
   1. Scarring related to past episiotomy
   2. Inflammation, lesions, growths occur with infection or cancer
   3. Fistulas result from trauma, infection, injury, spreading malignancy

q. Examination of cervix and vagina with speculum

1. Bluish color indicates pregnancy
2. Pale cervix indicates anemia
3. Cervix to right or left of midline may indicate pelvic mass, uterine adhesions, pregnancy
4. Projection of cervix > 3 cm into vaginal canal indicates pelvic or uterine mass
5. Transverse or star shaped cervical lacerations indicate trauma and tearing of cervix
6. Enlarged cervix associated with infection
7. Redness around cervical os and easy bleeding occurs with ectropion (eversion of columnar epithelium lining of cervical canal)
8. Small, white or yellow, raised round areas on cervix are Nabothian cysts and may be normal or can become infected
9. Cervical polyps may originate from cervix or endometrium

r. Palpation of cervix, uterus, ovaries
   1. Retroversion or retroflexed uterus
   2. Pain upon movement of cervix suggests pelvic inflammatory disease (PID)
   3. Softening of uterine isthmus (Hegar's sign), softening of cervix (Goodell's sign), uterine enlargement are objective signs of pregnancy
   4. Firm irregular nodules continuous with uterine surface are likely to be myomas (fibroids)
   5. Palpable smooth compressible adnexal masses on one or both sides occur with ovarian tumors
   6. Profuse menstrual bleeding occurs with endometrial polyps, dysfunctional uterine bleeding (DUB), use of intrauterine device
   7. Irregular bleeding associated with endometrial polyps, DUB, uterine or cervical carcinoma, oral contraceptives
   8. Postmenopausal bleeding occurs with endometrial hyperplasia, estrogen therapy, endometrial cancer

FOCUSED STUDY TIPS

- Discuss with classmates privacy issues as they relate to health assessment interviews and physical assessments of male and female reproductive functioning. Describe specific nursing interventions to create a private and safe environment.
- Supplemental female and male sex hormones are utilized to treat medical conditions of the opposite sex. Describe when and why.
- Practice a health assessment interview for the opposite sex with a classmate or friend. Monitor your comfort level with questioning. Identify levels of comfort that need improvement.

CASE STUDY

A client comes to the clinic with the complaint of impotence. What questions should the nurse ask regarding the client's medical history? His sexual history? What other factors may contribute to this complaint?

CARE PLAN CRITICAL THINKING ACTIVITY

Describe differences between the health assessment interview for men and the health assessment interview for women. What nursing interventions can make the client more comfortable during this interview?

NCLEX TEST QUESTIONS

1. The nurse would expect a client with balanitis to complain of
   a. vaginal discharge.
   b. pain with urination.
   c. spontaneous urethral discharge.
   d. back pain.
2. Which client is at the highest risk for developing balanitis?
   a. 1-year-old with intact foreskin
   b. circumcised 40-year-old
   c. 12-year-old with intact foreskin
   d. circumcised 6-year-old
3. In the area of human sexuality, nurses may encounter problems in relating to their clients. A major barrier or problem the nurse should be aware of is
   a. lack of knowledge in human sexuality.
   b. the nurse's personal attitudes toward human sexuality.
   c. lack of appropriate referrals in this area.
   d. lack of proficiency in sexual history taking.
4. A 14-year-old presents to the clinic for a birth control method. She attends the class that describes the methods available to her. After class, she asked the nurse, "Which method is best for me to use?" The best response is
   a. "You are so young, are you sure you are ready for the responsibilities of a sexual relationship?"

   b. "Because of your age, we need your parents' consent before you can be examined and then we'll talk."
   c. "Before I can help you with that question, I need to know more about your sexual activity."
   d. "The physician can best help you with that after your physical examination."
5. When assessing the male child with hypospadias, the nurse would observe for
   a. the absence of a testicle.
   b. a urethral opening along the ventral surface of the penis.
   c. a herniation into the scrotal sac.
   d. a smaller-than-normal penis.
6. Assessing a client with benign prostatic hypertrophy, which complaint has the greatest priority for intervention?
   a. urinary retention
   b. burning with urination
   c. dribbling of urine
   d. decreased urine stream
7. Which of the client phone calls to the urology clinic should be returned first?
   a. 28-year-old man, with burning upon urination, greenish-yellow penile discharge
   b. 68-year-old man, complaining of inability to void for 2 days

c. 45-year-old man, with weak stream of urine, worsening over last 6 months

d. 52-year-old man, with foul-smelling dark-colored urine for past 2 days

8. When counseling a female client who has frequent urinary tract infections, the nurse would instruct her to
   a. drink several glasses of milk per day.
   b. eat foods that increase the alkalinity of urine.
   c. wipe from front to back after urination.
   d. limit sexual intercourse.

9. A nurse enters the private room of a male client and realizes he is masturbating. The appropriate response is to:
   a. set limits on his behavior in the hospital.
   b. apologize for intruding on the client's privacy.
   c. tell the client his behavior is inappropriate.
   d. ignore the behavior and continue with the intervention planned when entering the room.

10. A nurse counseling a 12-year-old can help her understand that her puberty growth spurt will:
    a. begin after she has become sexually mature.
    b. begin before she has become sexually mature.
    c. last throughout her adolescent years.
    d. last longer than her brother Mark's growth spurt.

CHAPTER 47

NURSING CARE OF MEN WITH REPRODUCTIVE SYSTEM DISORDERS

LEARNING OUTCOMES

After completing this chapter, you will be able to:

- Apply knowledge of normal male anatomy, physiology, and assessments when providing care for men with reproductive system disorders (see Chapter 46).
- Explain the pathophysiology of disorders of the male reproductive system.
- Discuss risk factors for cancers of the male reproductive system.
- Discuss the collaborative care, with related nursing implications, for men with disorders of the reproductive system.
- Provide appropriate nursing care for the man having prostate surgery.
- Use the nursing process as a framework for providing individualized care to men with disorders of the reproductive system.

KEY TOPICS

- Disorders of male sexual expression
- Disorders of the penis
- Disorders of the testes and scrotum
- Disorders of the prostate gland
- Male breast disorders
- Nursing care of men with reproductive system disorders

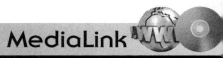

MediaLink

www.prenhall.com/lemone

Additional resources for this chapter can be found on the Student CD-ROM accompanying this textbook, and on the Companion Website at www.prenhall.com/lemone. Click on Chapter 47 to select the activities for this chapter.

CD-ROM
- Audio Glossary
- NCLEX Review

Companion Website
- More NCLEX Review
- Case Study
  Benign Prostatic Hyperplasia (BPH)
- Care Plan Activity
  Radical Prostatectomy
- MediaLink Application
  Prostate Cancer Prevention

LECTURE OUTLINE

I. Disorders of Sexual Expression
  A. Man with Erectile Dysfunction
    1. Inability of male to attain and maintain an erection sufficient to permit satisfactory sexual intercourse
    2. Impotence is used to describe
      a. Total inability to achieve erection
      b. Inconsistent ability to achieve erection
      c. Ability to sustain only brief erections
    3. Estimated 10 million men in U.S. have erectile dysfunction; most > 65
    4. Pathophysiology: Age-related changes
      a. Cellular and tissue changes in penis
      b. Decreased sensory activity
      c. Hypogonadism
      d. Effects of chronic illness (70%)
        1. Diabetes
        2. Kidney disease
        3. Chronic alcoholism
        4. Atherosclerosis and vascular disease
    5. Collaborative Care: Growing concern with aging of population and increased willingness of men and partners to verbalize and seek assistance with sexual concerns
    6. Diagnostic Tests
      a. Blood chemistry, testosterone, prolactin, thyroxin, PSA: identify metabolic and endocrine problems
      b. Nocturnal penile tumescence and rigidity (NPTR)
        1. Differentiate between psychogenic and organic causes of impotence
        2. Tests performed in sleep laboratory or portable devices for home use
      c. Cavernosometry and cavernosography of corpora to evaluate arterial inflow and venous outflow of penis
    7. Medications
      a. Oral medication: sildenafil (Viagra)
        1. Interferes with breakdown of biochemical involved with smooth muscle relaxation of corpus cavernosum necessary to produce erections
        2. Enhances effect of nitric oxide released during sexual stimulation
      b. Injectable medications (into penis)
        1. Papaverine: relaxes arterioles and smooth muscles inducing tumescence (swelling) and erection

    2. Prostaglandin E: acts as papaverine with fewer side effects
    3. Alprostadil (Caverject): or may be used as urethral minisuppository
      c. Hormone replacement therapy: treatment for androgen deficiency
        1. Testosterone injection (200 mg IM every 3 weeks)
        2. Topical patches
      d. Transdermal medications including nitroglycerine paste applied directly to penis
    8. Mechanical Devices: Vacuum constriction device (VCD)
      a. Draws blood into penis with a vacuum
      b. Traps it with constricting band at base of penis
      c. Single small band ("O-ring") left to maintain erection
    9. Surgery Procedures
      a. Revascularization procedures: usually only temporary results since insufficiency not corrected
      b. Implantation of prosthetic devices
        1. Semi-rigid rods: penis always in state of semi-erection
        2. Self-contained penile implant: penis flaccid until man compresses pump at head of penis, which transfers fluid to cylinder within penis
        3. Inflatable penile implant: penis flaccid until man compresses pump in scrotum and fluid transferred from abdominal reservoir to penis
    10. Nursing Diagnoses
      a. Sexual Dysfunction
      b. Situational Low Self-esteem
  B. Man with Ejaculatory Dysfunction
    1. Premature ejaculation
      a. Psychogenic or due to diabetes
      b. May respond to
        1. Wearing condoms to decrease sensitivity
        2. Utilizing relaxation and guided imagery techniques
        3. Utilizing constrictive rings at base of penis
    2. Delayed ejaculation: may occur with hypogonadism, or along with inability to ejaculate, may be due to effects from medications including antihypertensives, antidepressants, anxiolytics, narcotics

3. Retrograde ejaculation: may occur with age or treatment for prostatic or testicular cancer

II. Disorders of Penis
  A. Man with Phimosis or Priapism
    1. Phimosis: constriction of foreskin so it cannot be retracted over glans penis
      a. May be congenital or related to chronic infections under foreskin
      b. Prevents adequate hygiene and may lead to malignant changes
      c. May cause problems with urination and sexual activity
    2. Paraphimosis: foreskin is tight and constricted and not able to cover glans penis
      a. Glans is engorged and edematous, painful
      b. May result from long-term retraction of foreskin as with urinary catheterization of uncircumcised male
      c. Severe phimosis or paraphimosis may require surgical circumcision or treatment of infection with antibiotics
      d. May cause problems with urination and sexual activity
    3. Priapism: involuntary sustained painful erection not associated with sexual arousal
      a. May result in ischemia and fibrosis of erectile tissue with high risk of subsequent impotence
      b. May cause problems with urination and sexual activity
      c. Primary priapism occurs with tumors, infection, trauma
      d. Secondary priapism caused by
        1. Blood disorders (leukemia, sickle cell anemia, thrombocytopenia)
        2. Neurologic disorders (spinal cord injuries, stroke)
        3. Renal failure
        4. Risk with use of intracavernous injection therapy
      e. Treatment
        1. Conservative: iced saline enemas, intravenous ketamine to induce anesthesia or spinal anesthesia
        2. Aspiration of blood from corpus through dorsal glans followed by catheterization and pressure dressings
        3. Surgery to create vascular shunts
      f. Nursing Care
        1. Assessing penis
        2. Monitoring urinary output
        3. Providing pain control

  B. Man with Cancer of Penis
    1. Description
      a. Rare in U.S.
      b. Cause is unknown but risk factors include
        1. Phimosis
        2. Viral HPV and HIV infections
        3. Exposure to ultraviolet light
      c. Most cases are squamous cell carcinoma
    2. Manifestations
      a. Nodular or wart-like growth on glans or foreskin
      b. Tumor is slow growing and spreads to inguinal lymph nodes
      c. Lesions are painless but involve ulceration and bleeding
    3. Diagnostic Tests: Biopsy of lesion and suspicious inguinal lymph nodes
    4. Treatment
      a. After staging, small lesions may be treated with fluorouracil cream, external-beam radiation, laser therapy, surgical excision
      b. Large lesions require partial or total amputation of penis

III. Disorders of Testes and Scrotum
  A. Man with Benign Scrotal Mass
    1. Hydrocele
      a. Collection of fluid within tunica vaginalis from slight enlargement to size of grapefruit
      b. Differentiation by transillumination or ultrasound of scrotum
      c. May be secondary to trauma, infection, tumor
      d. May be treated by aspiration and agent injected into scrotal sac to sclerose tunica vaginalis and prevent reoccurrence
      e. Not associated with infertility
    2. Spermatocele
      a. Mobile painless mass forms when efferent ducts in epididymis dilate and form a cyst
      b. Results from leakage of sperm due to trauma or infection
      c. Not associated with infertility
      d. Treatment not usually necessary
    3. Varicocele
      a. Abnormal dilation of vein within spermatic cord caused by incompetent, congenitally missing valves that allow blood to pool in spermatic cord veins

b. Soft mass, which may be painful, occurs post puberty on left side usually

c. May interfere with spermatogenesis and cause infertility

d. Diagnosis by sonography

e. May be treated by ligation of spermatic vein or occluding it with sclerosing agent of balloon catheter

B. Man with Epididymitis

1. Infection of inflammation of structure that lies along posterior border of testis; occurs in sexually active men < 35 years

  a. Infection

    1. Sexually transmission of *C. trachomatis, N. gonorrhoeae*

    2. *E. coli, H. influenzae, Cryptococcus,* tuberculosis transmitted through unprotected anal intercourse

    3. Men older than 35 usually develop condition associated with urinary tract infection or prostatitis

  b. Chemical epididymitis, associated with inflammatory response to reflux of urine into ejaculatory ducts because of urethral strictures, or increased abdominal pressure from heavy lifting

2. Infection spreads by ascending the vas deferens from infected urethra or bladder

3. Early Manifestations

  a. Pain

  b. Local edema, progressing to erythema and edema of entire scrotum, especially on side of involved epididymis

4. Complications

  a. Abscess formation

  b. Infarction of testis

  c. Infertility

5. Diagnostic Tests: Culture of specimen from urethral swab or epididymal aspiration

6. Treatment

  a. Severe cases are treated with intravenous antibiotics and hospitalization

  b. Less severe cases are treated with outpatient antibiotics

  c. Sexual partners should be treated with antibiotics if organism is sexually transmitted

7. Nursing Care

  a. Symptomatic relief: ice packs, scrotal support

  b. Resolution may take weeks to months

c. Long-term effects include possible infertility

C. Man with Orchitis

1. Acute inflammation or infection of testis

2. Occurs as infection complication of epididymitis or systemic illness, commonly with mumps

  a. Sudden onset 3–4 days after swelling of parotid glands with high fever, unilateral or bilateral scrotal redness, swelling and pain

  b. Complication is atrophy of testis with irreversible damage to spermatogenesis

3. May occur as inflammation association with vasectomy, scrotal surgeries, and trauma

4. Treatment is supportive and symptomatic

  a. Antibiotics, if indicated

  b. Bed rest, scrotal support and elevation

  c. Hot or cold compresses

  d. Analgesics for pain

D. Man with Testicular Torsion

1. Twisting of spermatic cord with scrotal swelling and pain

  a. Circulation is blocked

  b. Results in vascular engorgement and ischemia

  c. Potential medical emergency

2. Occurs spontaneously, after trauma, physical exertion

3. Diagnosis made by history and physical examination; testicular scanning

4. Treatment

  a. Detorsion of testicle and fixation to scrotum as soon as possible

  b. Orchiectomy is indicated if testicle is significantly damaged or necrotic

E. Man with Testicular Cancer

1. Description

  a. Accounts for only 1% of cancers in males but is most common cancer in men between ages of 15 and 35

  b. Germ cell tumors are most common with spread to other organs by vascular and lymphatic channels before large masses occur in scrotum

2. Cause unknown but risk factors include

  a. Cryptorchidism (undescended testicle)

  b. Genetic predisposition

  c. Disorders of testicular development

  d. Maternal estrogen administration during pregnancy

3. Manifestations

  a. Painless hard nodule classic presenting manifestation

b. Metastatic manifestations may include edema of lower extremities, back pain, cough, hemoptysis, dizziness
4. Collaborative Care: Focus is on diagnosis, staging and treatment
5. Diagnostic Tests
   a. Serum studies for tumor markers such as human chorionic gonadotropin (hCG), alpha-fetoprotein (AFP)
   b. Serum lactic acid dehydrogenase (LDH) elevation; significantly with metastatic disease
   c. Liver function tests, x-rays, and CT scans of chest and abdomen to determine metastasis
6. Medication: Platinum-based combination chemotherapy is highly effective in treating the disease and has significantly improved survival rates
7. Surgery
   a. Radical orchiectomy is treatment used in all forms and stages
   b. Modified retroperitoneal lymph node dissection that preserves nerves necessary for ejaculation
8. Radiation Therapy: with early cancer may be used for treatment of retroperitoneal lymph nodes the most frequent site for distant metastasis; other testicle is carefully shielded
9. Health Promotion: all men should perform monthly testicular self-examination beginning at age 15
10. Nursing Diagnoses
    a. Knowledge Deficit (about testicular cancer and treatment)
    b. Ineffective Sexual Patterns (potential infertility)
11. Home Care
    a. Education and support for treatment, effects on sexual function
    b. Continued medical surveillance for 5–10 years after treatment
IV. Disorders of Prostate Gland
   A. Man with Prostatitis
      1. Prostatitis is term given to describe disorders involving infection or inflammation of the prostate gland
      2. Acute bacterial prostatitis
         a. Most often caused by ascending infection from urethra or reflux of infected urine: common organisms include *Pseudomonas, Klebsiella, Chlamydia*
         b. Manifestations

1. Increased temperature, malaise, muscle and joint pain
2. Urinary frequency and urgency, dysuria and discharge
3. Dull aching pain in perineum, rectum or lower back
4. Rectal exam reveals enlarged painful prostate
3. Chronic bacterial prostatitis
   a. History of recurrent urinary tract infections
   b. Manifestations: urinary urgency and frequency, dysuria, low back pain, perineal discomfort
4. Chronic prostatitis/chronic pelvic pain syndrome
   a. Inflammatory prostatitis
      1. Cause unknown, possibly autoimmune
      2. Manifestations include low back pain, urinary manifestations, pain in genitals and rectum, decreased libido, painful ejaculations
      3. No bacteria in urine but abnormal inflammatory cells are present in prostatic secretions
   b. Noninflammatory prostatitis (prostatodynia)
      1. Similar manifestations as with inflammatory prostatitis
      2. Urine and prostatic secretions show no evidence of bacteria or inflammation
5. Diagnostic Tests
   a. Urine and prostatic secretions are examined and cultured for blood cells and bacteria
   b. X-ray and ultrasound studies are used to visualize pelvic structures
6. Medications
   a. Bacterial prostatitis is treated with appropriate antibiotics; chronic prostatitis is treated with long-term antibiotics
   b. Inflammatory prostatitis is treated with NSAIDs for pain and anticholinergics for urinary symptoms
   c. Noninflammatory prostatitis (prostatodynia) is treated with muscle relaxants or alpha-adrenergic blocking agents
7. Nursing Care
   a. Education to increase fluid intake to 3 liters daily and to void often

b. Local heat and sitz baths may relieve pain and irritation
B. Man with Benign Prostatic Hyperplasia (BPH)
1. Age-related non-malignant enlargement of prostate gland that causes urinary dysfunction; begins at age 40–45 and continues affecting over half of males over age 75
2. Cause is unknown; risk factors include
  a. Age, family history
  b. Race, ethnicity (highest in African American men)
  c. Hormonal factors
3. Begins as small nodules in the inner layers of prostate; gradually enlarge and compress urethra causing partial or complete obstruction of outflow of urine from urinary bladder; detrusor muscles of bladder hypertrophy to compensate
4. Manifestations
  a. From obstruction: weak urinary stream, increased time to void, hesitancy, incomplete bladder emptying, postvoiding dribbling
  b. From irritation: frequency, urgency, incontinence, nocturia, dysuria, bladder pain
  c. Chronic urinary retention may occur resulting in overflow incontinence with any increase in intra-abdominal pressure
5. Complications
  a. Bladder diverticula
  b. Urinary tract infections
  c. Hydroureter, hydronephrosis, renal insufficiency
6. Treatment: determined by severity of manifestations and presence of complications
7. Diagnostic Tests
  a. Urinalysis: detect bacteria, WBC's, RBC's
  b. Renal function assessment: creatinine
  c. Prostate-specific antigen (PSA): rule out prostate cancer; level corresponds to volume of both benign and malignant prostate tissue
  d. Digital rectal examination (DRE): BPH prostate is asymmetrical and enlarged
  e. Post-voiding residual urine: over 100 mL is considered greater than normal
  f. Uroflowmetry: measuring urine flow rate; < 10mL/second indicates obstruction
  g. International Prostate Symptom Score: questionnaire that assesses frequency and difficulties with urination
8. Medications
  a. Finasteride (Proscar)
    1. Antiandrogen agent that causes enlarged prostate to shrink
    2. Significant side effects include
      a. Impotence
      b. Decreased libido
    3. Crushed tablets should not be handled by pregnant woman or could harm male fetus
  b. Alpha-adrenergic antagonists terazasin (Hytrin), tamsulosin (Flomax)
    1. Relieve obstruction and increase flow of urine
    2. May cause orthostatic hypotension
9. Surgery
  a. Men who are having significant problems or complications are candidates for surgery
  b. Procedures
    1. Transurethral resection of prostate (TURP): scope inserted through urethra; prostate tissue is removed and electrocautery is used to control bleeding; client may have continuous urinary irrigation post-operatively to control clotting
      a. Complications: postoperative hemorrhage, clot retention, inability to void, urinary tract infection
      b. Later complications: incontinence, impotence, retrograde ejaculation
    2. Transurethral incision of prostate (TUIP): Laser used to make small incisions in smooth muscle where prostate is attached to bladder; gland is split, reducing pressure on urethra
    3. Open prostatectomy: used with very large prostate
10. Phytotherapy: use of plants, including saw palmetto berry
11. Nursing Diagnoses
  a. Knowledge Deficit
  b. Urinary Retention
  c. Risk for Infection
  d. Risk for Imbalanced Fluid Volume (post TURP)

12. Home Care
    a. May be discharged home with indwelling catheter
    b. Client and family will need teaching, and possibly home care referral

C. Man with Prostatic Cancer
   1. Most common type of cancer and second leading cause of death in North America; primarily disease of older males
   2. Prognosis
      a. If diagnosed early is curable
      b. When cancer is confined to prostate at diagnosis, 5-year survival rate is 100%
      c. Death occurs secondarily to the debility of the multiple sites of skeletal metastasis, especially to vertebrae (compression fractures of spine)
   3. Pathophysiology
      a. Cause unknown, but androgens believed to play role in development
      b. Most primary cancers are adenocarcinomas
      c. Metastasis by lymph and venous channels is common
   4. Manifestations
      a. Early: asymptomatic
      b. Urinary: similar to BPH: urgency, frequency, hesitancy, dysuria, nocturia, hematuria, blood in ejaculate
      c. Metastasis: bone pain (may be initial manifestation)
   5. Risk Factors
      a. Age, race (African Americans)
      b. Genetic and heredity factors
      c. Vasectomy
      d. Dietary factors: diet high in fat and red meats, low in Vitamin A, Vitamin D, lycopene, selenium
      e. Low exposure to sunlight
   6. Diagnostic Tests
      a. DRE: prostate gland is nodular and fixed
      b. PSA levels are used to diagnose and stage prostate cancer and monitor treatment; normal levels are < 4 ng/mL; majority of men with prostate cancer have PSA > than 10 ng/mL
      c. Transrectal ultrasonography (TRUS):
      d. Prostatic biopsy (needle biopsy or transrectal ultrasound-guided biopsy): necessary to diagnose prostate cancer
      e. Bone scan, MRI, CT scans: determine metastasis
   7. Treatments
      a. Dependent on grade and stage of cancer

      b. Dependent on age, general health, and preference of client
   8. Surgery
      a. TURP: early disease in older men
      b. Radical prostatectomy
         1. Removal of prostate, prostatic capsule, seminal vesicles, portion of bladder neck
         2. Clients often have residual effects: impotence, urinary incontinence
      c. Retropubic prostatectomy: commonly done procedure since allows for good visualization, bleeding control and access to pelvic lymph nodes
      d. Perineal prostatectomy: done with clients who are poor surgical risks
      e. Suprapubic prostatectomy: rarely done due to difficult control of bleeding
      f. Men with urinary sphincter insufficiency may be treated with surgically implanted artificial urinary sphincter
   9. Radiation Therapy
      a. May be used as primary treatment for prostate cancer; may be delivered external beam or brachytherapy: interstitial implants of radioactive seeds
      b. Less risk of complications (impotence, rectal damage) with interstitial radiation
      c. Use palliatively for clients with metastatic disease reducing size of metastasis, controlling pain, restoring function (relieving spinal cord compression)
   10. Hormonal Manipulation: androgen deprivation therapy used to treat advanced prostate cancer in which tumor cells are androgen dependent
      a. Orchiectomy
      b. Administration of female hormonal agents
   11. Health Promotion
      a. Increase public awareness about early detection of prostate cancer
      b. Yearly PSA and DRE beginning at age 50
      c. Men in high risk groups (African descent, first-degree relative, diagnosed at younger age): testing at age 45
   12. Nursing Diagnoses
      a. Urinary Incontinence following treatment for prostatic cancer; stress incontinence, urge incontinence

b. Sexual Dysfunction
c. Acute/Chronic Pain
13. Home Care
 a. Address educational needs related to the type of treatment
 b. Continuing supervision under medical care
 c. Specific client needs including home health or hospice referrals

V. Male Breast Disorders
 A. Man with Gynecomastia
  1. Abnormal enlargement of male breast thought to result from high ratio of estradiol to testosterone
  2. Usually bilateral; if unilateral biopsy needed to rule out breast cancer
  3. Conditions that increase estrogen activity or decrease testosterone production contribute to gynecomastia
   a. Conditions that increase estrogen production
    1. Obesity
    2. Testicular tumors
    3. Liver disease
    4. Adrenal carcinoma

   b. Conditions that decrease testosterone production
    1. Tuberculosis
    2. Hodgkin's disease
    3. Injury or orchitis
  4. Medications associated with gynecomastia include digitalis, opiates and chemotherapeutic agents
  5. Treatment may include surgery to remove excess subcutaneous tissue
 B. Male with Breast Cancer
  1. Rare cancer and etiology is unknown; most tumors are estrogen-receptor positive
  2. Treatment includes surgery: modified radical mastectomy, node dissection, staging
  3. Radiation, chemotherapy, or hormonal therapy (tamoxifen)
  4. Castration is successful, palliative measure
  5. Nursing care involves assisting client and family deal with cancer diagnosis as well as diagnosis that may be source of embarrassment

FOCUSED STUDY TIPS

- Ask your instructor to arrange for you to observe a circumcision. During class, discuss the advantages and disadvantages of circumcision. Identify religious and social differences of opinion. List factors that need to be included in decision making for circumcision.
- Create a chronological timeline for males from birth to 90 years old. Insert on the timeline age-related reproductive disorders for which men are at risk.
- Research drugs used to treat men with erectile dysfunction. Identify assessment information necessary before these drugs are utilized. Describe common side effects and potential complications of their use.

CASE STUDY

Discuss postoperative care of a client with a penile implant. What nursing interventions are implemented? What teaching must be completed before discharge from the hospital, and who should be included in this teaching? What community resources might be necessary for the client?

CARE PLAN CRITICAL THINKING ACTIVITY

Incontinence is a common, yet disturbing, complication of treatment of prostate cancer. Describe how the nurse prepares the client for this potential complication.

NCLEX TEST QUESTIONS

1. The client experiencing prostatitis would most likely have which symptoms?
 a. spontaneous penile discharge, dysuria, and pain with ejaculation

 b. painful blisters and craterlike lesions, enlarged groin nodes, fever
 c. brownish rash on palms, painful craterlike lesions, malaise, and fever

d. perineal pain, pain upon voiding, low abdominal pain, and low back pain

2. The 23-year-old client has been diagnosed with testicular cancer. Which of the following should be included in his teaching plan?
   a. Future fertility is not affected by treatment.
   b. Impotence often results from needed treatments.
   c. Sperm banking should be done prior to treatment.
   d. Sexual interest will increase as a result of treatment.

3. When discharging a client from the hospital after a transurethral resection of the prostate (TURP) for benign prostatic hyperplasia (BPH), which of the following is essential to teach the client?
   a. The indwelling catheter will be removed by the physician in about 2 days.
   b. The color of the urine may become red and contain small clots.
   c. Pain in the lower abdomen is to be expected; take aspirin or ibuprofen (Advil).
   d. Drink plenty of fluids, especially water, and avoid caffeine and alcohol.

4. The parent of a newborn with epispadias is asking how this happened. The best answer would be:
   a. "The defect happens early in fetal development."
   b. "The alcohol you drank caused the defect."
   c. "Because you smoked, the penis did not form correctly."
   d. "You had a deficiency of folic acid that caused this."

5. The client is scheduled for a transurethral resection of the prostate (TURP) to treat his benign prostatic hypertrophy (BPH) and asks the nurse how his prostate became enlarged. The best response is:
   a. "Prostate enlargement happens to most men as they age and their hormones change."
   b. "Your prostate has become cancerous, which is really quite a rare occurrence."
   c. "Because of your diet, your prostate gland quit working and became larger."
   d. "Your chronic constipation put excessive force on the prostate and it enlarged."

6. The client with benign prostatic hyperplasia has undergone transurethral resection of the prostate (TURP) and is asking why he needs continuous bladder irrigation (CBI). The nurse's best response would be:
   a. "The irrigation prevents blood from clotting and blocking the catheter."
   b. "Your bladder needs to be kept full to promote healing after this surgery."
   c. "The urine would be very concentrated without the irrigation."
   d. "The saline running through the bladder helps keep you hydrated."

7. When performing perineal care on an uncircumcised male's penis, the nurse should return the foreskin to its natural position to prevent:
   a. an abnormal erection response.
   b. localized swelling and edema.
   c. potential urinary tract infection.
   d. embarrassment of the client.

8. In gathering data on an elderly male client the nurse suspects that the likely cause of his urinary retention and diminished force of urinary stream is:
   a. benign prostatic hyperplasia (BPH).
   b. urinary tract infection.
   c. voluntary urinary retention.
   d. anticholinergic medications.

9. Which of the following medications would the nurse be most likely to review in the discharge instructions of a client who has undergone a prostatectomy?
   a. antiviral medication
   b. antacid preparations
   c. stool softeners
   d. vitamin supplements

10. Which client is most likely to be diagnosed with testicular cancer?
    a. 25-year-old with sudden onset of testicular pain that started when he was lifting weights
    b. 18-year-old with unilateral painless hard nodule and dull ache in scrotum and pelvis
    c. 40-year-old with increasing rectal pain, low back pain, and low grade temperature
    d. 50-year-old with nocturia, hesitant and weak urinary flow, whose father had lung cancer

CHAPTER 48

NURSING CARE OF WOMEN WITH REPRODUCTIVE SYSTEM DISORDERS

LEARNING OUTCOMES

After completing this chapter, you will be able to:

- Apply knowledge of normal female anatomy, physiology, and assessments when providing nursing care for women with reproductive system disorders (see Chapter 46).
- Explain the pathophysiology of disorders of the female reproductive system.
- Describe the physiologic process of menopause.
- Discuss risk factors for cancers of the female reproductive system.
- Discuss the collaborative care, with related nursing implications, for women with disorders of the reproductive system.
- Provide appropriate nursing care for women having diagnostic tests and gynecologic surgery.
- Provide accurate information to women about health-promoting behaviors that prevent disorders of the female reproductive system or facilitate their early diagnosis.
- Use the nursing process as a framework for providing individualized care to women with disorders of the reproductive system.

KEY TOPICS

- The perimenopausal woman
- Menstrual disorders
- Structural disorders of the female reproductive system
- Disorders of female reproductive tissue
- Disorders of the female breast
- Disorders of female sexual expression
- Nursing care of women with reproductive system disorders

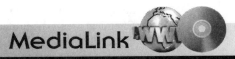

MediaLink

LECTURE OUTLINE

I. The Perimenopausal Woman
   A. Menopause: term used to signify permanent cessation of menses
      1. Perimenopausal period, or climacteric, is the period of time when reproductive function gradually ceases; usually lasts several years
      2. Begins with decline of estrogen production and extends until one year after final menstrual period: person is postmenopausal
      3. Most women stop menstruating between ages of 48–55
      4. By definition, a woman who has a follicular stimulating hormone (FSH) level > 30 mIU/mL, or who has not menstruated for one year, is menopausal
      5. Surgical menopause occurs when ovaries are removed in premenopausal women
      6. Chemical menopause often occurs during cancer chemotherapy when cytotoxic drugs arrest ovarian function
   B. Physiology
      1. As ovarian function decreases production of estradiol decreases and estrone becomes major ovarian estrogen; progesterone production is also markedly reduced
      2. Manifestations
         a. Breast tissue, body hair, skin elasticity, subcutaneous fat decreases
         b. Reproductive organs decrease in size
         c. Vasomotor instability may occur: hot flashes, palpitations, dizziness, headaches, insomnia, frequent awakening, night sweats
         d. Irritability, anxiety, depression
      3. Long-term Changes
         a. Imbalance in bone remodeling and osteoporosis
         b. Risk for cardiovascular disease
         c. Risk for breast cancer
      4. Collaborative Care
         a. Symptom relief
         b. Minimizing postmenopausal health risks
      5. Diagnostic Tests: Levels of FSH and LH rise and remain elevated
      6. Hormone Replacement Therapy (HRT)
         a. Used to alleviate unpleasant manifestations
            1. Believed to reduce risk of CHD, osteoporosis, Alzheimer's disease
      2. Research shows estrogen plus progestin increased risk of breast cancer, strokes, and heart attacks (risk of colon cancer and hip fracture decreases)
         b. Side effects: nausea, vomiting, weight gain, breast tenderness and engorgement, vaginal bleeding
         c. Contraindications
            1. Current endometrial cancer; past history of estrogen-dependent breast, ovarian, or cervical cancer
            2. Hypertriglyceridemia
            3. Active thrombotic disorders or inherited clotting disorders
            4. Acute or chronic liver disease or kidney failure
            5. Unexplained vaginal bleeding
            6. Pregnancy
      7. Selective Estrogen Receptor Modulators (SERMs): Alternative to HRT to prevent osteoporosis, i.e., raloxifene (Evista)
      8. Complementary Therapies
         a. Aromatherapy
         b. Herbs
         c. Supplements of vitamin E and soy
         d. Meditation
      9. Health Promotion
         a. American Cancer Society recommends cancer-related check-up every year after age of 40
         b. Screenings for cervical, breast, and colorectal cancer
         c. Health practices that decrease risk for cancer
      10. Nursing Diagnoses
         a. Knowledge Deficit: Health recommendations
            1. Calcium intake: 1200 mg day
            2. Weight bearing exercise
            3. Yearly mammograms, clinical breast examinations, Pap tests
            4. Monthly breast self-examinations
         b. Ineffective Sexuality Pattern
         c. Situational Low Self-esteem
         d. Disturbed Body Image
II. Menstrual Disorders
   A. Woman with Premenstrual Syndrome (PMS)
      1. Description
         a. Complex of manifestations: mood swings, breast tenderness, fatigue, irritability, food cravings, depression

b. Limited to 3–14 days before menstruation and relieved by onset of menses

c. Estimated to affect 25–40% of all women with mild to moderate manifestations

2. Premenstrual dysphoric disorder (PMDD): PMS is disabling condition; peak seen in women in mid-30's

3. Pathophysiology: Hormonal changes
   a. Altered estrogen-progesterone ratio
   b. Increased prolactin levels and rising aldosterone levels
   c. Increased production of aldosterone (sodium and water retention)
   d. Decreased levels of monamine oxidase in brain, associated with depression
   e. Decreased levels of serotonin, leading to mood swings

4. Collaborative Care
   a. If no organic cause is identified, goal is to relieve manifestations and assist client to develop self-care patterns to deal with episodes of PMS
   b. Treatment includes self-monitored record of manifestations, good health habits including regular exercise, avoiding caffeine, diet low in simple sugar and high in lean proteins

5. Medications
   a. Suppression of ovulation with gonadotropin-releasing hormone (GRH) agonists, oral contraceptives, danazol
   b. Progesterone and NSAIDs used to relieve cramping
   c. Diuretics to relieve bloating
   d. Selective serotonin reuptake inhibitors: fluoxetine (Prozac), sertraline (Zoloft), paroxetine (Paxil) to manage mood

6. Complementary Therapies
   a. Diet high in complex carbohydrates and low in simple sugars and alcohol
   b. Reduced sodium intake; increased intake of calcium, magnesium, vitamin E
   c. Restricted use of caffeine
   d. Adequate exercise and rest
   e. Techniques for relaxation and stress management

7. Nursing Diagnoses
   a. Acute Pain
   b. Ineffective Coping

8. Home Care
   a. Education of client regarding PMS is physiological response and not a pathological process

b. Active involvement to reduce manifestations

B. Woman with Dysmenorrhea
1. Pain or discomfort associated with menstruation
2. Pathophysiology
   a. Primary (no specific pelvic pathology): excessive production of prostaglandins stimulate uterine contractions causing uterine ischemia and pain; range is mild cramping to severe muscle spasms
   b. Secondary dysmenorrhea related to underlying organic conditions such as endometriosis, fibroid tumors, pelvic inflammatory disease, ovarian cancer
3. Diagnostic Test
   a. Pelvic examination: Pap smear, cervical and vaginal cultures
   b. FSH and LH levels to assess function of pituitary gland; correlated to time of menstrual cycle
   c. Progesterone and estradiol levels: assess ovarian function
   d. Thyroid function tests (T_3 and T_4)
   e. Vaginal or pelvic ultrasonography to detect any space-occupying lesions
   f. CT scan or MRI to detect any pelvic lesions
   g. Laparoscopy: diagnose structural defects and blockages
   h. Dilation and curettage (D&C): obtain tissue for evaluation or relieve dysmenorrhea and heavy bleeding
4. Medications
   a. Analgesics
   b. NSAIDs
   c. Oral contraceptives
5. Complementary Therapies
   a. Similar to those for client with PMS
   b. Local heat on abdomen
6. Nursing Care
   a. Education regarding controlling manifestations
   b. Self-care measures

C. Woman with Dysfunctional Uterine Bleeding (DUB)
1. Vaginal bleeding that is usually painless but abnormal in amount, duration, or time of occurrence
2. Types
   a. Amenorrhea: absence of menstruation
      1. Primary: absence of menses by age 16; 14 if no development of secondary sex characteristics

2. Secondary: absence of menses for at least 6 months in previously menstruating female
   3. Causes may include hormonal imbalances, excessive athletic training, anorexia nervosa, bulimia
   b. Oligomenorrhea: scant menses
   c. Menorrhagia: excessive or prolonged menstruation
   d. Metrorrhagia: bleeding between menstrual periods; Mittleschmerz (midcycle spotting with ovulation) is not considered metrorrhagia
   e. Postmenopausal bleeding: causes include endometrial polyps, endometrial hyperplasia, uterine cancer
3. Predisposing factors include: stress, extreme weight changes, use of oral contraceptives, or intrauterine devices (IUDs), postmenopausal status
4. Causes usually related to hormonal imbalances or pelvic neoplasms, benign or malignant
5. Pathophysiology
   a. Progesterone deficiency with relative estrogen excess results in endometrial hyperplasia
   b. Anovulation (absence of ovulation): associated with both estrogen and progesterone deficiencies
   c. Stress can cause hormonal imbalances
6. Collaborative Care
   a. Careful history and physical exam
   b. Client should keep menstrual history and chart basal body temperature several months to determine if ovulation is occurring
7. Diagnostic Tests
   a. CBC
   b. Thyroid function tests: T_3, T_4, TSH
   c. Endocrine studies to evaluate pituitary and adrenal function
   d. Serum progesterone levels
   e. Pap smear
   f. Pelvic ultrasound to identify cysts
   g. Hysteroscopy to detect abnormalities of uterine cavity
   h. Endometrial biopsy
8. Medications: Hormonal agents including oral contraceptives, progesterone; progestins, oral iron supplements
9. Surgery
   a. Therapeutic D&C (Dilation and Curettage): cervical canal dilated and uterine wall scraped; corrects excessive or prolonged bleeding

b. Endometrial ablation: endometrial layer of uterus is permanently destroyed using laser surgery or electrosurgical resection; menstruation and reproduction are ended
   c. Hysterectomy: removal of uterus when medical management not successful or malignancy present
      1. Premenopausal women ovaries are left in place
      2. Postmenopausal women total or panhysterectomy is performed which involves removal of uterus, fallopian tubes and ovaries
      3. Abdominal approach: incision made in abdomen and offers larger surgical view
      4. Vaginal approach: uterus removed through vagina; no surgical scar
10. Nursing Diagnoses
    a. Anxiety
    b. Sexual Dysfunction
11. Home care: Education and teaching regarding planned therapeutic interventions

III. Structural Disorders
A. Uterine Displacement
   1. Classifications according to direction of displacement
      a. Retroversion: backward tilting of uterus toward rectum
      b. Retroflexion: bending of uterine corpus in backward manner toward the rectum
      c. Anteversion: exaggerated forward tilting of uterus
      d. Anteflexion: folding of uterus upon itself
      e. Prolapse includes classifications
         1. First degree: mild, prolapse involves < half of corpus into vagina
         2. Second degree: moderated descent of entire uterus into vaginal canal; cervix is at introitus
         3. Third degree (procidentia): complete prolapse of uterus outside body with inversion of vaginal canal
         4. Cystocele: herniation of bladder into vagina
         5. Rectocele: herniation of rectum into vagina
   2. Pathophysiology
      a. Displacement can be congenital or acquired

b. Flexion disorders are related to scarring and inflammation of pelvic inflammatory disease (PID), endometriosis, pregnancy, tumors

c. Downward displacement into vagina results with weakened pelvic muscles, attributed to stretching of supporting ligaments and muscles during pregnancy and childbirth

3. Manifestations
   a. Backache
   b. Menorrhagia
   c. Dysmenorrhea
   d. Dysparuenia
   e. Heavy or dragging feeling in pelvis
   f. Stress incontinence
   g. Difficulty moving bowels

4. Collaborative Care
   a. Focus includes identification of cause, correction or minimizing condition, pain relief, prevent or treat infection, and education of the client
   b. Treatment includes teaching the client Kegel exercises to strengthen the weakened pelvic muscles

5. Surgery: Procedures to repair structural disorders
   a. Anterior colporrhapy: repair of cyctocele includes shortening pelvic muscles to tighten support of bladder
   b. Marshall-Marchetti-Krantz: resuspension of urinary bladder in correct anatomic position
   c. Posterior colporrhaphy: repair of rectocele includes shortening pelvic muscles to tight support for the rectum
   d. Prolapsed uterus may be surgically repositioned; in postmenopausal women, hysterectomy is often performed

6. Pessary
   a. Movable device inserted into vagina to provide temporary support for uterus or bladder
   b. Pessary is removed, cleaned, and reinserted

7. Nursing Diagnoses
   a. Stress Incontinence
   b. Anxiety

8. Home Care
   a. Education as determined by client needs including Kegel exercises
   b. Woman who has had surgery for resuspension of bladder may be discharged with indwelling urinary catheter or be instructed in self-catheterization procedure

B. Woman with a Vaginal Fistula
   1. Fistula: abnormal opening or passage between 2 organs or spaces
      a. Vesicovaginal fistula: fistula between urinary bladder and vagina: incontinent leakage of urine through vagina
      b. Rectovaginal fistula: fistula between rectum and vagina; incontinent leakage of stool or flatus through vagina
   2. Causative factors include complication of childbirth, surgery, or radiation therapy for gynecological cancer
   3. Diagnostic Tests
      a. Pelvic examination
      b. Dye instillation into urine and observe for leakage
      c. Urine and vaginal cultures
   4. Treatment
      a. Treatment of any infections
      b. Small fistula may resolve spontaneously or surgical repair
   5. Nursing Care: education regarding importance of careful perineal cleansing including perineal irrigation and sitz baths

IV. Disorder of Female Reproductive Tissue
   A. Woman with Cysts or Polyps
      1. Cyst is fluid-filled sac; polyp is highly vascular solid tumor attached by pedicle or stem; both may occur in vulva, cervix, endometrium, ovaries
      2. Types
         a. Bartholin's gland cysts: common, caused by infection or obstruction of Bartholin's gland
         b. Cervical polyps: common, occur > age 40, develop at vaginal end of cervix
         c. Endometrial cysts and polyps: cysts are caused by endometrial overgrowth and often filled with old blood (called "chocolate cysts") and associated with endometriosis; polyps are intrauterine growths
         d. Ovarian cysts: 2 types which regress spontaneously after several menstrual cycles
            1. Follicular cysts
            2. Corpus luteum cysts
         e. Polycystic Ovary Syndrome (POS): endocrine disorder with insulin resistance; early onset of diabetes type II, breast and endometrial cancer

1. Characterized by numerous follicular cysts
2. Anovulation, elevated estrogen, androgen and LH levels
3. Irregular menses or amenorrhea
4. Hirsutism, obesity and infertility
   3. Diagnostic Tests
      a. Serum hormone levels
      b. Pregnancy test
      c. Laparoscopy to visualize ovarian cysts
      d. Ultrasonography or x-ray examination to differentiate cysts from tumors
   4. Medications
      a. Antibiotics for any infections
      b. Oral contraceptives: regulation of ovarian hormones, treatment of functional ovarian cysts
         1. Clomiphene (Clomid, Serophene) to induce ovulation
         2. Dexamethasone to suppress adrenal androgens
   5. Surgery: Dependent on the condition
      a. Drain abscesses
      b. Remove polyps or cysts
      c. Restore ovulation
   6. Nursing Care
      a. Relieve pain
      b. Follow treatment plan
      c. Prevent recurrence or complications
      d. Educate regarding self-care
B. Woman with Leiomyoma (fibroid tumors)
   1. Description
      a. Benign tumors originating from smooth muscle of uterus
      b. Most common type of pelvic tumor
      c. More common in African American women
      d. Usually develop in uterine corpus as
         1. Intramural: embedded in myometrium present as enlargement of uterus
         2. Subserous: beneath serous lining and project into peritoneal cavity; may compress ureter or bladder
         3. Submucous: beneath endometrial lining and more likely to cause bleeding, infection, necrosis
   2. Cause not understood but associated with estrogen stimulation; most shrink with menopause
   3. Manifestations: large tumors crowd other organs causing
      a. Pelvic pressure
      b. Pain
      c. Dysmenorrhea

d. Menorrhagia and fatigue
e. Urinary urgency and frequency
   4. Diagnostic Tests: include ultrasound and laparoscopy
   5. Treatment
      a. Treatment depends on
         1. Size and location
         2. Severity of manifestations
         3. Client age and childbearing status
      b. Medication
         1. Leuprolide acetate (Lupron) used to decrease size of tumor
         2. Gonadotropin-releasing hormone (GRH) agonists
      c. Surgery
         1. Myomectomy: removal of tumor without removing uterus
         2. Hysterectomy: large tumors and perimenopausal women
         3. Uterine fibroid embolization: catheter guided to fibroid's blood supply and particles used to embolize artery and cause fibroid to slough off
   6. Nursing Care: Educate client to continue with medical follow-up
C. Woman with Endometriosis
   1. Description
      a. Condition in which multiple small implantations of endometrial tissue develop throughout pelvic cavity
      b. Affects 10–15% of women in childbearing age
      c. More common in those postponing childbearing
   2. Risk Factors
      a. Early menarche, short menstrual cycles
      b. Menses > 7 days
      c. Increased menstrual flow and pain
      d. First degree relatives with condition
   3. Cause is unknown; theories include hormonal or inflammatory changes, retrograde menstruation, spread through vascular or lymphatic routes
   4. Pathophysiology
      a. Abnormally located endometrial tissue responds to cyclic ovarian hormonal stimulation and bleeding occurs at sites of implantation
      b. Scarring, inflammation, adhesions develop progressively
      c. Implants regress during pregnancy and atrophy with menopause unless woman takes HRT

    d. Scarring can interfere with ability to conceive

  5. Manifestations

    a. Abdominal and back pain

    b. Dysmenorrhea

    c. Dyspareunia

    d. Infertility

  6. Diagnostic Tests

    a. Pelvic ultrasound

    b. CBC

    c. Laparascopy to visualize implants for definitive diagnosis

  7. Medications

    a. Pain control with NSAIDs, analgesics

    b. Hormonal therapy

      1. Oral contraceptives, progesterone to suppress ovulation

      2. Danazol (Danocrine) to induce amenorrhea and involution of endometrial tissue (causes masculinizing effects)

      3. GRH used to elevate levels of estrogen and progesterone and minimize bleeding

  8. Surgery

    a. Laparoscopy with laser ablation (excision or removal) of endometrial implants

    b. Total hysterectomy for refractory endometriosis

  9. Nursing Care

    a. Pain relief

    b. Education regarding fertility

D. Woman with Cervical Cancer

  1. Cancer of cervix has a decreased death rate since screening with Papanicolaou smear over last 30 years; death rates are twice the rate for African-American women in comparison to white women

  2. Most cervical cancers are squamous cell carcinomas that begin in cervical epithelium

  3. Pathophysiology

    a. Cervical carcinoma in situ (precancerous dysplasia) is associated with human papillomavirus (HPV) infection; strong association with *Chlamydia trachomatis*; precursor lesions spontaneously regress (60%); persist (30%); undergo malignant (10%)

    b. Squamous cell cancers spread by direct invasion to vaginal wall, pelvic wall, bladder, rectum

  4. Manifestations

    a. Preinvasive cancer limited to cervix and rarely causes symptoms

    b. Invasive cancer cause

      1. Bleeding after intercourse or between menstrual periods

      2. Increasing vaginal discharge after cancer progresses

      3. Advanced disease: referred pain in back or thigh, hematuria, bloody stools, anemia, weight loss

  5. Risk Factors

    a. Infection of external genitalia and anus with HPV

    b. First intercourse before 16 years of age

    c. Multiple sex partners or male partners with multiple partners

    d. History of sexually transmitted infections, HIV infection

    e. Smoking, poor nutrition, family history, exposure to DES

  6. Diagnostic Tests

    a. Pap smear primary screening tool

      1. If atypical cells are found, test is repeated

      2. Abnormal cells are described regarding cell changes, such as infectious, inflammatory, atrophic

    b. Colposcopy and cervical biopsy of suspicious area

    c. Loop diathermy technique (loop electrosurgical excision procedure—LEEP) for diagnosis and treatment of dysplastic lesions

    d. MRI or CT scan of pelvis, abdomen, and bones if metastasis suspected

  7. Treatments

    a. Surgery

      1. Laser surgery with colposcopy, if cancer limited to cervical epithelium

      2. Cryosurgery use of probe to freeze tissue causing sloughing for noninvasive lesions

      3. Conization: performed to treat microinvasive carcinoma

      4. Hysterectomy: invasive lesions

      5. Radical hysterectomy: also include fallopian tubes, lymph nodes, and ovaries

      6. Pelvic exenteration: removal of all pelvic contents including bowel, vagina, and bladder, if cancer recurs without lymph involvement; involves creation of ileal conduit and colostomy

b. Radiation therapy: used to treat invasive cancer; includes external beam therapy or intracavity cesium irradiation

c. Chemotherapy may be used if cancer does not respond to other treatments

8. Health Promotion

a. American Cancer Society recommends annual screening with Pap test at age of 18 or when beginning sexual activity

b. After 3 consecutive negative tests may be performed less frequently

c. Nurses educate women regarding risk factors and connection between sexual activities and cervical cancer

9. Nursing Diagnoses

a. Fear

b. Impaired Tissue Integrity

10. Home care

a. Education indicated according to treatment: surgery, radiation, chemotherapy

b. Referral to home health agencies and cancer organizations

E. Woman with Endometrial Cancer

1. Description

a. Most frequently diagnosed pelvic cancer in U.S.

b. Peak incidence in postmenopausal women ages late 50's–early 60's

c. With early diagnosis and treatment 5-year survival rate is about 90%

2. Pathophysiology

a. Tumors are adenocarcinomas, which are slow to grow and metastasize

b. Cancers develop in endometrial lining; endometrial hyperplasia is a precursor

c. Begins in fundus, invades vascular myometrium and spreads throughout reproductive tract

d. Target areas for metastasis are lungs, liver, bone

3. Manifestations

a. Abnormal painless vaginal bleeding: menorrhagia or metrorrhagia; any bleeding in postmenopausal women is abnormal

b. Later: pelvic cramping, bleeding after intercourse, lower abdominal pressure

c. Late: lymph node enlargement, pleural effusion, abdominal masses, ascites

4. Risk Factors

a. Prolonged estrogen stimulation with hyperplasia

b. Obesity

c. Anovulatory menstrual cycles, decreasing ovarian function, estrogen-secreting tumors, estrogen therapy without progesterone

d. Diabetes mellitus, HPT, polycystic ovary disease

e. Use of Tamoxifen

5. Diagnostic Tests

a. Vaginal ultrasonography: determine endometrial thickening: hypertrophy or malignant changes

b. Endometrial biopsy or D&C for definitive diagnosis

c. Transvaginal ultrasound: measure endometrial thickness

d. Laparoscopy to determine stage of cancer

e. X-ray, MRI, bone scan to determine extent of metastasis

6. Treatment (based on results of staging)

a. Surgery: treatment of choice

1. Total abdominal hysterectomy (includes ovaries and fallopian tubes)

2. More advanced cancers may be treated with radical hysterectomy with node dissection

b. Medications

1. Progesterone therapy for recurrent disease, especially for women with well-differentiated tumors

2. Chemotherapy: cisplatin or combination therapy for disseminated disease

c. Radiation: External and internal preoperatively or adjuvant treatment in advanced cases

7. Health Promotion

a. All perimenopausal and postmenopausal women should have annual pelvic examinations

b. High risk groups endometrial biopsies every 2 years

c. Any postmenopausal bleeding should be investigated medically

d. Effective management of diabetes and HPT

8. Nursing Diagnoses

a. Acute Pain related to abdominal hysterectomy surgery

b. Disturbed Body Image

c. Ineffective Sexual Patterns

9. Home Care: Education and support regarding specific treatment and

prognosis, pain control measures, and community resources

F. Woman with Ovarian Cancer
  1. Description
    a. Second most common cancer
    b. Most lethal: 14000 women die in U.S. yearly
    c. Peak age is 40–80
    d. More common in white females than black
  2. Pathophysiology
    a. Most tumors are epithelial; cancer spreads by local shedding of cancer cells into peritoneal cavity and direct invasion of bowel and cancer
    b. Spreads through blood and lymph to involve liver and lungs
    c. Lymph node involvement blocks lymph drainage from abdomen resulting in ascites
  3. Manifestations
    a. Early stages: none; begins as vague, mild indigestion, urinary frequency, abdominal bloating, constipation
    b. Abnormal vaginal bleeding if hormone-stimulating tumor or tumor erodes vaginal wall; pelvic pain
    c. Late-stage: enlarged abdomen with ascites
  4. Risk Factors
    a. Family history: 50% risk if 2 or more close relatives have ovarian cancer; also inherited risks with breast-ovarian cancer syndrome; family cancer syndrome
    b. High-fat diet; use of powders with talc in genital area
    c. Prior use of fertility drugs, HRT, diet low in fruit and vegetables
  5. Collaborative Care
    a. Surgery to determine stage and remove tumor
    b. Often disease is well-advanced prior to diagnosis
  6. Diagnostic Tests
    a. Research being done on test of protein patterns reflecting presence of disease
    b. Laparoscopy: definitive diagnosis and organ involvement
    c. Pap smears: abnormal in 30% of women
    d. CA125: tumor marker highly specific to epithelial ovarian cancer
    e. Transvaginal or abdominal ultrasonography: used to measure ovarian size but cannot differentiate between benign or malignant ovarian masses
    f. CT scan and x-ray to determine areas of metastasis
  7. Treatment
    a. Surgery: treatment of choice
      1. Usually total hysterectomy with bilateral salpingoophorectomy and removal of omentum
      2. May remove one ovary if early disease and woman desires children
    b. Chemotherapy
      1. To achieve remissions; not curative
      2. Treatment includes use of cychophosphamide, cisplatin or paclitaxel (Taxol)
    c. Radiation: External or intracavity implants used palliatively
  8. Nursing Care: Education and support during treatment and dealing with generally poor prognosis
  9. Home Care
    a. Assist with client and family members to have examinations and follow up to find ovarian cancer early and obtain treatment
    b. Long-term use of oral contraceptives may decrease risk
    c. Education regarding follow-up for early signs, but regular pelvic examinations should be done since early cases are asymptomatic
    d. Referrals to home care, hospice, cancer support organizations as need indicates

G. Woman with Cancer of Vulva
  1. Description
    a. Cancer occurs in women aged 60–70
    b. Prognosis depends on degree of involvement, general health status of woman, and ability to withstand treatment
    c. Early disease without lymphatic involvement has 5 year survival rate of 85–90%
    d. Cause is unknown
  2. Pathophysiology
    a. Most cancers are epidermoid or squamous cell carcinomas
    b. Most often labia majora is primary site
    c. Spreads by direct extension and metastasis through lymphatic system
  3. Risk Factors
    a. Associated with sexually transmitted disease, especially HPV

b. Herpes simplex type 2 infection
c. Advanced age, diabetes, history of leukoplakia
4. Manifestations
   a. Lesions found on routine examination or self-examination; lesions have discoloration from white macular patches to red painless sores; may seem to grow outward, inward or appear wart-like
   b. Pruritis; women often have history prolonged vulvar irritation
   c. Late signs include perineal pain and bleeding, dysuria
5. Diagnostic Tests
   a. Biopsy of lesion
   b. Metastasis is investigated with chest x-ray, CT scans, MRI
6. Treatment
   a. Surgery: preferred treatment
      1. Early, noninvasive lesions: laser surgery, cryosurgery, electrocautery
      2. More advanced lesions are treated with vulvectomy: removal of vulva, labias, clitoris and prepuce
      3. Subcutaneous tissue and regional lymph nodes are included with radical vulvectomy if disease is more invasive
   b. Radiation: if lymph nodes are involved
   c. Chemotherapy: to treat metastasis
7. Nursing Care
   a. Dealing with treatment and cancer diagnosis
   b. Client may be at high risk for infection and impaired healing
   c. Skin care, nutrition
V. Disorders of Female Breast
   A. Woman with Benign Breast Disorder
      1. Description
         a. Breast tissue responds to changes in hormones, nutrition, physical and environmental stimuli
         b. Most women notice increased tenderness and lumpiness in breasts prior to menses
         c. Half of women who menstruate regularly find a lump in their breast, 80% of these lumps are not cancerous
      2. Fibrocystic Changes (FCC)
         a. Physiologic nodularity and breast tenderness that fluctuates with menstrual cycle; most common ages 30–50
         b. Two forms

1. Nonproliferative form (cystic or fibrous): do not increase risk for breast cancer
2. Proliferative form (giant cysts or proliferative epithelial lesions): do increase risk for breast cancer
      c. Manifestations
         1. Unilateral or bilateral pain and tenderness in upper outer breast quadrant
         2. May feel lumpy prior to menses
         3. Nipple discharge may be present
         4. Multiple mobile cysts form
         5. Fluid aspirated from cysts may be milky white to yellow, brown or green; blood tinged fluid is suspicious of malignancy
      3. Intraductal Disorders
         a. Intraductal papilloma
            1. Tiny wart-like growth on inside of mammary duct
            2. Causes nipple discharge which can be clear and sticky or bloody
            3. Discharge must be investigated for malignancy
            4. Most common in women in 30–40s
         b. Mammary duct ectasia
            1. Palpable lumpiness beneath areola
            2. Sticky, thick nipple discharge (green, greenish brown, bloody)
            3. Burning and itching around nipple
            4. Occurs in perimenopausal women
            5. Must be investigated for malignancy
      4. Collaborative Care
         a. Confirm diagnosis with testing
         b. Biopsy may be necessary for diagnosis
      5. Diagnostic Tests
         a. Mammography
         b. Analysis of nipple discharge
         c. Ductography
         d. Biopsy
      6. Treatment
         a. Cyst aspiration may relieve pain
         b. Well-fitting bra worn day and night
         c. Eliminating xanthines (coffee, tea, cola, chocolate) from diet
         d. Aspirin, mild analgesics, local heat or cold, vitamin E
         e. Hormonal therapy is controversial in treatment
      7. Nursing Care: Involves education and emotional support through diagnostic and treatment procedures

B. Woman with breast cancer
1. Most commonly occurring cancer in women and second leading cause of death of American women
2. Causes include environmental, hormonal, reproductive, and hereditary factors
3. Pathophysiology
   a. Begins as single transformed cells and is hormone dependent
   b. Classified as noninvasive or invasive
   c. Multiple types of breast cancer
      1. Most are adenocarcinomas and arise in terminal section of breast ductal tissue
      2. Infiltrating ductal carcinoma: most common, 70% of cases
      3. Inflammatory carcinoma of breast is most malignant form
      4. Paget's disease is rare type involving infiltration of nipple epithelium
   d. May metastasize through vascular or lymphatic systems and commonly involves bone, brain, lung, liver, skin, lymph nodes
   e. Staging cancer according to tumor size, lymph node involvement, and whether distant metastasis has occurred
4. Manifestations
   a. Nontender lump in breast (upper outer breast quadrant)
   b. Abnormal nipple discharge, rash around nipple, nipple retraction or change in nipple position, dimpling of skin
   c. Detection on mammography
5. Risk Factors
   a. Age
   b. Genetic factors, family history
   c. History of previous breast cancer, proliferative fibrocystic disease, previous chest radiation as with treatment for Hodgkin's disease
   d. Women who begin menstruating prior to age of 12 and have menopause after age 50
   e. Use of oral contraceptives
   f. Not having children or having after age of 30; not breastfeeding
   g. Using HRT more than 5 years
   h. Obesity, drinking alcohol, high-fat diet
6. Diagnostic Tests
   a. Clinical breast examination by trained health professional
   b. Mammogram: low dose x-ray of breast; some controversy regarding frequency recommendation, but American Cancer Society recommends annual screening starting at age 40
   c. Percutaneous needle biopsy to define cystic masses, fibrocystic changes; specimens for cytologic examination
   d. Stereotactic biopsy using mammography and computer to guide needle
   e. Excisional biopsy removes entire lump
   f. Ductal lavage and nipple aspiration withdraws fluid to analyze abnormal cells
7. Treatment
   a. Determined by
      1. Woman's age
      2. Stage of cancer
      3. Trend includes conservative surgery combined with chemotherapy, hormone therapy or radiation
   b. Medications
      1. Tamoxifen (Nolvadex)
         a. Oral medication that interferes with estrogen activity
         b. Used as
            1. Adjuvant for early stage breast cancer
            2. Treatment of advanced breast cancer
            3. Preventive treatment for women at high risk for breast cancer
      2. Chemotherapy is standard of care for cases with axillary node involvement
      3. Immunotherapy for tumors that are receptive positive
   c. Surgery
      1. Mastectomy: various types
         a. Radical mastectomy: removal of entire breast, underlying chest muscles, and axillary lymph nodes
         b. Simple mastectomy: removal of entire breast
         c. Segmental or lumpectomy: removal of tumor and surrounding margin of breast tissue; not suitable for multicentric neoplasms or large tumors
         d. Modified radical mastectomy: removal of breast and axillary node dissection

2. Axillary node dissection performed with all invasive breast carcinoma as part of staging; may cause lymphedema, nerve damage
3. Sentinel node biopsy: involves injecting radioactive substance or dye into region of tumor and dye is traced to first (sentinel) lymph node which is most likely to contain cancer; if sentinel node is positive more nodes are removed
4. Breast reconstruction
    a. May be performed at time of mastectomy or afterward
    b. Types
        1. Placement of submuscular implant
        2. Use of tissue expander to be followed later by implant
        3. Transposition of muscle and blood supply from abdomen or back
5. Postmastectomy exercises to regain function and promote lymph drainage when sufficient healing has taken place
    a. Wall climbing
    b. Overhead pulleys
    c. Rope turning
    d. Arm swings
   d. Radiation Therapy
    1. Used post surgery to destroy any remaining cancer cells
    2. Used preoperatively to shrink large tumor
    3. Commonly used in combination with lumpectomy
    4. Palliatively for pain control or prevention of fractures
    5. Experimentally used as single concentrated dose during surgery: intraoperative radiotherapy
8. Nursing Care
    a. Breast cancer is not one disease but many
    b. Education and support through diagnosis, treatment
    c. Assist client and family to deal with fear and threat of death
    d. Post operative care and education since short hospital stay
9. Health Promotion: American Cancer Society 2002 recommendations
    a. Monthly breast self-examination (BSE) beginning at age of 20 (after menstrual period)
    b. Clinical breast examination every 3 years age 20–39 years
    c. Clinical breast examination and mammogram yearly at age 40
10. Nursing Diagnoses
    a. Anxiety
    b. Decisional Conflict
        1. Facilitate client contact with treatment team: surgeon, oncologist, plastic surgeon, and other health professionals
        2. Assist verbalizing concerns
    c. Anticipatory Grieving: Educate client that feelings of grief are normal and individual
    d. Risk for Infection: Education regarding postoperative and/or radiation care
    e. Risk for Injury: Education regarding interventions to prevent lymphedema for those with lymph node dissection
    f. Body Image Disturbance
        1. Information regarding reconstructive surgery or breast prosthesis
        2. Appropriate referral to support groups; one to one counseling
11. Home Care
    a. Education regarding self-care needs including continuing with medical care and treatment plan
    b. Diet and rest, postmastectomy exercises
    c. Available support groups and breast cancer resources
    d. Referrals for prostheses, home care, hospice as indicated
VI. Disorders of Sexual Expression
   A. Sexual Response Cycle
    1. Four phases
        a. Excitement
        b. Plateau
        c. Orgasm
        d. Resolution
    2. Nurses should be able to discuss sexual concerns of women and make appropriate referrals
   B. Types
    1. Dyspareunia: painful intercourse
        a. Organic (vaginismus, imperforate hymen, vaginal scarring)
        b. Psychogenic (anxiety-fear-guilt cycle) in nature
    2. Inhibited Sexual Desire
        a. May relate to childhood teaching
        b. Cultural and religious influences

c. Fear of pregnancy or sexually
transmitted disease
d. Depression
3. Orgasmic dysfunction
a. Physiologic (illness, medications
depressing CNS)
b. Psychogenic

C. Nursing Care
1. Discussion, which may include partner,
should include onset, duration, and
context of problem
2. Referral for counseling according to
client's preference

FOCUSED STUDY TIPS

- Create a chronological timeline for a female from birth to 90 years old. Insert on the timeline age-related reproductive disorders for which the female is at risk.
- Compare and contrast disorders of male sexual expression and female sexual expression. Define their similarities and their differences. Describe how these factors affect nursing practice.
- In class, discuss different religious, social, and cultural attitudes toward sexual expression. Identify information useful to nursing practice. Solicit information from male and female classmates.

CASE STUDY

Removal of the lymph nodes during mastectomy puts the client at risk for the long-term complications of lymphedema and infection. Describe in detail what teaching the nurse will do to enable the client to prevent these long-term potential complications.

CARE PLAN CRITICAL THINKING ACTIVITY

When completing a health assessment interview, the client states that she may be going through menopause. What data does the nurse review? What additional questions will the nurse ask? What objective and subjective data must the physician have to determine if menopause has begun? What laboratory tests will aid in the diagnosis?

NCLEX TEST QUESTIONS

1. Which of the following would probably be ordered for the client suffering from primary dysmenorrhea?
a. meperidine hydrochloride (Demerol)
b. propanolol (Inderal)
c. acetaminophen and codeine phosphate (Tylenol #3)
d. naproxen (Naprosyn)

2. Which of the following statements by a female client indicates that instruction in methods to prevent urinary tract infection (UTI) was understood?
a. "I should limit intake of water so I won't need to urinate so often."
b. "I should only wear nylon underpants."
c. "I should drink 8 to 10 glasses of fluid per day."
d. "I should void every 6 hours while I am awake."

3. A 45-year-old client has just been admitted to the hospital for an abdominal hysterectomy following a diagnosis of uterine cancer. Results of lab tests

indicate that the client's WBC is 9800/cu mm. The most appropriate intervention is to
a. call the operating room and cancel the surgery.
b. notify the surgeon immediately.
c. take no action as this is a normal value.
d. call the lab and have the test repeated.

4. The nurse is teaching a postmenopausal client about the use of calcium to prevent the effects of osteoporosis. The client asks, "Why do I have to take vitamin D with my calcium?" Which of the following is the nurse's best response?
a. "Vitamin D prevents osteoporosis."
b. "Vitamin D increases intestinal absorption of calcium."
c. "You are most likely to be deficient in vitamin D."
d. "Calcium and vitamin D supplementation is the only way to prevent osteoporosis."

5. A nurse is caring for a client who has had an abdominal hysterectomy. The client expresses

concern about developing thrombophlebitis. Which nursing intervention will minimize the effects of venous stasis?

a. gentle leg massage

b. a pillow under the knees in a position of comfort

c. sitting at the bedside with the feet flat on the floor

d. early ambulation around the nursing unit

6. A female client experiences swelling from her left shoulder to her fingertips within 24 hours after her left modified radical mastectomy with node dissection. The nurse explains to the client that this results most directly from

a. elevating her left arm on pillows.

b. decreased lymph drainage due to node removal.

c. widespread metastasis of her cancer.

d. blood and fluid collected under her incision.

7. Teaching has been effective when the client diagnosed with endometriosis describes the condition as

a. collections of endometrium outside the uterus.

b. endometrium growing among the myometrium.

c. small, solid tumors within the uterine wall.

d. tiny pockets of blood throughout the pelvis.

8. The client with endometriosis is most likely to make which statement?

a. "I've been alternating between diarrhea and constipation."

b. "I haven't been able to get pregnant in 7 years of trying."

c. "I get urinary tract infections about every other month."

d. "I have green vaginal discharge and pain with intercourse."

9. Which of the following symptoms indicates dysfunctional uterine bleeding?

a. monthly intervals of menstrual bleeding

b. complete irregular menstrual bleeding lasting more than 10 days

c. absence of menarche by age 14

d. pain with ovulation

10. Pelvic inflammatory disease (PID) is an inflammatory condition of the pelvic cavity and may involve the ovaries, Fallopian tubes, vascular system, or pelvic peritoneum. The nurse explains to the client that the most common cause of PID is

a. tuberculosis bacilli.

b. *Streptococcus.*

c. *Staphyloccoccus.*

d. gonorrhea.

CHAPTER 49

NURSING CARE OF CLIENTS WITH SEXUALLY TRANSMITTED INFECTIONS

LEARNING OUTCOMES

After completing this chapter, you will be able to:

- Apply knowledge of normal anatomy, physiology, and assessments when providing nursing care for the client with a sexually transmitted infection (STI) (see Chapter 46).
- Explain the pathophysiology and manifestations of the most common STIs.
- Identify diagnostic tests and collaborative care used to diagnose and treat STIs.
- Describe teaching to prevent and control STIs.
- Use the nursing process as a framework for providing individualized care to clients with STIs.

KEY TOPICS

- Overview of sexually transmitted infections (STIs)
- Infections of the external genitalia
- Urogenital infections
- Nursing care of clients with STIs

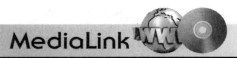

MediaLink

www.prenhall.com/lemone

Additional resources for this chapter can be found on the Student CD-ROM accompanying this textbook, and on the Companion Website at www.prenhall.com/lemone. Click on Chapter 49 to select the activities for this chapter.

CD-ROM
- Audio Glossary
- NCLEX Review

Companion Website
- More NCLEX Review
- Case Study
  Syphilis
- Care Plan Activity
  Gonorrhea

LECTURE OUTLINE

I. Sexually Transmitted Infection (STI)
   A. Definition and Background
      1. Any infection transmitted by sexual contact: vaginal, oral, anal intercourse
      2. Also referred to as sexually transmitted diseases (STDs) or venereal disease (VD)
      3. Epidemic proportions in U.S. and continue to increase worldwide; estimates are more than two-thirds of persons are < age 25

4. Viral STI's are considered incurable (HIV, genital warts, genital herpes)
5. Women and infants are disproportionately affected
      a. Transmission of STI occurs more easily from male to female
      b. Greater risk for complications such as pelvic inflammatory disease (PID) and genital cancers

6. Factors influencing escalating incidence of STI's
   a. Oral contraceptive availability: decreases unplanned pregnancy but not sexually transmitted infections; in fact predisposes women due to less acidic vaginal environment that occurs with oral contraceptives
   b. STIs such as syphilis, herpes simplex virus, chancroid facilitate HIV transmission; immunosuppression of HIV infection potentiates infectious process of other STIs
7. Highest incidence in persons with multiple sexual partners and persons of color living in lower socioeconomic urban areas; this may be related to drug abuse and limited access to medical care
8. All states require reporting of specific STIs to state and federal agencies: syphilis, gonorrhea, AIDS; some states require reporting of Chlamydia

B. Characteristics of STIs
   1. Most can be prevented by use of latex condoms
   2. Transmission occurs during heterosexual and homosexual activities
   3. Sexual partners of infected person must be treated for complete effective treatment
   4. Frequently same client has 2 or more STIs

C. Complications of STIs
   1. PID
   2. Ectopic pregnancy
   3. Infertility
   4. Chronic pelvic pain
   5. Neonatal illness
   6. Death: most serious STI is HIV which is incurable and frequently fatal

D. Prevention and Control
   1. Most effective way to prevent STI is to avoid sexual intercourse with affected partner
   2. Testing for STI including HIV prior to having intercourse
   3. Use of condoms decreases likelihood of transmission of STI
   4. Injecting drug users can decrease risks
      a. Following drug-treatment program
      b. Not sharing needles
      c. Using clean needles
      d. Cleaning used needles with bleach and water
   5. Sex partners of persons with STI should be identified and contacted

II. Types of STI
   A. Vaginal Infections
      1. May be caused by yeasts, protozoa, bacteria
      2. Male partner does not usually have manifestations
      3. Risk Factors
         a. Use of oral contraceptives or broad-spectrum antibiotics
         b. Obesity
         c. Diabetes
         d. Pregnancy
         e. Unprotected sexual activity
         f. Multiple sexual partners
         g. Poor personal hygiene
      4. Preventive Measures
         a. Avoid frequent douching
         b. Avoid wearing nylon underwear and/or tight pants
         c. Avoid unprotected sexual activity
         d. Avoid sex with multiple partners
      5. Pathophysiology
         a. Growth of microorganisms is favored by altered pH
         b. Changes in normal flora
         c. Low estrogen levels
      6. Specific Types of Infections
         a. Bacterial vaginosis (nonspecific vaginitis)
            1. Causative organism: *Gardnerella vaginalis* and others
            2. Manifestations: vaginal discharge: thin, whitish-gray with foul, fishy odor
            3. Complications: PID, preterm labor, premature rupture of membranes, postpartum endometritis
            4. Treatment: client and partner: metronidazole hydrochloride (Flagyl), clindamycin (Cleocin)
         b. Candidiasis (moniliasis, yeast infection)
            1. Causative organism: *Candida albicans*, which is normal vaginal flora, but problematic when multiplies rapidly
            2. Causative factors: increased estrogen levels, antibiotics, diabetes mellitus, fecal contamination
            3. Manifestations: odorless thick, cheesy vaginal discharge; pruritis and irritation of vulva, dysuria, dyspareunia

4. Initial presenting symptom for many HIV-positive women is vaginal candidiasis, which is difficult to treat
5. Miconazole nitrate vaginally
c. Trichomoniasis
   1. Causative organism: *Trichomonas vaginalis* (protozoan)
   2. Males are asymptomatic
   3. Manifestations: frothy green-yellow vaginal discharge with strong odor, itching and irritation of genital area
   4. Complications: premature rupture of membranes
   5. Treatment of client and partner: metronidazole hydrochloride (Flagyl)
7. Diagnostic Tests: Vary with suspected organism
   a. Culture of vaginal secretions, microscopic examination
   b. Glucose tolerance tests, if indicated
   c. HIV screening, if indicated
8. Nursing Care
   a. Education of client regarding control of infection
   b. Education of client regarding treatment of sexual partner
9. Nursing Diagnoses
   a. Knowledge Deficit
      1. Discussion of disease transmission and prevention
      2. Complete treatment to prevent recurrent or reinfection
   b. Acute Pain
B. Infections of External Genitalia
   1. Genital Herpes (herpes simplex genitalis)
      a. Common infectious genital ulceration in U.S.
         1. Considered epidemic
         2. Affects 1 million individuals
         3. Currently incurable
      b. Potential complications for women: infection of newborn during delivery; possibly increased incidence of cervical cancer
      c. Manifestations
         1. Majority of persons are asymptomatic
         2. Incubation period is 3–7 days
         3. Painful red papules appear in genital area
            a. Males: lesions on glans or shaft of penis

b. Females: lesions on labia, vagina, cervix; with anal intercourse lesions appear in and around anus
4. Papules form small painful blisters filled with clear fluid containing virus particles; blisters break, shed virus and create patches of painful ulcers lasting 6 weeks or longer if they become infected; touching blisters will spread infection to other areas of body
5. First outbreak lasts 12 days and recurrent infection episodes last 4–5 days; time in between is called latency in which client is infectious but without symptoms
6. Prodromal symptoms include itching, tingling, burning, throbbing where lesions commonly appear and pain in legs, groin, buttocks; may be more infectious
d. Collaborative Care
   1. Symptom relief
   2. Stopping spread of infection
e. Diagnostic Tests
   1. Presumptive diagnosis based on history and physical exam, including lesions and patterns of recurrence
   2. Definitive diagnosis made by isolation of virus in tissue culture; should be obtained within 48 hours of appearance of blisters
f. Medications
   1. Acyclovir (Zivorax) helps reduce length and severity of first episode and is treatment of choice; orally for 7–10 days until lesions heal, available in intravenous form
   2. Other antivirals used for resistant strains
g. Nursing Diagnoses
   1. Acute Pain: keep lesions clean and dry
   2. Sexual Dysfunction: manage condition and prevent spread to partners, children
   3. Anxiety
      a. Need Pap smears every 6 months
      b. Vaginal delivery if woman without manifestations
h. Home Care
   1. Education to recognize prodromal symptoms and trigger events

2. Abstain from sexual contact from time prodromal symptoms appear until 10 days after all lesions have healed

2. Genital Warts (condyloma acuminatum or venereal warts)
   a. Description
      1. Caused by human papilloma virus (HPV)
      2. Transmitted by all types sexual contact
      3. Incubation period 6 weeks–3 months
      4. Several types
      5. Associated with cervical dysplasia and vaginal, vulvar, penile, and anal cancers
      6. Chronic condition
   b. Manifestations
      1. Most persons have no symptoms
      2. Some have single or multiple painless, cauliflower-like growths in vulvovaginal area, perineum, penis, urethra, anus
      3. Women: may occur in vagina or cervix and is only apparent during pelvic examination
   c. Complications
      1. Obstruction of urethra
      2. Bleeding
      3. Transmission of virus to fetus during pregnancy or delivery (causes respiratory papillomatosis in infant)
   d. Collaborative Care
      1. Treatment directed at wart removal
      2. Relief of symptoms
      3. Teaching to prevent recurrence and future transmission (chronic condition)
   e. Diagnostic Tests
      1. Diagnosis made by clinical appearance or Pap smear specimens
      2. If positive, test for syphilis and gonorrhea
      3. If lesions bleed, biopsies done to rule out malignancies
   f. Treatment
      1. Topical agents include podofilox or podophyllin, which have serious side effects and are contraindicated during pregnancy
      2. Cryotherapy
      3. Electrocautery
      4. Surgical excision
      5. Carbon dioxide laser surgery

   g. Home Care
      1. Educate to follow treatment plan
      2. Prevention of recurrence
      3. Annual Pap smears, since increased risk of cervical cancer

C. Urogenital Infections
   1. Chlamydia
      a. Description
         1. Causative organism is *Chlamydia trachomatis*
         2. Bacterium is viral in nature
         3. Spread through any sexual contact and to neonate through the birth canal
         4. Estimated to affect 3 million persons yearly in U.S.
      b. Chlamydia syndromes include acute urethral syndrome, nongonococcal urethritis, mucopurulent cervicitis, and PID
      c. Manifestations
         1. Incubation period 1–3 weeks; may be present months to years without noticeable symptoms
         2. Males: exhibit dysuria, urinary frequency and discharge; complications include epididymitis, prostatitis, sterility, Reiter's syndrome
         3. Females: invades cervix and ascends into upper reproductive tract showing PID (endometritis, salpingitis, chronic pelvic pain); major cause of infertility and ectopic pregnancy
      d. Diagnostic Tests
         1. Culture of tissue from female endocervix and urethra; male urethra
         2. Test for antibodies to chlamydia
         3. Polymerase chain reaction (PCR) or ligase chain reaction (LCR): specific tests on urine and vaginal swab specimens
      e. Treatment
         1. Men and non-pregnant women: single oral dose of zaithromycin (Zithromax) or doxycycline twice per day for 7 days
         2. Pregnant women: erythromycin or ofloxacin twice per day for 7 days
      f. Home Care
         1. Education regarding treatment
         2. Refer partners for examination and treatment

3. Use of condoms
2. Gonorrhea
   a. Description
      1. Disease caused by Neisseria gonorrhoeae
      2. Spread by direct sexual contact or during delivery through birth canal to newborn
      3. Most reportable communicable disease in U.S.
   b. Pathophysiology
      1. Incubation is 2–8 days post exposure
      2. Targets female cervix, male urethra
      3. Without treatment disseminates to other organs
         a. Males: prostate, epididymis, periurethral glands
         b. Females: PID; neonate: infections affecting eye, upper respiratory tract, anorectal infection
   c. Manifestations
      1. 20% males and 80% females are asymptomatic until advanced disease
      2. Male: dysuria; serous, milky or purulent discharge, regional lymphadenopathy
      3. Female: dysuria, urinary frequency, abnormal menses, increased vaginal discharge, dyspareunia
      4. Anal and rectal gonorrhea: pruritis, mucopurulent rectal discharge, rectal bleeding and pain, constipation
      5. Gonococcal pharyngitis: fever, sore throat, enlarged lymph glands
   d. Complications
      1. PID leading to internal abscesses, chronic pain, ectopic pregnancy, infertility
      2. Neonate: blindness, infection of joints, septicemia
      3. Epididymitis and prostatitis: infertility
      4. Spread of infection to blood and joints
      5. Increased susceptibility to HIV transmission
   e. Collaborative Care
      1. Eradication of pathogen
      2. Prevention of reinfection or transmission
   f. Diagnostic Tests
      1. Analysis of fluid specimen from infected area
      2. Urinalysis
      3. Gram stain of specimen
   g. Treatment
      1. Many strains are penicillin-resistant
      2. Treatment with ciprofloxacin (Cipro), ofloxacin (Flocin), ceftriaxone (Rocephin) intramuscularly
      3. Often client is also treated for chlamydial infection
      4. Sexual partners should also be tested and treated
   h. Home care
      1. Complete prescribed treatment including completing medication and returning for follow-up visit to health care practitioner
      2. Referral of sexual partners
      3. Prevention of recurrence of disease
3. Syphilis
   a. Description
      1. Complex systemic STI caused by spirochete *Treponema pallidum*
      2. May infect almost any body tissue or organ
      3. Transmitted from open lesions during sexual contact
      4. May also be transmitted by infected blood or saliva
   b. Remains problem in many urban centers with high rates among drug users, transients, homeless
   c. Pathophysiology
      1. Incubation period: average 21 days
      2. Spirochete enters through break in skin or mucous membrane, spreads through blood and lymphatic system
      3. Clinical stages
         a. Primary syphilis: appearance of chancre and regional enlargement of lymph nodes; chancre appears at site of inoculation such as genitals, anus, mouth; remains highly contagious
         b. Secondary syphilis: occurs 2 weeks–6 months after initial chancre; skin rash especially on palms of hands and soles of feet; mucous patch in mouth, sore throat, generalized

lymphadenopathy, condyloma in genital area or mouth, flu-like symptoms, alopecia; lasts 2–6 weeks, remains highly contagious

  c. Latent and tertiary syphilis: begins 2 or more years after initial infection; no symptoms and client is not contagious except through blood; one third of persons progress to tertiary stage; with HIV progression is more rapid

  d. Manifestations of late stage syphilis

    1. Rapid onset of infiltrating tumors (gummas) in skin, bones, liver; client usually seeks treatment

    2. Diffuse inflammatory response affecting CNS and cardiovascular system causing irreversible damage

 d. Collaborative Care

  1. Inactivate spirochete

  2. Educate client to prevent reinfection and further transmission

  3. Referral of sexual partners for testing and treatment

 e. Diagnostic Tests: Diagnosis is complex since disease is similar to other conditions

  1. VDRL and RPR: test antibody production; persons with syphilis are positive in 4–6 weeks; not specific to syphilis

  2. FRA-ABS (fluorescent treponemal antibody absorption) test: specific for *T. pallidum* and will confirm diagnosis

  3. Immunofluorescent staining: specimen from lesions is tested and examined for presence of *T. pallidum*

  4. Darkfield microscopy: specimen from chancre examined for presence of *T. pallidum*

 f. Treatment

  1. Primary and secondary syphilis: benzathine penicillin G, intramuscularly single dose

  2. Syphilis of undetermined length: 3 doses of the penicillin at weekly intervals

  3. Doxycycline is used for clients allergic to penicillin

 g. Home care

  1. Education

  2. Referring partners for testing and treatment

  3. Abstaining from sex for minimum 1 month post treatment

  4. Prevent further reinfection or transmission

  5. Follow-up testing

4. Client with Pelvic Inflammatory Disease (PID)

 a. Term used to describe infection of pelvic organs: fallopian tubes (salpingitis); ovaries (oophoritis); cervix (cervicitis), endometrium (endometritis), pelvic peritoneum, pelvic vascular system

 b. Caused by one of several infectious agents; 80% of infections are from gonorrhea or chlamydia and both agents are often present together

 c. Estimates are 1 million cases yearly in U.S.

 d. Complications

  1. Infertility

  2. Ectopic pregnancy

  3. Pelvic abscesses

  4. Chronic abdominal pain

  5. Premature hysterectomy

  6. Depression

 e. Prognosis depends on

  1. Number of episodes

  2. Promptness of treatment

  3. Modification of risk-taking behaviors

 f. Manifestations

  1. Fever

  2. Purulent vaginal discharge

  3. Severe lower abdominal pain

  4. Pain upon cervical movement

  5. Some clients have mild manifestations and do not recognize them

 g. Diagnostic Tests: Clinical picture and history

  1. CBC with differential: shows markedly elevated WBC

  2. Sedimentation rate: increased

  3. Laparoscopy or laparotomy: reveals inflammation, edema, hyperemia of fallopian tubes, generalized pelvic involvement, abscesses, scarring

 h. Medications

1. Combination antibiotic therapy with 2 broad-spectrum antibiotics administered orally, or intravenously if client is acutely ill (doxycycline, cefoxitin, cleocin, gentamicin, ofloxacin, ceftriaxone, Flagyl)
2. Analgesics
3. Intravenous fluids if indicated
   i. Nursing Care: Hospitalized clients are often on bedrest in semi-Fowlers

position to promote drainage and localize infectious process
   j. Nursing Diagnoses
      1. Risk for Injury
      2. Knowledge Deficit
   k. Home Care
      1. Teach client to complete treatment and prevent re-infection
      2. Discuss possibility of infertility

FOCUSED STUDY TIPS

- Almost all clients with STIs experience anxiety. Create a list of specific nursing interventions that minimize anxiety for these clients.
- Visit a Planned Parenthood clinic. Identify resources available for the prevention of STIs. Describe how you will utilize this information in your nursing practice.
- Visit the laboratory of your clinical facility. Ask to review the policy and procedure for reporting STIs. Describe to a classmate why reporting of STIs is necessary for local and national health.

CASE STUDY

J. R., a male client, presents to the clinic complaining of penile discharge, urinary frequency, and burning during urination. What objective and subjective data are necessary for the nurse to obtain to determine risk factors for sexually transmitted infections? What laboratory tests might the physician order?

CARE PLAN CRITICAL THINKING ACTIVITY

Certain behaviors are associated with the transmission of STIs. How would the nurse present these behaviors to a group of teenagers? When asked by this same group how STIs can be prevented, what would be the best response?

NCLEX TEST QUESTIONS

1. A client reports to the clinic with complaints that a sexual partner from last year has been diagnosed with syphilis. The nurse would expect the client to have
   a. had a painless sore that healed and a rash on the palms of the hands.
   b. negative VDRL, negative RPR, and positive FTA-ABS.
   c. night sweats, cough, low-grade fever, and elevated WBC.
   d. vaginal discharge, dysuria, and pain with orgasm.

2. A male client has been diagnosed with *Chlamydia trachomatis* infection. The plan of care should include
   a. instructions to take all of the doxycycline (Vibra-tabs) as ordered.

   b. encouragement to use condoms with most episodes of intercourse.
   c. obtaining the names of sexual contacts if client desires.
   d. teaching of testicular self-exam (TSE) for diagnosis.

3. Which statement indicates that the teaching for the client with genital herpes simplex virus 1 (HSV1) infection has been effective?
   a. "When I feel a recurrence starting, I'll begin taking my medication."
   b. "When I am finished with this medication, I'll be cured of the infection."
   c. "The medication will help me feel better but doesn't affect the infection."
   d. "I'm guaranteed I'll never have another infection if I take my medication."

4. Female clients with *Chlamydia trachomatis* infections will most likely present with which signs and symptoms?

   a. painful blisters on the perineum and high fever of sudden onset

   b. painless craterlike lesion on the labia that lasts 6 weeks

   c. rapidly progressing pruritic rash on labia and buttocks

   d. yellow-green vaginal discharge, dysparunia, pelvic pain

5. The nurse has instituted contact precautions on a client with herpes infection. These precautions would not include

   a. special particulate (HEPA) filter mask.

   b. private room or double room with a client with the same illness.

   c. gloves when providing client care and changing gloves following contact procedures.

   d. gown if clothing will come in contact with the client, environmental surfaces, or items in the room.

6. The client with a new diagnosis of genital herpes simplex virus 2 (HSV2) wants to know how she contracted the infection. The nurse's best answer is based on which of the following?

   a. Inanimate objects can harbor HSV2 for several hours.

   b. HSV2 is found only in the genital tract and not orally.

   c. Sexual contact is the most common mode of transmission.

   d. Immune system suppression is needed to contract the infection.

7. A young male college student came to the clinic suffering from genital herpes. Which of the following interventions would be most appropriate?

   a. Encourage him to maintain bed rest for several days.

   b. Monitor temperature every 4 hours.

   c. Instruct him to avoid sexual contact during acute phases of illness.

   d. Encourage him to use antifungal agents regularly.

8. When counseling a teenager about STDs, what information about genital warts should be included?

   a. Condom use with partners will prevent spread of the virus.

   b. Present partners need to be evaluated for lesions but cannot be assumed to be the source of transmission.

   c. Lesion eradication will decrease viral transmission.

   d. Lesions associated with genital warts may become malignant.

9. A 19-year-old female client is 24 weeks pregnant and has just been diagnosed with herpes genitalis. When developing a counseling plan for her, the nurse should emphasize that she:

   a. must avoid having intercourse for the rest of the pregnancy.

   b. should avoid using condoms to prevent the spread of lesions.

   c. may need a cesarean delivery if the lesions are active at the time of delivery.

   d. should wear undergarments made only of cotton.

10. In planning discharge instructions for a client newly diagnosed with genital herpes, the nurse knows that which of the following drugs would be effective in treating genital herpes?

    a. penicillin (Bicillin)

    b. rifampin (Rifadin)

    c. acyclovir (Zovirax)

    d. ribavarin (Virazole)

Answer Key for NCLEX Test Questions

Chapter 1

1. Answer: c; Cognitive level: Application; Nursing process: Planning; Client need: Safe, effective care environment; Rationale: The ANA standards of clinical nursing practice (1998) allow objective evaluation of nursing licensure and certification, institutional accreditation, quality assurance, and public policy.
2. Answer: a; Cognitive level: Application; Nursing process: Planning; Client need: Safe, effective care environment; Rationale: An advance directive, or living will, is a document in which a client formally states preferences for health care in the event that he or she later becomes mentally incapacitated.
3. Answer: b; Cognitive level: Analysis; Nursing process: Planning; Client need: Safe, effective care environment; Rationale: A major component of the educator role of the nurse today is discharge planning. Discharge planning maintains continuity of care after the client leaves the health care setting. **4.** Answer: d; Cognitive level: Knowledge; Nursing process: Planning; Client need: Health promotion and maintenance; Rationale: HIV infection ranks as the fifth cause of death among 25- to 44-year-olds and is the leading cause of death for black men of this age.
5. Answer: d; Cognitive level: Application; Nursing process: Implementation; Client need: Safe, effective care environment; Rationale: Delegation is carried out when the nurse assigns appropriate and effective work activities to other members of the health care team. The nurse retains accountability for the activities that are performed. **6.** Answer: a; Cognitive level: Analysis; Nursing process: Planning; Client need: Health promotion and maintenance; Rationale: Chronic problems affecting the homeless include high blood pressure, chronic respiratory problems (including tuberculosis), heart and peripheral vascular disorders, and malnutrition. **7.** Answer: d; Cognitive level: Application; Nursing process: Implementation; Client need: Psychosocial integrity; Rationale: The nurse, as a client advocate, must first establish that the client is competent. If the client is competent, the situation, the

alternatives, and the potential harm from refusal must be carefully explained.

Chapter 2

1. Answer: b; Cognitive level: Application; Nursing process: Planning; Client need: Psychosocial integrity; Rationale: Work training programs following illness or injury are examples of a tertiary prevention measure. The tertiary level focuses on stopping the disease process and returning the affected individual to a useful place in society within the constraints of any disability. **2.** Answer: c; Cognitive level: Application; Nursing process: Assessment; Client need: Physiological integrity; Rationale: A handicap is the total adjustment to disability that limits functioning at a normal level (Stanhope & Lancaster, 1995). **3.** Answer: d; Cognitive level: Application; Nursing process: Assessment; Client need: Health promotion and maintenance; Rationale: Tuberculosis and diabetes mellitus are among the leading causes of illness among Native Americans in the United States.
4. Answer: d; Cognitive level: Application; Nursing process: Planning; Client need: Health promotion and maintenance; Rationale: The older adult has increased incidence of chronic illness and increased potential for serious illness or death from infectious illnesses.
5. Answer: c; Cognitive level: Application; Nursing process: Planning; Client need: Health promotion and maintenance; Rationale: Accidents are the leading cause of injury and death in people between ages 15 and 24 (CDC, 1999). **6.** Answer: c; Cognitive level: Application; Nursing process: Planning; Client need: Health promotion and maintenance; Rationale: Cancer is the third leading cause of death in adults between ages 25 and 64 in the United States, with one-third of cases occurring between ages 35 and 64. The middle-aged adult is at risk for cancer as a result of increased length of exposure to environmental carcinogens.
7. Answer: b; Cognitive level: Application; Nursing process: Implementation; Client need: Health

promotion and maintenance; Rationale: Substance abuse is a major cause for concern in the young adult population.

Chapter 3

1. Answer: d; Cognitive level: Application; Nursing process: Planning; Client need: Health promotion and maintenance; Rationale: Medicare is a federal health insurance plan for acute-care needs of the disabled and those over the age of 65. This plan covers some services provided in hospitals, long-term facilities, and the home.   **2.** Answer: d; Cognitive level: Application; Nursing process: Planning; Client need: Safe, effective care environment; Rationale: Medicare is homecare's primary source of funding.   **3.** Answer: b; Cognitive level: Application; Nursing process: Planning; Client need: Safe, effective care environment; Rationale: Age and functional disability are the primary predictors of need for home care services. About half of all home care clients are over the age of 65.   **4.** Answer: a; Cognitive level: Application; Nursing process: Implementation; Client need: Safe, effective care environment; Rationale: When preparing clients for discharge to home, the nurse focuses on safety and survival first.   **5.** Answer: d; Cognitive level: Application; Nursing process: Implementation; Client need: Physiological integrity; Rationale: Most of the home health nurse's time is spent teaching.
6. Answer: d; Cognitive level: Application; Nursing process: Implementation; Client need: Safe, effective care environment; Rationale: Palliative care is alleviating or controlling symptom.

Chapter 4

1. Answer: d; Cognitive level: Application; Nursing process: Assessment; Client need: Physiological integrity; Rationale: Pain is a subjective experience. It is helpful if the client can freely describe his perception of pain.   **2.** Answer: a; Cognitive level: Knowledge; Nursing process: Assessment; Client need: Physiological integrity; Rationale: Constipation is one of the most common side effects of narcotic analgesics and a common problem for the terminally ill client. Poor dietary intake and inactivity also contribute to constipation.   **3.** Answer: c; Cognitive level: Application; Nursing process: Assessment; Client need: Physiological integrity; Rationale: Autonomic responses to pain may result in increased blood pressure, tachycardia, rapid respirations, perspiration, and dilated pupils.   **4.** Answer: d; Cognitive level: Application; Nursing process: Implementation; Client need: Physiological integrity; Rationale: A TENS unit

is most commonly used to relieve chronic benign pain and acute postoperative pain.   **5.** Answer: a; Cognitive level: Analysis; Nursing process: Assessment; Client need: Physiological integrity; Rationale: Precipitating factors of pain include sleep deficits, anxiety, temperature extremes, excessive noise, anxiety, fear, depression, and activity.
6. Answer: d; Cognitive level: Application; Nursing process: Implementation; Client need: Safe, effective care environment; Rationale: Clients may refuse medication, but nurses are responsible for the client's safety, plan of care, and the legal status of their licenses. They must provide and document the teaching provided to the client regarding the actions of the drug and reasons for its use.   **7.** Answer: a; Cognitive level: Application; Nursing process: Planning; Client need: Safe, effective care environment; Rationale: Pain medication needs to be given early in the pain cycle so it will reach its peak effectiveness as the pain begins to intensify.

Chapter 5

1. Answer: c; Cognitive level: Application; Nursing process: Planning; Client need: Physiological integrity; Rationale: Isotonic solutions have the same concentration of solutes as plasma.   **2.** Answer: a; Cognitive level: Application; Nursing process: Assessment; Client need: Physiological integrity; Rationale: Early manifestations of hyperkalemia include diarrhea, colic, anxiety, parethesias, irritability, and muscle tremors and twitching.   **3.** Answer: b; Cognitive level: Application; Nursing process: Planning; Rationale: Acid-base balance is evaluated primarily by measuring arterial blood gases (ABGs). *Blood gases* are utilized to identify acid-base disorders and their probable cause, to determine the extent of the imbalance, and to monitor treatment.   **4.** Answer: d; Cognitive level: Application; Nursing process: Implementation; Client need: Physiological integrity; Rationale: Whenever possible, IV potassium should be administered via a central line because rapid blood flow through central veins dilutes the KCl (potassium chloride) solution, decreasing discomfort of administration.   **5.** Answer: c; Cognitive level: Application; Nursing process: Implementation; Client need: Physiological integrity; Rationale: Continuously monitor ECG when administering IV calcium to clients taking digitalis due to increased risk of digitalis toxicity.   **6.** Answer: c; Cognitive level: Application; Nursing process: Planning; Client need: Physiological integrity; Rationale: Common causes of hypocalcemia are hypoparathryroidism resulting from surgery (parathyroidectomy, thyroidectomy, radical neck dissection, and acute pancreatitis). **7.** Answer: d; Cognitive level: Application; Nursing process: Implementation; Client need: Physiological integrity; Rationale: A fluid challenge may be done to evaluate fluid volume when urine output is low and cardiac or renal function is questionable.

Chapter 6

1. Answer: c; Cognitive level: Application; Nursing process: Assessment; Client need: Safe, effective care environment; Rationale: In shock, there is decreased blood volume to the kidneys. This manifests as decreased urinary output, or oliguria. **2.** Answer: c; Cognitive level: Application; Nursing process: Implementation; Client need: Safe, effective care environment; Rationale: The shock position is necessary to maintain vital signs. The other interventions may be needed also but are not initial interventions. **3.** Answer: d; Cognitive level: Application; Nursing process: Implementation; Client need: Physiological integrity; Rationale: Wound management follows the stabilization of hemodynamics. **4.** Answer: b; Cognitive level: Application; Nursing process: Planning; Client need: Physiological integrity; Rationale: Colloid solutions used to treat shock include 5% albumin, 25% albumin, hetastarch, plasma protein fraction, and dextran. **5.** Answer: c; Cognitive level: Application; Nursing process: Planning; Client need: Safe, effective care environment; Rationale: Colloid products reduce platelet adhesiveness and have been associated with reductions in blood coagulation. Consequently, the client's prothrombin time (PT), INR, platelet count, and activated partial thromboplastin time (PTT) should be monitored when these solutions are administered. **6.** Answer: b; Cognitive level: Application; Nursing process: Implementation; Client need: Physiological integrity; Rationale: Inotropic drugs are given to increase cardiac output and improve tissue perfusion only after fluid volume restoration. **7.** Answer: a; Cognitive level: Application; Nursing process: Implementation; Client need: Physiological integrity; Rationale: When neuro status deteriorates, the airway must be ensured to avoid compromising oxygenation or aspiration. The other goals are appropriate after airway patency is ensured.

Chapter 7

1. Answer: c; Cognitive level: Application; Nursing process: Assessment; Client need: Physiological integrity; Rationale: It is important to have preoperative vital signs so the client's progress can be monitored to ensure that his/her postoperative condition is stable. **2.** Answer: d; Cognitive level: Application; Nursing process: Assessment; Client need: Physiological integrity; Rationale: Tachycardia (increased pulse rate) is a symptom or manifestation of atelectasis, which is a common postoperative respiratory complication. **3.** Answer: b; Cognitive level: Application; Nursing process: Planning; Client need: Physiological integrity; Rationale: Opioid analgesics, such as morphine and meperidine (Demerol) are considered the foundation for managing moderate to severe postoperative pain. They are administered IV in the early postoperative period for greater efficacy. **4.** Answer: c; Cognitive level: Application; Nursing process: Assessment; Client need: Physiological integrity; Rationale: Outpatient surgical centers must verify the client's ability to urinate before discharge from the center. **5.** Answer: d; Cognitive level: Application; Nursing process: Implementation; Client need: Physiological integrity; Rationale: Under normal circumstances, the client should be able to stand at the bedside 8 hours after surgery. Standing facilitates bladder emptying for men. **6.** Answer: c; Cognitive level: Analysis; Nursing process: Evaluation; Client need: Physiological integrity; Rationale: Successful teaching can be validated when the client is able to repeat information. A surgical description is irrelevant, application of the bag is taught postoperatively, and acceptance of the surgery is an emotional issue, not a physical issue. **7.** Answer: c; Cognitive level: Application; Nursing process: Implementation; Client need: Physiological integrity; Rationale: Use of an incentive spirometer postoperatively prevents the common respiratory complication of pneumonia and atelectasis.

Chapter 8

1. Answer: c; Cognitive level: Application; Nursing process: Assessment; Client need: Physiological integrity; Rationale: Along with neutrophils, a shift to the left is common in acute infection. This means that there are more immature neutrophils in circulation than normal, indicating an appropriate bone marrow response. **2.** Answer: c; Cognitive level: Application; Nursing process: Planning; Client need: Physiological integrity; Rationale: Aminoglycosides are bactericidal and especially effective against gram-negative organisms. **3.** Answer c; Cognitive level: Knowledge; Nursing process: Assessment; Client need: Safe, effective care environment; Rationale: Interferon is best described as a by-product of protein metabolism within the body. **4.** Answer: d; Cognitive level: Application; Nursing process: Implementation; Client

need: Physiological integrity; Rationale: Administering vaccines in the dominant arm of clients helps minimize local reactions because use and movement of the arm facilitate absorption of the solution.   **5.** Answer: a; Cognitive level: Application; Nursing process: Assessment; Client need: Physiological integrity; Rationale: Aminoglycosides are ototoxic and nephrotoxic. Frequent monitoring of serum creatinine levels will detect impaired renal functioning.
6. Answer: c; Cognitive level: Application; Nursing process: Implementation; Client need: Psychosocial integrity; Rationale: Frequent visits from family members will minimize social isolation. Keeping a door open or taking items into a strict isolation room is a violation of isolation policy and procedure.
7. Answer: a; Cognitive level: Application; Nursing process: Implementation; Client need: Safe, effective care environment; Rationale: Sensitivity studies identify pharmaceuticals that inhibit the growth of particular microorganisms.

Chapter 9

1. Answer: c; Cognitive level: Application; Nursing process: Implementation; Client need: Safe, effective care environment; Rationale: With a Type I hypersensitivity response, managing the client's airway takes highest priority, followed by maintaining cardiac output.   **2.** Answer: a; Cognitive level: Application; Nursing process: Implementation; Client need: Physiological integrity; Rationale: The blood transfusion needs to be stopped immediately since the client is experiencing early signs of a transfusion reaction. The doctor is notified immediately to provide further treatment.   **3.** Answer: d; Cognitive level: Knowledge; Nursing process: Assessment; Client need: Physiological integrity; Rationale: An autograft, a transplant of the client's own tissue, is the most successful type of tissue transplant. Skin grafts are the most common examples of autografts.   **4.** Answer: c; Cognitive level: Application; Nursing process: Implementation; Client need: Physiological integrity; Rationale: Slow-acting or antirheumatic drugs include Plaquenil and penicillamine. They are prescribed to treat autoimmune disorders when NSAIDs (nonsteroidal anti-inflammatory drugs) and corticosteroids are not effective or well tolerated by the client.   **5.** Answer: d; Cognitive level: Application; Nursing process: Assessment; Client need: Physiological integrity; Rationale: Kaposi's sarcoma is often the presenting symptom of AIDS. It is the most common cancer associated with the disease.   **6.** Answer: a; Cognitive level: Application Nursing process: Planning; Client need: Health

promotion and maintenance; Rationale: Immunotherapy, also called hyposensitization or desensitization, has been shown to be effective in preventing anaphylactic responses to insect venom. With weekly or biweekly subcutaneous injections of the allergen, the client develops IgG antibodies to the allergen that block the allergic IgE-mediated response.
7. Answer: c; Cognitive level: Application; Nursing process: Planning; Client need: Physiological integrity; Rationale: Potential complications of plasmapheresis include those associated with the placement of intravenous catheters, shifts in fluid balance, and alterations of blood clotting.

Chapter 10

1. Answer: d; Cognitive level: Application; Nursing process: Planning; Client need: Health promotion and maintenance; Rationale: The most important step in controlling cancer is educating the public about cancer and the warning signs of many cancers. Early diagnosis and treatment will result.   **2.** Answer: d; Cognitive level: Application; Nursing process: Planning; Client need: Physiological integrity; Rationale: Alkylating agents affect production of DNA, which inhibits cell growth and division.
3. Answer: d; Cognitive level: Application; Nursing process: Implementation; Client need: Physiological integrity; Rationale: The most effective deterrent to nausea and vomiting is to offer high-calorie and high-protein dietary supplements.   **4.** Answer: a; Cognitive level: Application; Nursing process: Planning; Client need: Health promotion and maintenance; Rationale: The cervix is the most common site, and squamous cell cancer is the most common cell type in females.   **5.** Answer: d; Cognitive level: Application; Nursing process: Assessment; Client need: Health promotion and maintenance; Rationale: BSE (breast self-examination) is a primary prevention method for early cancer detection. MRI is utilized to diagnose, and sigmoidoscopy and colonoscopy are useful preventative measures but fall below BSE in prevention priority.   **6.** Answer: d; Cognitive level: Application Nursing process: Implementation; Client need: Physiological integrity; Rationale: A change in bowel or bladder habits is one of the seven early warning signs of cancer.   **7.** Answer: c; Cognitive level: Application; Nursing process: Implementation; Client need: Health promotion and maintenance; Rationale: Avoiding smoking is a primary cancer preventive behavior. Smoking is the cause of approximately 75% of lung cancers in the United States. Tobacco is a known carcinogen.

Chapter 11

1. Answer: d; Cognitive level: Application; Nursing process: Implementation Client need: Psychosocial integrity; Rationale: Sitting quietly at the bedside offers respect for the dying client and allows the dying client to initiate communication of choice.   **2.** Answer: c; Cognitive level: Application; Nursing process: Planning; Client need: Health promotion and maintenance; Rationale: Finding regular relief for caregiving will provide the husband with respite care. The husband's caregiving will be more effective, and his health will improve if regular respite care is provided.
3. Answer: d; Cognitive level: Application; Nursing process: Implementation; Client need: Safe, effective care environment Rationale: Palliative treatment refers to end-of-life care utilizing measures that provide for the optimal comfort of the dying client.   **4.** Answer: c; Cognitive level: Application; Nursing process: Planning; Client need: Psychosocial integrity; Rationale: Gentle massage to improve circulation and shift edema is a comfort measured provided by nurses for clients nearing death. None of the other options are considered comfort measures.   **5.** Answer: b; Cognitive level: Application; Nursing process: Planning; Client need: Psychosocial integrity; Rationale: Kübler-Ross identifies five stages in the grief and loss process; the second stage is identified as denial.   **6.** Answer: a; Cognitive level: Application; Nursing process: Planning; Client need: Safe, effective care environment; Rationale: State nursing practice acts identify the scope of nursing practice for that area.

Chapter 12

1. Answer: c; Cognitive level: Application; Nursing process: Planning; Client need: Psychosocial integrity; Rationale: An acronym that can assist the client in recognizing behaviors that lead to relapse is HALT: **H**ungry, **A**ngry, **L**onely, and **T**ired.   **2.** Answer: b; Cognitive level: Application; Nursing process: Assessment; Client need: Physiological integrity; Rationale: Thiamine depletion is thought to cause the Wernicke-Korsakoff syndrome observed in chronic alcoholics. Severe cognitive impairment is a principal feature of Wernicke's encephalopathy and Korsakoff's psychosis.   **3.** Answer: c; Cognitive level: Application; Nursing process: Assessment; Client need: Physiological integrity; Rationale: Marijuana causes decreased spermatogenesis and testosterone levels in males and decreased levels of follicle-stimulating, luteinizing, and prolactin hormones in females.   **4.** Answer: d; Cognitive level: Application; Nursing process: Assessment; Client need: Safe,

effective care environment Rationale: Health care professionals have a higher risk for opiate abuse than other professionals due to the high accessibility to opiates in their line of work.   **5.** Answer: d; Cognitive level: Application; Nursing process: Assessment; Client need: Health promotion and maintenance; Rationale: Physiologic effects of chronic use of cannabis is airway constriction leading to bronchitis, sinusitis, asthma, and possible cancer.   **6.** Answer: d; Cognitive level: Application; Nursing process: Planning; Client need: Health promotion and maintenance; Rationale: Smoking during pregnancy leads to increased risks for infants such as low birth weight, spontaneous abortions, prenatal mortality, and sudden infant death syndrome.   **7.** Answer: c; Cognitive level: Application; Nursing process: Implementation Client need: Psychosocial integrity; Rationale: Verbalization of feelings in a nonthreatening environment may help the client develop insight.

Chapter 13

1. Answer: c; Cognitive level: Application; Nursing process: Assessment; Client need: Health promotion and maintenance; Rationale: Risk factors for skin cancer include male gender, age over 50, and extended exposure to sunlight.   **2.** Answer: d; Cognitive level: Knowledge; Nursing process: Assessment; Client need: Physiological integrity; Rationale: Melanin, a yellow-to-brown pigment, is present in larger amounts in persons with dark skin color than in those with light skin color.   **3.** Answer: a; Cognitive level: Application; Nursing process: Assessment; Client need: Health promotion and maintenance; Rationale: The equipment necessary for assessment of the skin includes a ruler (to measure lesions), a flashlight (to illuminate lesions), and disposable rubber gloves to protect the examiner.   **4.** Answer: b; Cognitive level: Application; Nursing process: Implementation; Client need: Health promotion and maintenance; Rationale: During a skin assessment, the examination should be conducted in a private room. The client removes all clothing and puts on a gown or drape. The areas to be examined should be fully exposed, but the client's modesty should be protected by keeping other areas covered.   **5.** Answer: c; Cognitive level: Application; Nursing process: Assessment; Client need: Safe, effective care environment; Rationale: Bruises are raised bluish or yellowish vascular lesions. Multiple bruises in various stages of healing suggest abuse.
6. Answer: b; Cognitive level: Application; Nursing process: Assessment; Client need: Health promotion and maintenance; Rationale: In dark-skinned clients, jaundice may be most apparent in the sclera of the

eyes.   **7.** Answer: c; Cognitive level: Application; Nursing process: Implementation; Client need: Physiological integrity; Rationale: Edema is assessed by depressing the client's skin over the ankle. A recording of "3+" indicates obvious pitting with swollen extremities.

Chapter 14

1. Answer: b; Cognitive level: Application; Nursing process: Assessment; Client need: Physiological integrity; Rationale: A Stage II decubitus is an area that is blistered, cracked, or abraded. The area surrounding the damaged skin is also reddened.   **2.** Answer: d; Cognitive level: Application; Nursing process: Implementation; Client need: Physiological integrity; Rationale: Frequent position change promotes circulation to pressure areas; gentle massage promotes circulation to the affected area.   **3.** Answer: c; Cognitive level: Application; Nursing process: Implementation; Client need: Physiological integrity; Rationale: Applying lotions with emollients in a thin layer over the skin and a thick layer over plaques usually helps to relieve pruritus for clients experiencing psoriasis.   **4.** Answer: a; Cognitive level: Comprehension Nursing process: Assessment; Client need: Physiological integrity; Rationale: Herpes zoster virus follows nerve pathways. Discomfort and pain are major problems for clients diagnosed with herpes zoster. Pain may last for weeks to months.
5. Answer: c; Cognitive level: Application; Nursing process: Planning; Client need: Physiological integrity; Rationale: Immunotherapy is a relatively new treatment modality for malignant melanoma.
6. Answer: c; Cognitive level: Application; Nursing process: Planning; Client need: Health promotion and maintenance; Rationale: For the client at risk for pressure ulcers, the goal is prevention. Existing ulcers require collaborative treatment to promote healing and restore skin integrity.   **7.** Answer: b; Cognitive level: Application; Nursing process: Planning; Nursing process: Physiological integrity; Rationale: Secondary bacterial infections may occur in any client with impaired skin integrity; if the client is immunocompromised, the risk is even greater.

Chapter 15

1. Answer: a; Cognitive level: Application; Nursing process: Planning; Client need: Physiological integrity; Rationale: Small, partial-thickness burns are not treated with skin grafting.   **2.** Answer: c; Cognitive level: Application; Nursing process: Implementation; Client need: Physiological integrity; Rationale: High-

calorie, high-protein diets are recommended to replace protein losses and to promote wound healing in clients with severe burns.   **3.** Answer: a; Cognitive level: Application; Nursing process: Implementation; Client need: Physiological integrity; Rationale: Because flexion is the natural resting position of joints and extremities, therapy includes maintaining burned joints in this anti-deformity position.   **4.** Answer: c; Cognitive level: Comprehension Nursing process: Planning; Client need: Physiological integrity; Rationale: Autografting is the process of transplanting skin from one part of the body to another part that has been injured; it is a method of permanent burn-wound closure.   **5.** Answer: c; Cognitive level: Application; Nursing process: Assessment; Client need: Physiological integrity; Rationale: Burn shock occurs within minutes of burn injury, causing fluid shifts from the intracellular and intravascular compartments into the Interstitium. It continues until capillary integrity is restored, usually within 24 to 36 hours following the injury.   **6.** Answer: b; Cognitive level: Application; Nursing process: Assessment; Client need: Physiological integrity; Rationale: Fluid replacement is necessary in all burn wounds that involve >20% Total Body Surface Area (TBSA).   **7.** Answer: c; Cognitive level: Application; Nursing process: Planning; Client need: Physiological integrity; Rationale: Edema in the upper airway peaks within the first 24 to 48 hours of the burn injury.

Chapter 16

1. Answer: a; Cognitive level: Comprehension; Nursing process: Planning; Client need: Physiological integrity; Rationale: Glucocorticoids are released in times of stress. An excess of glucocorticoids in the body depresses the inflammatory response and inhibits the effectiveness of the immune system.
2. Answer: c; Cognitive level: Application; Nursing process: Planning; Client need: Physiological integrity; Rationale: Overproduction of the thyroid hormone thyroxin increases the activity of the thyroid gland.
3. Answer: d; Cognitive level: Knowledge; Nursing process: Assessment; Client need: Physiological integrity; Rationale: Antidiuretic hormone (ADH) is also called vasopressin.   **4.** Answer: d; Cognitive level: Application; Nursing process: Evaluation Client need: Physiological integrity; Rationale: Trousseau's sign and Chvostek's sign are assessment techniques utilized to determine the presence of hypocalcemic tetany.   **5.** Answer: b; Cognitive level: Application; Nursing process: Assessment; Client need: Physiological assessment; Rationale: The two adrenal glands are pyramid-shaped organs that sit on top of the

kidneys. **6.** Answer: c; Cognitive level: Application; Nursing process: Assessment; Client need: Health promotion and maintenance; Rationale: The primary role of thyroid hormones is to regulate metabolism; they are also responsible for growth and development in children. **7.** Answer: b; Cognitive level: Application; Nursing process: Assessment; Client need: Physiological integrity; Rationale: The adrenal cortex secretes several hormones, all corticosteroids.

Chapter 17

1. Answer: d; Cognitive level: Application; Nursing process: Planning; Client need: Health promotion and maintenance; Rationale: Grave's disease is a disorder characterized by hyperthyroidism. **2.** Answer: c; Cognitive level: Knowledge; Nursing process: Assessment; Client need: Physiological integrity; Rationale: Acromegaly is the disorder in adults that results from excessive secretion of growth hormone. **3.** Answer: b; Cognitive level: Comprehension; Nursing process: Evaluation; Client need: Physiological integrity; Rationale: Cushing's syndrome is a chronic disorder in which hyperfunction of the adrenal cortex produces excessive amounts of circulating cortisol or ACTH. **4.** Answer: c; Cognitive level: Application; Nursing process: Planning; Client need: Physiological integrity; Rationale: Serum cortisol levels are decreased in adrenal insufficiency or Addison's disease. **5.** Answer: d; Cognitive level: Application; Nursing process: Assessment; Client need: Physiological integrity; Rationale: A deficit of calcium produces abnormal muscle contractions and is manifested by carpopedal spasms. **6.** Answer: b; Cognitive level: Knowledge; Nursing process: Evaluation; Client need: Physiological integrity; Rationale: Diabetes insipidus is the result of ADH insufficiency. **7.** Answer: a; Cognitive level: Application; Nursing process: Assessment; Client need: Physiological integrity; Rationale: The manifestations of SIADH occur as a result of water retention, hyponatremia, and serum hypoosmolality.

Chapter 18

1. Answer: b; Cognitive level: Application; Nursing process: Implementation; Client need: Safe, effective care environment; Rationale: The ADA (American Diabetes Association) recommends that if a diabetic client is unable to eat the usual foods, liquids and/or soft foods should be substituted. **2.** Answer: a; Cognitive level: Application; Nursing process: Implementation; Client need: Safe, effective care

environment; Rationale: Regular insulin begins to work 1/2 to 1 hour after administration. Meals mu given within 1/2 hour of administration of the insu **3.** Answer: d; comprehension; Nursing process: Assessment; Client need: Physiological integrity; Rationale: Clients with ketoacidosis are assessed for lethargy, which leads to coma as a result of metabolic acidosis. **4.** Answer: d; Cognitive level: Comprehension Nursing process: Planning; Client need: Safe, effective care environment; Rationale: Oral diabetic agents enhance hypoglycemic effects; insulin dosages may need to be reduced when utilizing oral diabetic agents. **5.** Answer: b; Cognitive level: Application; Nursing process: Assessment; Client need: Physiological integrity; Rationale: The diabetic experiencing ketoacidosis will manifest signs and symptoms of progressive dehydration; a goal of treatment of ketoacidosis is rapid rehydration and fluid resuscitation to prevent dehydration. **6.** Answer: d; Cognitive level: Comprehension; Nursing process: Assessment; Client need: Physiological integrity; Rationale: Peripheral neuropathies affect sensory functions. **7.** Answer: d; Cognitive level: Comprehension Nursing process: Planning; Client need: Physiological integrity; Rationale: The retinal capillary structure undergoes alterations in blood flow leading to retinal ischemia and blindness in clients with diabetes.

Chapter 19

1. Answer: a; Cognitive level: Comprehension; Nursing process: Planning; Client need: Physiological integrity; Rationale: Vitamin C is a water-soluble vitamin. **2.** Answer: d; Cognitive level: Application; Nursing process: Assessment; Client need: Health promotion and maintenance; Rationale: The client with inflammation of the gallbladder feels sharp pain on inspiration and stops inspiring. This is called Murphy's sign. (Murphy's sign is characterized by the client's voluntary limitation of inspiration to avoid pain related to gallbladder inflammation.) **3.** Answer: d; Cognitive level: Application; Nursing process: Implementation; Client need: Physiological integrity; Rationale: Of the items listed, orange juice contains the highest concentration of water-soluble vitamins. **4.** Answer: d; Cognitive level: Application; Nursing process: Implementation; Client need: Health promotion and maintenance; Rationale: Lentil rice soup is the best choice for increasing the protein content of the meal without compromising the lifestyle choice of the client. **5.** Answer: c; Cognitive level: Application; Nursing process: Assessment; Client need: Physiological integrity; Rationale: Inadequate caloric intake results in breakdown and loss of proteins that exceeds intake, resulting in a negative nitrogen balance.   **6.** Answer: a; Cognitive level: Application; Nursing process: Implementation; Client need: Physiological integrity; Rationale: Sunflower oil is a source of linoleic acid.   **7.** Answer: c; Cognitive level: Comprehension; Nursing process: Planning; Client need: Physiological integrity; Rationale: The energy value of foods is measured in kilocalories (kcal).

Chapter 20

1. Answer: a; Cognitive level: Application; Nursing process: Planning; Client need: Health promotion and maintenance; Rationale: According to U.S. guidelines, 2640 calories/day is the caloric requirement for a male whose IBW is 165 pounds.   **2.** Answer: d; Cognitive level: Comprehension; Nursing process: Planning; Client need: Physiological integrity; Rationale: VCLD (very low-calorie diets) are generally reserved for clients who are more than 35% overweight.
3. Answer: b; Cognitive level: Application; Nursing process: Assessment; Client need: Health promotion and maintenance; Rationale: Although body weight is most commonly utilized to identify obesity, measures of body fat are more accurate.   **4.** Answer: c; Cognitive level: Application; Nursing process: Planning; Client need: Physiological integrity; Rationale: Cutting caloric intake to 1300 calories/day will help the client to achieve her goal safely. A gradual, slow weight loss of no more than 1 to 2 pounds per week is recommended.   **5.** Answer: d; Cognitive level: Application; Nursing process: Assessment; Client need: Physiological integrity; Rationale: Thyroid disease is a potential cause of obesity. Fatigue, failure to lose weight with calorie reduction, dry skin, and amenorrhea are manifestations of thyroxine deficiency.   **6.** Answer: d; Cognitive level: Application; Nursing process: Assessment; Client need: Physiological integrity; Rationale: Anthropometry is the measurement of skinfold or fatfold thickness at various sites on the body.
7. Answer: c; Cognitive level: Application; Nursing process: Implementation; Client need: Physiological integrity; Rationale: Asking for immediate restoration of diet orders after NPO status of a client is the most aggressive example of a nursing intervention that will prevent the development of malnutrition.

Chapter 21

1. Answer: c; Cognitive level: Analysis; Nursing process: Implementation; Client need: Physiological integrity; Rationale: Normal saline is used for

irrigation of nasogastric tubes to prevent the potential complication of fluid and electrolyte imbalances.
2. Answer: d; Cognitive level: Application; Nursing process: Implementation; Client need: Physiological integrity; Rationale: Helicobacter pylori (H. pylori) is strongly associated with Type B gastritis and ulcers. It is not known exactly how H. pylori leads to ulcer formation.   **3.** Answer: d; Cognitive level: Application; Nursing process: Implementation; Client need: Physiological integrity; Rationale: Severe abdominal pain, increased heart rate, increased respiratory rate, and diaphoresis, along with a rigid abdomen and diminished or absent bowel sounds, are indicative of an ulcer perforation, a lethal complication. Emergency care includes establishing intravenous access for fluid replacement and notifying the physician.   **4.** Answer: a; Cognitive level: Analysis; Nursing process: Application; Client need: Physiological integrity; Rationale: Zantac is an H_2-receptor antagonist that reduces acidity of the stomach environment by blocking the ability of histamine to stimulate acid secretion by the gastric parietal cells. This action reduces both the volume and concentration of hydrochloric acid within the stomach.
5. Answer: a; Cognitive level: Analysis; Nursing process: Assessment; Client need: Physiological integrity; Rationale: Dumping syndrome is the most common problem associated with surgical procedures used to treat peptic ulcer disease. Manifestations include nausea with possible vomiting, and epigastric pain with cramping and borborygmi.   **6.** Answer: c; Cognitive level: Analysis; Nursing process: Implementation; Client need: Physiological integrity; Rationale: People who have experienced trauma are especially at risk for stress-ulcer development. An H_2-antagonist is generally prescribed for prophylactic measures to prevent ulcer formation.   **7.** Answer: d; Cognitive level: Analysis; Nursing process: Implementation; Client need: Physiological integrity; Rationale: Cimetidine (Tagamet) should be administered with meals and at bedtime. Antacids should not be administered 1 hour before or after histamine-blocking drugs to ensure absorption.
8. Answer: b; Cognitive level: Analysis; Nursing process: Implementation; Client need: Physiological integrity; Rationale: Ulcers are more common in people who smoke and who are chronic users of NSAIDs. The client should discuss non-NSAID therapy for the treatment of arthritis.   **9.** Answer: b; Cognitive level: Application; Nursing process: Assessment; Client need: Physiological integrity; Rationale: The inability to inject air into the tube may be an indication of displacement or occlusion. Regular irrigation with water and brushing as indicated will

help maintain tube patency. Blood may be expected following surgery, and the green bile-like substance is expected. **10.** Answer: c; Cognitive level: Application; Nursing process: Planning; Client need: Physiological integrity; Rationale: The presence of nausea may indicate the NG tube is occluded. Instillation of normal saline will determine patency of tube. Other measures may be necessary; however, determining patency of the tube is the priority.

Chapter 22

1. Answer: d; Cognitive level: Analysis; Nursing process: Assessment; Client need: Health promotion and maintenance; Rationale: Careful monitoring of the client with ascites is essential because the treatment for the ascites can cause further fluid shifts and electrolyte imbalances. Weight should be monitored daily using a consistent technique. Intake and output measurement is also important, but daily weight provides the most accurate assessment of fluid status. **2.** Answer: a; Cognitive level: Application; Nursing process: Implementation; Client need: Physiological integrity; Rationale: Physiologic responses to cirrhosis includes decreased production of clotting factors, lack of platelets, and increased fibrinolysis, all leading to altered coagulation. The client should be taught bleeding precautions. **3.** Answer: b; Cognitive level: Application; Nursing process: Implementation; Client need: Physiological integrity; Rationale: Medication to reduce the nitrogenous load is a cornerstone of therapy for cirrhosis, particularly for clients with high blood ammonia levels. Lactulose (Chronulac) suppresses metabolism of ammonia and aids in its elimination through feces. **4.** Answer: a; Cognitive level: Analysis; Nursing process: Assessment; Client need: Physiological integrity; Rationale: Laboratory values expected in pancreatitis include an elevated amylase, elevated lipase, elevated serum glucose, and decreased serum calcium levels. **5.** Answer: a; Cognitive level: Analysis; Nursing process: Planning; Client need: Physiological integrity; Rationale: Because the liver biopsy is an invasive procedure and the risk of bleeding exists, vital signs should be monitored routinely to assess for bleeding or shock. **6.** Answer: a; Cognitive level: Application; Nursing process: Implementation; Client need: Physiological integrity; Rationale: The client is exhibiting signs of airway occlusion and immediate nursing intervention is to release the esophageal balloon to preserve airway function. **7.** Answer: c; Cognitive level: Analysis; Nursing process: Assessment; Client need: Physiological integrity; Rationale: Hypoalbuminemia causes a decrease in plasma colloidal osmotic pressure.

This pressure normally holds fluid in the intravascular compartment; when plasma colloidal osmotic pressure decreases, fluid escapes into extravascular compartments. **8.** Answer: d; Cognitive level: Analysis; Nursing process: Assessment; Client need: Physiological integrity; Rationale: When calcium is deposited in fatty necrotic pancreatic tissue, the serum levels are decreased for 7 to 10 days. Decreased serum calcium levels are a sign of severe pancreatitis. Symptoms of hypocalcemia include numbness around the mouth and tingling in the hands and feet. **9.** Answer: c; Cognitive level: Analysis; Nursing process: Planning; Client need: Physiological integrity; Rationale: Steatorrhea is the presence of fat in the stool. Because of the disturbance in fat metabolism, clients with steatorrhea will need to be administered the fat-soluble vitamins A, D, and E in a water-soluble form. **10.** Answer: a; Cognitive level: Analysis; Nursing process: Assessment; Client need: Physiological integrity; Rationale: Obstruction of the common bile duct may result in bile reflux into the liver, producing jaundice, pain, possible hepatic damage, or pancreatitis.

Chapter 23

1. Answer: c; Cognitive level: Analysis; Nursing process: Assessment; Client need: Physiological integrity; Rationale: In a paralytic ileus, peristalsis stops as a result of either neurogenic or muscular impairment. The bowel lumen remains patent, but contents are not propelled forward. Bowel sounds are assessed to determine peristalsis. **2.** Answer: c; Cognitive level: Analysis; Nursing process: Assessment; Client need: Health promotion and maintenance; Rationale: The appropriate procedure for assessing a client's abdomen is to inspect the abdomen, auscultate bowel sounds, percuss the abdomen, and palpate the abdomen last. **3.** Answer: a; Cognitive level: Analysis; Nursing process: Assessment; Client need: Physiological integrity; Rationale: The pH level affects the enzymatic action of protein digestion. **4.** Answer: a; Cognitive level: Analysis; Nursing process: Assessment; Client need: Physiological integrity; Rationale: Steatorrhea is the presence of fat in the stool, which indicates a malabsorption of fat. **5.** Answer: a; Cognitive level: Application; Nursing process: Implementation; Client need: Physiological integrity; Rationale: Constipation affects older adults more frequently than younger people. The older adult is encouraged to increase dietary fiber intake to provide bulk and keep stools soft and easy to expel. Additionally, six to eight glasses of water per day, unless contraindicated, help maintain stool softness and bulk. **6.** Answer: c; Cognitive level: Analysis; Nursing process: Assessment; Client need: Physiological integrity; Rationale: The correct assessment technique is to inspect, auscultate, and then palpate the abdomen. **7.** Answer: a; Cognitive level: Analysis; Nursing process: Assessment; Client need: Health promotion and maintenance; Rationale: Surgical procedures such as an appendectomy are included in the client's past health history. Occupation and education are included in the client's social history. The father's history of cancer is included as part of the client's risk factors. **8.** Answer: b; Cognitive level: Application; Nursing process: Implementation; Client need: Physiological integrity; Rationale: Soluble fiber adds weight to feces, and insoluble fiber acts as a bulking agent to assist in the elimination process. Fiber also helps draw water into the fecal mass, softening the stool and making defecation easier. **9.** Answer: c; Cognitive level: Analysis; Nursing process: Assessment; Client need: Physiological integrity; Rationale: Early in the course of a mechanical obstruction, borborygmi and high-pitched tinkling bowel sounds are present, reflecting the small bowel's attempts to propel contents past the obstruction. **10.** Answer: b; Cognitive level: Analysis; Nursing process: Evaluation; Client need: Physiological integrity; Rationale: The recommended diet for bowel elimination is one that is low in refined foods, high in dietary fiber, and contains adequate fluids. Foods that have a high-fiber content are recommended. Exercise also promotes bowel elimination.

Chapter 24

1. Answer: b; Cognitive level: Analysis; Nursing process: Assessment; Client need: Physiological integrity; Rationale: Celiac disease is a chronic hereditary disorder characterized by sensitivity to the gliadin fraction of gluten, a cereal protein. Gluten is found in wheat, rye, barley, and oats. **2.** Answer: c; Cognitive level: Analysis; Nursing process: Assessment; Client need: Physiological integrity; Rationale: Foods that increase intestinal gas include salad items such as broccoli, Brussels sprouts, cabbage, cauliflower, corn, cucumbers, peas, radishes, and spinach. Though dairy products may increase intestinal gas, the client consumes milk each day for breakfast, and the increased flatus has only been experienced for the past 3 days. **3.** Answer: a; Cognitive level: Analysis; Nursing process: Evaluation; Client need: Physiological integrity; Rationale: Stress- and anxiety-reducing techniques such as meditation, visualization, and exercise may be helpful because there is a relationship between

irritable bowel syndrome and stress, anxiety, and depression. Cigarette smoking is discouraged. Reducing the intake of fresh fruits and vegetables may reduce excess gas and flatus. **4.** Answer: c; Cognitive level: Analysis; Nursing process: Implementation; Client need: Physiological integrity; Rationale: Extreme thirst, sunken eyeballs, and poor skin turgor indicate dehydration in the client. Measures to promote rehydration should be implemented immediately. Though the client with excessive diarrhea will likely experience electrolyte imbalances, the symptoms are indicative of dehydration. **5.** Answer: b; Cognitive level: Analysis; Nursing process: Assessment; Client need: Physiological integrity; Rationale: A high-fiber diet increases stool bulk, decreases intraluminal pressures, and may reduce spasm. Therefore, a high-residue diet with fiber is recommended for the client with diverticular disease. **6.** Answer: b; Cognitive level: Application; Nursing process: Implementation; Client need: Physiological integrity; Rationale: The management of a client with a bowel obstruction focuses on relieving the obstruction and providing supportive care. A nasogastric tube should be inserted immediately to reduce the possibility of aspiration of feculent vomit. **7.** Answer: c; Cognitive level: Application; Nursing process: Implementation; Client need: Physiological integrity; Rationale: Bulk-forming agents such as psyllium are the only laxatives that are safe for long-term use. The natural fiber creates bulk and draws water into the intestine, softening the stool mass. Psyllium should be mixed with a full glass of cool liquid just prior to administration. **8.** Answer: b; Cognitive level: Analysis; Nursing process: Planning; Client need: Physiological integrity; Rationale: Maintaining an adequate record of intake and output is important since the client is at increased risk for dehydration and hyponatremia because reabsorption of water will be diminished with an ileostomy. **9.** Answer: a; Cognitive level: Analysis; Nursing process: Assessment; Client need: Physiological integrity; Rationale: Continuous mild generalized or upper abdominal pain is the initial characteristic symptom of acute appendicitis. Over the next 4 hours, the pain intensifies and localizes in the right lower quadrant of the abdomen. On palpation, localized and rebound tenderness are noted at McBurney's point, halfway between the umbilicus and the right iliac crest. **10.** Answer: b; Cognitive level: Analysis; Nursing process: Assessment; Client need: Physiological integrity; Rationale: A sudden relief of pain as the distended and edematous appendix ruptures may indicate a perforation. This is a medical emergency and immediate intervention is necessary.

Chapter 25

1. Answer: a; Cognitive level: Analysis; Nursing process: Assessment; Client need: Physiological integrity; Rationale: Creatinine is the end product of creatine phosphate, found in skeletal muscle. Creatinine levels are directly proportional to renal excretory function.   **2.** Answer: b; Cognitive level: Analysis; Nursing process: Assessment; Client need: Physiological integrity; Rationale: The dilution or concentration of urine is largely determined by the action of antidiuretic hormone (ADH), which is secreted by the posterior pituitary gland. ADH causes the pores of the collecting tubules to enlarge, so that increased amounts of water move into the interstitial space. As the end result, water is reabsorbed and urine is more highly concentrated.   **3.** Answer: b; Cognitive level: Analysis; Nursing process: Assessment; Client need: Health promotion and maintenance; Rationale: The female has a short, straight urethra, which allows easier colonization of the bladder by bacteria normally found in the lower gastrointestinal tract.
4. Answer: a; Cognitive level: Application; Nursing process: Implementation; Client need: Physiological integrity; Rationale: The correct technique for a clean catch urine specimen is to have the client collect the urine specimen midstream of the void.   **5.** Answer: b; Cognitive level: Analysis; Nursing process: Evaluation; Client need: Physiological integrity; Rationale: Indication of normal renal perfusion is a urine output of at least 30 mL per hour. Postoperative clients are at risk for hypovolemia and decreased renal perfusion. Careful assessment of hourly urine output is essential for the postoperative client.   **6.** Answer: c; Cognitive level: Analysis; Nursing process: Assessment; Client need: Physiological integrity; Rationale: Normal serum creatinine level for an adult male is 0.6–1.2 mg/dL, and is slightly lower in the older adult. A 1.7 mg/dL level indicates a mild degree of renal insufficiency. Levels > 4 mg/dL indicate a severe impairment of renal function.   **7.** Answer: b; Cognitive level: Application; Nursing process: Implementation; Client need: Physiological integrity; Rationale: At the time the collection begins, the client is asked to void, and that specimen is discarded. All urine following the initial void is collected, including the last void when the 24-hour collection time is complete.   **8.** Answer: b; Cognitive level: Analysis; Nursing process: Evaluation; Client need: Physiological integrity; Rationale: The lungs eliminate or retain carbon dioxide, and the kidneys excrete or form bicarbonate. The kidneys regulate acid-base balance by secreting hydrogen ions into the renal tubular fluid, where it combines with bicarbonate ions

to form carbon dioxide and water. The water is eliminated in the urine, and the carbon dioxide diffuses into tubular cells, combines with water, and forms another bicarbonate and hydrogen ion. On the other hand, the respiratory response to changes in hydrogen ion concentration occurs within a matter of minutes, but is only about 50% to 75% effective.
9. Answer: d; Cognitive level: Analysis; Nursing process: Assessment; Client need: Physiological integrity; Rationale: The normal urine specific gravity is 1.001–1.030. An elevated urine specific gravity may be an indication of fluid volume deficit.   **10.** Answer: a; Cognitive level: Application; Nursing process: Assessment; Client need: Health promotion and maintenance; Rationale: Percussion of the kidneys helps assess pain or tenderness. Palpation is best performed by an advanced practitioner.

Chapter 26

1. Answer: b; Cognitive level: Application; Nursing process: Implementation; Client need: Physiological integrity; Rationale: Pyridium is a urinary tract analgesic that may be used to provide symptomatic relief of the pain, burning, frequency, and urgency associated with UTI. Pyridium does not treat the cause. The drug stains the urine reddish orange.
2. Answer: c; Cognitive level: Analysis; Nursing process: Assessment; Client need: Physiological integrity; Rationale: In older adults, acute urinary tract infection may be manifested by a change in behavior, an acute confusional state, incontinence, or a general deterioration in condition.   **3.** Answer: d; Cognitive level: Analysis; Nursing process: Assessment; Client need: Physiological integrity; Rationale: In an ileal conduit, a segment of ileum is separated from the small intestine and formed into a tubular pouch with the open end brought to the skin surface to form a stoma. The ureters are connected to the pouch. No fecal material should be present in the drainage appliance. The presence of fecal material requires immediate intervention.   **4.** Answer: a; Cognitive level: Analysis; Nursing process: Asssessment Client need: Physiological integrity; Rationale: The client with urinary retention is unable to empty the bladder completely. Catheterization is the immediate priority.
5. Answer: c; Cognitive level: Analysis; Nursing process: Assessment; Client need: Physiological integrity; Rationale: Increased fluid intake is contraindicated in the client with congestive heart failure. All medical history is considered when providing instructions to clients. Other measures may be implemented to help reduce the chance of urinary stones.   **6.** Answer: a; Cognitive level: Analysis;

Nursing process: Assessment; Client need: Physiological integrity; Rationale: Painless hematuria is the presenting sign in 75% of urinary tract tumors. Hematuria may be gross or microscopic. Ureteral tumors may cause colicky pain from obstruction. **7.** Answer: a; Cognitive level: Analysis; Nursing process: Assessment; Client need: Physiological integrity; Rationale: Dribbling after the first several voidings after the removal of a Foley catheter is considered normal. Urgency and frequency may indicate an infection. Urinary retention is abnormal. **8.** Answer: d; Cognitive level: Analysis; Nursing process: Evaluation; Client need: Physiological integrity; Rationale: Measures to reduce acidic urine includes avoiding excess intake of milk products, fruit juices other than cranberry juice, and sodium bicarbonate. Acidity of the urine inhibits bacterial growth. **9.** Answer: b; Cognitive level: Analysis; Nursing process: Assessment; Client need: Physiological integrity; Rationale: The typical presenting symptoms of cystitis include dysuria, urinary frequency and urgency, and nocturia. **10.** Answer: c; Cognitive level: Application; Nursing process: Assessment; Client need: Physiological integrity; Rationale: Urge incontinence is the inability to inhibit urine flow long enough to reach toilet after urge sensation. Stress incontinence is loss of urine associated with increased intra-abdominal pressure. Reflex incontinence is the involuntary loss of moderate volume of urine without stimulus or warning. Functional incontinence results from physiological, environmental, or psychosocial causes.

Chapter 27

1. Answer: a; Cognitive level: Analysis; Nursing process: Implementation; Client need: Physiological integrity; Rationale: Hyperkalemia is an indication of advancing renal failure. Manifestations of hyperkalemia include muscle weaknesses, paresthesias, and EGG changes. Determination of the effects of hyperkalemia on the heart should be performed immediately. **2.** Answer: b; Cognitive level: Analysis; Nursing process: Assessment; Client need: Physiological integrity; Rationale: Phosphate excretion is impaired in renal failure, leading to hyperphosphatemia. Calcium absorption is reduced because of impaired activation of vitamin D, contributing to hypocalcemia. **3.** Answer: c; Cognitive level: Application; Nursing process: Implementation; Client need: Physiological integrity; Rationale: Regulating the intake of fluids, proteins, and other substances normally eliminated in the urine can be effective in slowing or preventing the development

of uremia and other complications of chronic renal failure. **4.** Answer: a; Cognitive level: Analysis; Nursing process: Assessment; Client need: Physiological integrity; Rationale: Salt and water retention lead to edema and put the client at risk for heart failure and pulmonary edema, manifested by dyspnea and neck vein distention. The client in acute renal failure may void up to 400 mL/day. **5.** Answer: b; Cognitive level: Analysis; Nursing process: Evaluation; Client need: Physiological integrity; Rationale: Immunosuppressive drugs are used to minimize the rejection of organ transplants. Consequently, clients receiving immunosuppressive therapy are at increased risk of developing infections and neoplasms. **6.** Answer: b; Cognitive level: Application; Nursing process: Implementation; Client need: Physiological integrity; Rationale: When less dialysate is returned than has been instilled, the client has a net fluid gain. The physician is notified to evaluate the peritoneal catheter and client's fluid volume status. **7.** Answer: c; Cognitive level: Application; Nursing process: Assessment; Client need: Physiological integrity; Rationale: On assessment, a functional arteriovenous fistula has a palpable pulsation and a bruit on auscultation. **8.** Answer: d; Cognitive level: Analysis; Nursing process: Analysis Client need: Physiological integrity; Rationale: Fluid volume excess related to oliguria is the highest priority for the client with acute renal failure. Altered nutrition, activity intolerance, and risk for injury may be applicable and should be included in the client's plan of care. **9.** Answer: b; Cognitive level: Analysis; Nursing process: Assessment; Client need: Physiological integrity; Rationale: Hyperkalemia requires immediate intervention to prevent cardiac disturbances. Kayexalate, a potassium-binding exchange resin, may be administered either orally or by enema. This agent acts to remove potassium from the body by exchanging sodium for potassium, primarily in the large intestine. **10.** Answer: b; Cognitive level: Analysis; Nursing process: Planning; Client need: Physiological integrity; Rationale: The location of the incision in the upper abdominal region combined with the respiratory depressant effects of narcotic analgesics puts the postsurgical nephrectomy client at risk for respiratory complications. To allow optimal respiratory excursion, use semi-Fowler's position or side-lying positions as allowed and tolerated.

Chapter 28

1. Answer: d; Cognitive level: Analysis; Nursing process: Planning; Client need: Health promotion and maintenance; Rationale: Hypertension is a modifiable risk factor for coronary artery disease. Diet, exercise, and medications may be used to control hypertension. Age, gender, and family history are unmodifiable risk factors. **2.** Answer: b; Cognitive level: Analysis; Nursing process: Assessment; Client need: Health promotion and maintenance; Rationale: The palpated pulse of a client with a heart rate of 180 bpm and a blood pressure of 108/50 is expected to be weak and thready due to the tachycardia and decreased cardiac output. **3.** Answer: b; Cognitive level: Analysis; Nursing process: Assessment; Client need: Health promotion and maintenance; Rationale: Family history of heart disease is a nonmodifiable risk factor for coronary artery disease. Diabetes may be managed with diet, exercise, and medication; obesity may be managed with diet and exercise; and hyperlipidemia may be managed with diet, exercise, and medication. **4.** Answer: b; Cognitive level: Analysis; Nursing process: Evaluation; Client need: Physiological integrity; Rationale: Processed foods and canned meats and vegetables are high in sodium content and should be avoided by the client following a low-sodium diet. The client is instructed to monitor all food labels for hidden sodium content and to avoid adding additional salt in cooking. **5.** Answer: b; Cognitive level: Analysis; Nursing process: Assessment; Client need: Health promotion and maintenance; Rationale: Capillary refill that takes more than 3 seconds reflects circulatory compromise, such as hypovolemia. Serum electrolyte and arterial blood gas monitoring are invasive procedures. Echocardiography assesses cardiac structure and function. **6.** Answer: c; Cognitive level: Analysis; Nursing process: Assessment; Client need: Health promotion and maintenance; Rationale: To assess the client's initial rate and rhythm, the apical pulse should be counted for a full 60 seconds. This allows the opportunity to detect any murmurs, extra heart sounds, or dysrhythmias. **7.** Answer: c; Cognitive level: Analysis; Nursing process: Assessment; Client need: Physiological integrity; Rationale: Premature ventricular contractions (PVCs) are ectopic ventricular beats that occur before the next expected beat of the underlying rhythm. They are frequently associated with hypokalemia. **8.** Answer: b; Cognitive level: Analysis; Nursing process: Assessment; Client need: Physiological integrity; Rationale: Stimulation of the sympathetic nervous system results in the release of epinephrine from the adrenal medulla and the release of norepinephrine from the adrenal medulla and the sympathetic fibers. The result is an increased heart rate and increased cardiac output. **9.** Answer: c; Cognitive level: Analysis; Nursing process: Evaluation; Client need: Physiological integrity; Rationale: Animal

products such as red meats, organ meats, eggs, cheese, and dairy products are high in cholesterol. Vegetables, fruits, lean meats, and vegetable oils are recommended for a low-cholesterol diet. **10.** Answer: b; Cognitive level: Analysis; Nursing process: Assessment; Client need: Physiological integrity; Rationale: Orthopnea is experienced when the client cannot breathe effectively when lying down. Since the client is experiencing peripheral edema and orthopnea, he should be evaluated for pulmonary edema.

Chapter 29

1. Answer: b; Cognitive level: Analysis; Nursing process: Evaluation; Client need: Physiological integrity; Rationale: A decreased dietary intake of fat is recommended for the client with coronary artery disease. Butter, partially hydrogenated cooking oils, and fried foods such as chicken nuggets are high in fat. Tuna and other cold-water fish contain high levels of omega-3 fatty acids, which help decrease serum triglycerides, total serum cholesterol, and blood pressure. Dietary fiber should not be reduced. **2.** Answer: d; Cognitive level: Analysis; Nursing process: Implementation; Client need: Physiological integrity; Rationale: Nitroglycerin decreases myocardial work and oxygen demand through venous and arterial dilation, which in turn reduces preload and afterload. Hypotension is a common effect of nitroglycerin, therefore the blood pressure should be reassessed before administering further nitroglycerin. **3.** Answer: c; Cognitive level: Analysis; Nursing process: Evaluation; Client need: Physiological integrity; Rationale: A low-fat, low-cholesterol diet is suggested to help control cholesterol levels and promote weight reduction. Much saturated fat is found in whole-milk products and in red meats. Eating nonfat dairy products, fish, and poultry as primary protein sources can achieve a significant reduction in cholesterol. **4.** Answer: d; Cognitive level: Analysis; Nursing process: Evaluation; Client need: Physiological integrity; Rationale: Beta-blocking agents such as propranolol block the cardiac-stimulating effects of norepinephrine and epinephrine, preventing anginal attacks by reducing heart rate, myocardial contractility, and blood pressure, thus reducing myocardial oxygen demand. Abrupt withdrawal of beta-blocking agents may precipitate arrhythmias, hypertension, or myocardial ischemia. **5.** Answer: a; Cognitive level: Analysis; Nursing process: Evaluation; Client need: Physiological integrity; Rationale: Sublingual nitroglycerin is the drug of choice to treat acute anginal attacks. It acts within 1 to 2 minutes, decreasing myocardial work and oxygen demand. Headache is a common side effect of nitrate therapy. **6.** Answer: d; Cognitive level: Analysis; Nursing process: Planning; Client need: Physiological integrity; Rationale: Adenosine (Adenocard) is a Class V drug used to decrease conduction through the AV node and to treat supraventricular tachycardias. Lidocaine is used primarily in treating ventricular dysrhythmias. Bretylium is used primarily to treat ventricular tachycardia and ventricular fibrillation. Epinephrine is a vasopressor given for bradycardia. **7.** Answer: a; Cognitive level: Analysis; Nursing process: Assessment; Client need: Health promotion and maintenance; Rationale: Atrial fibrillation is characterized by disorganized atrial activity without discrete atrial contractions. A difference between apical and radial pulse rates indicates a decreased cardiac output. Other manifestations include hypotension, shortness of breath, fatigue, and angina. **8.** Answer: b; Cognitive level: Analysis; Nursing process: Implementation; Client need: Physiological integrity; Rationale: Bed rest is maintained as ordered after the cardiac catheterization in order to allow the arterial access site to seal, reducing the risk of bleeding. Immobilizing the affected extremity in an extended position helps reduce the risk of bleeding or thrombus formation. The client requires a clear explanation to promote understanding of the risks of getting up out of bed before the prescribed amount of time. **9.** Answer: c; Cognitive level: Analysis; Nursing process: Assessment; Client need: Physiological integrity; Rationale: Sudden cardiac death is usually caused by ventricular fibrillation and cardiac arrest. Nearly half of cardiac arrest victims die before reaching the hospital. **10.** Answer: a; Cognitive level: Analysis; Nursing process: Planning; Client need: Physiological integrity; Rationale: The client with atrial fibrillation is at high risk for thromboembolic formation. Embolization of organ systems is a constant threat and the incidence of stroke is high. Coumadin is the drug of choice as prophylaxis against clot formation.

Chapter 30

1. Answer: d; Cognitive level: Analysis; Nursing process: Assessment; Client need: Health promotion and maintenance; Rationale: Lung fields are assessed for the presence of rales, indicating pulmonary congestion. The client with pulmonary congestion may develop orthopnea, difficulty breathing while lying down. **2.** Answer: a; Cognitive level: Analysis; Nursing process: Assessment; Client need: Health promotion and maintenance; Rationale:

Dependent tissues tend to be most affected because of the effects of gravity; edema develops in the feet and legs of an upright client, in the sacrum of one who is reclining. **3.** Answer: c; Cognitive level: Analysis; Nursing process: Evaluation; Client need: Physiological integrity; Rationale: Jugular vein distention is a clinical manifestation of pulmonary edema and fluid volume excess. Non-distended jugular veins would be the most indicative sign of improvement in response to therapy. **4.** Answer: d; Cognitive level: Analysis; Nursing process: Assessment; Client need: Physiological integrity; Rationale: Furosemide (Lasix) is a loop diuretic. Diuretics promote potassium excretion, increasing the risk of hypokalemia—3.2 mEq/L is below the normal 3.5–5.0 mEq/L. **5.** Answer: d; Cognitive level: Analysis; Nursing process: Assessment; Client need: Physiological integrity; Rationale: The client with acute pulmonary edema usually presents with classic manifestations of the disorder. Dyspnea and shortness of breath are acute and severe; the client is highly anxious. Cyanosis is present, the skin is cool and clammy. A productive cough with pink, frothy sputum is also present. An S_3 gallop and crackles are auscultated. **6.** Answer: a; Cognitive level: Application; Nursing process: Implementation; Client need: Physiological integrity; Rationale: Digoxin (Lanoxin) exerts electrophysiologic effects on the heart by slowing conduction through the AV node and is often given for congestive heart failure and atrial fibrillation. This decreases the heart rate and reduces oxygen consumption. Digoxin is not administered if the pulse rate is below 60. **7.** Answer: c; Cognitive level: Analysis; Nursing process: Planning; Client need: Physiological integrity; Rationale: Signs of pacemaker malfunction include dizziness, fainting, fatigue, weakness, chest pain, or palpitations. **8.** Answer: d; Cognitive level: Application; Nursing process: Implementation; Client need: Physiological integrity; Rationale: For the client with pericarditis, elevate the head of the bed to Fowlers or high Fowler's position and assist the client to assume a position of comfort. This position reduces the work of breathing and decreases chest pain due to pericarditis. **9.** Answer: d; Cognitive level: Analysis; Nursing process: Assessment; Client need: Physiological integrity; Rationale: The client's apical pulse is at an acceptable rate. Pacing occurs when the client's heart rate falls below the pacemaker's programmed rate. The demand pacemaker for this client is set to pace at 72. **10.** Answer: a; Cognitive level: Analysis; Nursing process: Implementation; Client need: Physiological integrity; Rationale: Classic manifestations of aortic stenosis are dyspnea on exertion, angina pectoris, and exertional syncope. The client should be cautioned against strenuous exercise, stairs, or lifting to avoid syncope.

Chapter 31

1. Answer: b; Cognitive level: Analysis; Nursing process: Assessment; Client need: Health promotion and maintenance; Rationale: The blood pressure is measured with the client supine, legs dangling, and again with the client standing, obtaining each 2 minutes apart. A change from the horizontal to upright position normally causes a slight decrease (5 to 10 mm) in systolic blood pressure; the diastolic blood pressure normally remains unchanged or rises slightly. **2.** Answer: d; Cognitive level: Analysis; Nursing process: Planning; Client need: Physiological integrity; Rationale: Family history, ethnicity, and gender are nonmodifiable risk factors for hypertension. Obesity, stress, nutrition, and occupation are modifiable risk factors. **3.** Answer: b; Cognitive level: Analysis; Nursing process: Assessment; Client need: Physiological integrity; Rationale: Abdominal aortic aneurysms are associated with arteriosclerotic occlusive disease and hypertension. Most clients with abdominal aneurysms are asymptomatic but on examination have a pulsating mass in the mid and upper abdomen and a bruit over the mass. In clients who do complain of pain, the most common site is in the midabdominal or lower back area. **4.** Answer: b; Cognitive level: Analysis; Nursing process: Assessment; Client need: Health promotion and maintenance; Rationale: A positive Homan's sign, which is pain in the calf when the foot is dorsiflexed, may indicate the presence of a deep vein thrombosis; however, any condition of the calf can elicit a positive Homan's sign. The Homan's sign should not be assessed on a client suspected of having a deep vein thrombosis because there is a risk of detaching the thrombus from the vein wall as the calf muscle contracts. **5.** Answer: c; Cognitive level: Analysis; Nursing process: Planning; Client need: Physiological integrity; Rationale: Raynaud's disease is a condition in which the digital arteries respond excessively to vasospatic stimuli. Treatment focuses on keeping the hands warmed and free from injury, as wounds heal slowly and infections may be difficult to manage because of poor arterial circulation. **6.** Answer: d; Cognitive level: Analysis; Nursing process: Assessment; Client need: Health promotion and maintenance; Rationale: The peripheral pulses of the lower extremities are palpated at the popliteal, dorsalis pedis, and posterior tibia areas. **7.** Answer: d; Cognitive level: Analysis; Nursing process:

Assessment; Client need: Health promotion and maintenance; Rationale: The assessment findings suggest peripheral arteriosclerosis (peripheral vascular disease) in which there is a decreased blood supply to tissues, most commonly seen in the lower extremities. **8.** Answer: c; Cognitive level: Analysis; Nursing process: Assessment; Client need: Health promotion and maintenance; Rationale: A capillary refill greater than 3 seconds indicates compromised circulation. Notification of the primary health care provider for further evaluation is warranted. **9.** Answer: c; Cognitive level: Analysis; Nursing process: Assessment; Client need: Health promotion and maintenance; Rationale: Intermittent claudication is usually described as a cramping or aching sensation in the calves of the legs, the thighs, and the buttocks. Pain is a primary manifestation of peripheral arterial arteriosclerosis and arterial occlusion. **10.** Answer: b; Cognitive level: Analysis; Nursing process: Assessment; Client need: Health promotion and maintenance; Rationale: Varicose veins occur most commonly in the lower extremities. When the client is standing, the veins in the legs resemble vertical columns and must withstand the full force of venous blood pressure. On assessment, dilated veins beneath the skin of the upper and lower leg are obvious.

Chapter 32

1. Answer: c; Cognitive level: Analysis; Nursing process: Assessment; Client need: Physiological integrity; Rationale: The partial thromboplastin time (PTT) is increased in all types of hemophilia. People with hemophilia A are most often treated with factor VIII. Therapeutic results of the administration of factor VIII are evident by a decreased partial thromboplastin time (PTT). **2.** Answer: c; Cognitive level: Analysis; Nursing process: Assessment; Client need: Physiological integrity; Rationale: Because vitamin B_{12} is important for proper neurologic functioning, the client with a vitamin B_{12} deficiency may experience paresthesias (altered sensations, such as numbness or tingling) in the extremities. **3.** Answer: b; Cognitive level: Analysis; Nursing process: Planning; Client need: Physiological integrity; Rationale: Parenteral iron preparations are administered by deep gluteal intramuscular (IM) injection, using the Z-track method to decrease local irritation. **4.** Answer: a; Cognitive level: Analysis; Nursing process: Assessment; Client need: Physiological integrity; Rationale: During conditions causing decreased oxygen tension in the plasma, the hemoglobin S within the RBCs causes them to elongate, become rigid, and assume a crescent or sickle shape. As a result, the sickled cells tend to

clump together and obstruct capillary blood flow, causing ischemia and possible infarction of surrounding tissue, which causes pain. **5.** Answer: c; Cognitive level: Analysis; Nursing process: Planning; Client need: Physiological integrity; Rationale: Idiopathic thrombocytopenia purpura (ITP) is an acute or chronic condition in which the destruction of platelets is greatly accelerated. It is believed that the body's immune system destroys the platelets. Coricosteroids, such as prednisone, are administered to suppress the immune response and decrease the number of antibodies targeted for the platelets. Platelet transfusion may be necessary if platelet production has been impaired and the client is bleeding. Chemotherapy and bone marrow transplants are not included in the treatment of ITP. **6.** Answer: a; Cognitive level: Analysis; Nursing process: Implementation; Client need: Physiological integrity; Rationale: In the client with leukemia, changes in the white blood cells impair the immune system. This decreases the client's resistance to infection. The nurse must institute measures to prevent exposure to known or potential sources of infection. Because of the low platelet count, intramuscular injections and aspirin products are contraindicated. **7.** Answer: b; Cognitive level: Analysis; Nursing process: Planning; Client need: Physiological integrity; Rationale: Clients at risk for bleeding are instructed to avoid shaving with a regular razor, avoid rectal temperatures, and consume a diet that promotes the prevention of straining during bowel movement. Teeth may be brushed with a soft toothbrush or sponge. **8.** Answer: a; Cognitive level: Analysis; Nursing process: Implementation; Client need: Physiological integrity; Rationale: Gastrointestinal side effects of oral iron preparations may be decreased by taking iron with food.
9. Answer: b; Cognitive level: Analysis; Nursing process: Planning; Client need: Physiological integrity; Rationale: Parenteral replacement of vitamin B_{12} is required for clients with malabsorption disorders or who lack intrinsic factor. Parenteral replacement therapy must be continued for life to prevent recurring anemia. **10.** Answer: a; Cognitive level: Analysis; Nursing process: Assessment; Client need: Physiological integrity; Rationale: Bleeding from the puncture site is the most serious complication of a bone marrow biopsy or aspiration. After the procedure, the nurse applies pressure to the puncture site for 5 to 10 minutes and assesses vital signs. The puncture site is monitored for bleeding and infection for 24 hours.

Chapter 33

1. Answer: d; Cognitive level: Analysis; Nursing process: Planning; Client need: Physiological integrity;

Rationale: Vitamin K counteracts the effects of sodium warfarin (Coumadin) and should be limited in the client's diet. **2.** Answer: a; Cognitive level: Analysis; Nursing process: Assessment; Client need: Health promotion and maintenance; Rationale: Essential hypertension is a disorder characterized by blood pressure that persistently exceeds 140/90 mm Hg. A blood pressure reading of 132/84 indicates that the modifications have been successful. **3.** Answer: a; Cognitive level: Analysis; Nursing process: Planning; Client need: Physiological integrity; Rationale: Captopril (Capoten) is an antiotensin-converting enzyme (ACE) inhibitor that has potassium-sparing effects. The client should be encouraged to have potassium levels monitored and to avoid frequent consumption of foods that are high in potassium, such as oranges and bananas. **4.** Answer: d; Cognitive level: Analysis; Nursing process: Assessment; Client need: Physiological integrity; Rationale: Before administering sodium warfarin (Coumadin), the PT and INR results should be assessed by the physician to determine the need for discontinuation of the medication if excessively prolonged results are obtained. **5.** Answer: a; Cognitive level: Application; Nursing process: Implementation; Client need: Physiological integrity; Rationale: The nurse collaborates with the client in the management of hypertension by focusing on modifiable risk factors. Weight loss and sodium restriction are realistic goals that the client can be encouraged to achieve.
6. Answer: d; Cognitive level: Analysis; Nursing process: Assessment; Client need: Physiological integrity; Rationale: Uncontrolled moderate and severe essential hypertension may lead to cardiovascular complications, including left ventricular hypertrophy and congestive heart failure as a result of increased workload of the left ventricle. **7.** Answer: c; Cognitive level: Analysis; Nursing process: Assessment; Client need: Physiological integrity; Rationale: Intermittent claudication is manifested by complaints of pain and cramping after short periods of activity and is relieved by rest. **8.** Answer: b; Cognitive level: Analysis; Nursing process: Planning; Client need: Physiological integrity; Rationale: Protamine sulfate is the antidote for heparin and should be readily available for use during a continuous heparin infusion. Vitamin K is the antidote for Coumadin. Calcium gluconate is not administered as an antidote for bleeding caused by heparin.
9. Answer: b; Cognitive level: Application; Nursing process: Implementation; Client need: Health promotion and maintenance; Rationale: Marfan syndrome is inherited as an autosomal dominant trait. Therefore, there is a 2:4 chance of an offspring having the disorder if the partner doesn't have the disorder.

10. Answer: c; Cognitive level: Analysis; Nursing process: Planning; Rationale: The client should be acknowledged for the healthy lifestyle activities, while emphasizing that the strong family history of hypertension should not be ignored. Early detection is the key to prevention of complications.

Chapter 34

1. Answer: d; Cognitive level: Analysis; Nursing process: Assessment; Client need: Health promotion and maintenance; Rationale: Upon percussion of the lungs, hyperresonance is heard in clients with chronic asthma and pneumothorax **2.** Answer: a; Cognitive level: Application; Nursing process: Assessment; Client need: Physiological integrity; Rationale: When a client has respiratory difficulty in a supine position, the client is said to have orthopnea. Often, clients will use numerous pillows at night to avoid lying flat in bed. Determining the degree of respiratory difficulty during sleep may provide clues to actual or potential health problems. **3.** Answer: d; Cognitive level: Application; Nursing process: Assessment; Client need: Health promotion and maintenance; Rationale: When adventitious breath sounds are auscultated, the nurse should ask the client to deep breathe and cough to clear the airways. Following this activity, the nurse reassesses the lungs to better evaluate the lung sounds detected. **4.** Answer: a; Cognitive level: Analysis; Nursing process: Assessment; Client need: Physiological integrity; Rationale: Cheyne-Stokes respirations are a regular crescendo–decrescendo pattern with increasing then decreasing rate and depth of respirations followed by a period of apnea. **5.** Answer: c; Cognitive level: Analysis; Nursing process: Assessment; Client need: Physiological integrity; Rationale: A shift of the trachea to the left with no breath sounds on the right indicates a tension pneumothorax, which is a medical emergency requiring immediate intervention to preserve respiration and cardiac output. **6.** Answer: a; Cognitive level: Analysis; Nursing process: Assessment; Client need: Physiological integrity; Rationale: Wheezing, which is continuous, musical sounds, may be heard in clients with bronchitis, emphysema, and asthma, as well as other disorders causing problems with obstruction to airflow out of the lungs. **7.** Answer: c; Cognitive level: Analysis; Nursing process: Assessment; Client need: Physiological integrity; Rationale: A deviation of the trachea is indicative of a tension pneumothorax. This is a medical emergency which requires immediate intervention to preserve respiration and cardiac output. **8.** Answer: a; Cognitive level: Analysis; Nursing process: Assessment; Client need: Physiological

integrity; Rationale: Wheezing occurs as a result of obstruction to airflow out of the lung. A reduction in the degree of wheezing may indicate an improvement in the airway and reduction of obstruction; or it may indicate a worsening in the obstruction to airflow out of the lung. **9.** Answer: a; Cognitive level: Analysis; Nursing process: Assessment; Client need: Physiological integrity; Rationale: Pulmonary hypertension is a condition in which the pulmonary arterial pressure is elevated to an abnormal level. The normal mean arterial pressure in the pulmonary system is 12 to 15 mmHg. Chronic hypoxemia associated with chronic lung diseases may lead to pulmonary hypertension. **10.** Answer: d; Cognitive level: Analysis; Nursing process: Assessment; Client need: Health promotion and maintenance; Rationale: The nurse counts the infant's respiratory rate for 1 full minute because the rhythm of respirations is irregular in infants. Infants up to the age of 4 months are obligatory nose breathers.

Chapter 35

1. Answer: b; Cognitive level: Analysis; Nursing process: Assessment; Client need: Physiological integrity; Rationale: Daytime fatigue and sleepiness are clinical manifestations of sleep apnea. Frequent rest periods and activities should be planned according to how the client feels. **2.** Answer: c; Cognitive level: Analysis; Nursing process: Planning; Client need: Physiological integrity; Rationale: The client with posterior nasal packing is hospitalized because of potential respiratory complications. Hypoxemia is common. Monitoring respiratory function and oxygen saturation is the priority. **3.** Answer: c; Cognitive level: Analysis; Nursing process: Assessment; Client need: Physiological integrity; Rationale: The most notable manifestations of laryngeal cancer in the glottis are hoarseness or a change in the voice because the tumor prevents complete closure of the glottis during speech. **4.** Answer: d; Cognitive level: Analysis; Nursing process: Implementation; Client need: Physiological integrity; Rationale: Airway dryness leads to irritation of the nasal membranes. Supplemental humidity and an adequate fluid intake to maintain moist mucous membranes are suggested to reduce airway dryness. **5.** Answer: a; Cognitive level: Application; Nursing process: Implementation; Client need: Physiological integrity; Rationale: Anterior bleeding can usually be managed by simple first-aid measures such as applying pressure on the anterior portion of the nose for 5 to 10 minutes and applying ice packs to the nose and forehead to cause vasoconstriction. If applying pressure does not control the bleeding, pharmacological interventions, nasal packing, or surgery may be necessary. **6.** Answer: b; Cognitive level: Analysis; Nursing process: Implementation; Client need: Physiological integrity; Rationale: Most decongestant preparations cause vasoconstriction, which reduces the inflammation and edema of nasal mucosa and relieves nasal congestion. However, the duration of their effect is short, followed by vasodilation and rebound congestion.

7. Answer: c; Cognitive level: Analysis; Nursing process: Implementation; Client need: Physiological integrity; Rationale: The position that best promotes lung expansion and effective airway clearance is the Fowler's position. **8.** Answer: a; Cognitive level: Analysis; Nursing process: Planning; Client need: Safe, effective care environment Rationale: Clients with infectious diseases should be isolated if at all possible. In this case, the most appropriate assignment for the client is with another client with the same diagnosis. **9.** Answer: d; Cognitive level: Analysis; Nursing process: Planning; Client need: Physiological integrity; Rationale: Swelling is a potential complication following a tonsillectomy. Application of an ice collar reduces swelling and provides a mild analgesic effect. **10.** Answer: a; Cognitive level: Analysis; Nursing process: Assessment; Client need: Health promotion and maintenance; Rationale: Influenza is a highly contagious viral respiratory disease transmitted by airborne droplet and direct contact. Type A and type B influenza viruses are responsible for periodic epidemics, and Type C is more likely to be endemic, causing periodic minor illness.

Chapter 36

1. Answer: b; Cognitive level: Analysis; Nursing process: Planning; Client need: Physiological integrity; Rationale: Isoniazid and rifampin are known to cause vitamin B_6 and niacin deficiencies. Pyridoxine (vitamin B_6) is administered concurrently. **2.** Answer: c; Cognitive level: Analysis; Nursing process: Assessment; Client need: Physiological integrity; Rationale: The underlying pathology in adult respiratory distress syndrome (ARDS) is acute lung injury. The clinical manifestations of ARDS typically appear 24 to 48 hours after the initial insult. Dyspnea and tachypnea are the initial manifestations. **3.** Answer: c; Cognitive level: Analysis; Nursing process: Planning; Client need: Physiological integrity; Rationale: Planning; related to pulmonary hypertension in the cardiac client is essential because the pulmonary artery pressure rises significantly high before a systolic increase occurs. **4.** Answer: b; Cognitive level: Analysis; Nursing process: Implementation; Client need: Safe, effective care environment Rationale: As many as 75% to 80% of people with acquired immune

deficiency syndrome (AIDS) develop an opportunistic pneumonia caused by *Pneumocystis carinii,* a common parasite found worldwide. Immunity to P. carinii is nearly universal, except in immunocompromised people. **5.** Answer: d; Cognitive level: Analysis; Nursing process: Planning; Client need: Physiological integrity; Rationale: Pancreatic insufficiency and impaired enzyme secretion lead to maldigestion of proteins, carbohydrates, and fats. Pancreatic enzymes (pancrelipase) are taken with meals. **6.** Answer: a; Cognitive level: Analysis; Nursing process: Planning; Client need: Physiological integrity; Rationale: Increasing daily fluid intake promotes a decrease in viscosity of respiratory secretions. Chest physiotherapy and respiratory treatments promote airway clearance. **7.** Answer: b; Cognitive level: Analysis; Nursing process: Assessment; Client need: Safe, effective care environment Rationale: The client with active tuberculosis is placed in a private room with air flow control that prevents air within the room from circulating into the hallway or other rooms. A negative flow room and multiple fresh-air exchanges dilute the concentration of droplet nuclei within the room and prevent their spread to adjacent areas. **8.** Answer: a; Cognitive level: Analysis; Nursing process: Implementation; Client need: Physiological integrity; Rationale: Chronically high blood levels of carbon dioxide diminish the stimulatory effect of CO_2 on breathing; these clients are at increased risk for sleep apnea and for respiratory arrest with oxygen administration because oxygen suppresses their hypoxic drive to breathe. **9.** Answer: c; Cognitive level: Analysis; Nursing process: Assessment; Client need: Physiological integrity; Rationale: Clinical manifestations of pulmonary embolism include anxiety and apprehension, tachycardia, tachypnea, and diaphoresis. **10.** Answer: d; Cognitive level: Analysis; Nursing process: Assessment; Client need: Physiological integrity; Rationale: The water level should fluctuate with respiratory effort; if it does not, the system may not be patent or intact. Frequent assessment of the system is important to ensure appropriate functioning.

Chapter 37

1. Answer: b; Cognitive level: Analysis; Nursing process: Assessment; Client need: Health promotion and maintenance; Rationale: The normal capillary refill time is < or = 3 seconds. Longer capillary refill time may suggest compromised circulation caused by the leg cast. **2.** Answer: b; Cognitive level: Analysis; Nursing process: Assessment; Client need: Health promotion and maintenance; Rationale: The Romberg's test is performed by asking the client to stand with the feet together and eyes closed. There should be minimal swaying for up to 20 seconds. A positive Romberg's test may be seen in ataxia. **3.** Answer: a; Cognitive level: Analysis; Nursing process: Assessment; Client need: Health promotion and maintenance; Rationale: The immediate assessment is to determine the presence of pedal pulses. Sensation and bony deformities are included in the assessment. However, determining the presence of compromised circulation is the priority. **4.** Answer: b; Cognitive level: Application; Nursing process: Implementation; Client need: Health promotion and maintenance; Rationale: Ischemia-induced corpopedal spasm (positive Trousseau's sign) may be elicited by inflating a blood pressure cuff on the upper arm to 20 mm Hg above systolic blood pressure for 2 to 5 minutes. A positive Trousseau's sign is indicative of hypocalcemia. A positive Chvostek's sign is also indicative of hypocalcemia. Kernig's sign does not assess calcium status. **5.** Answer: b; Cognitive level: Analysis; Nursing process: Assessment; Client need: Physiological integrity; Rationale: An excess in serum magnesium depresses skeletal muscle contraction and central nervous system activity. A deficit results in increased irritability of the nervous system, cardiac dysrhythmias, and peripheral vasodilatation. **6.** Answer: c; Cognitive level: Analysis; Nursing process: Assessment; Client need: Physiological integrity; Rationale: During the remodeling phase, excess callus is removed and new bone is laid down along the fracture line. Eventually, the fracture site is calcified, and the bone is reunited. **7.** Answer: b; Cognitive level: Analysis; Nursing process: Assessment; Client need: Health promotion and maintenance; Rationale: Scoliosis is a lateral S-shaped curvature of the spine. Because of the asymmetry of the shoulders, clothing may not hang straight on the affected individual. Females usually complain that their dresses "don't hang straight." or that the hem of clothing is uneven. **8.** Answer: c; Cognitive level: Analysis; Nursing process: Assessment; Client need: Health promotion and maintenance; Rationale: Heberden's nodes and Bouchard's nodes are hard, nontender nodules on the dorsolateral parts of the distal and proximal interphalangeal joints, respectively. They are common in arthritis. **9.** Answer: c; Cognitive level: Analysis; Nursing process: Assessment; Client need: Physiological integrity; Rationale: Assessment; findings commonly associated with a hip fracture are pain and shortening of the affected lower extremity and external rotation. **10.** Answer: c; Cognitive level: Analysis; Nursing process: Assessment; Client need: Physiological integrity; Rationale: The systemic effects of hypercalcemia include neuromuscular changes secondary to decreased excitability at the myoneural junction. This results in muscle weakness and fatigue.

Deep tendon reflexes are hypoactive. Tetany and a positive Trousseau's sign are associated with hypocalcemia.

Chapter 38

1. Answer: b; Cognitive level: Analysis; Nursing process: Assessment; Client need: Physiological integrity; Rationale: Fat emboli occur when fat globules lodge in the pulmonary vascular bed or peripheral circulation. Fat embolism syndrome (FES) is characterized by neurologic dysfunction, pulmonary insufficiency, and a petechial rash on the chest, axilla, and upper arms. Long bone fractures and other major trauma are the principle risk factors for fat emboli. **2.** Answer: a; Cognitive level: Analysis; Nursing process: Assessment; Client need: Physiological integrity; Rationale: For traction to be successful, countertraction is necessary. In most instances, the countertraction is the client's weight. To ensure adequate countertraction, the weights must hang freely and must not touch the floor. The client's foot should not touch the footboard, and the foot of the bed should not be elevated. The rope should move freely through the pulleys. **3.** Answer: a; Cognitive level: Analysis; Nursing process: Implementation; Client need: Physiological integrity; Rationale: Stump dressings increase venous return, decrease edema, and help shape the stump for a prosthesis. With an above-knee amputation, a figure-eight bandage is started by wrapping the bandage around the waist and bringing the bandage down over the stump and back up around the hips. **4.** Answer: d; Cognitive level: Analysis; Nursing process: Assessment; Client need: Physiological integrity; Rationale: A hot spot palpated on a cast may indicate the presence of underlying infection. The nurse reports this finding immediately in order for appropriate interventions to be implemented. **5.** Answer: c; Cognitive level: Analysis; Nursing process: Assessment; Client need: Physiological integrity; Rationale: An early manifestation of compartment syndrome is pain. The peripheral pulse may be normal or decreased. **6.** Answer: c; Cognitive level: Analysis; Nursing process: Assessment; Client need: Physiological integrity; Rationale: Cold, pale fingers on a casted extremity indicate compromised circulation. Immediate intervention is necessary to preserve the limb. **7.** Answer: a; Cognitive level: Analysis; Nursing process: Implementation; Client need: Physiological integrity; Rationale: The client is instructed to avoid crossing legs, bending at hips, and sitting on low toilet seats to prevent dislocation of the hip. Walking and other exercises prescribed by the physician are encouraged. **8.** Answer: c; Cognitive level: Application; Nursing process: Implementation;

Client need: Physiological integrity; Rationale: A pillow should be placed between the client's legs when the client is at rest in bed or turning. A pillow supports the legs and prevents adduction during turning. Adduction may dislocate the hip.   **9.** Answer: c; Cognitive level: Analysis; Nursing process: Evaluation; Client need: Physiological integrity; Rationale: An ice pack should be applied continuously to the injured extremity for 24 hours. Ice causes vasoconstriction and decreases the pooling of blood in the injured area. Ice may also numb the tender area. The extremity is elevated 2 inches above the heart to promote venous return and decrease edema. Padding the ice pack with a towel or cloth promotes comfort. Some swelling is expected.   **10.** Answer: c; Cognitive level: Analysis; Nursing process: Planning; Client need: Physiological integrity; Rationale: Long bone fractures and other major traumas are the principle risk factors for fat emboli and are the major cause of death after fracture of a long bone.

Chapter 39

1. Answer: d; Cognitive level: Application; Nursing process: Implementation; Client need: Health promotion and maintenance; Rationale: Modifiable risk factors for osteoporosis include calcium deficiency, estrogen deficiency, smoking, and sedentary lifestyle. Unmodifiable risk factors include genetic factors, age, race, and female gender.
2. Answer: c; Cognitive level: Analysis; Nursing process: Planning; Client need: Health promotion and maintenance; Rationale: A regular exercise plan and adequate diet maintaining a daily calcium intake as prescribed are the priority discharge planning needs. Physical activity and weight-bearing exercises prevent or slow bone loss. Safety factors, medication administration, and proper body mechanics are important and should be included in the client's plan of care.   **3.** Answer: c; Cognitive level: Analysis; Nursing process: Evaluation; Client need: Health promotion and maintenance; Rationale: Duchenne's muscular dystrophy is inherited as a recessive single gene defect on the X chromosome (a sex-linked recessive disorder) and is, therefore, transmitted from the mother to the male children.   **4.** Answer: a; Cognitive level: Analysis; Nursing process: Assessment; Client need: Physiological integrity; Rationale: The most common complaint is localized pain of the commonly affected bones. The pain is usually due to metabolic bone activity, secondary degenerative osteoarthritis, fractures, or nerve impingement.   **5.** Answer: b; Cognitive level: Analysis; Nursing process: Evaluation; Client need:

Health promotion and maintenance; Rationale: Exercise programs are helpful in the management of low back pain provided that the client begins gradually and increases activity gradually as the recovery process continues.   **6.** Answer: b; Cognitive level: Analysis; Nursing process: Assessment; Client need: Physiological integrity; Rationale: Osteomyelitis is an infection of the bone. Clinical manifestations include high temperature with chills, abrupt onset of pain, and tachycardia, as well as swelling, erythema, and warmth at the involved site.   **7.** Answer: a; Cognitive level: Analysis; Nursing process: Planning; Client need: Health promotion and maintenance; Rationale: The discussion and teaching should focus on modifiable risk factors of sedentary occupation, lack of exercise, obesity, smoking, and sitting for long periods. The client's race, gender, and genetic factors are unmodifiable risk factors.   **8.** Answer: d; Cognitive level: Analysis; Nursing process: Assessment; Client need: Physiological integrity; Rationale: Serum alkaline phosphatase is the most frequently used laboratory test for Paget's disease. Alkaline phosphatase is an enzyme located in the plasma membrane of osteoblasts. As the disease progresses in clients with untreated Paget's disease, a steady rise of the phosphatase can be expected.   **9.** Answer: c; Cognitive level: Analysis; Nursing process: Implementation; Client need: Physiological integrity; Rationale: Pathologic fractures may occur at the tumor site because bone destruction can weaken the area. Supporting the limbs during position changes is one measure to reduce the incidence of fractures. Restricting activities is not necessary, pivot transfers are contraindicated, and calcium supplement does not prevent pathologic fractures.   **10.** Answer: a; Cognitive level: Analysis; Nursing process: Evaluation; Client need: Health promotion and maintenance; Rationale: The Milwaukee brace is worn 23 hours a day and is removed only for bathing. A smooth cotton T-shirt should be worn under the brace to reduce irritation of skin surfaces.

Chapter 40

1. Answer: c; Cognitive level: Analysis; Nursing process: Assessment; Client need: Physiological integrity; Rationale: In decorticate posturing, the upper arms are close to the sides; the elbows, wrists, and fingers are flexed; the legs are extended with internal rotation; and the feet are plantar flexed.   **2.** Answer: a; Cognitive level: Analysis; Nursing process: Assessment; Client need: Physiological integrity; Rationale: Maintenance of an awake and alert status is depended on the proper functioning of the reticular activating system and both cerebral hemispheres. **3.** Answer: b; Cognitive level: Analysis; Nursing process: Assessment; Client need: Physiological integrity; Rationale: Normal doll's eye movements are reflexive movements of the eyes in the opposite direction of head rotation; they are an indicator of brain stem function. An abnormal response is noted when the eyes fail to turn together and eventually remain fixed in the midposition as the head is turned. **4.** Answer: a; Cognitive level: Analysis; Nursing process: Assessment; Client need: Physiological integrity; Rationale: Decerebrate posturing is an abnormal posture in which the neck is extended, with the jaw clenched; the arms are pronated, extended, and close to the sides; the legs are extended straight out; and the feet are plantar flexed. **5.** Answer: d; Cognitive level: Analysis; Nursing process: Assessment; Client need: Physiological integrity; Rationale: With the client supine, the knees and hips are flexed, then the knee is straightened. With meningeal irritation, the client will be unable to extend the leg due to excessive pain. **6.** Answer: a; Cognitive level: Analysis; Nursing process: Assessment; Client need: Health promotion and maintenance; Rationale: Cranial nerve III is the oculomotor nerve. Testing pupillary light reflexes assesses this cranial nerve. **7.** Answer: c; Cognitive level: Analysis; Nursing process: Assessment; Client need: Physiological integrity; Rationale: Cranial nerve VIII is the acoustic nerve. Tinnitus may indicate toxicity to the acoustic nerve. **8.** Answer: b; Cognitive level: Analysis; Nursing process: Assessment; Client need: Physiological integrity; Rationale: A stiff, sore neck may indicate meningeal irritation. The client complaining of a stiff, sore neck, along with complaints of fever, nausea, chills, and malaise, should be evaluated immediately for the potential of meningitis. **9.** Answer: a; Cognitive level: Analysis; Nursing process: Assessment; Client need: Health promotion and maintenance; Rationale: Chvostek's sign is performed by tapping on the side of the client's face. Twitching of the nose or lip is a positive finding and indicates hypomagnesemia. **10.** Answer: b; Cognitive level: Analysis; Nursing process: Assessment; Client need: Physiological integrity; Rationale: The functional areas of the temporal lobe include smell, hearing, and auditory association.

Chapter 41

1. Answer: c; Cognitive level: Analysis; Nursing process: Planning; Client need: Physiological integrity; Rationale: Thickened and/or soft foods should be served in order to minimize the risk of aspiration.

Liquids are more easily aspirated. Prior to offering food or fluids, the gag reflex and ability to chew and swallow should be assessed. **2.** Answer: b; Cognitive level: Analysis; Nursing process: Planning; Client need: Physiological integrity; Rationale: Organisms can enter the body through the pin insertion site. Careful monitoring of the pin site for redness, edema, and drainage is essential. **3.** Answer: d; Cognitive level: Analysis; Nursing process: Assessment; Client need: Physiological integrity; Rationale: Clients with cord injuries at C-3 or above have paralysis of the respiratory muscles and cannot breathe without a ventilator **4.** Answer: c; Cognitive level: Application; Nursing process: Implementation; Client need: Physiological integrity; Rationale: Manifestations of autonomic dysreflexia include pounding headache, bradycardia, hypertension, flushed, warm skin with profuse diaphoresis above the lesion, and pale, cold, and dry skin below the lesion. The immediate intervention is to elevate the client's head to increase pooling of blood in the lower extremities and decrease venous return, thus decreasing blood pressure. Assess blood pressure every 2 to 3 minutes while at the same time assessing for stimuli that initiated the response, such as a full bladder. **5.** Answer: b; Cognitive level: Analysis; Nursing process: Assessment; Client need: Physiological integrity; Rationale: Aphasia, the inability to use or understand language, occurs as a result of left hemisphere CVA. Left-sided hemiplegia and neglect syndrome occurs with right hemisphere CVA. **6.** Answer: a; Cognitive level: Analysis; Nursing process: Planning; Client need: Physiological integrity; Rationale: Immediate postoperative assessment includes monitoring for signs of nerve-root compression by assessing leg strength, ability to wiggle toes, and ability to detect touch. Temperature, along with other vital signs, level of pain, and dressing are all important assessments to be implemented and should be included in the client's plan of care. **7.** Answer: c; Cognitive level: Application; Nursing process: Implementation; Client need: Physiological integrity; Rationale: Headache and stiff neck in a client with a known arteriovenous malformation may indicate intracranial hemorrhage due to vessel rupture. Immediate intervention is necessary to preserve neurological function and life. **8.** Answer: b; Cognitive level: Analysis; Nursing process: Assessment; Client need: Safe, effective care environment Rationale: The nurse assist the client by standing on the client's affected side and supporting the client by grasping the safety belt in the middle of the client's back or placing one arm around the client's waist and the other arm around the inferior aspect of the client's upper arm. **9.** Answer: a; Cognitive level: Application; Nursing process: Implementation; Client need: Physiological integrity; Rationale: A lumbar puncture is performed to inject the dye for a myelogram. Headaches may occur following a lumbar puncture. Encourage increased intake of oral fluids to replace the fluids withdrawn during the examination. Analgesics are administered as prescribed for postexamination pain, headache, or muscle spasm. **10.** Answer: d; Cognitive level: Analysis; Nursing process: Assessment; Client need: Physiological integrity; Rationale: A Swan-Ganz catheter is used for assessing cardiovascular status on a continuous basis.

Chapter 42

1. Answer: b; Cognitive level: Analysis; Nursing process: Planning; Client need: Physiological integrity; Rationale: Maintaining the head of the bed 30 degrees and maintaining alignment to avoid hyperextension or exaggerated neck flexion facilitates venous drainage from the cerebrum. **2.** Answer: a; Cognitive level: Application; Nursing process: Planning; Client need: Physiological integrity; Rationale: Teaching the importance of taking all medication until completely gone is a major focus of client teaching because some clients may think it is acceptable to stop the medication as soon as they feel better. **3.** Answer: c; Cognitive level: Application; Nursing process: Implementation; Client need: Physiological integrity; Rationale: The immediate priority during a seizure is protection from injury. The client's bedrails should be padded. Tongue blades are contraindicated during a seizure, and the client should be placed in the side-lying position to avoid aspiration. Oxygen may be administered once the client resumes breathing. **4.** Answer: c; Cognitive level: Application; Nursing process: Implementation; Client need: Physiological integrity; Rationale: Dexamethasone may be administered to reduce cerebral edema in the client with a head injury. The use of dexamethasone may lead to gastric ulcers, therefore prophylactic cimetidine is routinely ordered concurrently with dexamethasone. **5.** Answer: c; Cognitive level: Analysis; Nursing process: Assessment; Client need: Physiological integrity; Rationale: With an epidural hematoma, the client may lose consciousness with the initial injury, then have a brief lucid period before the level of consciousness rapidly declines from drowsiness to coma as the hematoma expands. **6.** Answer: d; Cognitive level: Analysis; Nursing process: Assessment; Client need: Physiological integrity; Rationale: Mannitol is an osmotic diuretic that draws fluid out of brain cells by increasing the osmolality of the blood. Increased diuresis indicates that the mannitol is exerting the desired effect. **7.** Answer: d; Cognitive level:

Analysis; Nursing process: Assessment; Client need: Physiological integrity; Rationale: Often, the earliest manifestations of a change in intracranial pressure are alterations in the level of consciousness and respirations. Assess vital sign trends because vital signs alone do not correlate well with early deterioration. **8.** Answer: d; Cognitive level: Analysis; Nursing process: Assessment; Client need: Physiological integrity; Rationale: Cushing's triad represents the brain stem's final effort to maintain cerebral perfusion. Manifestations are increased mean arterial pressure (MAP), increased pulse pressure, and bradycardia. **9.** Answer: d; Cognitive level: Application; Nursing process: Planning; Client need: Physiological integrity; Rationale: Clients sustaining a closed head injury should be monitored closely for the development of manifestations of increased cerebral edema leading to increased intracranial pressure. **10.** Answer: a; Cognitive level: Analysis; Nursing process: Assessment; Client need: Physiological integrity; Rationale: Because the client is at risk for injury with seizures, factors precipitating a seizure and any warning signs (aura) are assessed. Asking the client directly if there are any indications a seizure is coming on is the most effective method of determining if an aura exists.

Chapter 43

1. Answer: c; Cognitive level: Analysis; Nursing process: Planning; Client need: Physiological integrity; Rationale: Myasthenia gravis is a chronic, progressive neuromuscular disorder characterized by fatigue and severe weakness of skeletal muscles. Medication should be administered about 30 minutes prior to meals to enhance swallowing and chewing. Note the time of day when fatigued to assist in planning a meal schedule. **2.** Answer: d; Cognitive level: Analysis; Nursing process: Implementation; Client need: Psychosocial Integrity Rationale: Interventions vary with the clinical stage of the disorder. Clients who have Parkinson disease require substantial supportive care. The immediate intervention is to discuss with the client the concerns related to the diagnosis, nutritional therapy, and the effects of medications. Speech and physical therapy may be required to retain the optimal level of functioning possible; however, allowing the client the opportunity to discuss the diagnosis and learn about the nutritional and medication needs is the priority. **3.** Answer: a; Cognitive level: Application; Nursing process: Assessment; Client need: Physiological integrity; Rationale: Guillain-Barré syndrome is an acute demyelinating disorder of the peripheral nervous system characterized by progressive, usually rapid muscle weakness and paralysis. The disease is characterized by progressive ascending flaccid paralysis of the limbs, accompanied by paresthesias and numbness. The cause is unknown, but it is associated with prior viral respiratory or gastrointestinal infection. **4.** Answer: c; Cognitive level: Application; Nursing process: Implementation; Client need: Physiological integrity; Rationale: Nonintentional tremors associated with Parkinson disease may be controlled with purposeful, voluntary movement. The client is encouraged to hold an object or to engage in purposeful movement with the affected hand. Valium is not used in the treatment of symptoms of Parkinson disease. **5.** Answer: b; Cognitive level: Analysis; Nursing process: Assessment; Client need: Physiological integrity; Rationale: Uncoordinated movements, and swallowing and chewing problems, put the client with Huntington disease at high risk for aspiration. Foods that are small and thick enough to manage, such as thick soups, mashed potatoes, stews, and casseroles, are more readily tolerated and manipulated by the tongue than liquids. **6.** Answer: d; Cognitive level: Application; Nursing process: Implementation; Client need: Psychosocial Integrity Rationale: Both health care workers and family members need to remember that clients with Parkinson's disease require sufficient time for self-expression; an unhurried approach is recommended. **7.** Answer: b; Cognitive level: Analysis; Nursing process: Planning; Client need: Physiological integrity; Rationale: Botulism is food poisoning caused by ingestion of food contaminated with a toxin produced by the bacillus *Clostridium botulinum*. The toxins block the release of acetylcholine from nerve endings and thus cause respiratory paralysis from paralysis of skeletal muscles. **8.** Answer: a; Cognitive level: Application; Nursing process: Implementation; Client need: Physiological integrity; Rationale: Impaired chewing and swallowing can cause nutritional problems in the client with Parkinson disease. Interventions include providing foods of proper consistency as determined by the client's swallowing function. Food that is too liquid can be aspirated, so thickened foods are best. The client should eat or be fed in the upright position. **9.** Answer: c; Cognitive level: Application; Nursing process: Implementation; Client need: Physiological integrity; Rationale: Chorea is a severely altered gait with irregular, uncontrollable movement; the distal extremity is most affected. Headaches, dizziness, and seizures are not manifestations of Huntington disease. **10.** Answer: c; Cognitive level: Application; Nursing process: Implementation; Client need: Physiological integrity; Rationale: The client is injected with edrophonium

chloride (Tensilon), a short-acting anticholinesterase. In clients with myasthenia gravis, there is a significant improvement in muscle strength that lasts approximately 5 minutes.

Chapter 44

1. Answer: c; Cognitive level: Analysis; Nursing process: Assessment; Client need: Health promotion and maintenance; Rationale: A cloudy appearance of the lens and loss of red reflex are indicative of cataracts. The client should be referred for further evaluation. **2.** Answer: c; Cognitive level: Analysis; Nursing process: Assessment; Client need: Health promotion and maintenance; Rationale: With aging, the hair cells of the cochlea degenerate, producing a gradually progressive hearing loss. In presbycusis, hearing acuity begins to decrease in early adulthood and progresses as long as the individual lives. **3.** Answer: b; Cognitive level: Analysis; Nursing process: Assessment; Client need: Health promotion and maintenance; Rationale: The onset of macular degeneration typically occurs around age 65; it affects males and females equally. Macular degeneration is not associated with injury, allergies, or exposures. **4.** Answer: c; Cognitive level: Application; Nursing process: Implementation; Client need: Health promotion and maintenance; Rationale: Infants and children are more prone to acute otitis media because their eustachian tubes are shorter and straighter than those of adults. **5.** Answer: b; Cognitive level: Application; Nursing process: Implementation; Client need: Physiological integrity; Rationale: To avoid startling the blind client, staff and visitors are encouraged to announce themselves upon entering the client's room. The nurse should be made aware of this necessary action. **6.** Answer: d; Cognitive level: Application; Nursing process: Implementation; Client need: Health promotion and maintenance; Rationale: Clients with hypertension are encouraged to have regular eye examinations by an ophthalmologist to measure intraocular pressure. **7.** Answer: d; Cognitive level: Application; Nursing process: Implementation; Client need: Physiological integrity; Rationale: The immediate focus of the history is on the complaints of eye problems. The client should be allowed to discuss pertinent history but may require guidance to focus on the specific complaint. **8.** Answer: b; Cognitive level: Application; Nursing process: Assessment; Client need: Health promotion and maintenance; Rationale: The Weber test is performed to detect conductive or sensorineural hearing losses. The Trendelenburg test is performed to assess the musculoskeletal system. The Snellen test is performed to assess vision. The Allen test is performed to assess radial circulation before obtaining arterial blood gases. **9.** Answer: c; Cognitive level: Analysis Nursing process: Assessment; Client need: Physiological integrity; Rationale: Tinnitus is an early sign of aspirin toxicity. Gastritis and hematuria may indicate late signs of aspirin toxicity. **10.** Answer: b; Cognitive level: Analysis; Nursing process: Assessment; Client need: Physiological integrity; Rationale: Classic signs and symptoms of Ménière's disease include vertigo and nausea. The client may also complain of a feeling of fullness in the ears and a roaring or ringing sensation.

Chapter 45

1. Answer: d; Cognitive level: Application; Nursing process: Implementation; Client need: Health promotion and maintenance; Rationale: Conductive hearing loss occurs as a result of perforated tympanic membrane, disruption or fixation of the ossicles of the middle ear, fluid, scarring, or tumors of the middle ear. **2.** Answer: b; Cognitive level: Analysis; Nursing process: Assessment; Client need: Physiological integrity; Rationale: The visual distortion of straight lines is a typical manifestation of early macular degeneration. The client should be referred for immediate evaluation. **3.** Answer: c; Cognitive level: Analysis; Nursing process: Planning; Client need: Physiological integrity; Rationale: The client is instructed to avoid activities that promote edema or increase intraocular period in the postoperative period. Straining, lifting, bending over, and strenuous activity are avoided. **4.** Answer: d; Cognitive level: Application; Nursing process: Implementation; Client need: Physiological integrity; Rationale: The immediate priority of care for clients with chemical burns is flushing the affected eye with copious amounts of fluid. Normal saline is preferred; however, water may be used if saline is not available. **5.** Answer: d; Cognitive level: Application; Nursing process: Implementation; Client need: Physiological integrity; Rationale: The correct technique to apply drops to the ear of an adult client is to pull the pinna upward and back before instilling the drops. **6.** Answer: c; Cognitive level: Application; Nursing process: Planning; Client need: Physiological integrity; Rationale: The client is positioned so the area of detachment is inferior. For this client, the detachment is of the right eye, so place the client supine with the head turned to the right. This allows the contents of the eye to place pressure on the detached area, bringing the retina in closer contact with the choroid. **7.** Answer: c; Cognitive level: Application; Nursing process: Implementation; Client need: Safe, effective care environment Rationale: To avoid falls related to vertigo, the client should be instructed to remain in bed and not to get up without assistance. The call light should be in a readily accessible place for the client. **8.** Answer: b; Cognitive level: Application; Nursing process: Implementation; Client need: Physiological integrity; Rationale: If a foreign body is embedded in or sticking out of the eye, no attempt is made to remove it. The object should be immobilized and the eye protected with a metal eye shield until an ophthalmologist can see the client. **9.** Answer: d; Cognitive level: Application; Nursing process: Implementation; Client need: Health promotion and maintenance; Rationale: Facing the client directly when speaking is the most appropriate method of communicating with a client experiencing sensorineural hearing loss. Exaggerated pronunciation of words, speaking loudly, and one-word answers are not effective means of communication for this client. **10.** Answer: c; Cognitive level: Application; Nursing process: Implementation; Client need: Physiological integrity; Rationale: Miotics work by causing contraction of the sphincter of the iris, constricting the pupil. The net effect is to facilitate aqueous humor outflow by increasing drainage through the trabecular meshwork in open-angle glaucoma.

Chapter 46

1. Answer: b; Cognitive level: Analysis; Nursing process: Assessment; Client need: Health promotion and maintenance; Rationale: Balanitis (inflammation of the glands) is associated with bacterial or fungal infections. Symptoms include pain with urination. **2.** Answer: c; Cognitive level: Analysis; Nursing process: Assessment; Client need: Health promotion and maintenance; Rationale: Balanitis (inflammation of the glands) is associated with bacterial or fungal infections. An uncircumcised young male is more at risk for infections than a circumcised male or a 1-year-old. **3.** Answer: b; Cognitive level: Analysis Nursing process: Assessment; Client need: Health promotion and maintenance; Rationale: The assessment of the reproductive and urinary systems is often difficult for both the beginning nurse and the client and requires skill on the part of the nurse when asking questions about sensitive topics that the client may be hesitant to talk about. The nurse should recognize his or her own personal attitudes toward human sexuality in order to establish therapeutic communication with the client regarding sexuality. **4.** Answer: c; Cognitive level: Application; Nursing process: Implementation; Client need: Health promotion and maintenance; Rationale: Before discussing birth control methods, the client's sexual history and current activity must be assessed.

5. Answer: b; Cognitive level: Analysis Nursing process: Assessment; Client need: Health promotion and maintenance; Rationale: Hypospadias describes a urethral opening along the ventral surface of the penis. All newborn males should be assessed for the presence of hypospadias or epispadias, a urethral opening along the dorsal surface of the penis. **6.** Answer: a; Cognitive level: Analysis Nursing process: Planning; Client need: Health promotion and maintenance; Rationale: Urinary retention related to benign prostatic hypertrophy can lead to other complications such as urinary tract infection. The urinary retention must be relieved immediately. Burning, dribbling, and decreased urine stream also require intervention; however, urinary retention is the priority.
7. Answer: b; Cognitive level: Analysis; Nursing process: Planning; Client need: Health promotion and maintenance; Rationale: Inability to void for 2 days results in urinary retention, which may cause further complications such as a urinary tract infection. This client should be evaluated immediately. **8.** Answer: c; Cognitive level: Application; Nursing process: Planning; Client need: Health promotion and maintenance; Rationale: Urinary tract infections are common in the female because of the close proximity of the urinary urethra. Preventive measures include instructing the client to wipe from front to back after urination to avoid contamination from the rectal area. Hygiene after sexual intercourse should be explained. Eating foods that decrease the alkalinity of urine is encouraged, as is consuming adequate amounts of water. **9.** Answer: b; Cognitive level: Application; Nursing process: Implementation; Client need: Health promotion and maintenance; Rationale: Nursing staff must respect the client's need for privacy. Apologize for intruding on the client's privacy and return at a later time for planned interventions. **10.** Answer: b; Cognitive level: Analysis Nursing process: Planning; Client need: Health promotion and maintenance; Rationale: The growth spurt for pubescent females occurs before becoming sexually mature.

Chapter 47

1. Answer: d; Cognitive level: Analysis; Nursing process: Assessment; Client need: Physiological integrity; Rationale: Symptoms of prostatitis include pelvic, low back, or perineal pain and pain upon voiding. **2.** Answer: c; Cognitive level: Application; Nursing process: Planning; Client need: Health promotion and maintenance; Rationale: Preserving sperm in a bank prior to treatment may help relieve the client's fears about his ability to father children in the future but must be completed prior to initiating treatment with surgery, chemotherapy, or radiation

therapy. **3.** Answer: d; Cognitive level: Application; Nursing process: Planning; Client need: Physiological integrity; Rationale: Following a transurethral resection of the prostate, the client is encouraged to consume an adequate amount of fluids, especially water, to promote urine elimination. Since regaining full urinary control may take up to 1 year, caffeine and alcohol are discouraged because of the diuretic effects. **4.** Answer: a; Cognitive level: Application; Nursing process: Implementation; Client need: Physiological integrity; Rationale: Epispadias is a defect in which the urinary meatus is above the tip of the penis. The defect happens in early fetal development. The cause is unknown. **5.** Answer: a; Cognitive level: Application; Nursing process: Implementation; Client need: Physiological integrity; Rationale: As men age, their prostate gland enlarges. Changes in the androgen dihydrostestosterone (DHT) may also contribute to prostatic hyperplasia. **6.** Answer: a; Cognitive level: Application; Nursing process: Implementation; Client need: Physiological integrity; Rationale: Continuous bladder irrigation is performed to prevent the formation of blood clots, which could obstruct urinary output. Bladder distension resulting from output obstruction increases the risk of bleeding.
7. Answer: b; Cognitive level: Application; Nursing process: Implementation; Client need: Health promotion and maintenance; Rationale: The foreskin should be returned to its natural position in order to prevent swelling and edema. The foreskin, if left retracted, may form a tourniquet effect on the penis, causing swelling and edema, which may further lead to compromised circulation to the penis. **8.** Answer: a; Cognitive level: Analysis; Nursing process: Assessment; Client need: Health promotion and maintenance; Rationale: Benign prostatic hyperplasia (BPH) is the most common disorder in the aging male client. Clinical manifestations include urinary retention, diminished force of urinary stream, and hesitancy in initiating voiding, postvoid dribbling, nocturia, frequency, and urgency. **9.** Answer: c; Cognitive level: Analysis Nursing process: Planning; Client need: Physiological integrity; Rationale: Clients should be instructed to keep bowel movements regular and soft to avoid pressure on the prostate area. Mild laxatives or stool softeners may be taken as ordered.
10. Answer: b; Cognitive level: Analysis; Nursing process: Assessment; Client need: Health promotion and maintenance; Rationale: Testicular cancer is the most common cancer in men between the ages of 15 and 35, and it is the third leading cause of cancer death in young men. The classic presenting symptom of testicular cancer is a painless hard nodule. An occasional manifestation includes dull ache in pelvis or scrotum.

Chapter 48

1. Answer: d; Cognitive level: Analysis; Nursing process: Planning; Client need: Physiological integrity; Rationale: Dysmenorrhea may be treated with analgesics, prostaglandin inhibitors such as NSAIDs, or oral contraceptives. NSAIDs such as naproxen are the likely beginning choice.   **2.** Answer: c; Cognitive level: Analysis Nursing process: Evaluation; Client need: Physiological integrity; Rationale: Preventive measures for urinary tract infections include drinking 8 to 10 glasses of fluid per day, wearing cotton panties, and voiding every 2 to 4 hours while awake.
3. Answer: c; Cognitive level: Application; Nursing process: Implementation; Client need: Physiological integrity; Rationale: A WBC count of 9800/cu mm is a normal laboratory value. No intervention is necessary.
4. Answer: b; Cognitive level: Application; Nursing process: Implementation; Client need: Health promotion and maintenance; Rationale: Postmenopausal clients are at risk for osteoporosis. Vitamin D increases intestinal absorption of calcium.
5. Answer: d; Cognitive level: Analysis; Nursing process: Planning; Client need: Physiological integrity; Rationale: Clients undergoing abdominal surgery are at risk for developing thrombophlebitis. Measures to reduce the chance of the thrombophlebitis include early ambulation. The client should dangle legs the evening of surgery, then be assisted to ambulate as tolerated.   **6.** Answer: b; Cognitive level: Application; Nursing process: Implementation; Client need: Physiological integrity; Rationale: Swelling and edema following a radical mastectomy with node dissection occur as a result of decreased lymph drainage due to node removal. Measures to reduce edema include elevating the affected arm on a pillow and encouraging range-of-motion exercises.   **7.** Answer: a; Cognitive level: Analysis Nursing process: Evaluation; Client need: Health promotion and maintenance; Rationale: Endometriosis is a condition in which multiple, small, usually benign implantations of endometrial tissue develop throughout the pelvic cavity.   **8.** Answer: b; Cognitive level: Analysis Nursing process: Assessment; Client need: Health promotion and maintenance; Rationale: Endometriosis causes scarring, inflammation, and adhesions, which interfere with fertility and is responsible for 30% to 45% of all cases of female infertility.   **9.** Answer: b; Cognitive level: Analysis; Nursing process: Assessment; Client need: Health promotion and maintenance; Rationale: Excessive or prolonged menstruation, menorrhagia, is a type of dysfunctional uterine bleeding. Complications resulting from menorrhagia include excessive blood loss, fatigue, anemia, hemorrhage, and sexual dysfunction.   **10.** Answer: d; Cognitive level:

Application; Nursing process: Implementation; Client need: Physiological integrity; Rationale: The most common cause of pelvic inflammatory disease is gonorrhea. Other common organisms include *Chlamydia trachomatis, Escherichia coli,* and *mycoplasma hominis.*

Chapter 49

1. Answer: a; Cognitive level: Analysis Nursing process: Assessment; Client need: Physiological integrity; Rationale: Manifestations of syphilis include a chancre sore that heals, followed by a rash on palms and soles.   **2.** Answer: a; Cognitive level: Application; Nursing process: Planning; Client need: Physiological integrity; Rationale: Health teaching for the client with a chlamydial infection includes focusing on the need to comply with the treatment regimen (taking all antibiotics as prescribed), referral of sexual partners for examination and necessary treatment, and the use of condoms to avoid reinfection.
3. Answer: a; Cognitive level: Analysis Nursing process: Evaluation; Client need: Physiological integrity; Rationale: The client is taught to recognize prodromal symptoms of recurrence and factors that seem to trigger recurrences. Abstinence from sexual contact from the time prodromal symptoms appear until 10 days after all lesions have healed is necessary to prevent transmission of the disease. There is no cure for herpes.   **4.** Answer: d; Cognitive level: Analysis Nursing process: Assessment; Client need: Physiological integrity; Rationale: Female clients infected with *Chlamydia trachomatis* may be asymptomatic or will present with yellow-green vaginal discharge, dysparunia, and pelvic pain.
5. Answer: a; Cognitive level: Analysis; Nursing process: Assessment; Client need: Safe, effective care environment Rationale: Contact precautions for a client with herpes infection includes a private room or rooming with a client with the same illness, gloves when providing client care, and gowning if clothing will come in contact with the client, environmental surfaces, or items in the client's room. HEPA filter masks are not required since the virus is not transmitted via the airborne route.   **6.** Answer: c; Cognitive level: Application; Nursing process: Implementation; Client need: Health promotion and maintenance; Rationale: Genital herpes simplex virus 2 is spread by vaginal, anal, or oral–genital contact.
7. Answer: c; Cognitive level: Application; Nursing process: Implementation; Client need: Health promotion and maintenance; Rationale: Clients infected with genital herpes are instructed to recognize prodromal symptoms of recurrence and factors that

seem to trigger recurrences. Abstinence from sexual contact from the time prodromal symptoms appear until 10 days after all lesions have healed. Antifungal agents are not effective. **8.** Answer: b; Cognitive level: Application; Nursing process: Planning; Client need: Health promotion and maintenance; Rationale: Genital and anal warts are caused by the human papillomas virus (HPV). HPV is transmitted by all types of sexual contact and is most commonly found in young, sexually active adults and is associated with early onset of sexual activity and multiple sexual partners. Present partners should be evaluated for lesions, but they may not be the source of transmission.

9. Answer: c; Cognitive level: Analysis; Nursing process: Planning; Client need: Health promotion and maintenance; Rationale: Transmission of genital herpes from mother to neonate occurs during passage through the birth canal. The nurse should discuss with women of childbearing age that cesarean delivery can prevent transmission of infection to the neonate. **10.** Answer: c; Cognitive level: Analysis; Nursing process: Planning; Client need: Physiological integrity; Rationale: Acyclovir (Zovirax) helps reduce the length and severity of the first episode and is the treatment of choice for genital herpes.